# YOUR HEALT

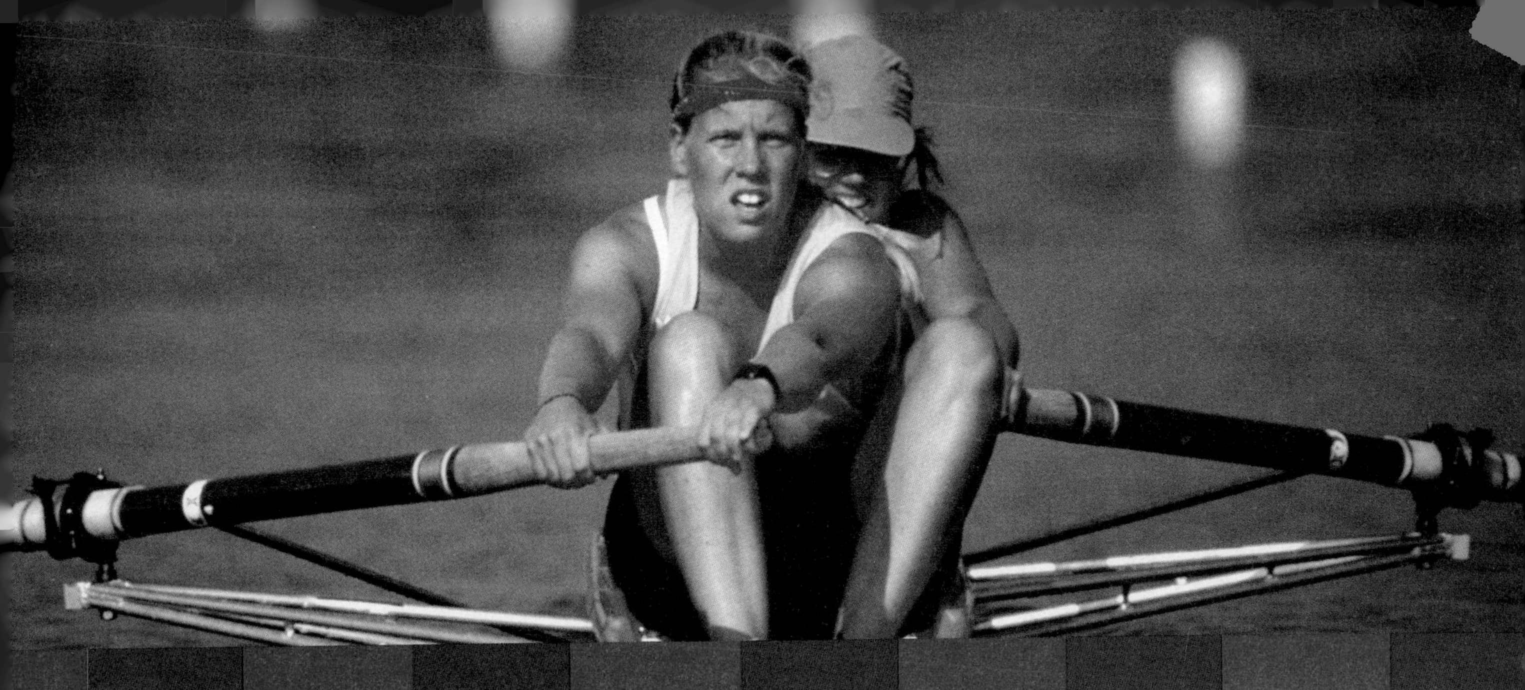

# YOUR HEALTH

Dianne Hales

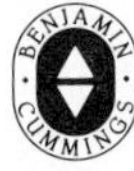


The Benjamin/Cummings Publishing Company, Inc.

Redwood City, California ■ Menlo Park, California ■ Reading, Massachusetts
New York ■ Don Mills, Ontario ■ Wokingham, U.K. ■ Amsterdam ■ Bonn
Sydney ■ Singapore ■ Tokyo ■ Madrid ■ San Juan

Sponsoring Editor: Pat Coryell
Developmental Editor: Devra Lerman
Production Supervisor: John Walker
Associate Marketing Manager: Stacy Treco
Copy Editor: Toni Murray
Text Designer: Bruce Kortebein Design Office
Cover Designer: Rudolphe M. Zehntner
Cover Photographer: David Madison
Artists: Edith Allgood, Mary Burkhardt, Carey Crockett,
Lisa French, Linda Harris-Sweezy, Fran Milner
Photo Researcher: Darcy Lanham
Composition and Film: Graphic Typesetting Service

Photograph credits are listed in the back of the book.



**Library of Congress Cataloging-in-Publication Data**

Hales, Dianne R., 1950–
Your health / Dianne Hales.
p. cm.
Includes bibliographical references and index.
ISBN 0-8053-2770-3
1. Health. I. Title.
RA776.H149 1991
613—dc20

90-25381
CIP

ABCDEFGHIJ—VH—9543210

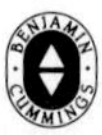

The Benjamin/Cummings Publishing Company, Inc.
390 Bridge Parkway
Redwood City, California 94065

## DEDICATION

To the joys of my life:
Bob and Julia.
With all my love,
D. H.

# PREFACE

## If you have your health, you have everything.

This statement sums up the promise of *Your Health.* Designed to help readers live more fully, more happily, and more healthfully, *Your Health* is not just a book to be read; it is a tool students can use to make the most of their health and their lives.

Health involves every aspect of living—psychological, emotional, spiritual, physical, behavioral, environmental, and social. *Your Health* provides the basic knowledge and understanding of all these areas that students need for a lifetime of well-being. Every chapter emphasizes practical information they can use immediately, whether they're trying to cope with an emotional problem, eat more nutritiously, get in shape, improve their relationships, practice safer sex, avoid harmful habits, or prevent long-term health risks.

*Your Health* is a book about and for students—about their minds and bodies, their needs and wants, their past and their potential. Its goal is to show students that they have more control over their lives and well-being than anything or anyone else does. Now and in the future, their health is their most important asset—and one of their greatest responsibilities. *Your Health* helps them face that responsibility by developing their decision-making skills.

*Your Health* talks directly to students but never talks down to them. Its tone is friendly; its style is easy to read. Real-life examples and case histories help readers see the connections between what they read and how they live.

*Your Health* has been created by the same team that produced the four editions of the leading college health textbook, *An Invitation to Health.* We realized that some instructors want the same positive approach, accurate information, and consistent emphasis on behavioral change that *An Invitation to Health* offers, but in a more concise book.

*Your Health* is shorter than *An Invitation to Health* (by about 145 pages) and zeroes in on practical applications of knowledge and on the issues that most touch students' lives. With a simpler vocabulary and writing style, it is the ideal length and level for brief health or wellness courses and classes that highlight the essentials of personal health.

Like its concept, the design of *Your Health* is innovative. Throughout the book, dynamic full-color photographs and colorful graphics make the text visually enticing for students. With dramatic images and bright colors, *Your Health* is as fresh and exciting to the eye as it is to the mind.

## INSIDE YOUR HEALTH

To involve readers right from the start, *Your Health* begins with a "Wellness Inventory" that assesses every dimension of well-being. Its six sections, divided into eighteen chapters, present key concepts in health in a logical, comprehensive manner. Here is a brief outline of what *Your Health* offers:

## SECTION I YOUR MIND

### 1. Making the Most of Your Health

Key topics: Defining health, the promise of wellness, the mind-body-spirit connection, spiritual health, taking charge of your life, making choices and changes, the payoffs of prevention.

### 2. Taking Care of Your Mind

Key topics: Psychological wellness, personality theories, self-understanding, decision-making, challenges of daily living, psychological problems (including eating disorders, phobias, panic attacks, depression, and suicide), seeking help, feeling better.

**3. Meeting the Challenges of Stress**
Key topics: Understanding stress and its sources, its impact on the body, techniques for defusing stress, stress management, relaxation skills, tackling test stress.

## SECTION II YOUR BODY

**4. Eating Wisely and Well**
Key topics: Healthful eating, the basic food groups, eating to prevent disease and boost good health, nutritional controversies, controlling weight, overcoming obesity, beyond dieting.

**5. The Joy of Fitness**
Key topics: Shaping up, flexibility, aerobic fitness, muscular strength and endurance, the benefits of exercise, designing a fitness program, the dangers of steroids, preventing injuries.

## SECTION III YOUR SEXUALITY

**6. Your Relationships**
Key topics: Communication skills, living alone, at home or with a partner, dating, choosing a mate, marriage, two-career couples, parenthood, new forms of family ties, building better relationships.

**7. Sexual Health and Behavior**
Key topics: Women's and men's sexual health, sexual development, gender differences, homosexuality, bisexuality, sexual activities, safer sex, overcoming sexual problems, sexual assault.

**8. Reproductive Choices**
Key topics: The beginning of life, a comprehensive guide to birth control options, abortion, the process of pregnancy, giving birth, infertility, adoption.

## SECTION IV YOUR LIFESTYLE

**9. Drug Use and Abuse: Recognizing the Risks**
Key topics: Understanding drug use, misuse and abuse, the making of a drug habit, prescription and non-prescription drugs, psychoactive drugs (including the latest research on cocaine, crack, crank, ice, marijuana, and other illegal drugs), overcoming addiction.

**10. Alcohol: Responsible Drinking**
Key topics: Changes in drinking patterns, moderate drinking, how alcohol affects the body and brain, hangovers, warning signs of a drinking problem, alcoholism, children of alcoholics, recovery.

**11. Tobacco: Breaking a Deadly Addiction**
Key topics: Who smokes and why, how tobacco affects the body, chewing tobacco, snuff, pipes, passive smoking, quitting.

## SECTION V YOUR HEALTH RISKS

**12. Your Options for Health Care: Making Wise Choices**
Key topics: The basics of self-care, knowing when to seek care, finding health professionals, getting the most out of medical services, paying for care, alternative therapies, quackery.

**13. Cardiovascular Disease: Beating the Number One Killer**
Key topics: How the heart works, the dangers of high blood pressure and high cholesterol, lowering the risk of heart attacks, new treatments for heart disease, preventing strokes.

**14. Cancer, Major Illnesses, and Accidents: Beating the Odds**
Key topics: What causes cancer, the most common cancers, the importance of prevention, new treatments and new hope, diabetes, epilepsy, other chronic illness, avoiding accidents, safety rules.

**15. Immunity and Infectious Diseases: Protecting Yourself**
Key topics: Agents of infection, the immune system, common infectious diseases (including the most recent warnings on measles and Lyme disease), immune system problems, HIV infection/AIDS, sexually transmitted diseases (including chlamydia, herpes, human papilloma virus, chancroid, syphillis, gonorrhea, lice, and crabs).

## SECTION VI YOUR FUTURE

**16. The Environment's Impact**
Key topics: Polluted air, hazards of indoor pollution, new questions about safe drinking water, chemical pollutants, noise as an environmental hazard, radia-

tion risks, overpopulation, social health problems (including violence, spouse abuse, and child abuse).

### 17. Growing Older and Feeling Better

Key topics: Living longer and better, challenges of old age, longevity, how long you might live, issues of an aging society.

### 18. The Final Chapter: Coming to Terms with Death

Key topics: Defining death, how we respond to death, preparing for life's end, grief, practical arrangements, the meaning of death.

## FEATURES

### Strategies for Change

To help students translate what they read into action, *Your Health* features behavioral strategies within the text of every chapter. Examples include "Helping Others Change Bad Habits" (p. 8), "Conquering Shyness" (p. 19), "Coping with Change" (p. 41), "Eating Light and Right" (p. 83), "Choosing a Contraceptive" (p. 176), "How to Drink Without Getting Drunk" (p. 231), "What to Do If You Have an STD" (p. 352), and "Protecting Yourself from Indoor Air Pollution" (p. 361).

### Self-Surveys

Every chapter includes a self-assessment so students can examine their health and behavior, identify problems, and make appropriate changes. For example, students can gauge their level of fitness in the Chapter 5 Self-Survey, "How Fit Are You?" (p. 98); they may confront a drinking problem by doing the Chapter 10 Self-Survey, "Do You Have a Drinking Problem?" (p. 238); and they may improve their conservation habits after going through the Chapter 16 Self-Survey, "Assessment of Environmental Sensitivity" (p. 362).

### Health Spotlights

In every chapter, we focus on a relevant topic that will help make the text material come alive for the students. Some Health Spotlights tell the story of individuals, such as "Diary of a Student with Anorexia" in the mental health chapter (p. 29) and "A Letter from a Gay Man to His Parents" in the sexuality chapter (p. 149). Others, such as "Avoiding Date Rape" (p. 159), "Coaddiction: Are You Helping a Drug User?" (p. 221), "Unclogging your Arteries," (p. 299) and "A Message About AIDS" (p. 343), explore major issues in health today.

### What Do You Think?

In this feature, we describe situations and pose questions that explore the ethical and emotional complexities of everyday health decisions. Among the topics covered are: Interracial dating (p. 128), homophobia (p. 160), the prosecution of pregnant women who use drugs (p. 196), drug testing (p. 223), consequences of drunk driving (p. 244), marketing cigarettes to teenagers, minorities, and women (p. 262), radical environmentalism (p. 372), and the right to die (p. 401).

### Health Headlines

The most up-to-date stories highlight relevant developments from one of the fastest-changing fields of science. Examples include: "Stress and Herpes: Breaking the Cycle" (p. 42), "Where Does Living Together Lead?" (p. 122), "HIV on Campus" (p. 147), "The Psychological Impact of Abortion" (p. 183), "Are Alcoholics Born or Made?" (p. 235), "Are Hospitals Hazardous to Health?" (p. 280), "Eat Less, Live Longer?" (p. 379), and "The State of the World" (p. 361).

### Hales Index

This feature presents health facts and statistics in a telegraphic way that will intrigue even casual readers. Among the questions that the Hales Index answers: How many people have ever suffered from shyness? (p. 27) What are the five most and least stressful cities in America? (p. 39) How many pounds of broccoli does the average American eat annually? How many pounds of ice cream? (p. 64) What percentage of married people say their spouses are their best friends? (p. 115) How many college men and women would lie to obtain sex? (p. 142) What percentage of American couples use contraception? (p. 174) How many drivers on the road at any given time are drunk? (p. 234) How many Americans get an STD every year? (p. 327) How much garbage does the average American household throw away in a week? In a year? (p. 359)

### Making This Chapter Work for You

Every chapter ends with this feature, which both summarizes the key points in the chapter and provides guidelines for putting that knowledge into action. This behavior-oriented summary highlights key points and underscores the message that, unlike other subjects, health can not simply be studied: It must be lived.

### References and Definitions

*Your Health* includes footnoted references and recommended readings for each chapter; they are pulled together at the end of the text for ease of use. The research is as up-to-date as possible. For students' convenience, we have included key definitions on pages where they occur, as well as a glossary at the back of the book.

### Your Health Care and Survival Guide

This book-within-a-book provides key information on safety, emergencies, and preventive health care. Its streamlined design helps readers quickly find what they need to know to prevent accidents, handle emergencies, solve everyday health problems, and recognize health warnings.

### Your Health Directory (The Yellow Pages)

This practical reference is a handy listing of the addresses and telephone numbers of agencies and hotline services that provide health information and assistance. Students can use this directory for many purposes, including gathering materials for term papers and finding out where to turn in crisis situations.

## MAJOR THEMES

Throughout every chapter, students will find messages that apply to every aspect of their health. Among the most important are the following:

- You can do more for your health than doctors can; your health is your personal responsibility.
- You are not simply a creature of body, mind, or spirit, but of all three. Psychological, physical, spiritual, social, and environmental health are all parts of wellness.
- You can take charge of your health by changing health behaviors.
- You can learn to manage stress and to control its impact on your life.
- Prevention is always the wisest course.
- The way that you use—or abuse—your body when you're young can determine how you'll feel in your later years.
- Rather than waiting for bad health habits to take their toll, you can delay or avoid many problems by adopting healthful behaviors.
- You can safeguard your health by learning how to be a wise health-care consumer.
- Your planet's health, like your own, is your personal responsibility.
- Making healthful choices, day by day, can enhance both the quality and the quantity of your years on earth.

## SUPPLEMENTARY MATERIALS

*Your Health* is accompanied by a complete supplements package to meet every teaching need.

### The Instructor's Guide

Written by Carolyn Parks of the University of Tennessee, and Deborah Fortune, Ph.D., of the University of North Carolina at Charlotte, the Instructor's Guide provides a wealth of suggestions for lecture preparation. It contains comprehensive, detailed lecture outlines that are annotated with suggestions for ways to place emphasis on certain topics. Each chapter includes discussion questions, classroom activities, controversial topics, homework assignments, a list of relevant films, videos, and cassettes, and a special section on minority health issues. A list of agencies to contact for additional information is placed at the end of every chapter. Self-assessment exercises are included in an appendix that also includes hand-outs designed to augment transparency presentations.

### The Test Bank

The Test Bank, written by Christopher Cooke of the University of North Carolina, features a wide variety of well-written and thoughtfully conceived test questions. There are approximately 60 true/false, multiple choice, completion, and matching questions per chapter. Questions are referenced to the text by page number and subject heading. Answers are supplied for all questions. The Test Bank is also available on **Benjamin/Cummings Testing Software** for the IBM PC, the IBM PS/2, the Apple II, and the Macintosh microcomputers, allowing instructors to format and edit tests easily and quickly.

### Transparency Acetates

More than 50 illustrations, charts, and tables are available from the text and other sources.

### Video Tapes

- A nutrition and fitness video is available to *all* adopters.
- A collection of additional videos that present lively coverage of current health topics is also available. See your Benjamin/Cummings representative for further information.

### The Newsletter

The bi-annual *Sexuality and Health* newsletter, published by Benjamin/Cummings, keeps you up-to-date on a wide variety of health topics. Available to college and university adopters at no charge.

## TO YOUR HEALTH

*Your Health* shows students how to become caretakers of their own health. It teaches them what they can do for themselves in order to achieve total wellness. it also takes the logical next step and shows them how to put health into action and take charge of their lives.

The responsibility for health ultimately remains with each individual. By providing the information and strategies students need to handle that responsibility, *Your Health* can help them live happier, fuller, more productive lives.

Our basic message to both instructors and students is simple: Since nothing is more important than your health, nothing may be more important than *Your Health.*

## REVIEWERS

This book and its supplements could not have come together without the attention of many health professionals giving me their advice and the benefit of their experience. My gratitude goes to reviewers Carolyn Allred, Central Piedmont Community College; Rick Barnes, East Carolina University; John Carter, The Citadel; Susanne Christopher, Portland Community College; Kelly Dodd, Johnson County Community College; Susan Hall, California State University—Northridge; Richard Kaye, Kingsborough Community College; Patricia McGuigan-Kenney, Pennsylvania State University; Jan Mittleider, College of Southern Idaho; and Barbara Ritsema, Montgomery College.

## ACKNOWLEDGEMENTS

*Your Health* owes its existence to its sponsoring editor, Pat Coryell, whose vision, energy, and commitment made this book possible. Devra Lerman brought insight, intelligence, and dedication to her role as editorial midwife on the project. The production supervisor, John Walker, was a model of grace, professionalism, and creativity under intense deadline pressure. Bruce Kortebein dazzled us with his brilliant text designs and intuitive sense of how this book should look. Debra Hunter, Grace Wong, Betsy Dilernia, Darcy Lanham, and Stacy Treco also played important roles in the making of *Your Health.* They, along with the rest of the talented staff at Benjamin/Cummings, have my deep appreciation and admiration. I consider it a privilege to work with them—and a pleasure to know them.

# SPECIAL FEATURES

## HEALTH SPOTLIGHT



## HEALTH HEADLINE

## SELF-SURVEYS



## HALES INDEX



## WHAT DO YOU THINK?

# BRIEF CONTENTS

# DETAILED CONTENTS

## SECTION I ■ YOUR MIND 1



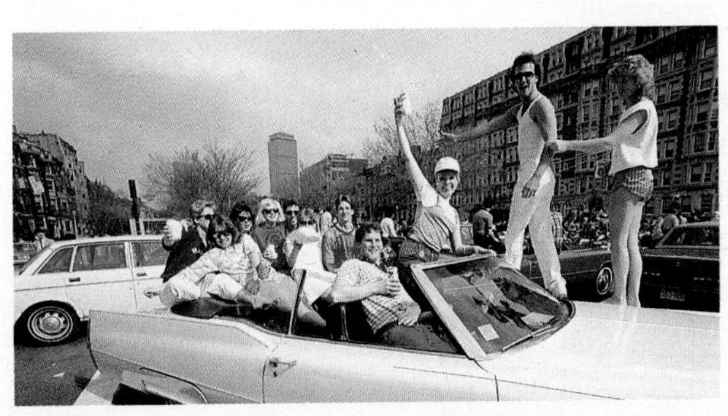

## CHAPTER 3 MEETING THE CHALLENGES OF STRESS 36



# SECTION II ■ YOUR BODY 55

## CHAPTER 4 EATING WISELY AND WELL 56

## CHAPTER 5 THE JOY OF FITNESS 88



# SECTION III ■ YOUR SEXUALITY 111

## CHAPTER 6 YOUR RELATIONSHIPS 112



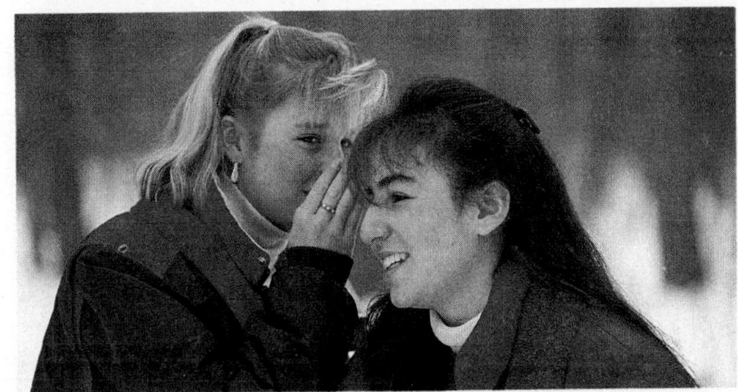

## CHAPTER 7 SEXUAL HEALTH AND BEHAVIOR 131



## CHAPTER 8 REPRODUCTIVE CHOICES 162

## SECTION IV ■ YOUR LIFE-STYLE 199

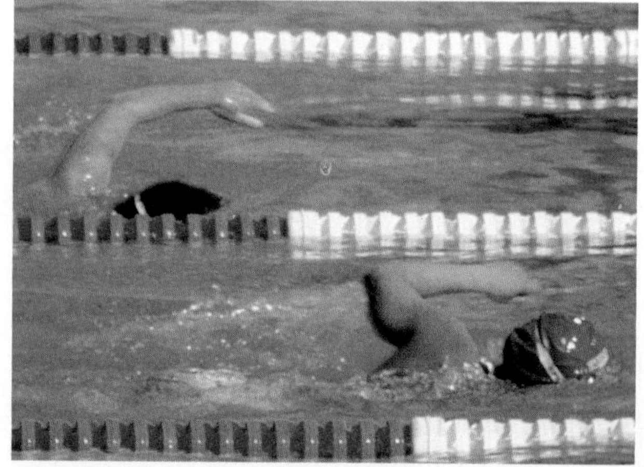

# WELLNESS INVENTORY

What does it mean to enjoy wellness? This book takes a holistic view of health by exploring the various dimensions of your life and well-being, and focusing on what you can do to make the most of all of them. This wellness survey can help you achieve this goal by highlighting those aspects of your life-style that can be improved.

This inventory was designed to educate rather than test. Each statement describes what is believed to be a wellness attribute. The higher your score, the more of these attributes you believe to be true for yourself. The information you gain by taking the wellness inventory can be valuable to you to facilitate your growth in the area of your choosing. There are no trick questions to test your consistency. All statements are worded so that you can tell what the more desirable answer is; this places full responsibility on you to answer each statement as honestly as possible. Remember, it's not your score, but what you learn about yourself that counts.

Set aside time for yourself to complete the inventory. Use the following scoring system throughout, recording your score in the boxes beside each statement:

2 = Yes, usually
1 = Sometimes, maybe
0 = No, rarely

Select the one answer that best indicates how true the statement is for you at this time. If you decide that a statement does not apply to you, or you don't want to answer it, you can skip it and not be penalized in your score. After you have responded to the statements in each section, compute your average score from that section, and transfer that number to the Wellness Inventory Wheel on the last page of this inventory. See the following example.

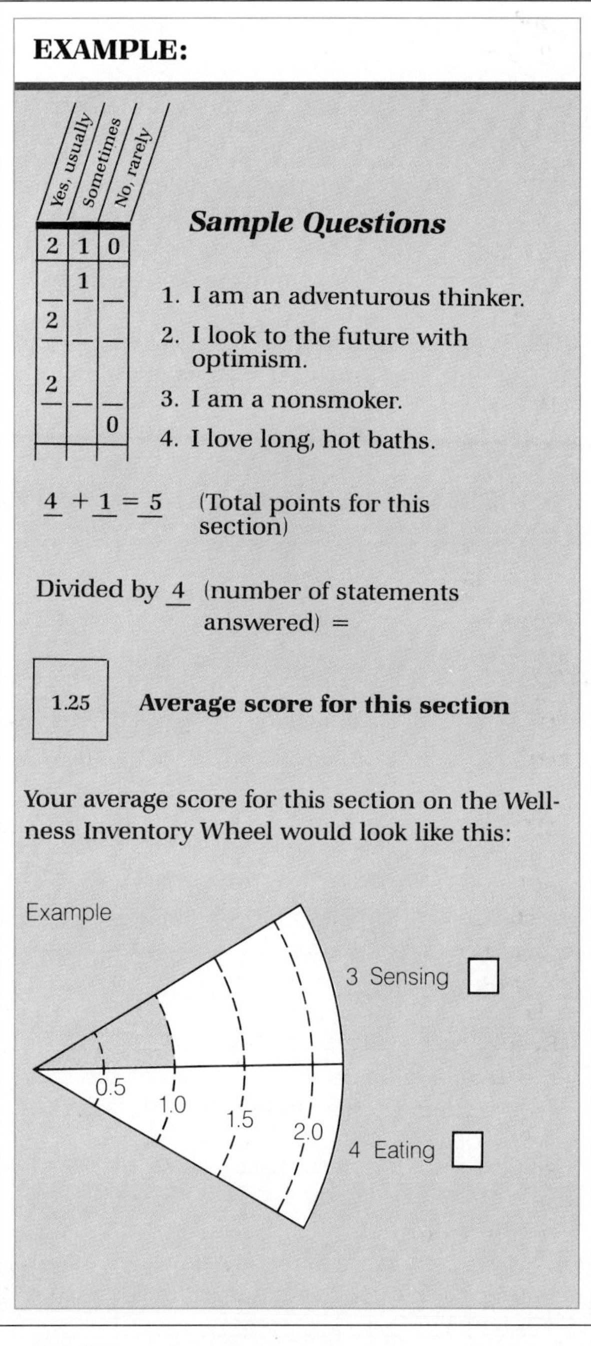

## SECTION 1 WELLNESS, SELF-RESPONSIBILITY, AND LOVE

| 2 (Yes, usually) | 1 (Sometimes) | 0 (No, rarely) | Statement |
|---|---|---|---|
| | 1 | | 1. I believe how I live my life is an important factor in determining my state of health, and I live it in a manner consistent with that belief. |
| | 1 | | 2. I vote regularly. |
| | | 0 | 3. I feel financially secure. |
| | 1 | | 4. I conserve materials/energy at home and at work. |
| 2 | | | 5. I protect my living area from fire and safety hazards. |
| | 1 | | 6. I use dental floss and a soft toothbrush daily. |
| 2 | | | 7. I am a nonsmoker. |
| 2 | | | 8. I am always sober when driving or operating dangerous machinery. |
| | 1 | | 9. I wear a safety belt when I ride in a vehicle. |
| 2 | | | 10. I understand the difference between blaming myself for a problem and simply taking responsibility for that problem. |

8 + 5 = 13 = Total points for this section

Divided by __ (number of statements answered) = 1.3 **Average score for this section** (Transfer to the Wellness Inventory Wheel on summary page)

## SECTION 2 WELLNESS AND BREATHING

| 2 | 1 | 0 | Statement |
|---|---|---|---|
| | | - | 1. I stop during the day to become aware of the way I am breathing. |
| 2 | | | 2. I meditate or relax myself for at least 15 minutes each day. |
| 2 | | | 3. I can easily touch my hands to my toes when standing with knees straight. |
| | 1 | | 4. In temperatures over 70°F (21°C), my fingers feel warm when I touch my lips.* |
| 2 | | | 5. My nails are healthy and I do not bite or pick at them. |
| | | - | 6. I enjoy my work and do not find it overly stressful. |
| | 1 | | 7. My personal relationships are satisfying. |
| | | - | 8. I take time out for deep breathing several times a day. |
| | 1 | | 9. I have plenty of energy. |
| | 1 | | 10. I am at peace with myself. |

6 + 4 = 10 = Total points for this section

Divided by __ (number of statements answered) = 1.0 **Average score for this section** (Transfer to the Wellness Inventory Wheel on summary page)

*If your hand temperature is below 85°F in a warm room, an overactive sympathetic nervous system could be to blame. You can learn to warm your hands with biofeedback and thereby relax.

## SECTION 3 WELLNESS AND SENSING

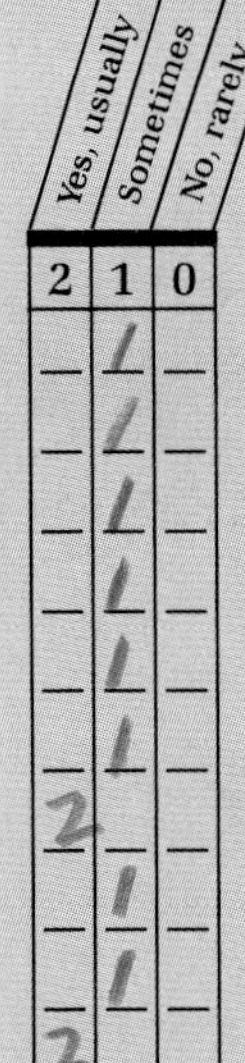

1. My place of work has largely natural lighting or full spectrum fluorescent lighting.
2. I avoid extremely noisy areas or wear protective ear covers.
3. I take long walks, hikes, or other outings to actively explore my surroundings.
4. I give myself presents, treats, or nurture myself in other ways.
5. I enjoy getting, and can acknowledge, compliments and recognition from others.
6. It is easy for me to give sincere compliments and recognition to other people.
7. At times I like to be alone.
8. I enjoy touching or hugging other people.
9. I enjoy being touched or hugged by others.
10. I get and enjoy backrubs or massages.

4 + 8 = 12 = Total points for this section

Divided by __ (number of statements answered) =

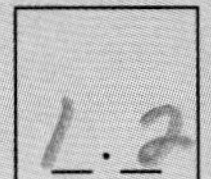

**Average score for this section** (Transfer to the Wellness Inventory Wheel on summary page)

## SECTION 4 WELLNESS AND EATING

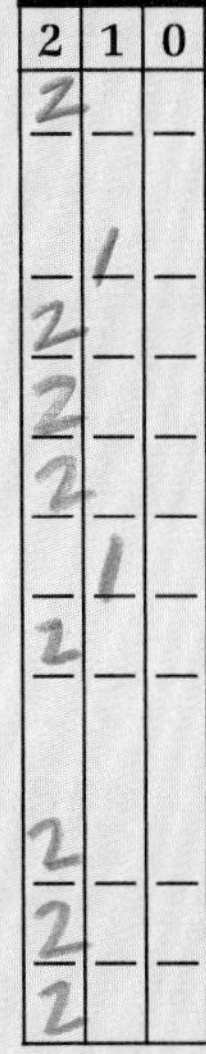

1. I am aware of the difference between refined carbohydrates and complex carbohydrates and eat a majority of the latter.
2. I think my diet is well balanced and wholesome.
3. I drink fewer than 5 alcoholic drinks per week.
4. I drink fewer than 2 cups of coffee or black (nonherbal) tea per day.
5. I drink fewer than 5 soft drinks per week.
6. I add little or no salt to my food.
7. I read the labels for the ingredients of all processed foods I buy and I inquire as to the level of toxic chemicals used in production of fresh foods—choosing the purest available to me.
8. I eat at least two raw fruits or vegetables each day.
9. I have a good appetite and am within 15% of my ideal weight.
10. I can tell the difference between "stomach hunger" and "mouth hunger," and I don't stuff myself when I am experiencing only "mouth hunger."*

16 + 2 = 18 = Total points for this section

Divided by __ (number of statements answered) = 1.8

**Average score for this section** (Transfer to the Wellness Inventory Wheel on summary page)

*"Stomach hunger" is a signal that your body needs food. "Mouth hunger" is a signal that it needs something else (attention/acknowledgement), which you are not getting, so it asks for food, a readily available substitute.

## SECTION 5 WELLNESS AND MOVING

| Yes, usually | Sometimes | No, rarely | |
|---|---|---|---|
| 2 | 1 | 0 | |
| | | | 1. I climb stairs rather than ride elevators. |
| | | | 2. My daily activities include **moderate** physical effort.* |
| | | | 3. My daily activities include **vigorous** physical effort.** |
| | | | 4. I run at least **one** mile three times a week (or equivalent aerobic exercise). |
| | | | 5. I run at least **three** miles three times a week (or equivalent aerobic exercise). |
| | | | 6. I do some form of stretching exercise for 10 to 20 minutes at least **three** times per week. |
| | | | 7. I do some form of stretching exercise for 10 to 20 minutes at least **six** times per week. |
| | | | 8. I enjoy exploring effective ways of caring for myself through the movement of my body. |
| | | | 9. I enjoy stretching, moving, and exerting my body. |
| | | | 10. I am aware of and respond to messages from my body about its needs for movement. |

__ + __ = __ = Total points for this section

Divided by __ (number of statements answered) = __.__

**Average score for this section**
(Transfer to the Wellness Inventory Wheel on summary page)

*Moderate includes rearing young chldren, gardening, scrubbing floors, walking briskly, etc.
**Vigorous includes heavy construction work, farming, moving heavy objects by hand, etc.

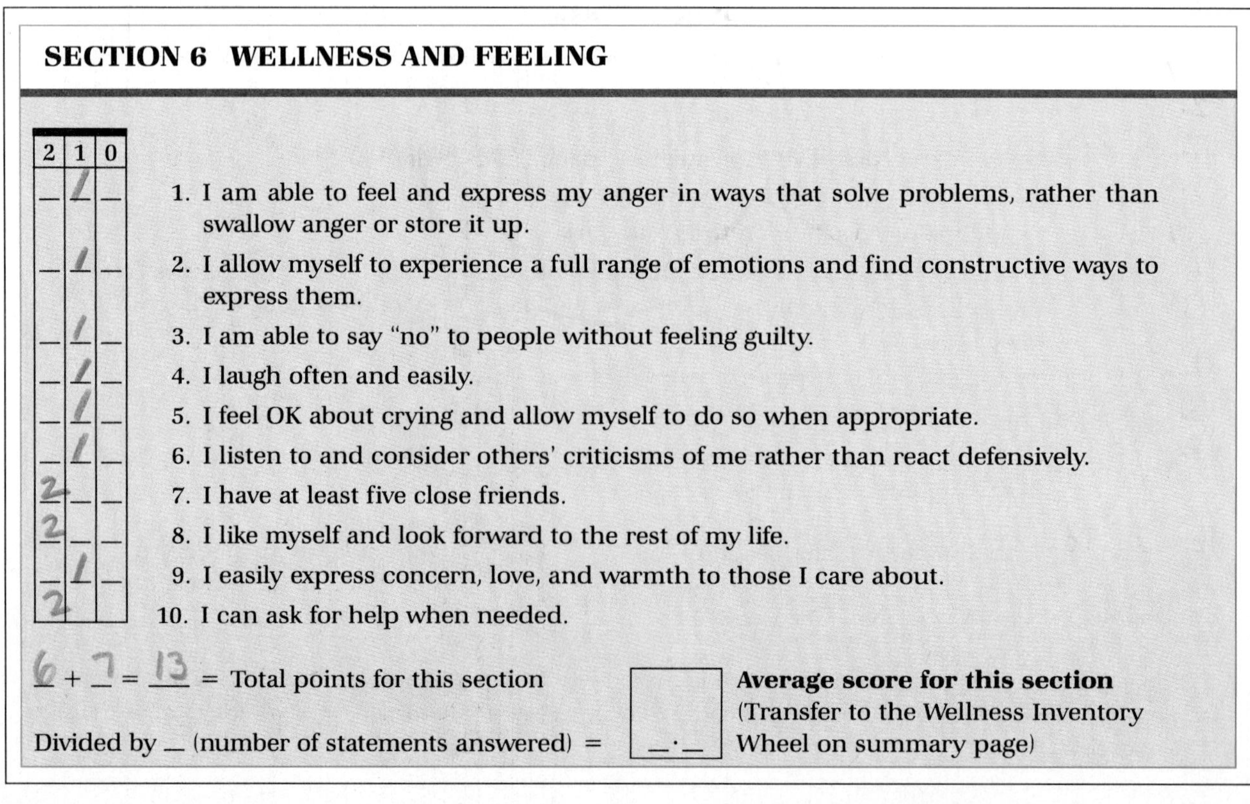

## SECTION 6 WELLNESS AND FEELING

| 2 | 1 | 0 | |
|---|---|---|---|
| | | | 1. I am able to feel and express my anger in ways that solve problems, rather than swallow anger or store it up. |
| | | | 2. I allow myself to experience a full range of emotions and find constructive ways to express them. |
| | | | 3. I am able to say "no" to people without feeling guilty. |
| | | | 4. I laugh often and easily. |
| | | | 5. I feel OK about crying and allow myself to do so when appropriate. |
| | | | 6. I listen to and consider others' criticisms of me rather than react defensively. |
| | | | 7. I have at least five close friends. |
| | | | 8. I like myself and look forward to the rest of my life. |
| | | | 9. I easily express concern, love, and warmth to those I care about. |
| | | | 10. I can ask for help when needed. |

__ + __ = __ = Total points for this section

Divided by __ (number of statements answered) = __.__

**Average score for this section**
(Transfer to the Wellness Inventory Wheel on summary page)

## SECTION 7 WELLNESS AND THINKING

Yes, usually | Sometimes | No, rarely

2 | 1 | 0

1. I am in charge of the subject matter and the emotional content of my thoughts; and am satisfied with what I choose to think about.
2. I am aware that I make judgements wherein I think I am "right" and others are "wrong."
3. It is easy for me to concentrate.
4. I am conscious of changes (such as breathing pattern, muscle tension, skin moisture, etc.) in my body in response to certain thoughts.
5. I notice my perceptions of the world are colored by my thoughts at the time.
6. I am aware that my thoughts are influenced by my environment.
7. I use my thoughts and attitudes to make my reality more life-affirming.
8. Rather than worry about a problem when I can do nothing about it, I temporarily shelve it and get on with the matters at hand.
9. I approach life with the attitude that no problem is too big to confront, and some mysteries aren't meant to be solved.
10. I use my creative powers in many aspects of my life.

_ + _ = _ = Total points for this section

Divided by _ (number of statements answered) = _._

**Average score for this section** (Transfer to the Wellness Inventory Wheel on summary page)

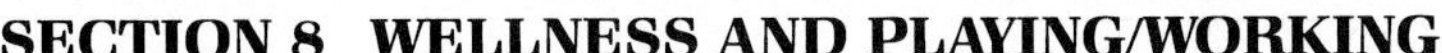

## SECTION 8 WELLNESS AND PLAYING/WORKING

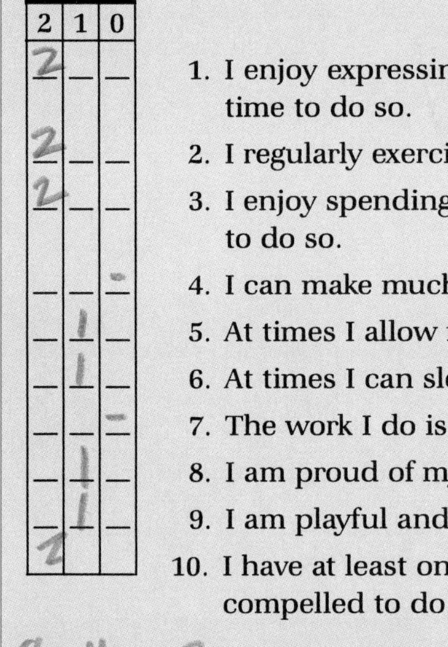

2 | 1 | 0

1. I enjoy expressing myself through art, dance, music, drama, sports, etc., and make time to do so.
2. I regularly exercise my creativity "muscles."
3. I enjoy spending time without planned or structured activities and make the effort to do so.
4. I can make much of my work into play.
5. At times I allow myself to do nothing.
6. At times I can sleep late without feeling guilty.
7. The work I do is rewarding to me.
8. I am proud of my accomplishments.
9. I am playful and the people around me support my playfulness.
10. I have at least one activity (hobby, sport, etc.) that I enjoy regularly but do not feel compelled to do.

_ + _ = _ = Total points for this section

Divided by _ (number of statements answered) = _._

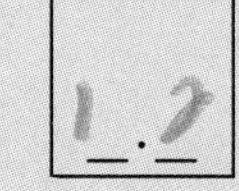

**Average score for this section** (Transfer to the Wellness Inventory Wheel on summary page)

## SECTION 9 WELLNESS AND COMMUNICATING

| Yes, usually 2 | Sometimes 1 | No, rarely 0 | |
|---|---|---|---|
| 2 | | | 1. In conversation I can introduce a difficult topic and stay with it until I've gotten a satisfactory response from the other person. |
| 2 | | | 2. I enjoy silence. |
| 2 | | | 3. I am truthful and caring in my communications with others. |
| | 1 | | 4. I assert myself (in a nonattacking manner) in an effort to be heard, rather than be passively resentful of others with whom I don't agree. |
| 2 | | | 5. I do not try to cover up my mistakes and apologize for them if appropriate. |
| | 1 | | 6. I am aware of my negative judgements of others and accept them as simply judgements—not necessarily truth. |
| | 1 | | 7. I am a good listener. |
| 2 | | | 8. I am able to listen to people without interrupting them or finishing their sentences for them. |
| | 1 | | 9. I can let go of my mental "labels" (i.e., this is good, that is wrong) and judgemental attitudes about events in my life and see them in the light of what they offer me. |
| | 1 | | 10. I am aware when I play psychological "games" with those around me and work to be truthful and direct in my communications. |

10 + 5 = 15 = Total points for this section

Divided by __ (number of statements answered) = 1.5 **Average score for this section** (Transfer to the Wellness Inventory Wheel on summary page)

## SECTION 10 WELLNESS AND SEX

| 2 | 1 | 0 | |
|---|---|---|---|
| | 1 | | 1. I feel comfortable touching and exploring my body. |
| | | | 2. I think it's OK to masturbate if one chooses to do so. |
| 2 | | | 3. My sexual education is adequate. |
| | 1 | | 4. I feel good about the degree of closeness I have with men. |
| | 1 | | 5. I feel good about the degree of closeness I have with women. |
| 2 | | | 6. I am content with my level of sexual activity. |
| | 1 | | 7. I fully experience the many stages of lovemaking rather than focus only on orgasm. |
| 2 | | | 8. I desire to grow closer to some other people. |
| | 1 | | 9. I am aware of the difference between needing someone and loving someone. |
| 2 | | | 10. I am able to love others without dominating or being dominated by them. |

8 + 5 = 13 = Total points for this section

Divided by __ (number of statements answered) = 1.3 **Average score for this section** (Transfer to the Wellness Inventory Wheel on summary page)

## SECTION 11 WELLNESS AND FINDING MEANING

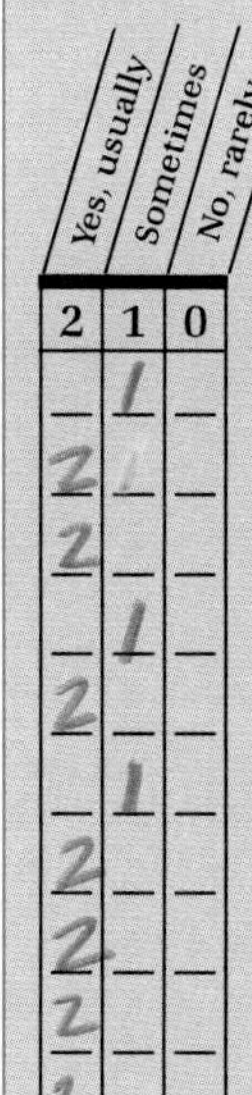


1. I believe my life to have direction and meaning.
2. My life is exciting and challenging.
3. I have goals in my life.
4. I am achieving my goals.
5. I look forward to the future as an opportunity for further growth.
6. I am able to talk about the death of someone close to me.
7. I am able to talk about my own death with family and friends.
8. I am prepared for my death.
9. I see my death as a step in my evolution.*
10. My daily life is a source of pleasure to me.

14 + 3 = 17 = Total points for this section

Divided by __ (number of statements answered) =

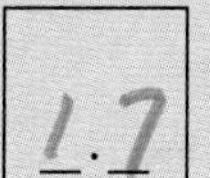


**Average score for this section** (Transfer to the Wellness Inventory Wheel on summary page)

*Seeing your death as a stage of growth and preparing yourself consciously is an important part of finding meaning in your life.

## SECTION 12 WELLNESS AND TRANSCENDING

| 2 | 1 | 0 | |
|---|---|---|---|
| | 1 | | 1. I perceive problems as opportunities for growth. |
| | 1 | | 2. I experience synchronistic events in my life (frequent "coincidences" seeming to have no cause-effect relationship). |
| 2 | | | 3. I believe there are dimensions of reality beyond verbal description or human comprehension. |
| | 1 | | 4. At times I experience confusion and paradox in my search for understanding of the dimensions referred to above. |
| | 1 | | 5. The concept of God has personal definition and meaning to me. |
| 2 | | | 6. I experience a sense of wonder when I contemplate the universe. |
| 2 | | | 7. I have abundant expectancy rather than specific expectations. |
| | 1 | | 8. I do not pressure others to accept my beliefs. |
| | | – | 9. I use the messages interpreted from my dreams. |
| | 1 | | 10. I enjoy practicing a spiritual discipline or allowing time to sense the presence of a greater force in guiding my passage through life. |

6 + 6 = 12 = Total points for this section

Divided by __ (number of statements answered) =

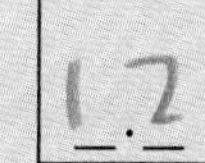


**Average score for this section** (Transfer to the Wellness Inventory Wheel on summary page)

## THE WELLNESS INVENTORY WHEEL

Transfer your average score from each section to the corresponding box around the Wheel below. Then graph your score by drawing a curved line between the "spokes" that define each segment. (Use the scale provided—beginning at the center with 0.0 and reaching 2.0 at the circumference.) Lastly, fill in the corresponding amount of each wedge-shaped segment.

When you have completed the Wellness Inventory, study the Wheel's shape and balance. How smoothly would it turn? What does it tell you? Are there any surprises in this for you? How does it feel to you? What don't you like about it? What do you like about it? Use it as a guide to furthering your wellness and have a great journey!

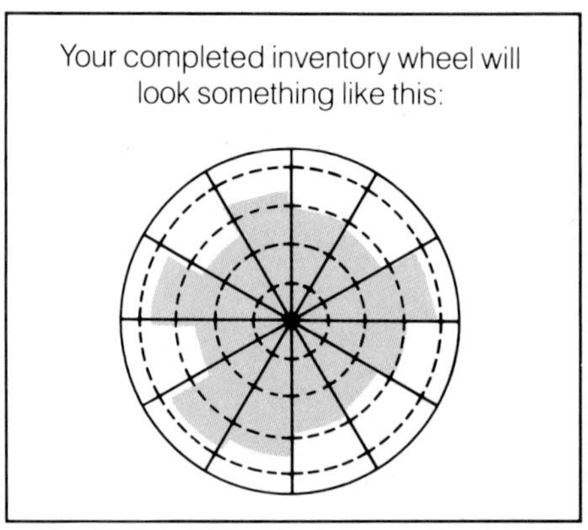
Your completed inventory wheel will look something like this:

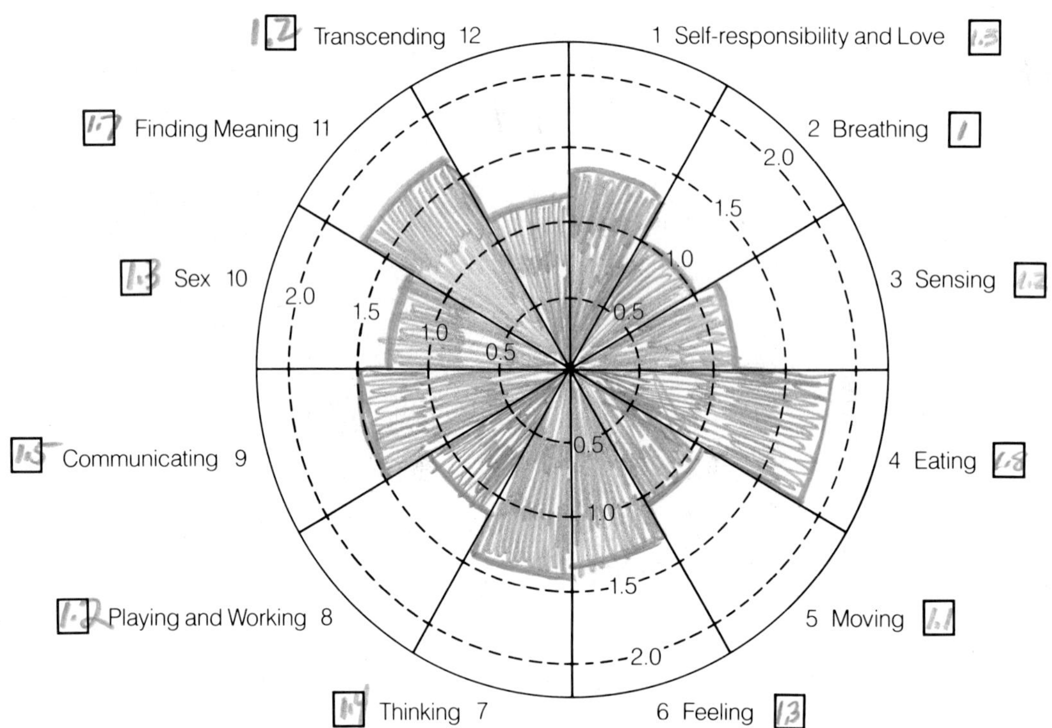


SOURCE: Abridged from the "Wellness Inventory" from the *Wellness Workbook* by J. W. Travis and R. W. Ryan, Ten Speed Press, Berkeley, California. 1988. For further information contact Wellness Associates, Box 5433, Mill Valley, CA 94941. This version of the Wellness Inventory does not include all footnotes contained in the original.

SECTION I

# YOUR MIND

Health involves every aspect of living—psychological, emotional, spiritual, environmental, and social. In this section you will learn about the feelings and thoughts that distinguish you from all others. You will discover that the life of your mind is complex and dynamic, rooted in the understanding of who you are and enriched by the quest to become all that you might be. You will learn not only about the challenges everyone must face, but about ways to meet them. And as you learn more about yourself, you will also learn about the people with whom you share your environment and your life.

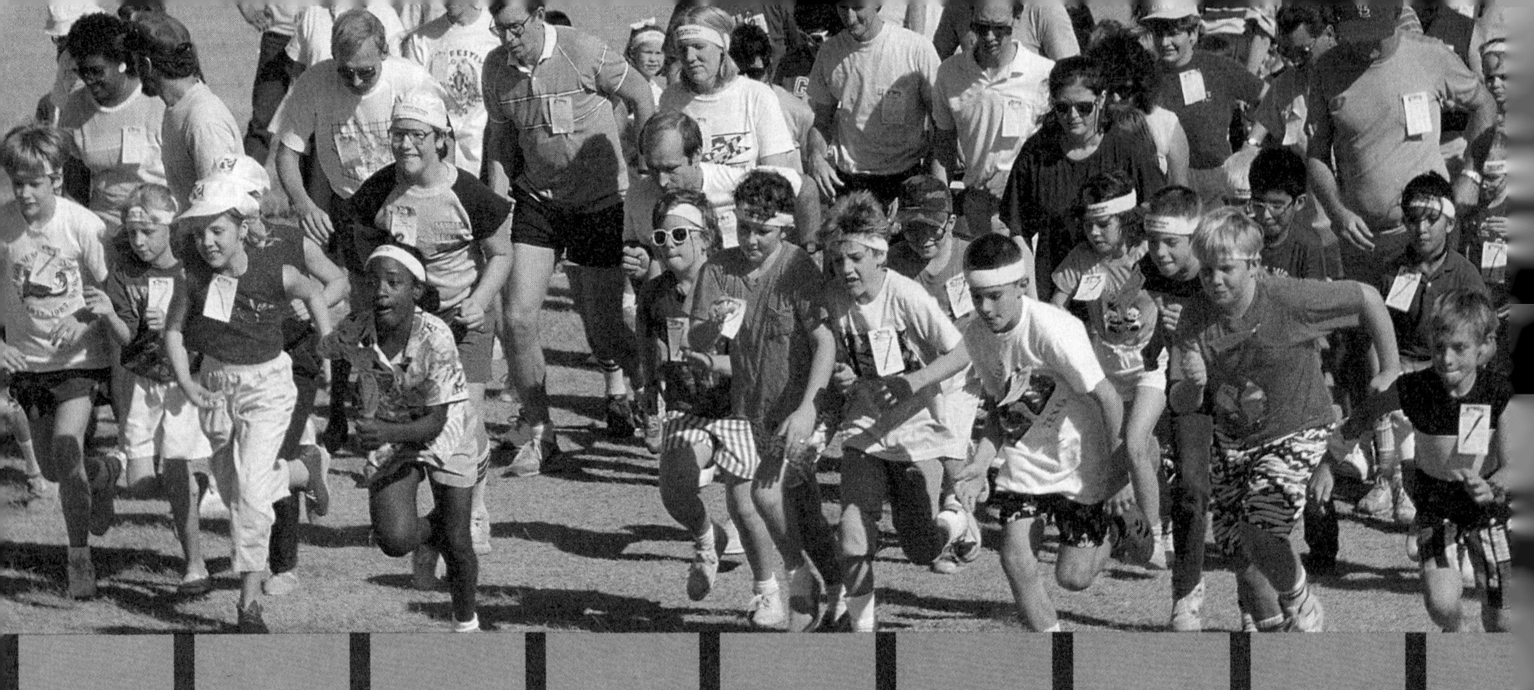

# 1 MAKING THE MOST OF YOUR HEALTH

In this chapter

What is health?

Taking charge of your life

Making this book work for you: Taking charge of your health

*How are you?* People may ask you that question dozens of times a day. "Fine," you answer without thinking. But how often do you ask yourself how you really are? How do you feel about yourself and your life? Are you eating well and working out regularly? Do you have close friends to share your triumphs and traumas? Do you smoke or drink heavily? Do you get regular health checkups? Are you aware of environmental threats to your health?

This book asks these questions and many more. It is a book about you: your mind and your body, your spirit and your social ties, your needs and your wants, your past and your potential. Its basic premise is simple: You have more control over your life and well-being than anything or anyone else does. Through the decisions you make and the habits you develop, you can influence how well—and perhaps how long—you will live. By providing the information and understanding you'll need to handle this responsibility, *Your Health* can help you live more fully, more happily, and more healthfully. The invitation to health that it extends to every reader is one offer you literally cannot afford to refuse; the quality of your life may depend on it.

## WHAT IS HEALTH?

**Health** means being sound in body, mind, and spirit. The World Health Organization defines it as "not merely the absence of disease or infirmity," but "a state of complete physical, mental, and social well-being."[1]

Health professionals view various states of good and ill health as points on a continuum (see Figure 1-1). At one end is early and needless death. At the other is optimal health, when you feel and perform at your very best. Individuals in the middle are neither sick enough to need medical attention nor well enough to live each day with zest and vigor. They may be aware of what they could do to feel better, but they lack the knowledge or commitment to reach their goals. On the negative side of the continuum, they may develop early signs of health problems. If ignored, these can become symptoms of serious illnesses that may prove disabling.

Health cannot be neatly divided into physical, mental, spiritual, and social elements. Therefore, this book takes a holistic approach, one that looks at the individual as a whole rather than part by part. It explores various dimensions of your life and focuses on what you can do to make the most of all of them. Holistic health practitioners emphasize self-responsibility in nutrition, stress management, physical fitness, preventive medical care, and environmental awareness—all major themes in this book.

### The Quest for Health

In the past, medical science focused on treating disease and improving living conditions, with remarkable success. Pneumonia, which claimed thousands of lives each year, is now usually curable. Appendicitis is rarely fatal. Syphilis, which once crippled millions, can be diagnosed and treated. Surgery can be performed with reasonable safety on any part of the body, including the heart, which was considered inoperable just a few decades ago. Sophisticated technology routinely corrects impaired vision and hearing.

As scientific knowledge has replaced superstitions about health, our level of well-being has improved

**health** Being sound in body, mind, and spirit.

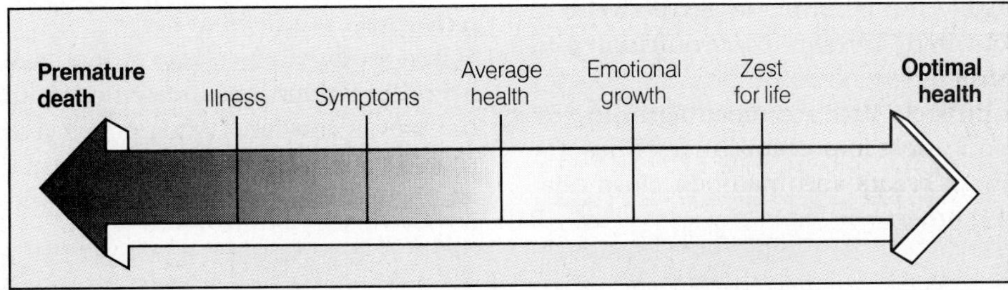


SOURCE: Hales, Dianne. *An Invitation to Health, Fourth Edition*, Benjamin/Cummings, 1989.

**FIGURE 1-1** The health-illness continuum.

dramatically. According to the National Center for Health Statistics, babies born in the United States in 1900 had a life expectancy of 49.2 years. Babies born in the 1990s are expected to live for about 75 years.[2] Our health standard is one of the highest in human history.

Do these statistics mean that all or most Americans are living healthfully? Unfortunately, no. Although we do not face the same health threats that our ancestors did, we still die earlier than we might. The nation's infant mortality rate, considered the best indicator of a society's health, is lower than ever before, but we still rank behind 21 other developed nations. Our children are more likely to be murdered, live in poverty, or come from broken homes than children in other industrialized countries.

Injury caused by accidents, suicides, and violent crime is the primary reason for death before age 40. Our most lethal illnesses are related to our life-styles. Though improved health services can make the difference between life and death (for example, in saving accident victims), even the most heroic medical efforts ultimately can't make up for decades of poor health habits. Certainly the potential for great gains in health exists. The question is whether you, as an individual, choose to make the most of your potential. If you decide to try, this book will show you how.

## The Promise of Wellness

In the traditional "illness" model of health, you are healthy as long as you are not sick. Increasingly, people want to do more than avoid becoming ill; they want to feel as well as they possibly can. **Wellness,** like health, ranges from an absence of physical symptoms to high-level wellness, which some health specialists describe as "an ever-expanding experience of purposeful, enjoyable living."[3] You can create this state of body, mind, and spirit by:

- knowing what your real needs are and how to meet them by communicating your emotions to other people
- acting assertively, not passively or aggressively
- nurturing your body through good nutrition and regular exercise
- engaging in projects that are meaningful to you and reflect your most important inner values
- knowing how to create and maintain close relationships with others

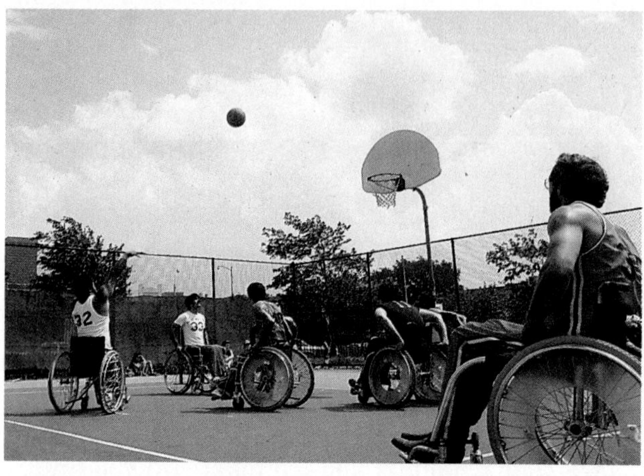

Disability does not always prevent people from leading full, active lives.

- responding to challenges in life as opportunities to grow in strength and maturity, rather than feeling beset by problems
- creating the life you really want, rather than just reacting to what seems to happen to you
- responding to troublesome symptoms in ways that improve your physical condition and increase your knowledge about avoiding similar problems in the future
- knowing your inner patterns—emotional and physical—and understanding the signals your body gives you
- trusting that your personal resources are your greatest strengths for living and growing

## Mind, Body, and Spirit

As Americans have become more active in their pursuit of wellness, they've realized that health consists of more than fitness. According to a recent Gallup poll reported in *American Health,* most recognize that a positive mental attitude and a sense of spiritual fulfillment are essential to true well-being.[4]

As this book uses the word, **spiritual** does not mean belonging to a particular religion. Its essential component is a belief in some meaning or order in the universe, a higher power that provides a greater significance to individual life.

In a study of 69 college students, which was published in *Psychology Today,* psychologists found that the active Christians, who derived great meaning from religion and saw God as their partner, were healthier and had fewer colds, headaches, ulcers, respiratory

**wellness** A state of optimal health.
**spiritual** Relating to the beliefs each of us has about the universe, human nature, and the significance of life and relationships.

## HALES INDEX

Life expectancy of a baby girl born in 1990: 83.4 years

Life expectancy of a baby girl born in 1905: 61.4 years

Life expectancy of a baby boy born in 1990: 76.1 years

Life expectancy of a baby boy born in 1905: 54 years

Number of Americans who put off medical treatment because they can't afford it: 1 in 4

Number of infants who die in their first year in Japan: 5 per 1,000 births

Number of infants who die in their first year in the United States: 10 per 1,000 births

Number of infants who die in their first year in the Soviet Union: 25 per 1,000 births

Country with the highest percentage of children affected by divorce: United States (23 percent)

Countries with the highest child poverty rates: United States and Australia (17 percent)

Number of Americans who participate in self-help groups: 20 million

Number of support groups in the U.S.: 500.000

SOURCES: **1, 2, 3, 4** Office of the Actuary, Social Security Administration. **5** "One in Four Pass Up Medical Care," *San Francisco Chronicle*, February 5, 1990. **6, 7, 8** U.S. Census Bureau's Center for International Research, 1990 study. **9, 10** U.S. Centers for Disease Control, February 1990. **11, 12** Franklin, Erica. "Help Yourself to Self-Help," *American Health*, April 1989.

problems, and other ailments than passive Christians, who were less involved with their religion, and questors, who were still searching for the truth. The active Christians were also more likely to pray—an activity that lessens tension, boosts optimism, and offers a sense of control over a situation.

Spiritual health can serve as a buffer against every form of stress, preserving hope and dignity in the bleakest of circumstances. One of the victims of the Holocaust left this testament to spirituality scratched on a wall in an abandoned house in Germany:

> I believe in the sun—even when it does not shine;
> I believe in love—even when it is not shown;
> I believe in God—even when he does not speak.

## TAKING CHARGE OF YOUR LIFE

For years skeptics predicted that the movement toward wellness that began in the 1970s would self-destruct, just as fads often do. It hasn't. As we approach the year 2000, the trend toward wellness is growing stronger every year. Taking charge of health has become especially important in a world that can seem harder to understand and control every day. And the way we define health has changed. In addition to taking responsibility for the way they look, feel, and live, Americans are working to take charge of every aspect of their lives—physical, psychological, emotional, spiritual, environmental, and social.[5]

To help you take charge of your life, each chapter of *Your Health* provides strategies for change, practical tips that you can use to enhance your own well-being. By applying them in your daily life, you can gain greater control of your body and your life.

### STRATEGY FOR CHANGE

**Making a Change**

- Set small, manageable goals. If you want to change the way you eat, start by changing just one meal a week. In a year you'll have a new way of eating, and you won't miss your old routine.
- Get support from friends, but don't expect them to supply all the willpower you need. In the long run your own commitment has to be strong enough for you to keep you on the right track.
- Focus on the immediate rewards of your new behavior. You may stop smoking so that you'll

HEALTH SPOTLIGHT

## Changing Your Life

Awareness of a bad habit is always the first step toward changing it. Once you identify a behavior you'd like to change, keep a diary for one or two weeks, noting what you do, when and where you do it, and what you're feeling at the time. If you'd like, enlist the help of friends or family to call attention to your behavior.

Sometimes awareness itself makes a difference. In a University of Hawaii study, simply keeping a diary led to permanent change in 15 percent of individuals seeking help for breaking bad habits. In another study, overweight women who wrote down type of food, quantity, and calories *before* eating meals or snacks consumed fewer calories and lost more weight than women who recorded the same information *after* eating.

Once you've identified the situations or people that trigger a behavior, develop a plan to avoid them. For instance, if you snack continuously when studying in your room, try working in the library, where food is forbidden.

Planning ahead is a crucial part of successful change. If you can't avoid certain situations, anticipate how you might cope with the temptation to return to your old behavior. Develop alternatives. See yourself walking past the desserts in the cafeteria or chewing gum instead of lighting a cigarette.

Some people find it helpful to sign a "contract," a written agreement in which they make a commitment to change, with their partner, parent, or health educator. Spelling out what they intend to do and why underscores what they're trying to accomplish.

Above all else, change depends on the belief that you can and will succeed. In several studies at Stanford University, the individuals most likely to reach a goal were those who believed they could. The more strongly they felt that they would change their behavior, the more energy and persistence they put into making the change.

A recent survey of 1,000 Americans showed that an individual's power to change may be greater than most people realize. Among the key findings:

- Positive feelings, not negative ones like fear, motivate most people to make changes.
- Individuals are about 10 times more likely to change on their own than to be helped by doctors or therapists.
- A sudden insight or unpredictable event is more likely to push someone to change than a carefully developed plan.
- For the majority of those who cut alcohol and cigarettes down or out, quitting was easier than they'd expected.
- Men and women are equally open to change. But the ones who welcome change most tend to be young and well educated.
- Generally, people make more important life changes in their twenties than at any other time.

SOURCES: Gurin, Joel. "Remaking Our Lives," *American Health*, March 1990. Lawrence Green, director of the Center for Health Promotion, University of Texas Health Sciences Center, Houston, April 20, 1987, speech. Hodgson, Ray and Peter Miller. *Self-Watching: Addictions, Habits, Compulsions: What to Do about Them.* New York: Facts on File, 1982.

live longer, but take note of every other benefit you notice: less coughing, more spending money, no more stale tobacco taste in your mouth.

- To boost your self-confidence, remind yourself of past successes you've had in making changes. Give yourself pep talks, praising yourself on how well you've done so far.
- Reward yourself regularly. Plan a pleasant incentive for every week you stick to your new behavior: a new album, an evening out with some friends, a call to someone you love.
- Expect and accept some relapses. The greatest rate of relapse occurs in the first few weeks after making a behavior change. During this critical time, get as much support as you can.

## HEALTH HEADLINE

### Medical Research: For Men Only?

**The scientific studies on which health professionals often base their recommendations and treatment suffer from a serious gender gap, according to a recent analysis of research subjects. Middle-aged white men often make up the entire population used to study how effective various preventive strategies, drugs, and other treatments are. For example, all the 22,071 physicians who participated in a study of aspirin's ability to prevent heart attacks were men. Other groups that have been missing from medical studies are the elderly, Asians, blacks, and other nonwhite minorities. Congress and federal agencies are studying ways to ensure more representative samples in future research studies.**

SOURCES: Cotton, Paul. "Is There Still Too Much Extrapolation from Data on White Middle-Aged Men?" *Journal of the American Medical Association*, vol. 263, no. 8, February 23, 1990. Cotton, Paul. "Examples Abound of Gaps in Medical Knowledge Because of Groups Excluded from Scientific Study," *Journal of the American Medical Association*, vol. 263, no. 8, February 23, 1990.

## The Payoffs of Prevention

In the present health care system, most of us play the role of Humpty-Dumpty. As long as we sit quietly on the wall, we're ignored. But when we fall, the medical equivalents of all the king's horses and all the king's men come running to put us back together again.

Imagine what our society would be like if we concentrated on preventing, rather than treating, disease. In 1990 the federal Centers for Disease Control reported that nine preventable diseases are responsible for more than half the deaths in this country—but research and treatment for these diseases get only 2 percent of the public health dollars spent by the states. The illnesses, ranging from heart disease and lung cancer to cervical cancer and cirrhosis, claim 1.1 million lives a year nationwide. At least one third could be prevented by elimination of smoking alone.[6]

According to the National Cancer Institute, changes in diet might prevent an additional 35 percent of unnecessary deaths. A simple act like buckling auto seat belts could save as many as 15,000 lives each year. Exercise also yields an impressive return on the time you invest in it: One hour of working out can buy two extra hours of life.

Preventive care has already scored some dramatic successes. The death rate for heart disease and stroke has been falling steadily, and should continue to decline as we enter the twenty-first century. Advances in scientific understanding and available therapy deserve some credit. But just as important, if not more so, are changes in life-style, including less smoking, fewer high-cholesterol foods, and increased exercise.

According to a study by researchers at the UCLA School of Public Health, devout Mormons—who abstain from tobacco, alcohol, caffeine, and drugs and eat a well-balanced diet—have some of the lowest death rates from cancer and heart disease ever reported. The 5,000 men in the study had half the expected number of cancer deaths; their wives had two-thirds the expected number.[7]

A healthful life-style not only pays off for individuals, but also for businesses. Several insurance companies now offer substantial premium discounts for nonsmoking employees of client corporations or for clients participating in fitness programs. Hundreds of corporations that have developed wellness programs for employees have cut down on absenteeism and boosted productivity; some award bonuses for losing weight or quitting cigarette smoking.

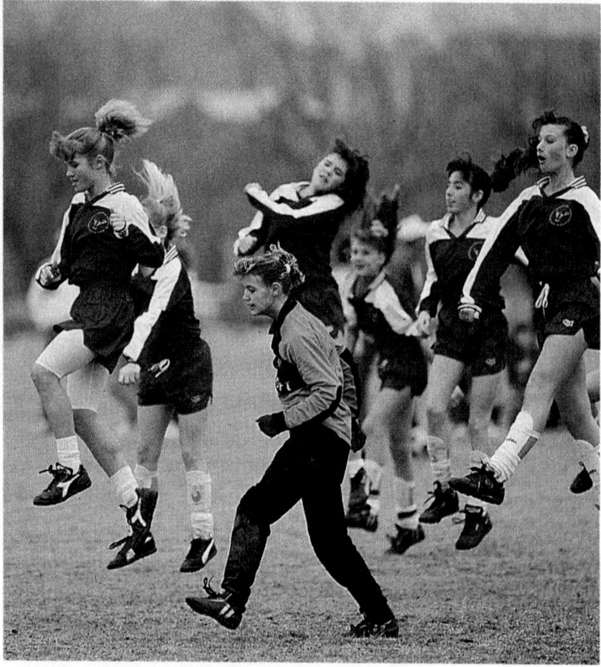

Enjoying activities with friends is a satisfying way to maintain good health.

## A New American Dream

As we approach the twenty-first century, Americans are changing the way they view their health and their lives. According to a recent Gallup poll commissioned by *American Health,* our definition of health is expanding to include basic quality-of-life issues, such as being loved and living in a safe environment, as well as medical concerns. Health has emerged as the starting point for living the good life, not as an end in itself. In fact, we now see health as a subject as big—and as full—as life itself.[8]

When asked to rate the items most important to health, at least three-quarters of the 800 adults polled included the following:

- *Attitude*—Being optimistic, having a sense of control, feeling full of energy
- *Environment*—Clean air and water
- *Stress Control*—Sleeping well, having fewer worries, less stressful relationships, time to relax
- *Relationships*—Having someone to love and supportive friends and family
- *Work*—Having a personally satisfying job

Though Americans still place a high value on avoiding illness, exercising, eating right, controlling weight, not smoking, and learning more about their bodies (see Table 1-1), we are now pursuing some-

### STRATEGY FOR CHANGE

### Helping Others Change Bad Habits

You can never change other people directly, but you can change the way you act toward them. If someone you love has a habit that's undermining his or her health, here's what you can do:

- Say how you feel. Using "I" statements, express your concerns, such as "I'm afraid you'll get cancer if you keep smoking," or "I worry that you're pushing yourself too hard."
- Don't accuse or attack. If you do, the other person will go on the defensive.
- Provide reasons to change. Gather articles and books, pass them along, and discuss them later.
- Ask what you can do to help with the change. The buddy system is one of the best possible motivators. Volunteer to start an exercise program or go on a diet along with your friend.
- Stop reinforcing bad habits. Don't pick up cigarettes or sweets just because you happen to be in the store. You're just making it easier for your friend not to change.
- Don't expect huge changes overnight. Habits are always a long time in the making and the breaking. Be realistic and think in terms of months, not weeks.
- Offer rewards. When your friend manages to go for a week or two without relapsing, plan a special outing together.

### HEALTH HEADLINE

**People Helping People**

**The number of self-help organizations in the U.S. They provide comfort, overcome addictions, soothe the spirit, and even extend the lives of cancer patients. Groups have organized around hundreds of different problems, including substance abuse, obesity, sexual disorders, failed relationships, and dozens of diseases. In addition, there are self-help groups for those living with people with any of these troubles. For listings of the National Self-Help Clearinghouse and specific self-help groups, see "Your Health Directory" at the back of this text.**

SOURCE: Franklin, Erica. "Help Yourself to Self-Help," *American Health,* April 1989.

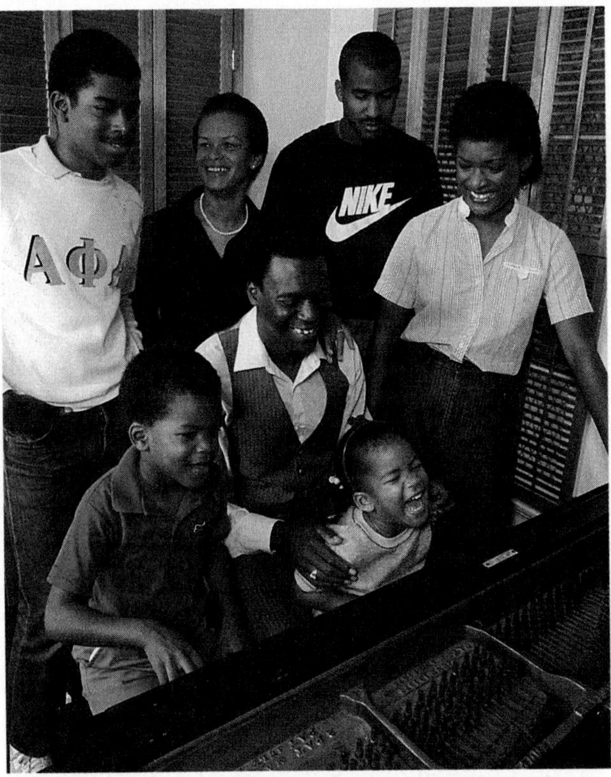


For most of us, people, relationships, and shared experiences are what give life meaning and richness.

**TABLE 1-1** America's Top Ten Health Concerns

1. Staying free of disease
2. Avoiding smoking
3. Living in an environment with clean air and clean water
4. Having someone to love
5. Having a positive attitude on life
6. Having supportive friends and family
7. Knowing how to cope with medical emergencies
8. Avoiding excess, such as eating or drinking too much
9. Eating a balanced, nutritious diet
10. Getting regular exercise

SOURCE: Yankelovich, Daniel and Joel Gurin. "The New American Dream," *American Health,* March 1989.

thing more: a sense of emotional and spiritual fulfillment as well as physical well-being. The editors of *American Health* have dubbed this goal "the new American dream." As they note, it's "a lot more complicated than the old one. We still want a lot of traditional things: strong families, rewarding careers, freedom from stress, a connection with nature. We've come to feel they're essential parts of our health . . . but today, the dream isn't just about material fulfillment, it's about enhancing personal capacity." That's what this book is about too.

## WHAT DO YOU THINK?

When Martin was 18, a car accident left him permanently paralyzed from the waist down. For months after he regained consciousness, Martin struggled to relearn everything: how to speak, how to feed himself, how to read and write. His hard work paid off, and he is now a college student with many friends and high hopes for a career in computer science. Do you consider him healthy? Can a person with a severe disability achieve high-level wellness? Why or why not?

One of these days Sharon plans to start taking better care of herself. But right now, between evening classes and a full-time sales job, she doesn't have time to cook balanced meals or work out every day. Besides, she keeps her weight down by skipping meals. Sharon's sure she could quit smoking her pack of cigarettes a day if she really tried. And if she drinks too much at parties, well, she deserves to relax once in a while. She'll worry about shaping up later, when it really matters. Would you describe Sharon as healthy? As long as she looks and feels okay, should she change her life-style? If she doesn't change, what will her health be like ten or twenty years from now?

According to the Department of Health and Human Services, a white baby will live six years longer than a black baby born on the same day in the United States. Black infants are more than twice as likely as white babies to die in their first year of life. Why is there such an enormous health gap between black and white Americans? What can we do, as a society and as individuals, to provide equal health opportunities for blacks and other minorities?

## MAKING THIS BOOK WORK FOR YOU

### Taking Charge of Your Health

Health is not merely the absence of illness, but a state of physical, mental, and social well-being. Now and in the future, your health is your most important asset—and responsibility.

Every day you make decisions that affect how well you feel and function. You decide what to eat, whether to drink or smoke, when to exercise, how to cope with a crisis. Beyond these daily matters, you decide when to see a doctor, what kind of doctor, and with what sense of urgency. The entire process of maintaining or restoring health depends on your decisions; it cannot start or continue without them.

No one says these choices are easy to make. Loneliness, pressure, financial strain, and the loss of loved ones are matters that weigh on all of us at one time or another. Yet there are signals to alert us to coming physical and emotional storms, and effective ways to handle them. These health self-defense techniques constitute the promise of this book.

Throughout every chapter, you will recognize some familiar themes—messages that apply to every aspect of your health. Among the most important are the following:

- You can do more for your health than doctors can; your health is your personal responsibility.
- You are not simply a creature of body, mind, or spirit, but of all three.
- You can take charge of your health by changing your health behaviors.
- You can learn to manage stress and to control its impact on your life.
- The way you use—or abuse—your body when you're young can determine how you'll feel in your later years.
- Rather than waiting for bad health habits to take their toll, you can delay or avoid many problems by adopting healthful behaviors.
- You can safeguard your health by learning how to be a wise health-care consumer.

*Your Health* focuses on you as an individual and on what you can do to make the most of your life. Yet you do not live out your days alone. For most of us, people, relationships, and shared experiences are what give life richness and meaning. Beyond these is the environment that shapes and is shaped by our existence.

At every stage of your life, your health will be affected by issues larger than your own experiences: by changes in values—in relationships, in the workplace, and in the home—and by dangers from pollution or unsafe consumer products. These issues can seem too big and too complex for you to solve. But you can maintain the sort of emotional awareness that will enhance your health and your ability to contribute to others' well-being. Ultimately, only you can identify what makes your life worthwhile.

*Your Health* places the responsibility for your good health where it belongs: with you. With the aid of your health instructors, this text can provide the basic information you need for a lifetime of well-being. But information isn't enough; action is the key. The habits you form now, the decisions you make, and the ways in which you live day by day will all shape your health and, therefore, your future.

This book can give you the understanding you'll need to make good decisions and establish a healthful life-style, but you cannot simply read and study health the way you study French or chemistry—you must decide to live it. Remember: Nothing is more important than your health.

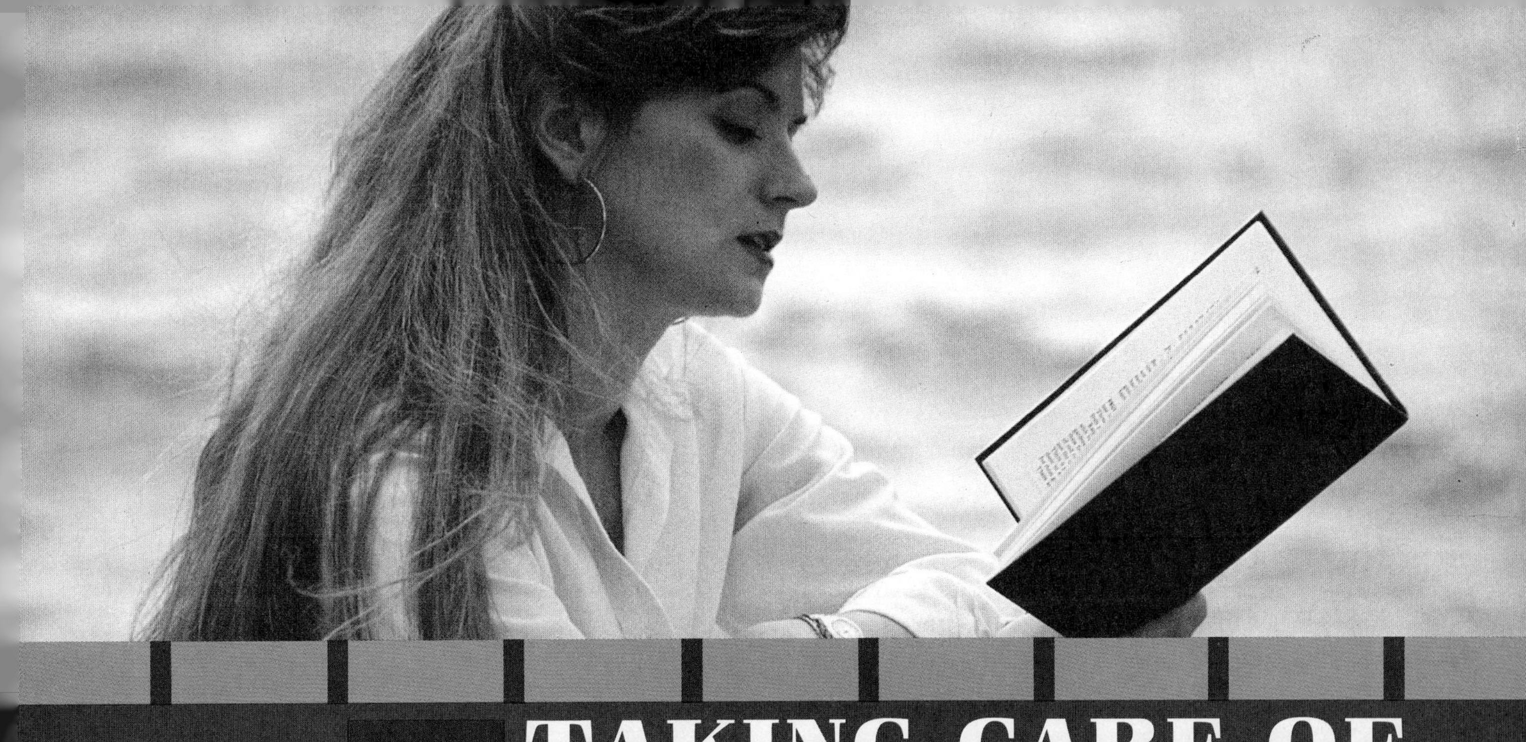

# 2 TAKING CARE OF YOUR MIND

In this chapter

The healthy mind

Your personality

Getting to know yourself

Challenges of daily living

Understanding problems of the mind

Major mental disorders

Seeking help

Types of therapy

Making this chapter work for you: Keeping your mind healthy

***Just as taking care of your body is essential for physical health, taking care of your mind is the key to psychological well-being.*** **This chapter explains what a healthy mind is, what you need for psychological wellness, and how you can cope with the normal ups and downs of everyday life. As you learn more about the mind, you may be able to cope better on your own and to recognize early warning signals that you or someone you love needs professional help.**

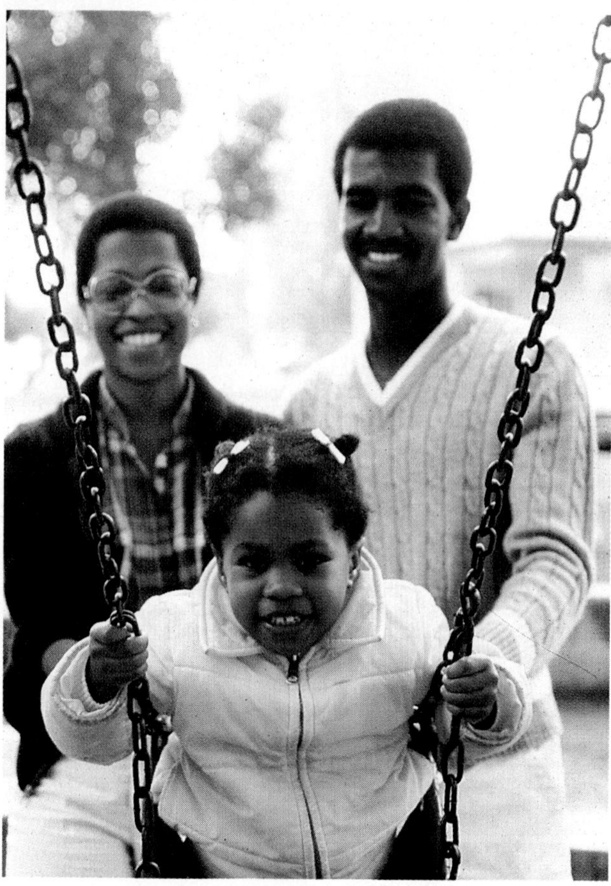

The experiences of childhood have a profound impact on adult life.

## THE HEALTHY MIND

Like physical well-being, **psychological health** is more than the absence of problems or illness. Psychological health refers to both emotional and mental states—that is, feelings *and* thoughts. Happy men and women in peak psychological health love and are loved, face life's challenges with confidence, and enthusiastically work to fulfill their potential. There is no single ideal for psychological health, however. The goal is not for all individuals to turn into identical robots, but for each individual to develop the unique possibilities within himself or herself.

In *Normality and the Life Cycle,* Dr. Daniel Offer and Dr. Melvin Sabshin list common characteristics of psychologically healthy men and women:

- reasonableness and balance
- a sense of self-worth
- the ability to love
- the capacity to make and maintain intimate relationships
- an acceptance of the limitations and possibilities of reality
- the pursuit of work suited to natural gifts and training
- a sense of fulfillment that makes the gestures of living worth the effort they require[1]

By considering how you match up to this list, you can begin to work toward wellness of mind as well as of body. No one has all the characteristics of good psychological health all the time, and the lack of any one factor does not indicate a psychological disorder.

**Emotional health** generally refers to feelings and moods: You may feel sad, happy, worried, excited, frustrated, fulfilled—sometimes all in the course of a single day. Emotionally healthy individuals are in touch with their feelings and can acknowledge and express them. In an analysis of major studies of emotional wellness, psychologist Deane Shapiro identified the following characteristics of emotionally healthy people:

- determination and effort to be healthy
- flexibility and adaptability to a variety of circumstances
- development of a sense of meaning and affirmation of life
- understanding that the self is not the center of the universe
- compassion for others
- ability to be unselfish in serving or relating to others
- depth and satisfaction in intimate relationships
- a sense of control over the mind and body so a person can make health-enhancing choices and decisions[2]

**psychological health** A state of emotional and mental well-being.
**emotional health** The ability to express and acknowledge one's feelings and moods.

**Mental health** describes the ability to perceive reality as it is, to respond to its challenges, and to develop rational strategies for living. Mentally healthy individuals are realistic in evaluating themselves and setting expectations.

Like physical disorders, mental problems can range from minor, temporary traumas to disabling, life-threatening illnesses. Psychiatrist Karl Menninger developed a continuum to represent the range of psychological states, from optimal mental health to severe mental illness (see Figure 2-1).

Menninger defined mental health in terms of self-control and the ability to cope with life's challenges. At the first level of dysfunction, a person may laugh too loudly, weep too often, feel tense, worry, or overreact to stress. It's normal to feel this way occasionally, but if these behaviors recur frequently, they interfere with our ability to function at our best.

As dysfunction progresses, individuals develop paralyzing fears (called phobias) and basic personality disorders, such as infantile behavior. As mental illness becomes more severe, individuals may become violent, lose touch with reality, and become incapable of rational thought.

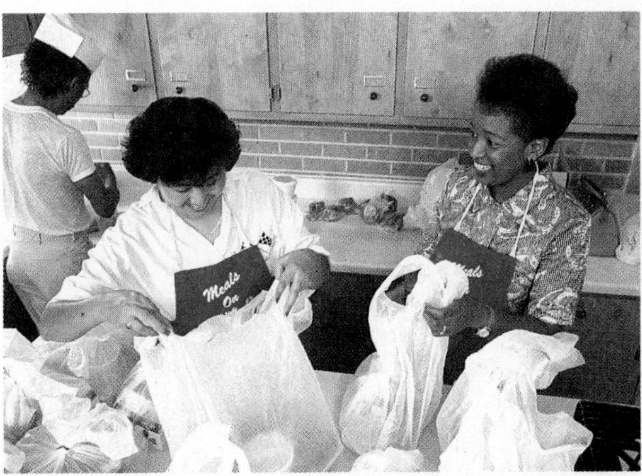

As adults, we must choose between the stagnation of satisfying only our personal needs, and the pursuit of meaningful and socially useful tasks.

## YOUR PERSONALITY

The person you are and the personality you develop reflect many influences: heredity, environment, cultural values, family expectations, role models, the experiences you've had, and the lessons you've learned from them. Because of the complex interaction of all these factors, it may be difficult to know why you are the way you are. Various theories about human personality can enrich your understanding.

### Theories of Personality

Sigmund Freud, a major figure in modern psychiatry, was the first person to explain and define the **psyche,** which is the sum of all mental activity, including both **conscious** functions (those of which you are aware, such as memorizing) and **unconscious** functions (those of which you're unaware, such as dreaming). Freud defined three aspects, or structures, of

**mental health** The ability to perceive reality as it is.
**psyche** The sum of mental activity, including the conscious and unconscious functions.
**conscious** In Freudian theory, the feelings, thoughts, and impressions of which a person is aware.
**unconscious** In Freudian theory, that part of mental activity, including repressed wishes and fears, of which a person is unaware.

Level of Dysfunction →

| Optimal mental health | Level 1 | Level 2 | Level 3 | Level 4 | Level 5 |
|---|---|---|---|---|---|
| Normal coping devices and ego control | Hyperreactions<br>Anxiety<br>Nervousness<br>Minor physical symptoms | Personality disorders<br>Phobias | Social offenses<br>Open aggression<br>Violent acts | Severe depression and despondency<br>Psychotic and bizarre behavior | Severe psychological deterioration<br>Loss of will to live |

SOURCE: Hales, Dianne. *An Invitation to Health, Fourth Edition,* Benjamin/Cummings, 1989.

**FIGURE 2-1** Menninger's continuum. With each increased level of dysfunction, a person shows increasingly maladaptive coping devices and the severity of mental illness increases.

the psyche: the **id,** which operates unconsciously, constantly seeking pleasure and satisfaction of instinctual, or built-in drives; the **ego,** which controls and regulates instinctual drives and puts the demands of reality before the pursuit of pleasure; and the **superego,** an internal "parent" that tells you what you should or shouldn't do.

Other schools of psychiatry have focused on different social and cultural factors in explaining personality development. Erik Erikson traced psychological development beyond puberty, into the social world. Unlike Freud, who emphasized the negative or abnormal aspects of human behavior, Erikson provided a picture of how the ego can develop successfully in a good environment. He identified various stages of ego development from birth to death, beginning with the development of trust, independence, initiative, and competence in childhood and continuing through ego identity, intimacy, and generativity (giving of oneself beyond home and family) in adulthood.

**Humanism** also focuses on what is unique, positive, and distinctive about human behavior and experience. Abraham Maslow, one of the most influential humanists, saw all men and women as essentially good and described people as personalities in the process of becoming. Maslow believed human needs progress from the basic necessities for survival (food, water, sleep, shelter, and sexual expression) to safety and security, love and affection, and self-esteem (see Figure 2-2). When individuals develop to the extent that they can satisfy all these needs, they achieve a state of wellness and fulfillment that Maslow called **self-actualization.**

Among the characteristics of self-actualized persons are:

- an adequate perception of reality and acceptance of it
- a high degree of acceptance of themselves and others, including a feeling of brotherly love
- a high level of independence based upon their own values
- a high level of creativity and inventiveness, including the ability to look for positive potential in problems
- a spontaneity in thinking, behavior, and emotions
- the ability to focus on tasks or missions rather than on themselves
- an appreciation of basic pleasures, such as nature, children, friends, and music

Self-actualization
Fulfillment of one's potential
Self-esteem
Respect for self, respect of others
Love and affection
Ability to give and receive affection; feeling of belonging
Safety-security
Ability to protect oneself from harm
Physiological needs
Fulfillment of needs for food, water, shelter, sleep, sexual expression

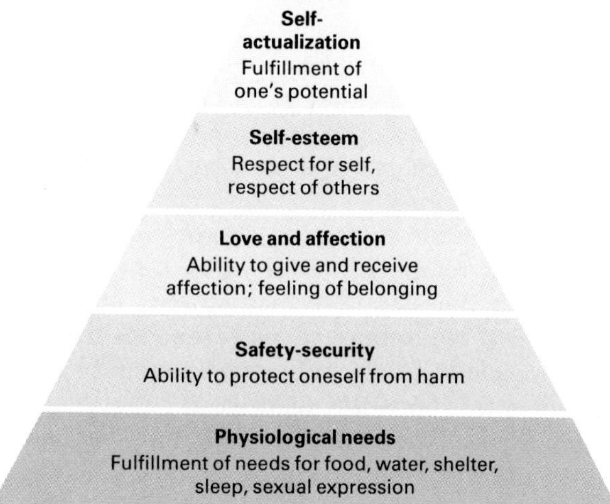

SOURCE: Hales, Dianne. *An Invitation to Health, Fourth Edition,* Benjamin/Cummings, 1989.

**FIGURE 2-2** Maslow's hierarchy of needs.

**Behaviorism** looks at human action in terms of **stimulus** (an environmental factor that can evoke a reaction in an organism) and **response** (the behavior or action caused by a stimulus). According to behavioral theory, each person is a blank slate at birth. **Positive conditioning** (rewarding someone for certain behavior) and **negative conditioning** (punishing someone for certain behavior) mold individuals so that they react to particular kinds of situations in characteristic ways. **Behavioral modification,** or behavioral therapy, uses positive and negative conditioning to help a person change a behavior. For

**id** In Freudian theory, one of the three divisions of the psyche; the primitive part of the unconscious, composed of unrestrained instincts for pleasure and survival.
**ego** In Freudian theory, one of the three divisions of the psyche; a person's consciousness or awareness of self.
**superego** In Freudian theory, one of the three divisions of the psyche; the internal voicing of messages from parents and society regarding morals, behavior, and goals.
**humanism** A philosophy concerned with human needs, human potential, and the importance of self-actualization.
**self-actualization** According to Abraham Maslow, a state of wellness and fulfillment that can be achieved after certain human needs are satisfied; living to one's full potential.
**behaviorism** A branch of psychology that views normal and abnormal behavior as the product of conditioned responses to stimuli.
**stimulus** An environmental factor able to evoke a response in an organism.
**response** A behavior or an action compelled by a stimulus.
**positive conditioning** teaching by means of rewards for desired behavior.
**negative conditioning** Teaching by means of punishment for undesired behavior.
**behavioral modification** An approach to psychological problems that focuses on a symptom and aims to eliminate it by rewarding desired behavior; by punishing unwanted behavior; or by gradual reconditioning, which eliminates the source of the problem.

example, if you are trying to quit smoking, you may plan a small reward for yourself to celebrate after each week without a cigarette.

## GETTING TO KNOW YOURSELF

Mental health begins with self-understanding and self-acceptance. You can gain insight into your own personality and behavior by learning about your needs, feelings, values, goals, decision-making methods, and coping mechanisms.

### Your Needs

Newborns are totally dependent—that is, they cannot survive without care. They depend on others for food, shelter, and protection, as well as for fulfillment of their emotional needs. In growing to maturity, children take on more responsibility and become more independent. But no one ever becomes totally self-sufficient. As adults, we easily recognize our basic physical needs, but we often fail to acknowledge our emotional needs. Yet they too must be met if we are to be as fulfilled as we possibly can be.

#### Self-esteem

Each of us wants and needs to feel significant as a human being with unique talents, abilities, and roles in life. A sense of self-esteem gives us confidence to dare to achieve at school or work and to reach out to others to form friendships and close relationships. Self-esteem is the little voice within that whispers, "You're worth it. You can do it. You're okay."

Your self-esteem is based, not on external factors like wealth or beauty, but on what you believe about yourself. It's not something you're born with or something anyone else can give to you. As children, early accomplishments—crawling, walking, forming words and sentences—earn the appreciation that pushes youngsters toward new tasks. As adults, we must consider ourselves worthy of love, friendship, and success if we are to be loved, to make friends, and to achieve our goals. Many adults have low self-esteem, and the struggle to accept themselves as they are—with their strengths *and* weaknesses—is often lifelong.

**HEALTH HEADLINE**

**Put on a Happy Face**

A smile can make you feel better, but a frown can bring you down, according to a new theory of how expression affects emotions. As facial muscles relax or tighten, says psychologist Robert Zajonc of the University of Michigan, they raise or lower the temperature of the blood flowing to the brain. The impact isn't great enough to overcome a very strong emotion, such as the profound sadness of grief, but it can influence everyday moods.

SOURCE: Goleman, Daniel. "Facial Expressions Can Help Create the Moods They Show," *New York Times*, July 18, 1989.

**STRATEGY FOR CHANGE**

**Affirmations for Self-esteem**

Believing in yourself is the first step to self-esteem. Affirmations are positive statements that help reinforce the most positive aspects of your personality and experience—statements such as "I am a loving, caring person" or "I am honest in expressing my feelings."

On a sheet of paper, list the things you would like to have or experience. Construct the statements as if you were already enjoying the situations you list, beginning each sentence with "I am," such as "I am feeling great about doing well in my classes," or "I am enjoying the opportunity to meet new people." Visualize each situation, and get in the habit of repeating these affirmations several times a day.

#### Independence

Both family and society influence our ability to grow toward independence. As we master increasingly difficult tasks, we develop confidence and a strong sense of self. Although we may always seek the opinions of others, we base decisions upon personal values and goals. In this sense our behavior is inner-directed rather than shaped by others. As independent individuals, we remain true to ourselves and our own values as we weigh the pros and cons of any decision, whether it concerns using or refusing drugs or choosing a career.

#### Love

You may not think of love as a basic need like food and rest, but it is essential for both physical and psy-

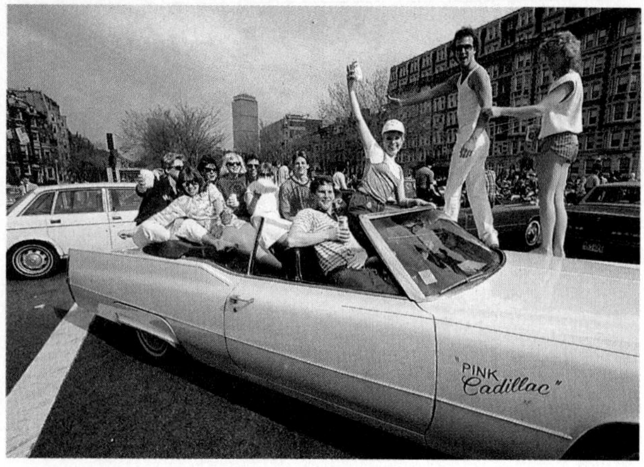


As we mature, we must make decisions about our values and our goals in life.

chological well-being. Although *being* loved is enough to get us started in a healthy life, as mature individuals we need to express love as well as to receive it, to remain separate and independent but join in a union with someone we value as much as ourselves. We move toward this state of loving as we gradually learn to love others and to find fulfillment by fulfilling the needs of others as well as our own needs.

## Your Feelings

What we feel from one day to the next is what our lives are all about. Our feelings act as signals leading us toward pleasure, goodness, and love and away from harm and hurt. They range from the joy of finding love, which fills us with warmth and excitement, to the cold, bleak despair of losing a cherished partner or parent. And they help us in ways we may never be able to put into words.

Sometimes we cut ourselves off from our feelings, if only because they are so powerful that they scare us. We can't always explain why we feel the way we do. And we may not want to admit, even to ourselves, that we're capable of negative feelings like jealousy and hatred as well as positive feelings like love and kindness.

Yet feelings are not good or bad in themselves. They are signals of what's going on psychologically inside our minds, just as blood pressure and temperature readings are indicators of what's going on inside our bodies. And feelings can affect us physically as well as psychologically. Negative feelings, such as frustration and anger, may undermine our health, whereas love, happiness, and other positive emotions may enhance and protect our well-being.

**values** The criteria by which people evaluate themselves, others, and the events in life.

### STRATEGY FOR CHANGE

**Getting in Touch with Your Emotions**

One good method for getting in touch with your feelings is to keep a personal journal. Reflect upon each day or week, and identify the most meaningful parts of it. If you find yourself worrying about a particular person or situation, record your concerns in detail. As you read your own notes, try to see the hidden reasons for your concern.

## Your Values

Your **values** are the standards by which you evaluate things, people, events, and yourself. They provide guidance in a complex, confusing world and, if understood and applied, help give life meaning and structure. For instance, you may place a high value on honesty and loyalty, and you may try to make these qualities part of your life. Nothing may distress you more than discovering that someone has lied to you or betrayed your trust.

There can be a huge difference in what people *say* they value and how they actually act. If you think through your own values, however, you can make sure you live in accordance with your beliefs.

### STRATEGY FOR CHANGE

**Being True to Yourself**

To learn more about what you value most, consider what you'd like to have written on your tombstone. In other words, how would you like to be remembered? Your honest answer should tell you what you value most. Now try to describe yourself, as you are today, in a brief sentence. Ask friends or family members for their descriptions of you. How would you have to change to become the person you want to be remembered as?

## Your Goals

We define ourselves not only by what we are now, but also by what we might become in the future. If you set your goals high, you may be able to attain more of your potential. But, at the same time, you have to be realistic about your abilities and opportunities. You may be a fine tennis player on the varsity team, but you have to be realistic in preparing for a career in sports. Are you good enough to play professionally? Or are you better at coaching others?

SELF-SURVEY

## How Do You See Yourself?

***Purpose***

This scale is designed to assist you in understanding your self-image. Positive attitudes toward yourself are important components of maturation and emotional well-being.

***Directions***

Read each statement carefully. Circle the letter in the columns on the right that corresponds to your response to each statement.

| **Self-Image Aspect** | **Rating** | | | |
|---|---|---|---|---|
| | STRONGLY AGREE | AGREE | DISAGREE | STRONGLY DISAGREE |
| 1. I feel that I'm a person of worth, at least on an equal plane with others. | A | B | C | D |
| 2. I feel that I have a number of good qualities. | A | B | C | D |
| 3. All in all, I am inclined to feel that I am a failure. | A | B | C | D |
| 4. I am able to do things as well as most other people. | A | B | C | D |
| 5. I feel I do not have as much to be proud of as others. | A | B | C | D |
| 6. I take a positive attitude toward myself. | A | B | C | D |
| 7. On the whole, I am satisfied with myself. | A | B | C | D |
| 8. I wish I could have more respect for myself. | A | B | C | D |
| 9. I certainly feel useless at times. | A | B | C | D |
| 10. At times I think I am no good at all. | A | B | C | D |

***Scoring***

Use the following table to determine the number of points to assign to each of your answers. To determine your total score, add up all the numbers that match the letter (A, B, C, or D) you circled for each statement.

| STATEMENT | A | B | C | D |
|---|---|---|---|---|
| 1. | 4 | 3 | 2 | 1 |
| 2. | 4 | 3 | 2 | 1 |
| 3. | 1 | 2 | 3 | 4 |
| 4. | 4 | 3 | 2 | 1 |
| 5. | 1 | 2 | 3 | 4 |
| 6. | 4 | 3 | 2 | 1 |
| 7. | 4 | 3 | 2 | 1 |
| 8. | 1 | 2 | 3 | 4 |
| 9. | 1 | 2 | 3 | 4 |
| 10. | 1 | 2 | 3 | 4 |

Total: ________ This is your self-esteem score. Classify your score by looking at the score ranges that follow.

| SCORE RANGE | CURRENT SELF-ESTEEM LEVEL |
|---|---|
| 40 | Highest self-esteem |
| 35–39 | High self-esteem |
| 30–34 | Above-average self-esteem |
| 20–29 | Below-average self-esteem |
| <20 | Low self-esteem |

***Interpretation***

The higher your score, the more positive your self-esteem.

High self-esteem means that individuals respect themselves, consider themselves worthy, but do not necessarily consider themselves better than others. They do not feel themselves to be the ultimate in perfection; but, on the contrary, recognize their limitations and expect to grow and improve.

Self-esteem is the most important variable in regard to human development and maturation. It is the master key that can open the door to the actualization of an individual's human potential.

SOURCE: Rosenberg, Morris. *Society and the Adolescent Self-Image.*

Don't underestimate your potential, but be honest. Look beyond yourself to your environment. What are the opportunities in the field that interests you most? Do you need a graduate degree? What about your financial obligations? Make a list of the things you need to do to meet your goals, and remember: The first steps toward meeting any goal are the most important.

## Your Decisions

Understanding the process by which you make a decision can help you understand more about yourself—and, in turn, help you make decisions that are better for you, now and in the future.

You may not even think of some of the choices you make every day—deciding what to wear, what to eat, and how to use your time, for example—as decisions. But you also make significant decisions—deciding whether to live with a boyfriend or a girlfriend, whether to cut class, whether to quit a job, or how to handle a conflict with your parents. Living is a continuous process of decision making. You can make better decisions if you plan and evaluate them.

### STRATEGY FOR CHANGE

#### Decision Making

Here is a framework for making choices that lead to better decisions:

1. *Determine your goal.* Define it, in words and on paper. Then test your definition against your own value system. Can you attain your goal and still be the person you want to be? Think awhile about where you're going.
2. *Identify your resources.* What resources do you have to meet the demands of your goal? Do you have the knowledge, skills, finances, time—whatever it takes? Find out from others who know. If there are problems, write them down. Be sure you're ready for the next step.
3. *Look for possible barriers.* How can you get what you need? Identify and select alternate plans. List solutions for any conflicts you foresee.
4. *Choose a plan.* When all the facts have been gathered, one approach usually stands out. Think it through, step by step, trying to anticipate what might go wrong.
5. *Try—and try again.* Embark on your first step, evaluate your performance, and continue to improve and refine your ideas. If you don't succeed with your first plan, formulate another.

## Your Coping Mechanisms

Most of us cope remarkably well by tackling problems head-on and taking action to solve them. In some cases we may take a day off to think through a difficult situation, talk the matter over with friends, or seek the advice of a counselor or trusted teacher.

However, under great stress or in circumstances that threaten our sense of self or self-esteem, we may not be capable of responding rationally and objectively. Without realizing it, we turn to psychological devices called **defense mechanisms,** which are ways of defending ourselves psychologically. Defense mechanisms can sometimes lead to unhealthy behavior, such as explaining to yourself when you overeat that you need the extra calories to cope with the extra stress in your life. The following are some of the most common defense mechanisms:

**Repression,** the underlying basis of all defense mechanisms, is the way we keep threatening impulses, fantasies, memories, feelings, or wishes from becoming conscious. For example, you might "not hear" the alarm clock the morning after a late night or you might "forget" an unappealing chore like putting out the garbage.

**Denial** is the flat refusal to accept a painful reality, such as the death of a loved one or the diagnosis of a debilitating disease. This is not an unusual temporary reaction, but it can indicate a serious emotional problem if it persists for a prolonged period after a shock.

**Rationalization** substitutes "good," acceptable reasons for the real motivations for behavior. For example, suppose you turned in a classmate who was cheating on an exam and rationalized your action by arguing that cheating is unfair to others. Your real reason for reporting the incident, however, might have been jealousy.

**Projection** attributes your own unacceptable feelings or impulses to someone else. For instance, if you want to break up a long relationship, you might project your own restlessness onto your partner

**defense mechanism** Any of several irrational processes that work unconsciously to enable a person to cope with a difficult situation or problem.
**repression** The act of pushing unhappy or painful thoughts out of the conscious mind and into the unconscious.
**denial** A refusal to accept reality.
**rationalization** The creation of logical explanations for beliefs or actions that are really motivated by unconscious desires.
**projection** Externalizing one's own anxieties, guilts, or aggressions and blaming them on other people or outside causes.

and convince yourself that he or she is the one who wants to call it quits.

**Reaction formation** occurs when you adopt attitudes and behaviors that are the opposite of what you really feel. For example, you may lavishly compliment an acquaintance whom you despise.

**Displacement** redirects feelings from their true object to a more acceptable substitute. For instance, instead of lashing out in anger at a teacher or coach, you might snap at your best friend.

Under stress, everyone occasionally falls back on some of these defense mechanisms. However, healthier individuals do not rely heavily on them. Instead they cope through more positive means, including the following:

**Altruism** simply means helping or giving to others, which can be a source of enormous gratification.

**Humor** enables us to express negative feelings without causing distress. It is one of the healthiest ways to cope.

**Suppression** involves a deliberate decision to ignore an unpleasant subject—to "keep a stiff upper lip."

**Sublimation** redirects any drives considered unacceptable into acceptable channels. For instance, some people sublimate anger through athletic competition.

## CHALLENGES OF DAILY LIVING

Only fairy-tale princes and princesses live happily ever after in a never-never land of endless bliss—and only they might want to. Real life is invariably more challenging and complex than any fantasy world, as well as more interesting and rewarding. In the course of your lifetime, you're certain to encounter many psychological challenges. The following pages focus on the difficulties most often cited by college students.

### Overcoming Shyness

In a survey of some 10,000 people of various ages and income levels, psychologist Philip Zimbardo of Stanford University found that 40 percent described themselves as shy and another 40 percent said they had conquered past shyness. According to Dr. Zimbardo's findings, shyness is a serious problem for as many as 2 million adults.[3]

As many as 10 to 15 percent of children may be born with a tendency to become shy.[4] Others become shy because they don't learn proper social responses or because they experience rejection or shame. As a result, they become excessively concerned about being watched and evaluated. Shyness can be treated or cured. Or you may be able to overcome shyness on your own, in much the same way as you might set out to stop smoking or lose weight. One common technique used by counselors is role playing. The shy person acts out situations that normally produce butterflies in the stomach, such as calling for a date. With practice and time, shy people can emerge from their shyness and take pleasure in interacting with others.

**STRATEGY FOR CHANGE**

**Conquering Shyness**

- Introduce yourself to a new person each day. Write down what you want to say, and rehearse on your own or with a friend.
- Use a mirror to practice making eye contact and smiling. Talk into a tape recorder, listen to yourself, and decide how to improve your speaking voice and volume.
- Observe and copy the behavior of people who handle social situations well, perhaps those who make clear what they want without being obnoxious.
- Ask someone you don't know very well if you can borrow money for a phone call or an apple or whatever. Arrange to pay the person back.
- Every two weeks, invite someone to accompany you on an inexpensive outing, such as a visit to a museum.
- Ask several people for directions and strike up a brief conversation with one of them.
- When you're with others, focus on them and what they're saying. Try not to think about how you look or what you're saying.

**reaction formation** Adopting a behavior pattern that, in fact, directly contradicts the desires of the unconscious.
**displacement** Substituting a person, thing, or image for something that has an emotional meaning.
**altruism** An unselfish concern for the welfare of others.
**humor** The ability to laugh at oneself to handle stress and disappointment.
**suppression** The conscious inhibition of certain thoughts or impulses.
**sublimation** The channeling of sexual energy or a socially unacceptable urge into socially acceptable activities.

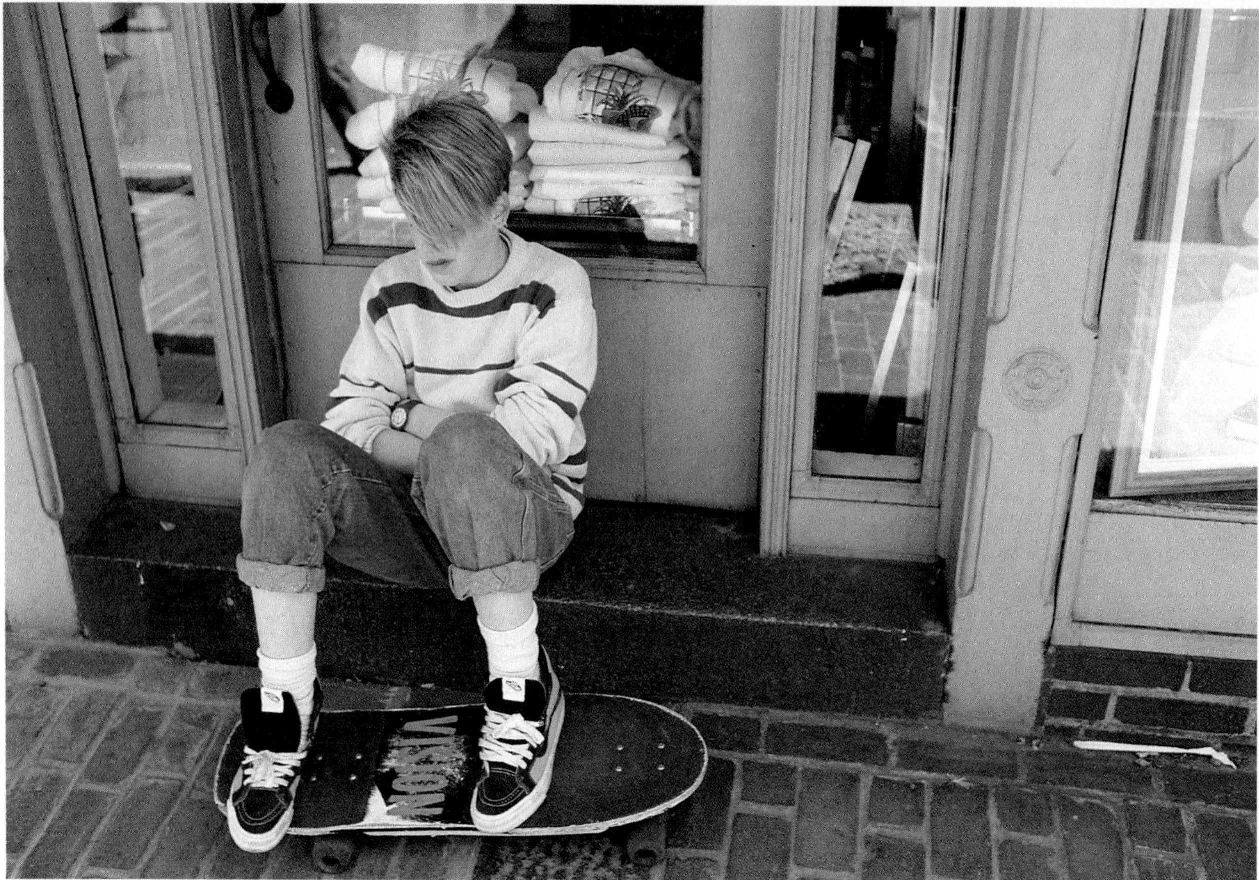


Children and teens are increasingly susceptible to depression.

## Overcoming Loneliness

Each of us has felt isolated at one time or another. Modern loneliness has been traced to the fast-paced nature of our society, to the breakdown of the family, and to patterns of urban living. With each new move or new job, we become strangers in a strange place. To combat loneliness, we may join groups, fling ourselves into projects and activities, or surround ourselves with people. The key to overcoming loneliness is developing resources to reach out to others and to fulfill our own potentials.

**STRATEGY FOR CHANGE**

**What to Do When You Feel Lonely**

- Learn to be by yourself. Enjoying your own company helps make you the sort of person others enjoy.
- Pursue some interests. Hike in the woods, perhaps, or join a singing group.
- Keep in touch with old friends, even when miles or years may separate you.
- Give of yourself as a volunteer. Nothing warms the spirit more than reaching out to those who need you.

## Overcoming Anxiety

In many situations you have good reason for experiencing **anxiety** (worry and apprehension). You may be concerned about an operation, a final exam, or a job interview. Many anxieties revolve around the people and values you cherish most. You may be so anxious about losing a friend or a lover that you try too hard to hold onto that person. You may try so hard to please a parent or a boss that you lose sight of your own values and needs.

Pinpointing the cause of anxiety may be difficult, even though you recognize its symptoms: a racing heart, a distracted mind, and a general edginess. Such anxiety can be the root of many problems. The best approach to reducing anxiety is finding out what is really provoking it. In its more severe forms, anxiety can be a total, paralyzing panic requiring professional treatment.

**anxiety** A feeling of apprehension and dread, with or without a known cause; may range from mild to severe and may be accompanied by physical symptoms.

## Overcoming the Blues

Everybody sings the blues now and then. You may feel sad, bad, down in the dumps, too weary to drag yourself out of bed. You'd rather be alone. Nothing interests or pleases you. You lose your appetite and your interest in sex. Although an occasional, temporary slide into sadness is normal, you should take steps to pull yourself back up as quickly as possible. If your spirits don't lift within two weeks, seek help. According to the National Institute of Mental Health, simply talking with a sympathetic person can help overcome mild depression.

**STRATEGY FOR CHANGE**

### What to Do When You're Down

- Stay active. Depression breeds inertia, so exercise can be the best preventive strategy. In studies of mildly depressed young people, regular aerobic exercise, such as walking or jogging, significantly improved mood.[5]
- Seek out pleasant activities—concerts, excursions, family outings, watching a splendid sunset. Find company. Call an old friend. Plan an outing with a group.
- Analyze recent events to identify possible sources of stress, such as changing roommates or taking on extra work.
- Talk to someone who cares about your feelings.
- Tune in to your "self-talk," the messages you're sending yourself, and identify unrealistically negative or critical thoughts.

## Overcoming Guilt

Guilt is one of the most common feelings, as well as one of the most powerful and potentially destructive. Unjustified, excessive guilt can sour your enjoyment of living and breed problems, such as self-punishment through drug abuse. Extreme guilt can develop into a self-loathing so intense that it may lead to depression and suicide.

However, guilt has a good side as well, for it allows you to recognize what you've done wrong and correct your errors. In short, guilt helps you recognize your responsibilities and fulfill them. If you never felt guilty, you might never learn in school, function in your job, or live in harmony with others.

**aggression** Forceful behavior with intent to dominate.
**assertiveness** The ability to be open and frank, especially in declaring one's rights.

**STRATEGY FOR CHANGE**

### Defusing Guilt

If you're plagued by guilt, take a long, inward look:

- Are you guilty because of something you did or failed to do? Have you broken—or do you think you've broken—some deeply held moral precept? Have you lied, cheated, broken a promise, violated some taboo, or hurt somebody? Are you hiding a secret? Have you betrayed a confidence?
- Once you've come up with some answers, think about them. Examine the principles behind your guilt, and decide whether they are your beliefs or beliefs handed down by your parents or society.
- Try not to judge yourself too harshly or to expect perfection. If you have done something wrong, accept it. Apologize if you can; correct the misdeed in whatever way possible. Tell yourself you've made a mistake, but it's history.
- Seek professional help if you can't put the problem behind you.

## Overcoming Anger

Like other feelings, anger can have positive as well as negative results—if you use your anger to solve problems rather than let it create new ones. When you get angry, remember to stick to the issue at hand. If it seems impossible to confront the situation directly, don't try to bottle up your feelings. Some people find that playing a hard game of tennis, running, or talking to a friend helps them cool off. Angry feelings are less likely to turn into aggressive actions if you can find a channel for their expression.

**Aggression** (attacks on other people), unlike anger, is not inevitable. Children learn to be aggressive from parents, friends, television, movies, and so on. Adults, too, seem influenced by how the media portray aggressive acts. A terrorist bombing or violent television murder sometimes triggers similar actions.

Whereas aggression is a response to anger and fear, **assertiveness** means recognizing your feelings and expressing them. You can change a situation you don't like by communicating your feelings and thoughts into words, by focusing on specifics, and by making sure you're talking with the person or persons directly responsible. Unlike aggression, assertiveness is a means of preventing anger and frustration from building up until they explode.

STRATEGY FOR CHANGE

**Cooling Off When You're Angry**

- Be clear about what's made you angry. The more specific you are in identifying what's made you mad, the easier it will be for you to deal with the problem.
- Once you know what you're angry about, tell the person or persons toward whom your anger is directed how you feel about the situation. If you can't do this, try to find a third party who will hear you out.
- Consider the other person's feelings. Ask how he or she feels about what you've said. This will help clarify the situation so that you're both aware of each other's perceptions of what happened.
- Take steps to prevent a repetition of the situation.

## UNDERSTANDING PROBLEMS OF THE MIND

Taking care of your psychological well-being is much like taking care of your physical health. Both depend on assuming responsibility for yourself—a responsibility that can never be taken lightly. In caring for your mind, you should be as conscientious as you are in tending to your body.

Mental illness, which some define simply as "misery requiring treatment," is a state of psychological impairment in which individuals cannot function normally. Whether mild, moderate, or severe, mental illness has nothing to do with personal weaknesses, willpower, or morality. Just like the body, the mind can become vulnerable, weaken, and develop illnesses. Yet, with treatment, the vast majority of psychologically troubled individuals can and do recover and return to full, happy, healthy lives.

### What Causes Mental Illness?

Many forms of mental illness are due to abnormalities in brain structure or chemistry. Some people may inherit a predisposition to certain mental disorders, such as depression. A traumatic experience, a childhood of abuse or neglect, or a parent's death may make a person more susceptible. Sometimes physical diseases, such as anemia (in which the blood contains too few oxygen-carrying red cells), cause psychiatric symptoms, such as depression. Because the body and mind are so interdependent, it's often difficult to pinpoint the origin of problems that involve both.

### Who Develops Psychological Problems?

According to the American Psychiatric Association, at any given time nearly one out of every five Americans—some 31 million to 41 million people—is suffering from a psychological disorder that requires professional treatment. Men and women are equally vulnerable to psychological disorders, but to different ones. Women are twice as likely as men to experience anxiety and depression; men are more likely than women to abuse drugs or alcohol.

You may develop such a problem yourself; without doubt, someone you know or care about will. The largest mental health survey ever, conducted by the National Institute of Mental Health and released in 1989, found that psychological disorders are as common as familiar health problems, such as high blood pressure.[6] Among the other findings of the survey were the following:

- One-third of all Americans will have a mental or drug-related problem at some point in their lives.
- People under 45 are more prone to mental illness than older individuals.
- Anxiety disorders, especially the intense fears known as phobias, are the most common problems.

## MAJOR MENTAL DISORDERS

In the past, therapists divided mental illness into two categories: **neurosis** (any symptom that an individual recognizes as unacceptable and distressing) and **psychosis** (gross impairment in perception of reality). Today, lay people continue to use these terms to describe varying degrees of impairment. A neurotic may be anxious, depressed, or obsessed, but he or she retains a solid footing in reality. A psychotic, however, has lost touch with reality.

The American Psychiatric Association's *Diagnostic and Statistical Manual of Mental Disorders, 3d Edition,* revised provides detailed descriptions of almost 300 different problems, including depressive disorders, anxiety disorders, and eating disorders.

---

**neurosis** A mental disorder in which emotional conflict is either expressed openly in anxiety or hidden by complex compensating mechanisms in the personality.

**psychosis** A mental disorder in which there is gross impairment in reality perception.

## Depressive Disorders

Everyone experiences mood swings, and feeling glad or sad is a normal part of life. However, a mood is considered abnormal if it is extremely prolonged and severe, disrupts daily activities, and is often accompanied by physical symptoms (such as sleep problems or changes in appetite or sexual interest). Severe mood disturbances, such as depressive disorders, can impair the ability to recognize reality and put the depressed person or others in danger.

### Risk Factors for Depression

Depression, characterized by an imbalance of crucial chemicals within the brain, can strike without warning or obvious reason. Some people seem biologically vulnerable. With others, environmental and psychological factors play a greater role. Although anyone can develop depression at any age, certain risk factors increase vulnerability:

- *Family History*—Two-thirds of depressed patients have family members who have also suffered depression.
- *Major Life Stresses*—Losses involving relationships typically pull women down; unhappily married, recently separated, or divorced women are especially vulnerable. Men are more prone to job-related depressions. Neglect, abuse, or separation from a parent because of illness or divorce can lead to childhood depression.
- *Physical Illness*—Depression can be a complication of many physical traumas and diseases, including stroke, epilepsy, head injury, anemia, mononucleosis, and some cancers. Medications—such as steroids, barbiturates, and antihypertension drugs—can also be culprits.
- *Substance Abuse*—Alcoholics and drug abusers have high rates of depression, and depressed individuals have high rates of substance abuse.
- *Gender*—Major depression is twice as common in women as in men, and milder mood disorders may occur 4 to 5 times more often in women. However, serious depression after childbirth, hysterectomy, or menopause is far less common than had been thought.[9]

### Major Depression

The disease of depression is every bit as real as diabetes or pneumonia and far more common than these illnesses. Depression traps one out of every five Americans in a cocoon of helplessness, hopelessness, and self-loathing. Occurring so frequently that it is sometimes called the common cold of mental health, depression may strike just once in a lifetime or may persist over many years.

Depression has been striking individuals earlier in life. Today's young people are about 10 times as likely to be depressed as their parents or grandparents. Although the average age for depression's onset is the late twenties, recent surveys indicate that 4 percent of school-age children and 8 percent of teens are depressed.[7] Teenage girls may now have the highest incidence of depression of any age group.

Only one out of every three depressed people seeks professional treatment. Those affected may not realize they're seriously ill, or the despair fostered by depression keeps them from getting help. Often, not even health professionals can spot depression. According to a report by psychiatrists at the University

**HEALTH HEADLINE**

### Rx: Reading

A good self-help book can help readers overcome psychological problems, including mild or moderate depression, anxiety, and stress. According to a 1989 study by psychologist Forrest Scogin, for many people the advice in high-quality manuals can be as effective as counseling. In another study of more than 400 psychologists, 36 percent said they regularly recommended books to their patients; 60 percent occasionally did so.

The most-recommended titles include *The Relaxation Response* (Avon) by Herbert Benson and Miriam Z. Klipper; *When I Say No I Feel Guilty* (Bantam) by Manuel Smith; *Feeling Good: The New Mood Therapy* (Morrow) by David B. Burns; and *How to Survive the Loss of a Love* (Bantam) by Melba Colgrove, Harold Bloomfield, and Peter McWilliams.

SOURCES: Goleman, Daniel. "Feeling Gloomy? A Good Self-Help Book May Actually Help," *New York Times*, July 7, 1989. McKee, Steve. "Bibliotherapy," *American Health*, December 1989.

of California, Los Angeles, in the *Journal of the American Medical Association,* doctors fail to recognize severe depression in half the patients who suffer it.[8]

Without treatment, depression can last for months and recur throughout a lifetime, shattering careers and relationships and undermining physical well-being. Depression can be as disabling as such serious illnesses as heart disease, arthritis, and diabetes. It can claim as well as cripple lives: 60 percent of those who commit suicide are depressed. Any person who, because of depression, has not been able to function normally for more than two weeks should see a qualified psychotherapist.

### Manic Depression

About one out of every 100 people suffers periods of depression that alternate with times of intense activity and elation. Individuals with manic, or bipolar, depression feel wonderful and energetic during manic periods, but their judgments and interpretations of the world are distorted. Lithium carbonate is a medication that prevents recurrences in about 70 percent of manics who use it.

### Seasonal Affective Disorder

For some people, the short gray days of winter trigger a form of depression that typically begins in October and persists until March. The victims of winter depression feel depressed and sluggish. They lose interest in sex and work; crave sweets and rich foods; and, unlike most depressives, gain rather than lose weight. Treatment consists of daily exposure to special lights that simulate sunlight.

### Depression Among Young People

The years touted as life's happiest are, for many young men and women, turning into the saddest.[10] Depression can be hard to spot in high school and college students because young people often "act out," or try to cover their feelings by becoming angry, running away, drinking, using drugs, or behaving aggressively at home or school. Unrecognized, untreated depression can deepen to a point at which teenagers feel death is the only way out. Teen suicides have tripled in the last 30 years (see the discussion of suicide later in this chapter).

### Overcoming Depression

When they do get help, about 90 percent of depressed patients improve within 3 to 6 weeks. Without treatment, an episode of depression can last for up to two years. (See the description of verbal and nonverbal therapies later in this chapter.)

**STRATEGY FOR CHANGE**

**If Someone You Love Is Depressed**

- Don't simply offer reassurances that things will look better soon. That sounds like a dismissal. Listen sympathetically.
- Be honest about your concerns.
- Discuss recent life events that could have triggered the depression.
- Keep your friend active.
- If you spot any hint of suicide, such as giving away prized possessions, take your loved one to a therapist without delay.

## Suicide

Recently, the suicide rate has soared among college students, women in their twenties, and racial minorities. Suicide is now the second leading cause of death among young adults between the ages of 15 and 24.[11] In the past, many suicides may have been reported as accidental deaths. Despite the increased reporting of suicides, however, experts believe that a higher percentage of people are actually taking their own lives.

### Risk Factors for Suicide

Researchers have looked for explanations for suicide by studying everything from phases of the moon to birth order in the family; yet they've found no conclusive answers. They have, however, identified certain characteristics that affect the likelihood of suicide:

- *Age*—In the past, the risk of suicide has increased with age, peaking among people in their late seventies. But in the last 30 years, the rate of suicide among adolescents and young adults has tripled.[12]
- *Sex*—Men commit suicide more frequently than women, but women attempt suicide 4 to 8 times as often as men. Men and women also choose different methods: Men tend to use knives and guns; women turn to poison and drugs.
- *Race*—The suicide rate is generally higher for whites, but it is rising among young blacks in ghettos. Native Americans have a suicide rate 5 times higher than that of the general population.
- *Marital Status*—Suicide rates are lowest among the married and highest among the separated, divorced, or widowed. In general, people who live alone are at higher risk.
- *Employment*—The unemployed are at higher risk than those working in or out of the home. Professionals (particularly male physicians) also have high suicide rates.

- *Physical Health*—People who commit suicide are more likely to be ill or to believe that they are. More than 80 percent see a doctor about a medical complaint within six months of suicide.
- *Mental Illness*—Depression, schizophrenia, and personality disorders are correlated with a high risk of suicide. One symptom in particular, hopelessness, is more highly correlated with suicide than depression itself.
- *Heavy Drinking*—This self-destructive behavior greatly increases suicide risk.
- *Previous Suicide Attempts*—Individuals who've tried to kill themselves are more than twice as likely to try again.
- *Loss*—Divorce, death of a loved one, or the end of other important relationships increases the risk.
- *Life Stresses*—Those who commit suicide tend to have experienced a high frequency of major life events—job changes, births, financial reversals, divorces, menopause, retirement—in the previous six months.
- *Interpersonal Conflict*—Long-standing, intense conflict with family members or other important people adds to the danger of suicide.

### Why Do People Kill Themselves?

Individuals on the verge of suicide are desperate. They cannot cope with their lives; they may feel ashamed, lonely, or helpless. Sometimes the reason for such feelings is physical, particularly among the elderly, who may be struggling with illness, pain, retirement, the loss of a spouse, or the threat of confinement to a nursing home. Pressure to succeed can drive young people to kill themselves. Suicidal children often grow up in families tormented by alcoholism or depression.

To depressed persons, suicide often seems a reasonable way of dealing with their profound sense that life is not worth living. Those who are painfully or terminally ill may think of suicide as a rational solution. For almost all, attempted suicide is a cry for help, a last attempt to communicate from a private hell.

According to the American Psychiatric Association, more than 5,000 young people kill themselves every year; as many as 500,000 may attempt suicide.[13] Often they feel no one needs them or cares. Many have suffered a loss: the end of a romance or friendship, the death of a loved one, their parents' separation or divorce.

### The Warning Signals of Suicide

Usually, a person considering suicide says or does something that should serve as a warning signal; three-fourths of suicide victims give verbal or behavioral clues to what they're planning. The most obvious clue is a previous attempt. Others are dramatic changes, for no apparent reason, in familiar routines of eating, drinking, or sexual activity.

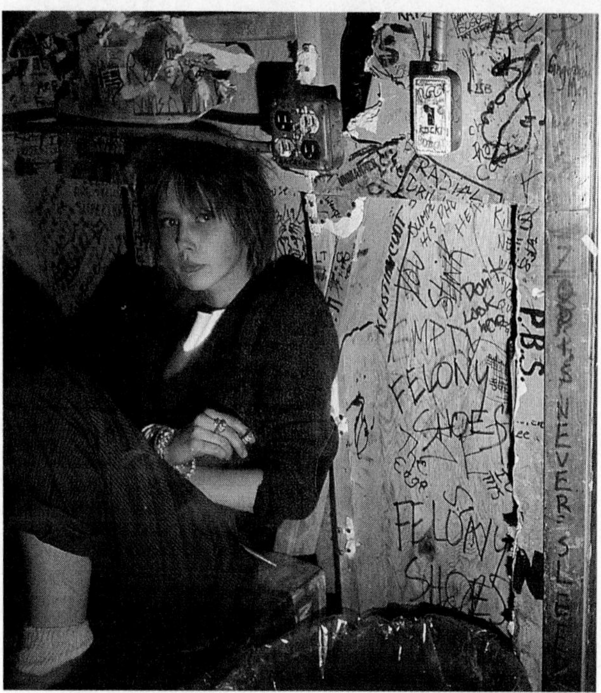

Loneliness and isolation may contribute to the high suicide rate among teens and young adults.

Among young people, the most frequent indications are:

- increased moodiness, seeming down or sad
- feelings of worthlessness or discouragement
- a withdrawal from friends, family, and normal activities
- changes in eating and sleeping habits
- specific suicide threats
- school compositions revealing a preoccupation with death
- persistent boredom
- a decline in the quality of schoolwork
- violent, hostile, or rebellious behavior
- running away
- the breaking off of friendships
- increased drug and alcohol use
- a failed love relationship
- an unusual neglect of personal appearance
- difficulty in concentrating
- a radical personality change
- complaints about physical symptoms, such as headache or fatigue

A teenager planning suicide may also:

- give verbal "hints" with statements such as "It's no use" or "Nothing matters anymore"
- give away favorite possessions, clean his or her room, or otherwise tie up loose ends
- suddenly become cheerful after a depression

**STRATEGY FOR CHANGE**

**Helping to Prevent Suicide**

If someone you know has talked about suicide, behaved unpredictably, or suddenly emerged from a severe depression into a calm, settled state of mind, don't rule out the possibility that he or she may attempt suicide. Instead:

- Encourage your friend to talk. Ask concerned questions. Listen attentively. Show that you take the person's feelings seriously and truly care.
- Don't offer trite reassurances or list reasons to go on living.
- Don't analyze the person's motives or try to shock or challenge him or her.
- Suggest solutions or alternatives to problems. Make plans.
- Encourage positive action, such as getting away for a while to gain a better perspective on a problem.
- Don't be afraid to ask whether your friend has considered suicide. The opportunity to talk about thoughts of suicide may be an enormous relief, and—contrary to a long-standing myth—will not fix the idea of suicide more firmly in a person's mind.
- Don't think that people who talk about killing themselves never carry out their threat. Most individuals who commit suicide give definite indications of their intent to die.
- If you feel that you aren't making any headway, suggest that both you and your friend talk to an expert.
- Stay close until you can get help. If you must leave your friend alone, negotiate with him or her. Have your friend promise that he or she won't do anything to harm himself or herself without first calling you. If your friend does call, get to him or her as soon as possible. Call for help immediately.

## Anxiety Disorders

General anxiety consists of excessive or unrealistic worry that persists for six months or longer. Anxious individuals may feel sore, restless, twitchy, exhausted, or tense. They may also complain of shortness of breath, fast heart rate, sweating, cold and clammy hands, dry mouth, dizziness, nausea, diarrhea, a "lump in the throat," hot flashes, chills, or frequent urination. They feel irritable, keyed up, or on edge. They cannot concentrate, and they have trouble sleeping. Symptoms usually develop when people are in their twenties or thirties. Anxiety affects men and women equally.

### Panic Attacks

An estimated 1 million Americans experience **Panic attacks,** intense episodes of fear, terror, and a sense of impending doom. Panic attacks resemble the body's normal response to life-threatening stress, but they come on suddenly—without warning or provocation. About one-third of all young adults have had at least one panic attack.[14]

During a panic attack most victims experience at least two or three of the following:

- a shortness of breath
- a racing heartbeat
- chest pain or discomfort
- a smothering, choking sensation
- dizziness, vertigo, or feelings of unsteadiness
- a tingling in the hands or "jelly" legs
- hot and cold flashes
- sweating
- a feeling of unreality
- faintness, trembling, shaking
- nausea, vomiting, diarrhea
- a fear of going crazy or dying

Panic attacks typically begin in adolescence or early adulthood. They tend to run in families, and recent studies suggest that biochemical factors as well as psychological ones (such as suppressed fear) may play an important role. Large amounts of caffeine sometimes trigger attacks.

Approaches to treating panic attacks vary. After three months of treatment with medications, about 90 percent of panic-attack sufferers improve, while 50 percent recover completely. Individual therapy and behavioral approaches can also reduce or eliminate attacks.

### Phobias

Everyone has dislikes and fears, such as being scared of the dark. A **phobia**—a persistent, irrational fear of

**panic attack** An intense experience of fear, terror, and a sense of impending doom.

**phobia** A persistent, irrational fear of a specific object, activity, or situation; produces a compelling desire to avoid what is feared.

## HALES INDEX

Number of Americans who develop a psychological problem during their lifetime: 1 in 3

Number of persons who've ever suffered from shyness: 19 in 20

Number of people in northern states who experience wintertime blues: 1 in 5

Number of men and women who suffer depression during their lifetime: 1 in 12

Number of Americans currently receiving psychotherapy: 34 million

Number of individuals who recover after therapy for a psychological disorder: 9 in 10

Number of troubled Americans who seek professional help for a psychological problem: 1 in 5

Percentage of Americans who've had an emotional problem in the last month: 15

Percentage of Americans who develop panic attacks during their lifetime: 1.5

Percentage of women under 30 with anorexia: 1

Percentage of women under 30 with bulimia: 3 to 5

SOURCES: **1, 2** Brody, Jane. "New Techniques Help Millions of Wallflowers Overcome Their Fears," *New York Times,* November 16, 1989. **3, 4, 5** National Institute of Mental Health. **6** American Psychiatric Association. **7, 8** Schroepfer, Lisa. "Emotional Ills Come Out of the Closet," *American Health,* April 1989. **9** Goleman, Daniel. "Doctors Cite Gains in Treating Panic Attacks," *New York Times,* January 30, 1990. **10, 11** Brody, Jane. "Bulimia and Anorexia," *New York Times,* February 22, 1990.

a specific object, activity, or situation—produces a compelling desire to avoid what is feared.

Phobias, which affect 5.1 to 12.5 percent of all Americans, are the most common psychiatric illness among women of all ages and the second most common illness among men over 25.[15] The most widespread phobias are agoraphobia—the fear of being in open or public places, such as department stores or in crowds—and simple phobias—which center on specific objects or situations, such as snakes or flying. Most phobias can be treated successfully by behavioral methods or drug therapy.

### Social Anxiety

"Social phobics" are more than supershy. They're gripped by an irrational fear that they will act in a way that is humiliating, even though they know the fear is excessive. Students with this form of people-panic may be overwhelmed by anxiety at the prospect of entering a crowded cafeteria, speaking in class, or going on a date.

Social phobia affects men and women equally. In one study, half of its victims avoided all social contacts outside the family, more than one-third abused alcohol, and some dropped out of school or were unable to work.[16] The first symptoms of social phobia usually appear in adolescence, but many social phobics delay seeking treatment for as long as 10 years. Various forms of psychotherapy, often coupled with medications, have proven very effective in treating social anxiety.

### Posttraumatic Stress Disorder

People who survive a trauma—rape, combat, earthquakes, plane crashes—may reexperience the event through painful nightmares or recollections that are characteristic of **posttraumatic stress disorder.** Trauma survivors may behave as if they were actually reliving the trauma. They may also suffer a kind of psychic numbing that prevents them from receiving pleasure from life's activities or developing close, tender relationships with others. Some survivors of traumas feel guilty about having survived when others did not.

## Eating Disorders

Increasing numbers of people—predominantly women in their teens and twenties—are practicing

**posttraumatic stress disorder** The repeated reliving of a trauma through nightmares or recollection.

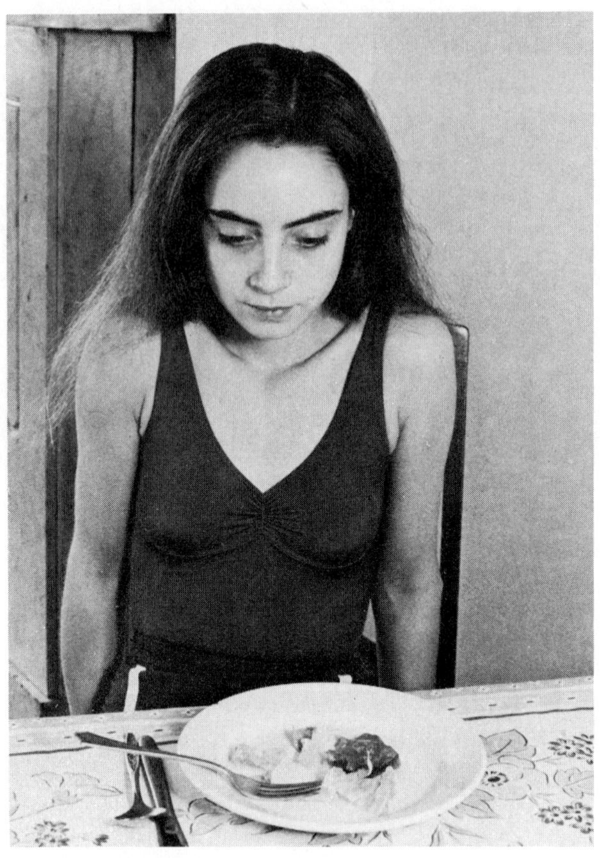

The anorexic struggles desperately to control weight to combat an underlying sense of helplessness.

bizarre and dangerous patterns of food consumption. The most prevalent are anorexia nervosa; bulimia nervosa; and a combination of these, called bulimarexia. Overeating in itself is not a psychiatric disorder, but it can be a symptom of emotional problems.

### Anorexia Nervosa

A disturbance in a person's sense of identity and autonomy can lead to **anorexia nervosa.** The anorexic struggles desperately to control weight to combat an underlying sense of helplessness. Anorexia may afflict as many as one out of every 100 young American women between the ages of 12 and 18.

About one third of all anorexics were mildly overweight when they first started dieting. Often a girl starts dieting to lose just a few pounds. But even though she eats less and loses weight, she still feels fat. Anorexia nervosa is potentially deadly. From 5 to 18 percent of its victims die because of malnutrition and starvation.

**Symptoms** Symptoms of anorexia nervosa include a refusal to maintain normal body weight; an intense fear of gaining weight or becoming fat; a distorted body image, so that the person feels fat even when emaciated; and in women, the absence of at least three menstrual periods.

### Bulimia Nervosa

The characteristics of **bulimia nervosa** are recurrent episodes of binge eating—rapid consumption of a large amount of food, usually sweets, in a short period of time—followed by self-induced vomiting or laxative abuse. Often, bulimics will stop only for sleep, social needs, or because of severe abdominal pain. They then induce vomiting to relieve guilt and control their weight. In severe cases, bulimics may spend hours every day gorging themselves and vomiting.

**Symptoms** Most bulimics look normal and are of normal weight. Symptoms include recurrent binge eating; a feeling of lack of control over eating behavior; a regular reliance on self-induced vomiting, laxatives, or diuretics; strict dieting or fasting; vigorous exercises to prevent weight gain; overconcern with body shape and weight.

### Bulimarexia

People with symptoms of both bulimia and anorexia nervosa, such as binge eating, vomiting, and self-starvation with severe weight loss, suffer from **bulimarexia.** The overlap between the two disorders is great. Between 40 and 50 percent of people with anorexia nervosa exhibit bulimic behavior.

### Causes and Treatment of Eating Disorders

A significant proportion of women with eating disorders have other psychological problems also, including depression and alcohol abuse. But eating disorders may have social as well as psychological causes, reflecting the cultural obsession with thinness as a symbol of strength, independence, achievement, and attractiveness.

Although bulimics are usually aware that vomiting

**anorexia nervosa** A psychological disorder in which refusal to eat and/or an extreme loss of appetite leads to malnutrition, severe weight loss, and possibly death.
**bulimia nervosa** Episodic binge eating, often followed by forced vomiting, and accompanied by a persistent overconcern with body shape and weight.
**bulimarexia** A psychological disorder that results in the self-starvation symptoms of anorexia nervosa and the binge-purge behaviors of bulimia.

HEALTH SPOTLIGHT

## Diary of a Student with Anorexia

| Day | Time and Place | Type of Food | Thoughts |
|---|---|---|---|
| Mon. | 8:00–9 A.M.<br>In class | 1 pack of gum | I need the gum to get me going. I wonder how many cavities I have. This is better than eating breakfast. I watched Jim eat and thought, "Wow! Is he consuming megacalories." I'm glad I'm not. |
| | 5:05 P.M.<br>Campus store | 1 apple | I wonder if anyone saw me buy this. They are probably thinking, "Boy, is she fat. That's all she should eat!" I'll have to exercise for a while. |
| Tues. | 10:00 A.M. | 2 packs of gum | I feel like a blimp today. I won't eat a lot. I wish I wouldn't eat so much gum. I can't help myself. It seems like I don't have any willpower. |
| | 3:30 P.M.<br>Dorm room | 1 apple, a few pieces of cauliflower, 1/2 piece of bread, 1/2 slice of cheese, 1 pack of gum | Drat, I blew it! Nothing more for me to eat. I'm mad at myself. I feel like I ate too much. I want to cry. I had a TV dinner in the oven, but I took it out—too many calories. |
| | Evening | | I did it again—I took 1/2 box of laxatives. Why did I do that? I know it won't help, because I need a whole box for it to do any good. |
| Wed. | Throughout the day and evening | 6 packs of gum | I'm going to go out tonight, so I'm not going to eat anything or my stomach will stick out. |
| Thurs. | 1:00 P.M.<br>Dorm room | 3 packs of gum<br>1 cup of popcorn<br>1 cup of spinach<br>1 tomato | I don't know why I ate that. Stop eating, you pig! |
| Fri. | 8:00–10:00 A.M.<br>In class<br>6:30 P.M.<br>Dorm room | 2 packs of gum<br><br>1/2 pear<br>1/2 cup of spinach<br>1 slice of cheese<br>1 soda cracker | I'm not doing very well today, but I have lost 4 pounds—so I feel a little better. I can't wait to go to bed so I can sleep all night and eat more tomorrow—especially gum. |
| Sat. | Throughout the day<br>11:00 P.M.<br>Came home from a party | 8 packs of gum<br>3 pieces of pizza<br>1 cup of spinach<br>1 piece of bread<br>5 soda crackers<br>1 bag of pretzels<br>1 cup of popcorn<br>2 pieces of cheese | I'm so hungry—I am going to eat and eat and eat. I'm really mad. I'm not hungry, but I can't stop eating. I asked my roommate to tell me to quit. She did and I quit. My stomach is gonna burst. |
| Sun. | Throughout the day<br>Dorm room | 4 packs of gum | I'm not going to eat very much today. I have to make up for last night! Boy, am I hungry. |
| | 6:30 P.M.<br>Dorm room | 1 pear | That is the best pear I've ever had. |
| | 9:00 P.M.<br>Dorm room | | I feel really scared. I thought about food all day today. I wish there were no such thing as food. I hate myself sometimes. |

SOURCE: Newman, Patricia and Patricia Halvorson. *Anorexia Nervosa and Bulimia.*

constantly, perhaps daily, is abnormal behavior, anorexics may deny they have a problem and resist treatment. However, once they acknowledge that they need help, they can get better. For anorexics, the first goal is to improve nutritional status, but all victims of eating disorders must understand what's going on in their minds as well as their bodies. Psychotherapists generally use a combination of techniques, which may include behavior therapy, insight-oriented psychotherapy, role playing, and family therapy.

## Schizophrenic Disorders

Among the most baffling of mental illnesses are the **schizophrenic disorders,** which profoundly distort an individual's sense of reality and significantly impair perceptions, thinking, emotions, speech, and physical activity. They affect 150 out of every 100,000 people and occur in every culture, in every part of the world. Schizophrenic disorders strike men and women equally, most often between the ages of 17 and 25. There are many types of schizophrenia and symptoms vary widely in intensity, severity, and frequency.[17]

**Symptoms** The first signs of schizophrenia are subtle: tension, difficulty sleeping or concentrating, social withdrawal. Over time, appearance and behavior deteriorate, and the person begins behaving bizarrely. The primary symptoms of full-blown schizophrenia include:

- Delusions, which are strange beliefs that have no basis in reality. A schizophrenic may think he or she is Jesus or the president, for example.
- Hallucinations in which the person sees things or hears voices and sounds that don't exist.
- Thought disorders in which the person strings together unconnected thoughts or makes up their own words.

Schizophrenia seems to worsen and improve in cycles known as remission and relapse. In remission, schizophrenics may appear normal, though they may remain unemotional. Contrary to many assumptions, schizophrenics are generally nonviolent.

**Causes** Scientists have many theories but no real answers about the causes of schizophrenia. Research indicates that people may inherit a susceptibility to the illness, which can be triggered by environmental factors, such as a viral infection that changes body chemistry, an abusive or violent childhood, or the traumas of adult life.

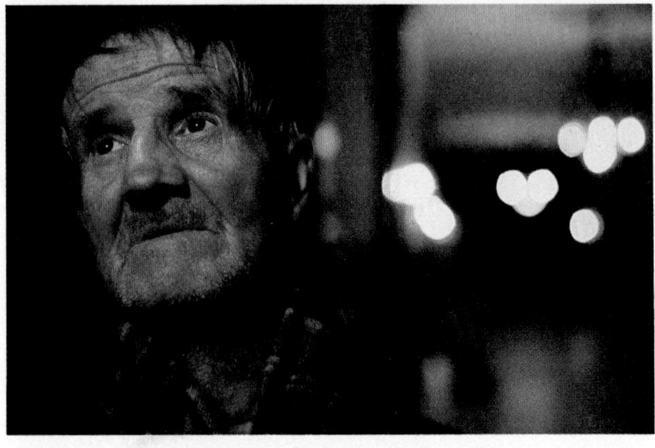

About 40 percent of the homeless are schizophrenics, some are incapable of making wise choices for themselves or of following a consistent program of treatment.

**Treatment** Schizophrenia cannot yet be cured. But, like diabetics, most schizophrenics who receive appropriate therapy can work, live with their families, and enjoy friends. Powerful drugs called antipsychotics reduce confusion, anxiety, delusions, hallucinations, and the other symptoms of schizophrenia.

Sadly, not all schizophrenics have the resources to get the care they need. These people often "fall between the cracks" of the social services system. About 40 percent of the homeless are schizophrenics. Without treatment, they may never be able to leave the streets and live productive lives.

# SEEKING HELP

An estimated 34 million Americans are currently receiving professional **psychotherapy** or counseling; millions more need such help.[18] Yet many people deny that they have a psychological problem, because they see such problems as a sign of weakness rather than an illness.

## When to Get Help

How can you know when you need professional help? According to mental health experts, common signals of trouble include the following:

- prolonged feelings of depression, hopelessness, helplessness, and despair

**schizophrenic disorders** A general term for a variety of mental disorders involving a highly distorted sense of inner and outer reality that significantly impairs a person's perceptions, thinking, speech, and physical activity
**psychotherapy** A treatment designed to produce a response by psychological means (suggestion, persuasion, reassurance, and support) rather than physical means.

- the inability to bounce back from a crisis within a few months
- thoughts of suicide
- a sense that life is out of control
- confusion or an inability to concentrate and think
- fears that people are out to get you
- difficulty getting along with people
- conflict in a relationship, marriage, or family
- the inability to stop destructive behavior, like gambling or drinking
- fears so intense they interfere with normal functioning
- emotional difficulty in coping with a physical illness
- frequent sexual problems
- persistent difficulty in sleeping

These symptoms don't mean that you're "crazy," but they do indicate that you need help in sorting out your life. Just as your body sometimes breaks down under the normal strain of day-to-day living, so too is your psyche vulnerable. Seeking help is the first step to feeling better and finding solutions to your problems.

### Where to Turn

As a student, your best contact for identifying local services may be your health education instructor or department. The health teachers can tell you about general and mental health services available on campus, community-based services, and special emergency services. On campus, you can also turn to the student health services or the office of the dean of student services or student affairs.

Within the community, you can turn to the city health department and neighborhood health centers; to local hospitals, which often have special clinics and services; and to local branches of national service organizations, such as United Way, Alcoholics Anonymous, other 12-step programs, and various support groups (see the listings in "Your Health Directory" in the appendix). You can call the psychiatric or psychological association in your city or state. Your family doctor may also be able to help.

The telephone book can also be helpful. Special programs are often listed either by the nature of the service, by the name of the neighborhood or city, or by the name of the sponsoring group. In large cities there are common names for types of services listed, which may be preceded by the city's name—the New York City Suicide Hot Line, for example. In addition to suicide prevention, available programs might include crisis intervention, violence prevention, child abuse prevention, drug treatment information, shelters for battered women, senior citizens' centers, and self-help and counseling services. Many services have special hot lines for coping with emergencies. Others provide information as well as counseling over the phone.

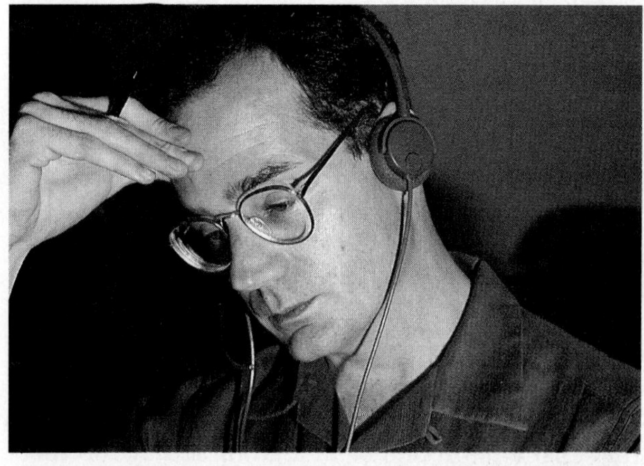

Hotline volunteers try to help individuals who may feel desperate and hopeless.

**STRATEGY FOR CHANGE**

#### How to Call for Help

- Briefly and clearly describe your type of problem, the primary thing that's bothering you, and where you live. Allow the health workers to ask for details.
- Be patient. Your call may be transferred, or you may be referred to other numbers before finding the correct person or facility. If your situation is an emergency, make that fact clear to the first person you talk to. If you cannot stay on the phone, give your location and specify the kind of help you need. For example, if someone is threatening to jump off a roof, ask for the police or fire department *and* for a professional counselor. Be sure to state your location clearly.
- Always ask to be referred elsewhere if your initial contact can't help you.
- When you reach the right person and if you are not in an emergency, ask what services are provided and at what cost, who is eligible, what the registration procedure is and how much time it involves, when and where your appointment will be and how to get there, and if there's anything you should bring (medicine, past records, addresses for past medical records, or specimens).

## TYPES OF THERAPY

Forget the couch. Chances are you won't find one in most therapists' offices. In the decades since Freud began probing the human mind, psychotherapy has evolved into a science. Today's therapists, though versed in Freudian theory, often combine several techniques, including talking therapies and nonverbal therapies.

### Talking Therapies

In the talking therapies, the patient interacts with the therapist one-on-one or in a group led by the therapist. The techniques used by the therapist depend on the therapist's background and the patient's problem. The most common types of talking therapy are psychodynamic therapy, brief psychotherapy, group therapy, and crisis intervention.

Psychodynamic therapy places great emphasis on childhood events. The therapist serves as an interpreter of experience, helping patients see how present feelings relate to early influences. One form of psychodynamic therapy, **psychoanalysis,** a technique pioneered by Freud, is a complex, lengthy process that deals with long-repressed feelings and issues.

**Brief psychotherapy** consists of short-term, structured treatments, generally ranging from 12 to 20 sessions over a period of 12 to 16 weeks (the time is agreed upon before treatment begins). The therapist takes a more active role than in open-ended, long-term therapy and focuses on a particular emotional problem causing acute distress. The two most frequent types of brief psychotherapy are:

- *Cognitive therapy,* in which the therapist's goal is to help a patient break out of a distorted way of thinking. For instance, a depressed student may feel rejected when a friend is late for their scheduled lunch. "No one likes to be with me," he concludes. In this situation, the therapist can help the patient break out of such negative thinking by pointing out that the friend had a legitimate excuse, apologized profusely, and made plans to get together again soon.
- *Interpersonal therapy,* which focuses on the patient's relationships. One 22-year-old woman sought help because of problems in her relationships with men. Constantly fearful of rejection, she felt a desperate need to please others. In the course of their focused sessions, the therapist helped her to trace these feelings to childhood experiences, including resentment of a younger sister who became their father's favorite and guilt when that sister was killed in an automobile accident.

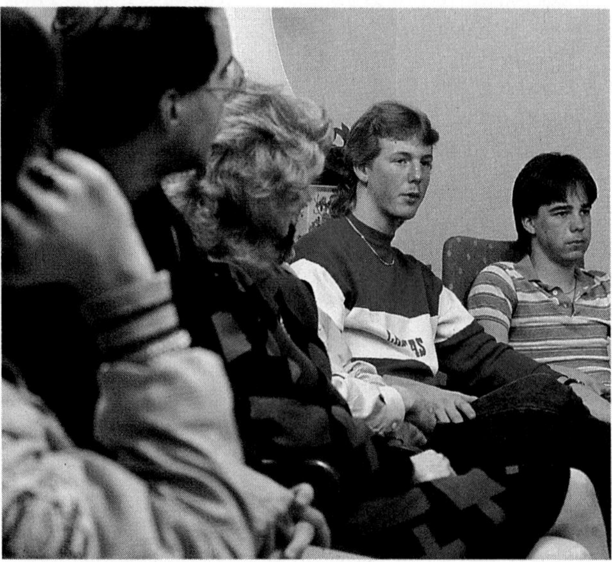

Therapy can provide a new way of looking at the world and of finding options you may not have guessed existed.

**Group therapy** works toward the same goals as individual psychotherapy: self-understanding, self-acceptance, and the modification of distressing behavior. Groups use a variety of methods from role playing to free conversation.

**Crisis intervention** is the psychiatric equivalent of emergency medical care—an immediate response to a dangerous, even deadly, situation. The crisis may be an intense wish to commit suicide, a drug overdose, or almost uncontrollable feelings of rage toward a child or spouse. Hot lines put callers in touch with a trained professional who can quickly determine what type of help they need most. See your local phone directory's Yellow Pages for listings.

**psychoanalysis** A system of psychotherapy, developed by Sigmund Freud, in which emotions, dreams, and behavior are analyzed in terms of repressed instinctual drives in the unconscious.

**brief psychotherapy** Short-term, structured treatments focusing on a specific emotional problem.

**group therapy** A treatment in which participants interact using a variety of therapeutic methods, such as role playing and free conversation, to achieve goals.

**crisis intervention** Immediate response to a dangerous situation.

**STRATEGY FOR CHANGE**

**Choosing a Therapist**

- Find out how often the therapist wants to see you. Once a week is the norm. Talk about fees and insurance coverage.
- Pay attention to the office atmosphere, and make sure you feel comfortable in the setting.
- Ask the therapist about credentials and length of practice. You may want someone who's very experienced or someone who seems more open to new ideas.
- Ask whether the therapist has had clients with problems similar to yours.
- Judge for yourself whether you feel you could work well together. Do you feel the therapist showed genuine concern? Do you feel that the therapist will take you seriously and treat you with respect? Do your instincts tell you this is someone you can trust with intimate details of your life? If not, feel no obligation. Ask for a referral to another therapist.
- If, after a few months, you don't feel that you're making progress in therapy, discuss this with your therapist. If you decide to leave therapy, ask for the name of another therapist with whom you might work better.

## Nonverbal Therapies

Some treatments rely on means other than the patient's own words to help resolve emotional problems.

### Behavioral Modification

Behavioral therapy focuses on a symptom, such as a fear of the outdoors, and aims to eliminate it by rewarding desired behavior, by punishing unwanted behavior, or by gradual reconditioning.

### Light Therapy

Seasonal affective disorder, the depression triggered by winter darkness, lifts for approximately 80 percent of SAD patients when they spend several hours a day in front of special fluorescent lights that mimic natural sunlight.

### Hypnosis

Hypnosis involves a unique type of concentration that is attentive, receptive, and well focused. The therapist structures this intense concentration in a way that helps a patient meet a particular goal, such as overcoming a phobia or breaking a bad habit. Hypnosis is most helpful in easing anxiety, overcoming phobias, curbing overeating, and coping with pain.

### Creative Therapies

Creative therapies can use any form of creativity, such as art or dance. Sometimes drawings express feelings and fears that cannot be put into words, particularly by children. Dance therapy, which encourages free, expressive movements, also can release pent-up emotions.

### Psychiatric Drugs

New psychiatric drugs have brought hope for indi-

**WHAT DO YOU THINK?**

Always shy, Carmen hated talking to strangers or meeting new people. When she went away to a college where she knew no one, she felt overwhelmed. Rather than going to mixers or tagging along when other students went out for pizza, she stayed in her room. A month after starting classes, she's become so self-conscious that, when someone talks to her, she turns away. What can Carmen do to overcome her shyness?

Yesterday afternoon your roommate came back from the grocery store with a box of jelly doughnuts, a large bag of potato chips, a pound of fudge, and a half gallon of ice cream. This morning you noticed the empty containers in the garbage pail. If you have reason to think your roommate might have gone on an eating binge, what would you do about it?

Ever since Tony's girlfriend broke up with him, he's been acting strangely. For days he locked himself in his room and played their favorite songs over and over again. He doesn't want to go out with his friends, and he looks as if he hasn't been eating or sleeping well. Several times he's mentioned how bad his old girlfriend would feel if "something" happened to him. If you were Tony's friend, what would be your primary concerns? If he confided that he had thought about killing himself but swore you to secrecy, what would you do?

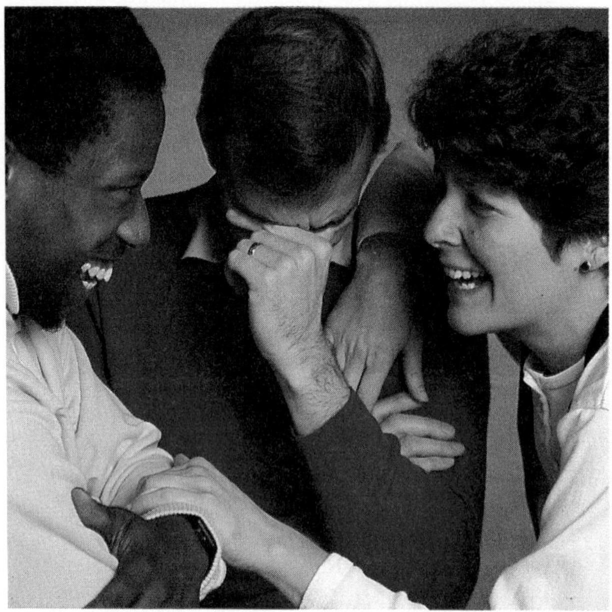

Sometimes the best therapy is also the cheapest and easiest—laughter releases tension and connects us with other people and brightens our mood.

viduals with depression, anxiety, and many other types of psychological disorders. Some help control disturbing symptoms, such as agitation. Antidepressant drugs correct the imbalance of brain chemicals that is typical of depression.

### Recovery

We accept recovery from influenza as normal. Afterward, we don't watch a man's body as if it were forever untrustworthy. We don't think of a woman as a failure because she has suffered an attack of appendicitis. Yet we think quite differently of the person who becomes mentally ill.

Unlike physical disease, mental illness is often seen as something immoral or bizarre, as a sign of failure, and as a permanent abnormality. We expect the body to master a disease like the flu in several days, but we think of mental illness as going on and on. However, mental illness does not have to go on indefinitely. A psychotic breakdown, a severe depression, even years of alcoholism can all have definite end points.

The stigma of psychological problems and illness is great. The reason may have less to do with the recovered person's former condition than with the so-called normal person's own fears about mental illness. Assuming that someone who has a psychological disorder can never be well again is unfair to friends, to family, and to yourself.

## MAKING THIS CHAPTER WORK FOR YOU

### Keeping Your Mind Healthy

**Emotional health and mental health are both components of psychological health: our ability to be in touch with our feelings and to perceive reality as it is. The psychologically healthy person is reasonable, self-aware, productive, and has a sense of reality, an appreciation of self and life, and the capacity to love others and maintain relationships. According to Karl Menninger, mental health can be viewed as a continuum ranging from the ideal, which is characterized by self-control and the ability to cope, to severe levels of dysfunction.**

**Sigmund Freud theorized that the psyche has both conscious and unconscious functions. Erik Erikson identified stages of ego development and maturation, from infancy to old age. Humanism views individuals as unique and self-defining, as more than the sum of their parts and functions. The humanist theorist Abraham Maslow proposed that human needs are the motivating factors in personality development. An individual who is able to satisfy basic physiological needs (for food, shelter, and sleep) as well as higher needs (for safety and security, love and affection, and self-esteem) is said to be self-actualized. Behavioral psychology views human behavior as a result of learned responses to various stimuli, not as a result of innate drives or needs.**

**Psychologically, we need to feel a sense of self-esteem, to achieve independence, and to love and be loved. Feelings are important clues to physical and psychological well-being. Values are the standards by which you evaluate yourself, other people, and the events in your life. Good decision-making requires self-knowledge and an ability to evaluate what is best for you. To cope with anxiety or conflict, you may use one or more of the following defense mechanisms: repression, denial, rationalization, projection, reaction formation, and displacement. Positive coping mechanisms include altruism, humor, suppression, and sublimation.**

**Among the common challenges that college students face are shyness (anxiety and fear in social situations), loneliness, anxiety (which may or may not have a specific cause), sadness, guilt, and anger.**

Mental illness can strike anyone at any age or stage of life. Depression, characterized by an imbalance of chemicals in the brain, may occur just once in a lifetime, or it can be a chronic condition. Risk factors include family history, life stresses, physical illness, substance abuse, and gender. Symptoms include lack of energy, sleep disturbances, and loss of interest in food, sex, and work. Depression is generally treated with psychotherapy, drug therapy, or a combination of both.

The percentage of suicides is growing, especially among young people and racial minorities. Factors that contribute to the likelihood of suicide include aging, gender, unemployment, solitary life-style, physical or mental illness, alcoholism, loss of an important relationship, and life stresses.

General anxiety—persistent, excessive, or unrealistic worry about past, future, or current events or situations—produces symptoms such as restlessness, tenseness, irritability, inability to concentrate, sweating, accelerated heart rate, dry mouth, diarrhea, and fatigue. Anxiety disorders include panic attacks, phobias, and posttraumatic stress disorder.

Anorexia nervosa is an eating disorder in which individuals try to control their weight to combat an inner sense of helplessness. Treatment consists of improved nutrition and behavioral and insight psychotherapy. In bulimia, the affected person goes on eating binges, consumes large amounts of foods, and then induces vomiting or uses laxatives to control his or her weight. Treatment consists of behavior modification techniques and psychotherapy. Bulimarexia includes symptoms of both bulimia and anorexia nervosa.

With treatment, most people with psychological problems can and do get better. The risk of not getting treatment is great, since individuals, pushed to the brink of despair by their suffering, may become convinced that killing themselves is the only answer. Psychological treatments include various types of talking therapies (including psychoanalysis, brief psychotherapy, group therapy, and crisis intervention) and nonverbal therapies (including behavioral therapy, light therapy, hypnosis, creative therapies, and drug therapy).

Among the practical applications of this chapter are some basic rules by which to live:

- Accept yourself. As a human being, you are, by definition, imperfect. Come to terms with the fact that you are a worthwhile person despite your inadequacies or mistakes.
- Respect yourself. Recognize your abilities and talents. Acknowledge your competence and achievements, and take pride in them.
- Trust yourself. Learn to listen to the voice within you, and let your intuition be your guide. No one knows you better than you do. Rely on your sense of self.
- Love yourself. Be happy to spend time by yourself. Learn to appreciate your company and to be glad you're you.
- Stretch yourself. Be willing to change and grow, to take risks and dare to be vulnerable.
- Look at challenges as opportunities for personal growth.
- Think not just of *where,* but of *who* you want to be. The goals you set, the decisions you make, the values you adopt now will determine how you feel about yourself and your life in the future.
- Take care of your body. Balanced nutrition and regular exercise can help you cope with everyday problems and prevent serious disorders. Your ideal, throughout your life, should be a healthy mind in a healthy body.

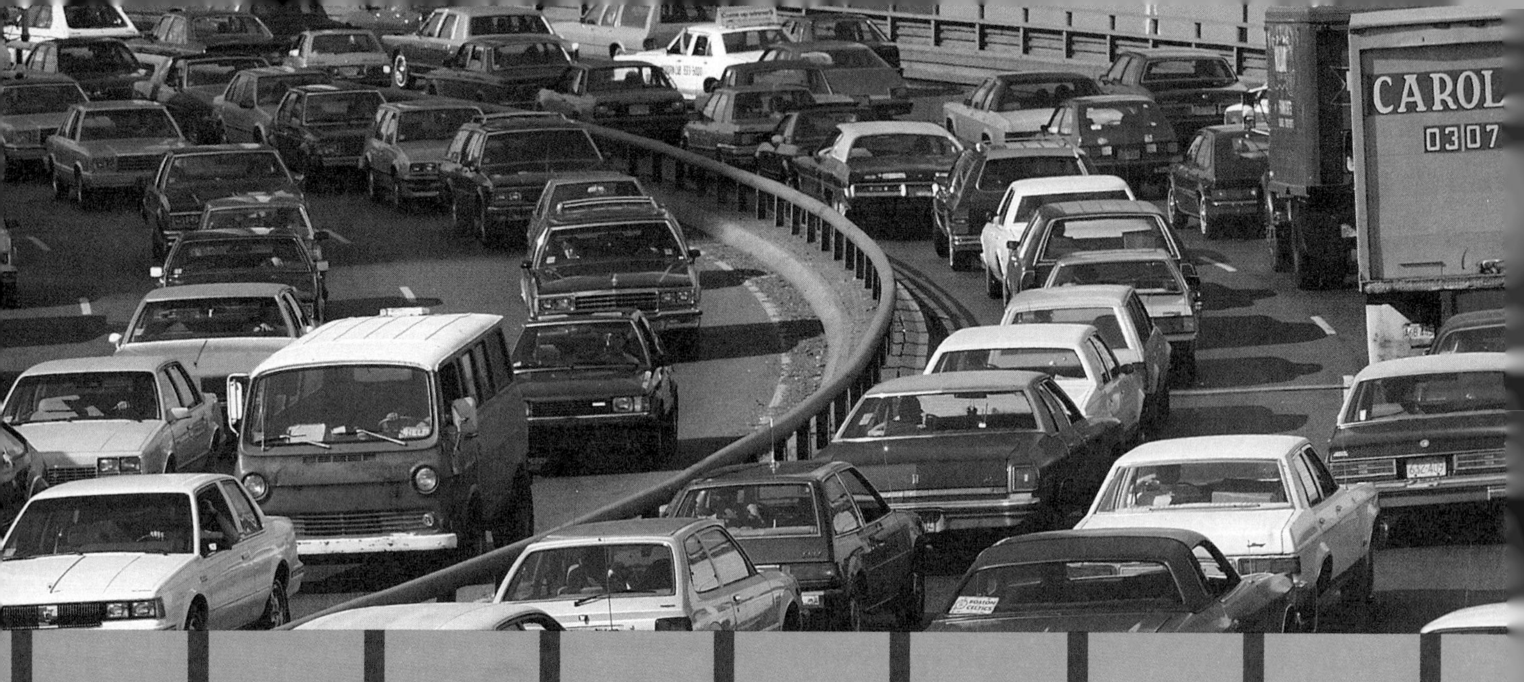


# 3 MEETING THE CHALLENGES OF STRESS

In this chapter

What is stress?

What causes stress?

The toll on the body

Stress-proofing yourself

Defusing stress

Making this chapter work for you: Learning to live with stress

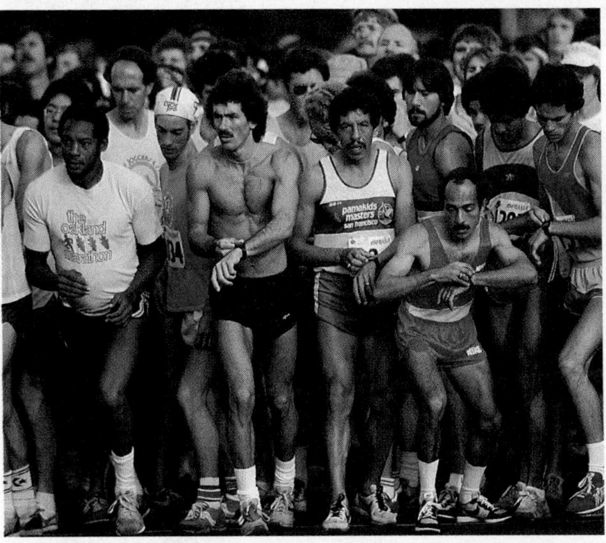

Competition can trigger stress or can be a good way of coping with stress.

*You know about stress.* You live with it every day: the stress of passing exams, preparing for a career, meeting people, facing new experiences. If you're an athlete, you know the stress of training and competition. If you have a job, you deal with the stress of meeting certain standards of performance. If you're a parent, you've agonized through the stress of a child's illness.

Stress knows no gender, no age, no ethnic or socioeconomic limits. Everyone has to deal with it. That isn't necessarily bad. An individual's response to stress, not the stressful situation itself, determines its impact. Face a crisis with a different outlook, be more flexible, find a way to enhance your sense of control, and you'll feel stimulated rather than stressed.

The stress-management skills in this chapter provide a good start. As you organize your time, release tension, and build up internal resources, you will begin to experience the sense of control that makes stress a challenge rather than an ordeal.

## WHAT IS STRESS?

Dr. Hans Selye, a pioneer in studying physiological responses to challenge, first used the word *stress* in its current psychological and physiological sense. He defined **stress** as "the nonspecific response of the body to any demand made upon it." In other words, the body reacts to stressors—the things that upset or excite us—in the same way, regardless of whether the stressor is positive or negative.

The stressor may be a fall on the stairs; a loud, unexpected sound; or a pop quiz, but the body's response is always the same. What you do about this physiological response determines the positive or negative impact of the stressor. Compare the responses of two people in "Health Spotlight: A Day in the Life of Chris and Pat" later in this chapter as they cope with the same situations, starting off with a stressor we've all faced: oversleeping for an early class.

Stress isn't always negative. Some of life's happiest moments—birth, reunions, weddings—are enormously stressful. We cry with the stress of frustration or loss; we cry, too, with the stress of love and joy. Selye coined the term **eustress** for positive stress (*eu* is a Greek prefix meaning good). Eustress challenges us to grow, adapt, and find creative solutions. **Distress** refers to the negative effects of stress that can deplete or even destroy life energy. Ideally, the level of stress in our lives is just high enough to motivate us to satisfy our needs and not so high that it interferes with our ability to reach our fullest potential.

### General Adaptation Syndrome

Our bodies constantly strive to maintain a stable and consistent physiological state. This is called **homeostasis.** Anything that disturbs this state triggers an **adaptive response**—an attempt to restore homeostasis.

Selye described the body's response to a stressor, whether threatening or exhilarating, as the **General Adaptation Syndrome** (**GAS**), which consists of three distinct stages:

1. *Alarm*—In the first stage, **alarm,** you feel your muscles, particularly in the face and neck, tighten. You may have a knot in the stomach. Your pulse

**stress** The nonspecific response of the body to any demands made upon it; may be characterized by muscle tension and acute anxiety or may be a positive force for action.
**eustress** A positive stress, which stimulates a person to function properly.
**distress** A negative stress, which may result in illness.
**homeostasis** The body's natural state of balance or stability.
**adaptive response** The body's attempt to reestablish homeostasis.
**General Adaptation Syndrome** (**GAS**) The sequenced physiological response to a stressful situation; consists of three stages—alarm, resistance, and exhaustion.
**alarm** The first stage of the General Adaptation Syndrome, or stress response, in which the body prepared for fight or flight.

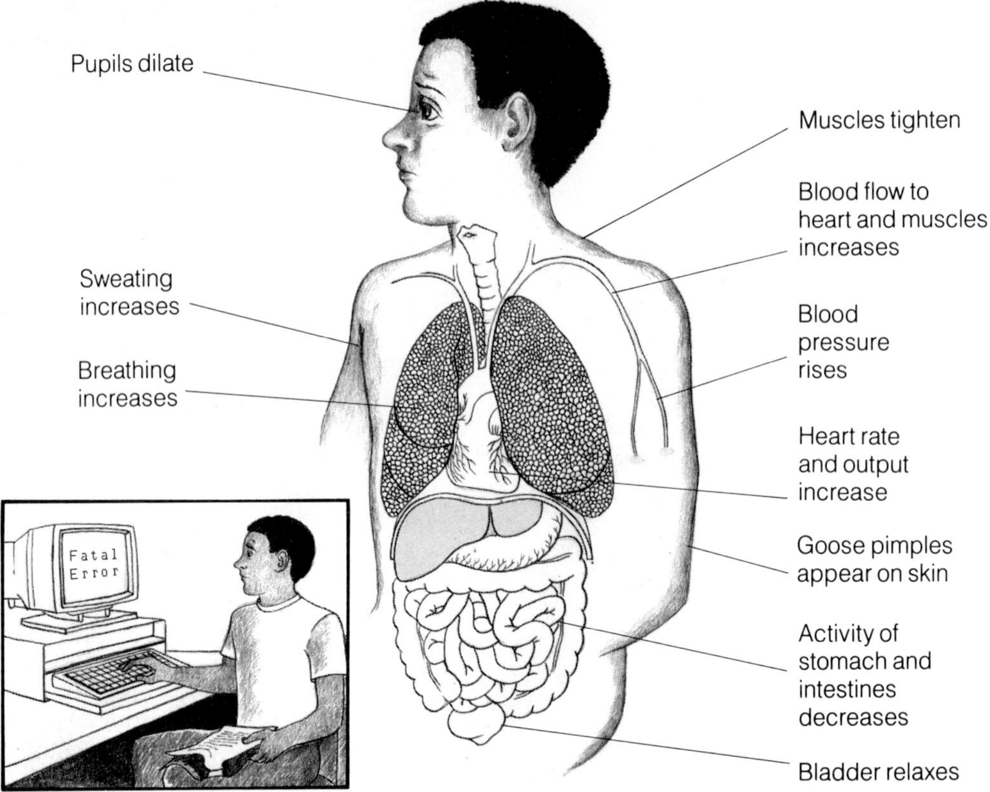


SOURCE: Hales, Dianne. *An Invitation to Health, Fourth Edition,* Benjamin/Cummings, 1989.

**FIGURE 3-1** Stressful situations can cause a physical response in virtually any part of the body.

is rapid, your mouth dry, your palms sweaty. Your body produces more of several powerful hormones that speed up the heart and increase blood pressure. At the same time, your muscles contract and your body makes its stored energy more available. You are prepared for fight or flight.

2. *Resistance*—After the initial alarm, the internal activities of your body return to normal; but it takes all your energy to keep up this normal state. At this stage, **resistance,** the energy focused on the stressor, changes from physical to mental.
3. *Exhaustion*—If the stress continues long enough, you can't keep up normal functioning. This stage is called **exhaustion,** and in it the signs of the first stage reappear. Even a small amount of additional stress at this point can cause a breakdown or, in some small animals, death.

Sometimes the GAS can save lives. Imagine stepping off a curb when suddenly a car turns the corner and speeds toward you. Your heart pounds; you feel your muscles tense. But you manage to jump faster and farther than you could have if you were relaxed.

Our bodies respond to stressors that aren't physical, such as not having enough money, in the same way they respond to physical stressors—even though neither fight nor flight will solve the problem. Weeks, even months, may pass, with no easing of the stress. Eventually we develop symptoms of the exhaustion stage. At that point, stress hits where it hurts: the head, the neck, the stomach, the heart, and the blood pressure (see Figure 3-1).

## Warning Signals of Stress Overload

How do you know when you're suffering from excessive stress? Usually your body, mind, and behavior provide clues, which you should never ignore:

- physical symptoms, including chronic fatigue, headaches, indigestion, diarrhea, and sleep problems
- frequent illness or worrying about illness
- self-medication, including use of nonprescription drugs
- problems concentrating on studies or work

**resistance** The second stage of the General Adaptation Syndrome, or stress response, in which the body's internal activities return to normal and the energy focused on the stressor changes from physical to mental.

**exhaustion** The final stage of the General Adaptation Syndrome, or stress response, in which the body can no longer maintain normal functioning.

## HALES INDEX

Hours a week that Americans spent on leisure in 1973: 26.2

Hours a week that Americans spent on leisure in 1989: 16.6

Average work week in 1973: 40.6 hours

Average work week in 1989: 46.8 hours

Percentage of women who describe themselves as "under a lot of stress": 57

Top source of stress among American men: Work overload on the job

Top source of stress among American women: Work overload at home

The five least stressful American cities:* State College, Pa., Grand Forks, N. Dak., St. Cloud, Minn., Rochester, Minn., McAllen/Pharr/Edinburg, Tex.

The five most stressful American cities:* Reno, Nev., Las Vegas, Nev., Miami, Fla., Lakeland/Winter Haven, Fla., Little Rock, Ark.

* Based on rates of alcoholism, suicide, divorce, and crime in a study conducted by Robert Levine, professor of psychology at California State University.

SOURCES: **1, 2, 3, 4** Tivnan, Edward. "Healing Time Sickness," *Psychology Today,* March 1989. **5** "National Survey of Women," press release sponsored by Within Vitamins, 1987. **6, 7** Kessler, Ronald and Elizabeth Schilling, "Effects of Daily Stress on Negative Mood," *Journal of Personality and Social Psychology,* November 1989. **8, 9** Levine, Robert. "City Stress Index," *Psychology Today,* November 1988.

- feeling irritable, anxious, or apathetic
- working or studying longer and harder than usual
- exaggerating, to yourself and others, the importance of what you do
- denying that any problem exists
- becoming accident-prone
- breaking rules, whether it's a curfew at home or a speed limit on the highway
- avoiding people
- going to extremes, such as drinking too much, spending a lot of money, or gambling

## WHAT CAUSES STRESS?

Our level of ongoing stress affects our ability to respond to a new day's stressors. Each of us has a breaking point for dealing with stress. A series of too-intense pressures or too-rapid changes can push us closer to that point. That's why it's important to anticipate potential stressors and plan how to deal with them.

### Life Changes

We experience change and stress at every stage of life. In childhood, we must cope with separation from parents when we begin school and learn how to make friends on our own. As teenagers, we must come to terms with the physical transformation of our bodies and with new responsibilities and freedoms. As young adults, we must set goals and directions for our lives and establish close supportive relationships.

After you graduate, you will face a never-ending series of changes as you become an employee, homeowner, spouse, or parent. By anticipating these potential stressors, you can plan ways in which to cope and reduce their impact.

Some of us are more vulnerable to life changes and crises than are others. For example, if your parents solved your problems for you, you may never have learned during childhood how to handle disappointment or frustration.

For any individual, too much change can cause enormous stress. In the 1960s, physicians Thomas Holmes and Richard Rahe, two stress experts, devised the Life Event Scale to evaluate individual levels of stress and potential for coping. The scale was based on life change units, estimates of each change's impact. The death of a partner or parent ranks high on the scale, but even changing apartments is considered a stressor. People who accumulate more than 300 life change units in a year are more likely to suffer serious health problems than those with fewer units. In general, younger people experience more life changes than older ones; factors such as sex, edu-

HEALTH SPOTLIGHT

## Test Stress

On the first day of class, the professor explains that the midterm will count for a quarter of your grade, a term paper for another quarter, and the final for half. "Great!" you think. "No need to worry about quizzes and class participation."

The midterm comes at the busiest of times. Poorly prepared, you barely manage a C−. You work extra hard on your term paper and earn a B+, but you know you have to keep a B average to qualify for financial aid.

In this course, as well as several others, everything hinges on the final exam. As the end of the semester approaches, you're tense, irritable, and preoccupied with the consequences of not doing well. Over and over again, you ask yourself, "What if I blow it?"

For many students, examination time is the most stressful part of the year. In studies at various colleges and universities, the incidence of colds and flus was found to soar during finals. The reason seems to be that stress depresses the levels of the protective immune cells that ward off viruses.

Students who don't come down with infections during exams often feel the impact of test stress in other ways. Many suffer headaches, upset stomachs, skin flare-ups, or insomnia. Some are so preoccupied with the possibility of failure that they can't concentrate on studying. Others, including many of the best and brightest students, "freeze up" during tests, and can't comprehend multiple-choice questions or write essay answers, even if they know the material.

As with other stressful situations, your feelings about confronting this situation—that is, *taking* a test, not the exam itself—determine the impact stress will have on you and your test performance. The students most susceptible to exam stress are those who believe they'll do poorly and who see tests as extremely threatening.

Often students' negative thoughts become a self-fulfilling prophecy: As they study, they keep wondering, "What good will studying do? I never do well on tests." As their fear increases, they try harder, pulling all-nighters. Fueled by caffeine and munching on sugary snacks, they become edgy and find it harder and harder to concentrate. By the time of the test, they're nervous wrecks, scarcely able to sit still and focus on the exam.

Can students do anything to reduce test stress and feel more in control? Yes, say researchers from Ohio State University. The key isn't studying more or better, but learning how to defuse stress through relaxation. In their study, one group of students was taught relaxation techniques—such as controlled breath-

cation, and social class also have a strong impact. Marriage seems to promote greater stability and fewer changes.

If you think you would score high on a student stress scale, think about the reasons your life has been in such turmoil. Are there any steps you could take to make your life more stable?

Of course, some changes, such as your parents' divorce or a friend's accident, may be beyond your control. Simply recognizing that fact seems to help reduce the stress. Keep in mind the words of the "Serenity Prayer," written by theologian Reinhold Niebuhr:

> God grant me the serenity
> To accept the things I cannot change,
> The courage to change the things I can,
> And the wisdom to know the difference.

ing, meditation, progressive relaxation, and guided imagery (described in this chapter)—a month before finals. The more the students used these "stress-busters," the higher their levels of immune cells during the exam period. The extra payoff was that they felt calmer and in better control during their tests.

Other effective ways of defusing test stress include the following:

- *Planning.* A month before finals, map out a study schedule for each course. Set aside a small amount of time every day or every other day to begin your review.
- *Thinking and talking positively.* Instead of dwelling on tests on which you did poorly in the past, focus on how well you might do if you are well prepared and confident.
- *Self-monitoring.* Watch yourself closely for signs of tension: headaches, digestive problems, temper flare-ups, muscle tightness. As soon as you spot a symptom, try to find a way to relieve it. Devote more time to your relaxation technique.
- *Taking extra good care of yourself.* Make sure you're eating regularly and wisely. Get enough sleep. Exercise often.
- *Regular stress breaks while studying.* Get up from your desk, breathe deeply, stretch, visualize a pleasant scene. You'll feel more refreshed than you would if you chugged another cup of coffee.
- *Using guided imagery.* Every day, as you practice your breathing or relaxation method, visualize yourself taking a final exam. Imagine yourself walking into the exam room feeling confident, opening up the test booklet, and seeing questions to which you know the answers.
- *Practicing.* You might ask your teacher if he or she is willing to give a mini-final to prepare students for the test situation. Or, you and your friends can make up tests for each other.
- *Expressing your feelings.* Talk to other students about their responses to exams. Chances are that many of them share your fears. Sometimes talking to your teacher or advisor can help.
- *Being satisfied with doing your best.* You can't expect to ace every test; all you can and should expect is your best effort. Once you've completed the exam, allow yourself the sweet pleasure of relief that it's over.

SOURCES: Kiecolt-Glaser, Janice and Ronald Glaser. "Stress, Health, and Immunity: Tracking the Mind-Body Connection." Presentation to the American Psychological Association, New York City, August 1987. Miller, Christina. "Afraid Stress Will Cause Sniffles? Relax," *American Heath,* January/February 1986.

## STRATEGY FOR CHANGE

### Coping with Change

- Seek accurate information about what's happening in your life. Knowledge can bring floating fears down to earth.
- Share worries with someone you trust, love, or respect. Be sure to talk out problems.
- Tune in to your "body talk." When you are under stress, you will get physical warning signals. Listen to your body, then ease up if necessary.
- Balance work and recreation. A set routine for relaxation will help.
- Avoid relying on alcohol and other drugs to help you cope.
- Avoid obsession with yourself. Doing some-

thing for others will take your mind off your concerns.
- Don't take yourself so seriously. You are human and make mistakes. Be able to laugh at yourself.
- Get enough rest, and sleep on a regular basis.

## Daily Hassles

In various recent studies, researchers have found that stress can come in little packages that eventually have a big effect. College students may feel pressure to perform well to qualify for good jobs or graduate schools. Others, struggling to meet steep tuition payments, must juggle a full course load with a part-time job. Some experience additional hassles because of constant bickering with parents or roommates.[1]

Psychologist Richard Lazarus has found that college students complain most about anxiety over wasting time, meeting high standards, and being lonely. Middle-aged men and women, by comparison, have primarily economic concerns, such as worries about prices and investments. But three hassles topped everyone's list: misplacing or losing things, trying to improve physical appearance, and having too much to do.[2]

### STRATEGY FOR CHANGE

#### Handling Hassles

When you're running low on money or time, the first thing you lose is perspective. A flat tire pushes you to the brink of tears. A rude comment sets off an ugly quarrel. To stop feeling hassled, just stop. Breathe deeply and slowly five times. Then ask yourself some questions:

- In a month will you remember what's made you so upset?
- If you had to rank this problem on a scale of 1 to 10, with worldwide catastrophe as 10, where would it rate?
- What are the most important things in your life: the person you love, your health, your family, your future career? Is this hassle a threat to any of them?
- If this were the worst thing to happen to you this year, would you feel lucky?
- Smile. Force the corners of your mouth upward if you must.
- Think of one simple thing that could make your life easier. What if you put up a hook to hold your keys so that you didn't spend 5 minutes searching for them every morning? Doing *something*, however small, will boost your sense of control.

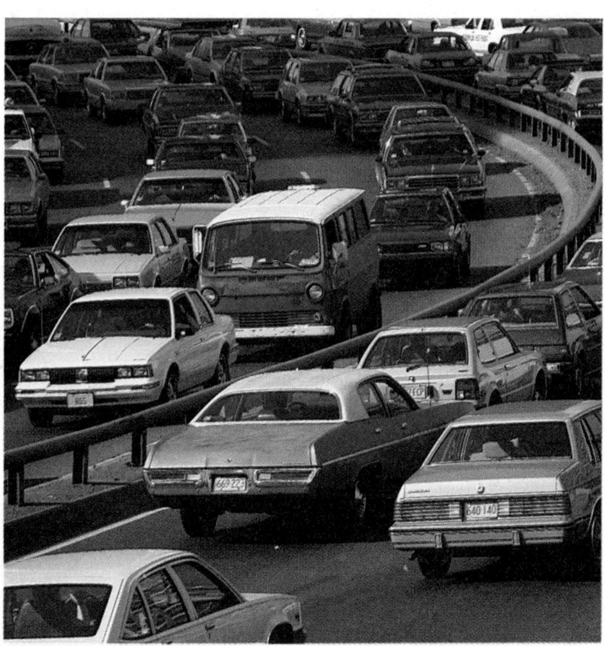

It's not just major crises that take a toll. Stress can also come in little packages, and the cumulative effect can be enormous.

### HEALTH HEADLINE

#### Stress and Herpes: Breaking the Cycle

Stress can trigger an episode of genital herpes, but the same techniques that defuse stress can prevent herpes outbreaks and reduce their length and severity. Researchers at the Geisinger Medical Center in Danville, Pennsylvania, found that herpes sufferers who learned relaxation, imaging, and other stress management techniques experienced only half as many outbreaks as those who simply attended support groups on the sexual and emotional difficulties of having herpes. When herpes did recur, the episodes were less severe and ended several days sooner.

SOURCE: Adelmann, Pamela. "Help for Herpes: Relax," *Psychology Today*, October 1989.

## Poor Time Management

Every day you make dozens of decisions, and the choices you make about how to use your time directly affect your stress level. If you have a big test on Monday and a term paper due Tuesday, you may plan to study all weekend. Then, when you're invited to a party Saturday night, you go. Although you set the alarm for 7:00 A.M. on Sunday, you don't pull yourself out of bed until noon. By the time you start studying, it's 4:00 P.M., and panic is building inside you.

One of the hard lessons of being on your own is learning that your choices and your actions have consequences. Stress is just one. But by thinking ahead, being realistic about your work load, and sticking to your plans, you can gain control over your time and your stress levels.

**STRATEGY FOR CHANGE**

**Managing Your Time**

- Keep a daily "to do" list. Rank items according to priorities: A, B, C. Evaluate the items. Should any Bs be As? Schedule your day to be sure the As get accomplished.
- Learn how to say no: Let the person know you understand his or her demands. Say no directly. Offer alternatives if you can.
- Try not to fixate on half-completed projects. Instead, divide large tasks, like a term paper, into smaller ones; reward yourself every time you complete a part.

## Social Stressors

Not all stressors are personal. In addition to daily hassles, you may experience stress as the result of discrimination because of race or physical disability; fear of violence in your neighborhood; or the threat of polluted air or water. (Chapter 16 discusses environmental stressors in depth.) Other common social stressors include isolation, unemployment, job stress, and burnout.

### Isolation

When University of California, Berkeley, epidemiologists S. Leonard Syme and Lisa Berkman examined the social support networks of 7,000 people in northern California, they found that those who were most isolated had death rates 2 to 3 times those of people with extensive social ties. In a 10-year study that followed 2,754 adults in Tecumseh, Michigan, University of Michigan researchers discovered that those with the fewest social contacts had 2 to 4 times the mortality rate of the others and died of a variety of diseases and accidents.[3]

### Unemployment

Every time the unemployment rate goes up 1 percent—from 5 to 6 percent, for example—suicide rates rise 4 percent and 4.3 percent more men and 2.3 percent more women are admitted to psychiatric hospitals for the first time. Many more people suffer lesser ills, including migraines, backaches, high blood pressure, and stomach ailments.[4]

### Job Stress

Americans' jobs are their primary source of stress, according to several recent reports. Insurance claims for job-related stress jumped throughout the 1980s, while claims for physical occupational troubles declined. When men and women in the Detroit area kept daily stress diaries for six weeks, conflict with coworkers emerged as the top tension in their lives.[5]

The most stressed workers are those at the bottom of the job ladder: writers, cooks, assembly-line workers. The reason they're stressed out: They have far less control over their work situation than the powerful executives calling the shots from the top.

### Workaholism and Burnout

Some people become so obsessed by their work and careers that they become workaholics, who live to work and love their work.[6] They may get so caught up in racing toward the top that they forget what they're racing toward and why. One consequence is **burnout,** a state of physical, emotional, and mental exhaustion brought on by constant or repeated emotional pressure.[7] It is particularly common in the helping professions, such as social work or nursing, in which men and women who've dedicated themselves to others may realize they have nothing left in themselves to give.

You can recognize the early signs of burn-out by monitoring yourself for symptoms, including the following:

- exhaustion
- sleep problems or nightmares
- increased anxiety or nervousness
- signs of muscular tension (headaches, backaches, and the like)
- increased use of alcohol or medication
- digestive problems, such as nausea, vomiting, or diarrhea
- loss of interest in sex
- frequent body aches or pain

---

**burnout** A state of physical, emotional, and mental exhaustion resulting from constant or repeated emotional pressure.

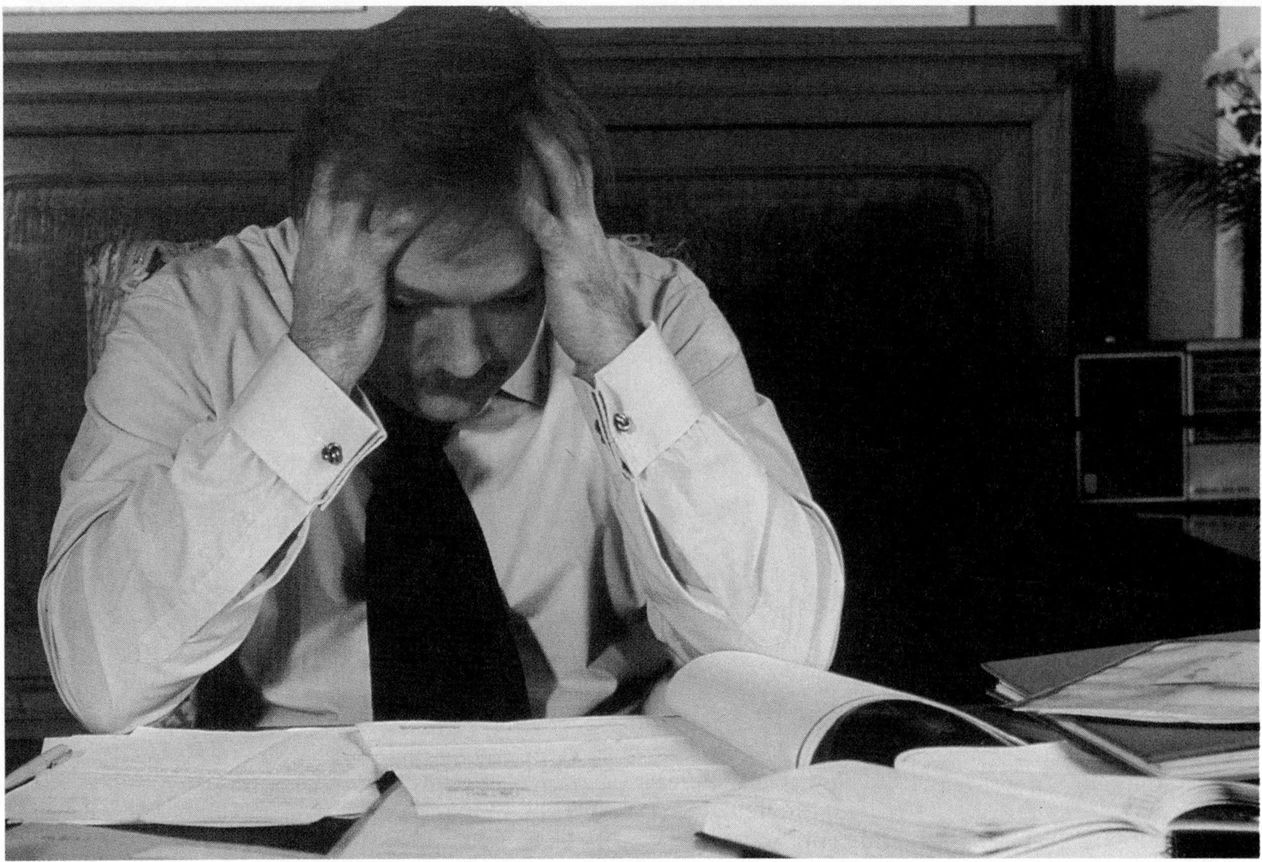

Burnout is a state of physical, emotional, and mental exhaustion.

- quarrels with family or friends
- negative feelings about everything
- at work: problems concentrating, job mistakes and accidents, feelings of depression, hopelessness, and helplessness

Teachers, doctors, counselors, air traffic controllers, professional athletes, executives, housewives, police officers—all become victims of burn-out, which may indeed be just a modern name for old problems such as depression. However, it is one stress response that has the potential for becoming an epidemic. The best way to avoid burnout is learning to cope well with smaller, day-to-day stresses. Then tiny frustrations won't smolder into a blaze that may be impossible to put out.

**STRATEGY FOR CHANGE**

**Preventing Burnout**

- Develop healthy life-style habits, which will enhance your resistance to stress and increase your ability to cope.
- Reach out and build a network of supportive friends, family members, neighbors, and coworkers.
- Learn to recognize situations that you cannot change so that you don't waste energy trying to change them.
- Draw a line between your personal life and your professional responsibilities. Don't let problems with one affect the other.
- Practice at least one stress-management technique (exercise, meditation, relaxation, or the like) regularly.
- Be nice to yourself. For example, reward yourself with a new tape or compact disc if you feel good about your performance on a test or on the job. Accept others' compliments.
- Develop positive addictions, such as exercise, instead of negative addictions, such as smoking or drinking. But remember that even a good behavior like exercise, carried to extremes, can hurt rather than help.

## Illness

Do you remember the way you felt the last time you had a bad cold? It wasn't just your throat that ached or your head that throbbed; you probably felt as bad psychologically as you did physically. Just as the mind

HEALTH SPOTLIGHT

## A Day in the Life of Chris and Pat

| Potential Stress | Chronic Stress Response (Chris) | Healthy Stress Response (Pat) |
|---|---|---|
| Oversleeps, rises at 7:30 | ACTION: Gulps coffee, skips breakfast, tears button off shirt getting dressed.<br>THOUGHTS: Oh, no! I'll miss my 8:00 class. I can't be absent again. It's the third time!<br>RESULT: Leaves home anxious and hungry. | ACTION: Phones classmate, asks her to take notes for him and explain lateness to prof. Eats breakfast.<br>THOUGHTS: I'll get the notes and ask the prof for help if I have to.<br>RESULT: Leaves home feeling okay. |
| Stuck behind slow driver | ACTION: Flashes lights, honks, curses, bangs on wheel with fist, passes on curve, nearly crashes.<br>THOUGHTS: Damn slow driver! I ought to run him off the road. | ACTION: Turns on radio and listens to music.<br>THOUGHTS: This is frustrating, but maybe I can think about ideas for my history term paper. |
| 10:00 class | ACTION: Sits in back, works on assignment for another class, doesn't hear question asked by teacher.<br>THOUGHTS: What a waste of time. I've got to study for my economics test. Why is the teacher always calling on me anyway? | ACTION: Listens and participates in class.<br>THOUGHTS: I'm glad I made this class. I'll bet the final includes a lot of this stuff. |
| Noon | ACTION: Skips lunch, has coffee in library, spills it on study notes.<br>THOUGHTS: My notes are ruined! I'll have to stay up all night reading the book. | ACTION: Eats lunch with classmates, relaxes, talks about sports and movies.<br>THOUGHTS: There's a lot more to school than just the classes. I really enjoy meeting new people. |
| Afternoon | ACTION: Forgets that oral presentation of ideas for history paper was scheduled for today's class, can give only vague thoughts. Is told to come up with solid outline by tomorrow.<br>THOUGHTS: That means I really will be up all night! How can they expect so much of me? | ACTION: Talks with teacher about some of the ideas mulled over in the car, is encouraged to research one, and works up an outline over the next week.<br>THOUGHTS: I'll have to schedule some research time at the library this weekend. |
| Evening | ACTION: Gets home from library late, eats fast-food hamburger in car, stomach upset, drinks six cups of coffee. Stays up until 4:00, studying. | ACTION: Gets home and runs a few miles, eats dinner, studies until 10:00. Asleep by 11:00. |
| Next morning | Wakes up late again, feels awful, blanks out on test. | Wakes up on time, goes over notes after breakfast, feels calm during test. |

SOURCE: Adapted from Farquhar, John W. *The American Way of Life Need Not Be Hazardous to Your Health.*

can have profound effects on the body, the body can have an enormous impact on the emotions. Whenever we come down with the flu or a migraine, we feel under the weather emotionally. A chronic disease like diabetes, which requires constant monitoring, has an even greater impact.

## THE TOLL ON THE BODY

Stress is a problem of excess. As one physician puts it, your body may react to a dime's worth of stress with a dollar's worth of energy. It doesn't matter whether the stress is good or bad, big or small; your body reacts in the same way.

Although stress can be the spice of life, it can also be the kiss of death. Just as it can undermine psychological contentment, it can erode physical well-being. Stress may be our number one health enemy and the greatest single contributor to disease.

### Heart Disease

In the 1970s, cardiologists Meyer Friedman and Ray Rosenman suggested that excess stress may be the most important factor in the development of heart disease.[8] They compared their patients to coronary-free individuals of the same age and developed two general categories: Type A and Type B. Hardworking, aggressive, and competitive, Type As never had time for all they wanted to accomplish, even though they usually tried to do several tasks at once. Type Bs were more relaxed, though not necessarily less ambitious or successful. (Of course, people who are extremely Type B may never accomplish anything.) In their research, Type A behavior was the major contributing factor in the early development of heart disease.

More recent research indicates that Type As who suffer heart attacks can cut their risk of death in half by modifying their behavior. Of the 862 participants in one recent study in the *American Heart Journal,* those who received counseling to change Type A traits had half the number of heart attacks as those who received only advice on diet, exercise, and treatments. The reformed Type As also reported other benefits, including improved relationships at home and work, increased productivity, less impatience, better perspective on problems, greater sensitivity to other people, and calmer responses to stress.[9]

### High Blood Pressure

People who react coolly to stress may seem upset but experience few physiological changes. In contrast, "hot" reactors to stress experience a flood of the powerful chemicals associated with the classic GAS stress response.[10] One of the most dangerous aspects of hot reacting is a dramatic rise in blood pressure as often as 30 to 40 times a day. As a result, blood pressure climbs higher for a longer time—and the higher the pressure and the longer it remains high, the greater the risk of developing chronic high blood pressure and heart disease.

### Immunity

The powerful chemicals triggered by stress dampen or suppress the **immune system,** the network of organs, tissues, and white blood cells that defend against disease. Impaired immunity makes the body more susceptible to many diseases, including infections (from the common cold to tuberculosis) and disorders of the immune system itself.

Traumatic stress, such as losing a loved one through death or divorce, impairs immunity for as long as a year. Even minor hassles take a toll. Under exam stress, students experience a dip in immune function and a higher rate of infections. (Refer to "Health Spotlight: Test Stress" in this chapter.)

### Digestive System

Did you ever get "butterflies" in your stomach before giving a speech in class or before a big game? The digestive system is, as one psychologist quips, "an important stop on the tension trail." In one study of college students, researchers at the University of North Carolina, Chapel Hill, found that stress and ineffective ways of dealing with it may trigger the bouts of stomach pain, bloating, diarrhea, or constipation known as irritable bowel syndrome.[11]

You don't have to avoid spicy foods to avoid problems, but pay attention to *how* you eat: Eating on the run, gulping food, or overeating result in poorly chewed foods, an overworked stomach, and increased abdominal pressure. The combination of bad eating habits and stress can add up to real pain in the stomach.

### Headaches

The most common type of headache is a **tension headache,** caused by involuntary contractions of

**immune system** The group of organs and tissues that protect the body from disease.

**tension headache** Pain and discomfort caused by involuntary contractions of the scalp, head, and neck muscles.

the scalp, head, and neck muscles. **Migraine headaches** are the result of constriction (narrowing) then dilation (widening) of blood vessels within the brain; chemicals leak through the vessel walls, inflame nearby tissues, and send pain signals to the brain. Surveys of college women show that Type A behavior can trigger both types of headaches. Stress can also be a culprit. The best strategy is preventive: a "relaxercise" a day, such as progressive relaxation or biofeedback, which are described later in this chapter. Breathing and relaxation techniques, usually coupled with medication, can relieve headaches after they strike.

### Skin Problems

If you break out the week before an exam, you already know that skin can be exquisitely sensitive to stress. Among the conditions worsened by stress are acne, psoriasis, herpes, hives, and eczema.

## STRESS-PROOFING YOURSELF

Although stress is a very real threat to emotional and physical well-being, it's important to keep in mind that it's not just what happens to you that matters, but how you handle it. In a 1989 study, researchers found that people who developed ulcers did not have more stressful events in their lives than others, but that they viewed these events much more negatively.[12] The inability to feel in control of stress, rather than stress itself, is the most damaging," says psychologist Joan Borysenko, director of the Mind-Body Clinic at Harvard University. "That's why the best preventive strategy is learning to manage stress."[13]

Sometimes becoming aware of potential stresses can help. Psychologist David Elkind describes three daily stress situations:[14]

- *Stresses That Are Foreseeable and Avoidable*—These range from going to a horror movie to getting so behind in your class assignments that you might fail the course. To cope better with this type of stress, explore your options. You can certainly choose not to go to the movies. As for your schoolwork, you can not do it and flunk, do it immediately, or procrastinate for a few more days. Obviously, getting the work done is most likely to reduce the pressure you feel.
- *Stresses That Are Neither Foreseeable nor Avoidable*—These can range from the serious, such as a bad accident, to the small, such as a delayed flight. There's nothing you can do to change the situation, and so you have to accept it. Simply realizing that fact can ease your anxiety.
- *Stresses That Are Foreseeable but Not Avoidable*—An exam is a good example of a stress you can anticipate but not avoid. However, you can make matters better by developing good study and work habits. Pay attention in class. Do homework assignments promptly. Allow time for reviewing before a test.

**STRATEGY FOR CHANGE**

**A Stress Diary**

You can use a diary to become aware of stress in your life:

- Note what stress symptoms you feel (tight stomach, headache, and so on), what you are doing and with whom, your thoughts or feelings at the moment, and your response to the stress.
- When you look at the weekly log of stresses, think how you might eliminate some stress-inducing situations.
- If you feel stressed because you always seem to be late for class, start planning your schedule better. Allow yourself a margin of half an hour between classes, and use the extra time to study.
- If certain people tend to trigger stress, analyze your relationships with them. Are you trying to suppress anger at them? Do you have to see them often? Can you see them less?
- Writing down pent-up feelings in a journal may yield an additional payoff: better immune function. In experiments at Southern Methodist University in Dallas, students who wrote about traumatic events and their emotional responses showed strikingly improved immune responses, even six weeks afterward, and reported few medical visits.[15]

### Reaching Out

When confronting stress, we have two options: We can either fight against it or we can adapt (adjust to the new situation or challenge). **Adaptation** is usually the better response, and one of the most effective ways of adapting is by working with others. Selye

**migraine headache** A severe headache resulting from the dilation of blood vessels in the head; sometimes accompanied by vomiting and nausea.
**adaptation** Any change in structure, form, or behavior to suit a new situation.

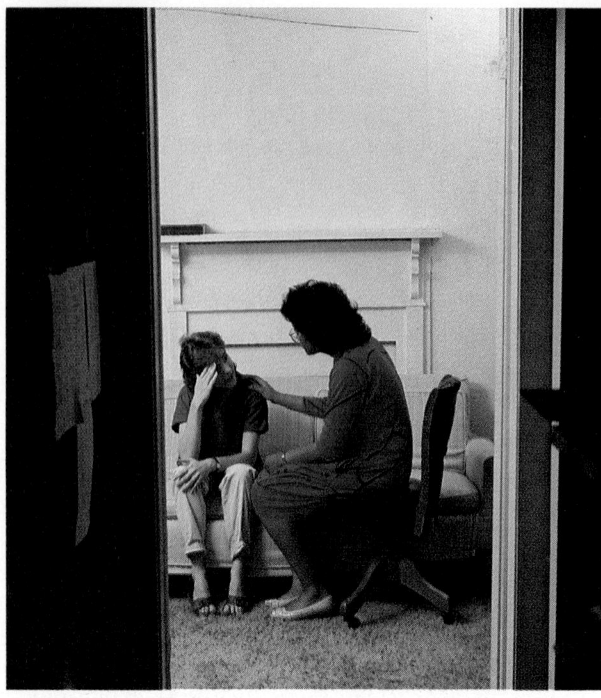

One of the most effective ways of adapting to stress is working with others.

describes this sort of cooperation with others for the self's sake as **altruistic egotism,** whereby we satisfy our own needs while helping others satisfy theirs. By helping others, we earn their help and enhance our belief that life is worth living.

### Individual Adaptation

Within the framework of your world, you can organize your life to avoid the smaller stresses that fray the nerves and sap energy. For example, living close to where you study or work can save you the stress of a long commute. To limit the constant assault of new information, listen to the news once a day rather than staying tuned to an all-news station. Try spending some time every day in total quiet—no television, no tape deck, no radio, no telephone.

### Positive Emotions

Just as negative stress responses can make us ill, positive emotions can decrease the effects of daily stress. One of the best preventive and curative medicines may be laughter. In his best-selling book, *Anatomy of an Illness as Perceived by the Patient,* Norman Cousins gives partial credit for his recovery from a painful disease to reruns of Marx Brothers movies and "Candid Camera."

Other important positive emotions are love, affection, and friendship. Statistics show that married people live longer, healthier lives than single people. In one study, Italian-American men suffered less heart disease than expected given the incidence of smoking and obesity. Much of the credit for their good health was given to the strong family ties in these men's lives.

**STRATEGY FOR CHANGE**

**Feeling Positive**

- Be optimistic. If you always look for what's wrong about yourself or your life, you'll find it—and feel even worse. You've heard the cliché about a glass being either half-full or half-empty, depending on the perspective of the beholder. Focus on one area in your life and identify positive aspects.
- Laugh. In one study, students who reported using humor as a way of coping with stress felt happier and healthier, their bodies churning out more of the cells that fight off viruses.[16]
- Have faith. Seeing your problems in a larger context can help you find the inner strength you need to deal with them one by one. If you believe that life has a greater meaning than mere daily survival, you may find stress less of a burden.
- Pray. According to several recent studies, active, meaningful prayer can reduce stress and produce a sense of control over life.[17]

## DEFUSING STRESS

Because stress can be deadly, be mindful of when you sense stress becoming too great. Screen yourself for signs of excessive stress, including anxiety and depression. As you learn about various approaches to combat stress, choose the ones that seem to suit you and experiment until you find one or two that you like best. With time and practice, you should see clear benefits.

### Breathing Techniques

You can use controlled breathing to help focus your thoughts, and to create a feeling of well-being. Here are some guidelines:

1. With your eyes open, focus on your breathing.

**altruistic egotism** A way of adapting in which a person cooperates with others by giving help and, in return, receives help as well as a sense of self-worth.

2. Take five slow, deep breaths, pulling air down into your lower abdomen and breathing out through your mouth. Concentrate on your breathing. If your mind wanders, empty it of all other thoughts.
3. As you breathe in, see yourself inhaling warm, soothing air.
4. As you breathe out, visualize yourself exhaling tension and stress and calming yourself.

### Relaxation

Relaxation produces a state that is the opposite of stress. Progressive muscular relaxation works by intentionally increasing and then decreasing tension in the muscles. Sit in a quiet, comfortable setting, as you would for the preceding breathing exercise. Clench and release various muscles, beginning with those of the hand, for instance, and then proceeding to the arms, shoulders, neck, face, scalp, chest, stomach, buttocks, genitals, and so on, down each leg to the toes.

Herbert Benson, a Harvard cardiologist, has developed a simple approach for soothing the stress in your body. His approach is called the relaxation response:

1. Sit quietly in a comfortable position.
2. Close your eyes.
3. Deeply relax all your muscles, beginning at your feet and progressing up to your face. Keep them relaxed.
4. Breathe through your nose. Become aware of your breathing. At the end of your exhale, say the word *one* silently to yourself, establishing this pattern: Breathe in . . . out, "one"; in . . . out, "one." Breathe easily and naturally.
5. Continue for 10 to 20 minutes.
6. Do not worry about whether you are successful in achieving a deep level of relaxation. Maintain a passive attitude and permit relaxation to occur at its own pace. When distracting thoughts occur, try to ignore them by not dwelling upon them, and return to repeating the word *one.* Practice the technique once or twice a day—but not within 2 hours after any meal, because the digestive processes seem to interfere with the relaxation response.

### Visualization/Guided Imagery

Relaxation and visualization require practice and, in some cases, instruction by qualified health professionals. However, the following tips can help you calm down and focus your mind on bolstering your immune system:

1. Sit or lie down in a comfortable position, with shoes off, clothing loose, lights dimmed, eyes closed.
2. Take a deep breath, filling your abdominal region, as well as your upper chest, with air. Slowly let the air out. Repeat, breathing deeper and feeling yourself relax.
3. Repeat a simple word or phrase (some people use a prayer) to yourself. Concentrate on this phrase, banishing all distracting thoughts.
4. Beginning with the top of your head, tense and relax the muscles in your body.
5. Conjure up a vivid image of a tranquil, quiet, safe place, and see yourself in that setting.
6. Sketch, in your mind or on paper, your perception of what your internal defenders look like. Make your image as personal and detailed as possible.
7. Practice this procedure 10 to 20 minutes a day.

### Meditation

Most forms of meditation have common elements: sitting quietly for 15 to 20 minutes once or twice a

## HEALTH HEADLINE

### Does Stress Bring on the Munchies?

**If you scarfed down a pint of ice cream the night before finals, don't blame stress. According to a study at the Uniformed Services University of the Health Sciences, most people under stress eat fewer sweets, rather than more, compared to those not under stress.**

**When men and women watched a pleasant travel video and a disturbing tape of bloody accidents, they snacked less during the upsetting video. The only exception: Women who were worried about their weight before the study. But, like all the men, women who weren't particularly diet conscious ate fewer sweets during the accident tape.**

SOURCE: Fischman, Ben. "Unsweetened Stress," *Psychology Today,* March 1989.

SELF-SURVEY

## Are You Stressed Out?

The Student Stress Scale represents an adaptation of Holmes and Rahe's Life Event Scale. It has been modified for teaching purposes to apply to college-age adults and should be considered a rough indication of stress levels and health consequences.

In the Student Stress Scale, each event, such as beginning or ending school, is given a score that represents the amount of readjustment a person has to make in life as a result of the change. In some studies, people with serious illnesses have been found to have high scores on similar scales.

To determine your stress score, add up the number of points corresponding to the events you have experienced in the past 12 months.

| | Event | | Points |
|---|---|---|---|
| 1. | Death of a close family member | ______ | 100 |
| 2. | Death of a close friend | ______ | 73 |
| 3. | Divorce between parents | ______ | 65 |
| 4. | Jail term | ______ | 63 |
| 5. | Major personal injury or illness | ______ | 63 |
| 6. | Marriage | ______ | 58 |
| 7. | Firing from a job | ______ | 50 |
| 8. | Failure of an important course | ______ | 47 |
| 9. | Change in health of a family member | ______ | 45 |
| 10. | Pregnancy | ______ | 45 |
| 11. | Sex problems | ______ | 44 |
| 12. | Serious argument with close friend | ______ | 40 |
| 13. | Change in financial status | ______ | 39 |
| 14. | Change of scholastic major | ______ | 39 |
| 15. | Trouble with parents | ______ | 39 |
| 16. | New girl- or boyfriend | ______ | 37 |
| 17. | Increase in work load at school | ___✓___ | 37 |
| 18. | Outstanding personal achievement | ______ | 36 |
| 19. | First quarter/semester in college | ______ | 36 |

day, concentrating on a word or image, breathing slowly and rhythmically. In Transcendental Meditation, the meditation process is essentially identical to the relaxation exercise, the main difference being that the meditator silently chants a phrase, or mantra, instead of the word *one*. Christians and Jews who use prayers stay with meditation longer than those reciting a meaningless phrase.

If you wish to try meditation, it often helps to have someone guide you through your first sessions. If you want to try it on your own, this step-by-step guide will introduce you to meditation:

1. Breathe deeply three times, allowing your breath to rise from your abdomen into your upper chest.
2. Exhale slowly through your mouth.
3. Imagine a white beam of light over the top of your head.

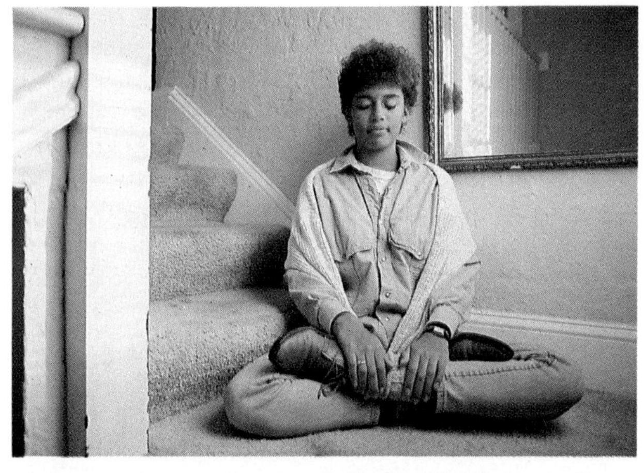

Meditation is one way to release stress. It involves sitting quietly for 15 to 20 minutes, concentrating on a single word or image, and breathing slowly and rhythmically.

| Item | | Points |
|---|---|---|
| 20. Change in living conditions | ______ | 31 |
| 21. Serious argument with an instructor | ______ | 30 |
| 22. Lower grades than expected | ______ | 29 |
| 23. Change in sleeping habits | ______ | 29 |
| 24. Change in social activities | ______ | 29 |
| 25. Change in eating habits | ______ | 28 |
| 26. Chronic car trouble | ______ | 26 |
| 27. Change in the number of family get-togethers | ______ | 26 |
| 28. Too many missed classes | ______ | 25 |
| 29. Change of college | ______ | 24 |
| 30. Dropping of more than one class | ______ | 23 |
| 31. Minor traffic violations | ______ | 20 |

Total ______

Here's how to interpret your score. If your score is 300 or higher, you are at high risk for developing a health problem. If your score is between 150 and 300, you have a 50-50 chance of experiencing a serious health change within two years. If your score is below 150, you have a 1-in-3 chance of a serious health change.

The following can help you reduce your risk:

- Watch for early signs of stress, such as stomachaches or compulsive overeating.
- Avoid negative thinking.
- Arm your body against stress by eating nutritiously and exercising regularly.
- Practice a relaxation technique regularly.
- Turn to friends and relatives for support when you need it.

SOURCE: Mullen, Kathleen and Gerald Costello. *Health Awareness Through Self-Discovery.*

4. Allow the light to begin slowly pouring into the top of your head, warming, energizing, and filling your insides.
5. Allow your muscles to be supported by the warm light.
6. Allow the light to move slowly from your head, down through your neck, shoulders, and arms until it fills your whole chest cavity, abdomen, hips, genitals, buttocks, legs, and feet. As it moves, feel the tension drain away from each part of your body.
7. Continue breathing deeply and slowly.
8. As the light flows through your body, allow blocked energy to be pushed slowly out your hands and dissipate into the atmosphere.

During this process, your body will feel light, tingly, relaxed and warm. There may be ripples of energy through the muscles. Relax, continue breathing, and enjoy the release of blocked energy. Open your eyes; sit quietly for a few minutes.

## Biofeedback

Quite simply, **biofeedback** is feedback, or information, about some activity that has just taken place within the body. An electronic monitoring device attached to the body detects a change in an internal function and communicates it back to the person through a tone, light, or meter. By paying attention to this feedback, most people can gain some control over functions previously thought to be beyond con-

**biofeedback** Information about some activity that has just taken place in the body.

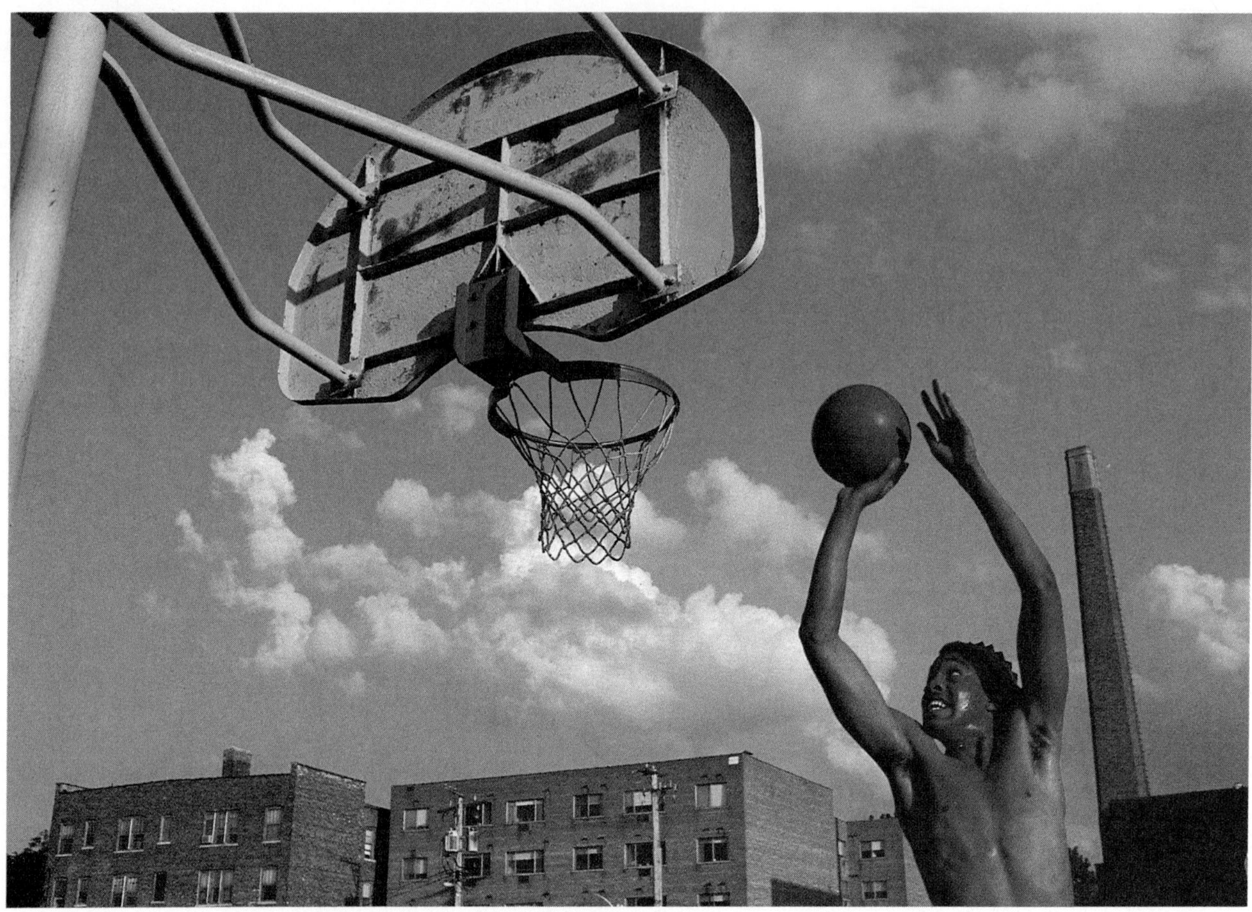

Channelling stress into physical activity can be a source of pleasure and relaxation.

scious control, such as body temperature, heart rate, muscle tension, and brain waves.

Biofeedback consists of three stages:

1. developing increased awareness of a body state or function
2. gaining control over it
3. transferring this control to everyday living without use of the electronic instrument

The goal of biofeedback for stress reduction is a state of tranquillity usually associated with the brain's production of alpha waves (which are slower and more regular than normal "waking" waves). After several training sessions, most people can produce alpha waves more or less at will.

### Exercise

Exercise helps defuse stress in a way that seems paradoxical: It causes the same physiological symptoms—increased blood pressure, faster heart rate, and so on—as a stressful situation, though not as intense. In this way, it conditions your body to cope with stress when you're in a sudden jam.

**STRATEGY FOR CHANGE**

**Sweating Away Stress**

- Choose an exercise that you truly enjoy.
- Exercise for at least 20 to 30 minutes three to five times a week.
- Schedule your workout for a time when you usually feel tense, such as the end of the day.
- If possible, choose a pleasant setting.
- Don't push too hard or try to go faster or farther than before. Repeat words like *smooth* and *steady* to yourself.

### Eating Right

A well-balanced, nutritious diet is essential to help your body cope with stress. If you skip breakfast, snack

## WHAT DO YOU THINK?

Stress-reduction workshops with titles like, "Massage for Relaxation," "Test-taking Tips," and "Cramming Techniques" have become popular on campuses around the country. At UCLA, students learn to visualize themselves calmly answering difficult exam questions. At New York University, a group called Peers' Ears offers student-to-student counseling. Do you think such programs help? Are any such programs available at your school? Would you participate in them? Why or why not?

Malcolm is working his way through college by helping out at his friend's auto body shop. Lately he's been getting less than 5 hours of sleep a night and wolfing down pizza and hamburgers between classes. His stomach's always upset, he's exhausted all the time, and he's had a cold that he hasn't been able to shake for weeks. What could Malcolm do to lower his stress load?

Jasmine never thought of herself as religious, but one day she stepped inside the college chapel just to find a quiet place to think. When she left, she felt refreshed and filled with a sense of inner peace. Ever since she's made these visits part of her routine and has started attending some weekend services. Yet she doesn't want her friends to find out. Can you understand her mixed feelings? What roles do faith and prayer play in her life—and in yours?

compulsively, and go on and off crash diets, you're undermining your body's stress defenses—and a stress-vitamin supplement is no substitute for wise food choice.

*How* you eat may matter as much as *what* you eat. If you wolf down a hamburger and fries in the car on your way to class, you're setting yourself, and your stomach, up for some problems. Unchewed foods are difficult to digest, and overloading your stomach can create heartburn and painful pressure.

Rather than stuffing yourself two or three times a day, eat several smaller, more nutritious meals. Chapter 4 provides the information you need to plan such meals. Every college cafeteria offers nutritious items like low-fat yogurt or salad, and you should get in the habit of carrying an apple with you to eat in case of an attack of the munchies.

### STRATEGY FOR CHANGE

#### What Not to Do

In trying to manage the stress in your life, do *not*:

- use drugs or alcohol
- smoke
- blame other people for your stress
- try to avoid hassles by avoiding people
- take work home with you every night and weekend
- become overly involved in your work or a hobby to avoid confronting a problem
- isolate yourself by arguing with others

## MAKING THIS CHAPTER WORK FOR YOU

### Learning to Live with Stress

**Stress is the physiological and psychological response to any demand placed on us or our bodies, whether the stress is positive or negative. The physiological response to stress is called the General Adaptation Syndrome (GAS), and it consists of three stages: alarm, resistance, and exhaustion.**

**Stressors include life changes; daily hassles; poor time management; social stressors such as isolation, unemployment, and work problems; and disease. If not dealt with, stress can lead to physical, emotional, and mental exhaustion and contribute to heart disease, high blood pressure, immune disorders, headaches, digestive diseases, skin problems, and other ailments.**

**Stress-management techniques such as stress planning and cooperation with others can lessen the impact of stress. Often the best responses to stress are adapting to circumstances that can't be changed and cooperating with others so that everyone's needs are met. You can also reduce the impact of stress by reorganizing your life to avoid as many small stressors as possible and by regular doses of laughter, love, and affection.**

**Breathing and relaxation techniques—visualization and guided imagery, and meditation—are stress-management methods in which you sit quietly in a**

relaxed state, breathing slowly and rhythmically while silently reciting a specific word or focusing on an image. Regular exercise and good nutrition can contribute to your well-being and ability to manage stress.

You can start applying stress-management techniques immediately. You may want to begin by doing some relaxation or awareness exercises. They will give you the sort of quiet peace of mind you need to focus on larger issues, goals, and decisions.

However, you needn't see stress as a problem to solve on your own. Reach out to others. Share your smiles and laughs. As you build friendships and intimate relationships, you may find that some irritating problems are easier to put into perspective. Don't be afraid to laugh at yourself and to look for the comic aspects of a situation. Sometimes it is possible to laugh your cares away.

In addition, you might try some of the approaches that psychologist Suzanne Kobasa suggests for transforming yourself from helpless to hardy.[18] Her recommendations include:

- *Focusing.* Take a strain inventory of your body every day to determine where things aren't feeling quite right. Ask yourself, "What's keeping me from feeling terrific today?" Focusing on problem spots, such as stomach knots or neck tightness, increases your sense of control over stress.
- *Reconstructing stressful situations.* Think about a recent episode of distress, and then write down three ways it could have gone better and three ways it could have gone worse. You'll be able to see that the situation wasn't as disastrous as it might have been, and you'll find ways to cope better in the future.
- *Self-improvement.* When your life feels out of control, turn to a new challenge. You might try volunteering at a nursing home, going for a long-distance bike trip, or learning a foreign language. As you work toward your new goal, you'll realize that you can still cope and achieve.

Stress always involves an interaction between a life situation and a person's ability to cope. Perhaps one of the best ways to think of it is captured by the Chinese word for crisis, which consists of two characters: one means danger; the other, opportunity.

SECTION II

# YOUR BODY

Your health is basically up to you. This section provides information on the tools you have at hand to make your body feel better—stronger, more energetic, slimmer and trimmer. By learning how to eat wisely and well and how to become physically fit, you can get started on a lifelong journey of becoming all you can be.

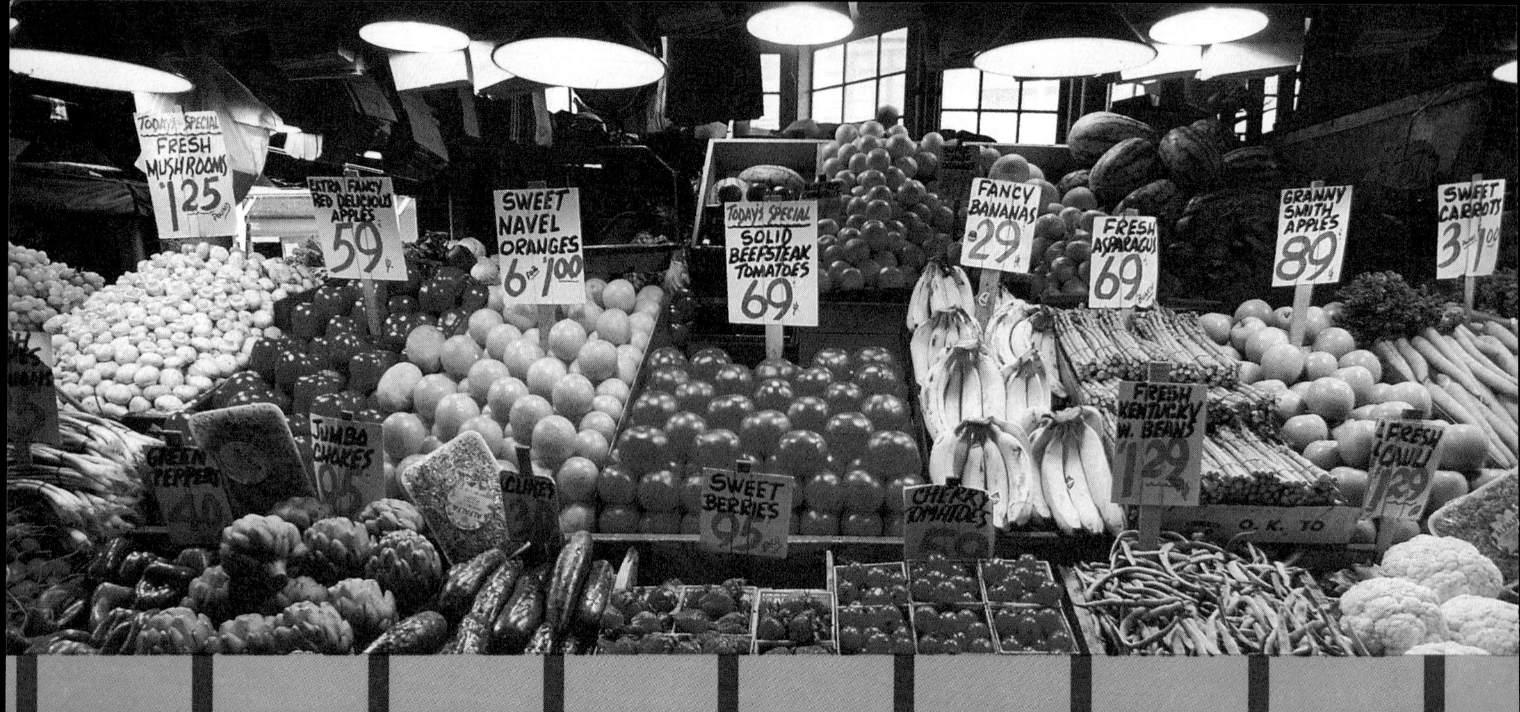


# 4 EATING WISELY AND WELL

**In this chapter**

**What makes food healthful?**

**Eating right: The four basic food groups**

**Eating to prevent heart disease and cancer**

**Eating for good health**

**Weight control**

**Obesity**

**Beyond dieting**

**Making this chapter work for you: Feeding yourself for a healthy future**

*Once eating was simple.* Now you hear about so many new claims and controversies that you may not know which foods are safe to put on your plate. Americans are trying to choose what they eat with greater care than in the past (see Table 4-1), but often we are so confused about what we should or shouldn't be eating that we're not sure how to eat wisely or well.

Food affects not only wellness, but weight. The eating habits you develop now may determine whether you ever develop weight problems. Men and women who become fat in their twenties and thirties tend to stay that way. This chapter translates the latest information on nutrition and weight control into basic advice you can use to eat well *and* feel well.

**TABLE 4-1** How Americans Have Changed Their Diets

| PERCENTAGE OF AMERICANS IMPROVING THE WAY THEY EAT | |
|---|---|
| Eating less fat | 46 |
| Eating more fruit and vegetables | 44 |
| Cutting down on candy and sweets | 40 |
| Eating less cholesterol | 35 |
| Cutting down on salt | 32 |
| Eating less red meat | 31 |
| Eating more chicken and fish | 22 |
| Cutting down on caffeine | 13 |
| Eating more health foods | 9 |
| Taking more vitamins | 7 |

SOURCE: Gurin, Joel. "Eating Goes Back to Basics," *American Health*, March 1990.

## WHAT MAKES FOOD HEALTHFUL?

We eat to live, and eating well helps us live well. We all need the same **nutrients**—proteins, fats, carbohydrates, vitamins, and minerals that form muscles, bones, and other tissues and provide energy for work and play—but in different amounts, depending on age, sex, size, health, and level of activity. **Nutrition** is the science that explores the interactions between our bodies and the food we eat. To understand why you should eat more of certain foods and less of others, you need to know about the nutrients that are the basic building blocks of good health.

### Protein

The framework for your muscles, bones, blood, hair, and fingernails is **protein.** Except for water content, over half of your body is made up of protein, which is essential for growth and repair. Some proteins also help regulate various body processes by serving as hormones, enzymes, or protective antibodies.

The National Academy of Sciences' recommended dietary allowance (RDA) for protein is 0.8 gram per kilogram of weight—an average of 63 grams a day for men and 50 grams a day for women. If you're like most Americans, you're eating twice as much protein as you need. Only about 12 to 15 percent of your daily calories should come from protein sources. Extra protein, like other excess calories, is stored as fat.

The best-known sources of protein are meat, poultry, fish, eggs, and dairy products. You can also get plenty of protein without eating any meat or dairy products. Legumes (beans, peas, and lentils) are 11 percent protein, just slightly less than an egg (13 percent protein).

Not all protein sources are created equal. **Complete proteins**—such as milk, meat, and fish—provide all the essential amino acids the body needs to synthesize its own proteins. **Incomplete proteins**—such as legumes and nuts—may have relatively low levels of one or two essential amino acids but fairly high levels of others. By combining **complementary proteins,** you can make sure that your body makes the most of the nonanimal proteins you eat (see Figure 4-1).

### Carbohydrates

Our bodies and brains need **carbohydrates** for their basic fuel: glucose. **Simple carbohydrates** (sugars) and **complex carbohydrates** (starches) both have 4

**nutrient** A food element essential to life and that the body cannot produce on its own.
**nutrition** A science devoted to the study of the need for, and effects of, food on organisms.
**protein** A substance that is basically a compound of amino acids; one of the essential nutrients.
**complete protein** A protein that contains all the amino acids needed by the body for growth and maintenance.
**incomplete protein** A protein that lacks one or more of the amino acids essential for protein synthesis.
**complementary protein** An incomplete protein that, when combined with another incomplete protein, provides all the amino acids essential for protein synthesis.
**carbohydrate** An organic compound—such as starch, sugar, or glycogen—composed of carbon, hydrogen, and oxygen; a source of bodily energy.
**simple carbohydrate** A sugar; like all carbohydrates, provides the body with glucose.
**complex carbohydrate** A starch found in cereals, fruits, and vegetables.

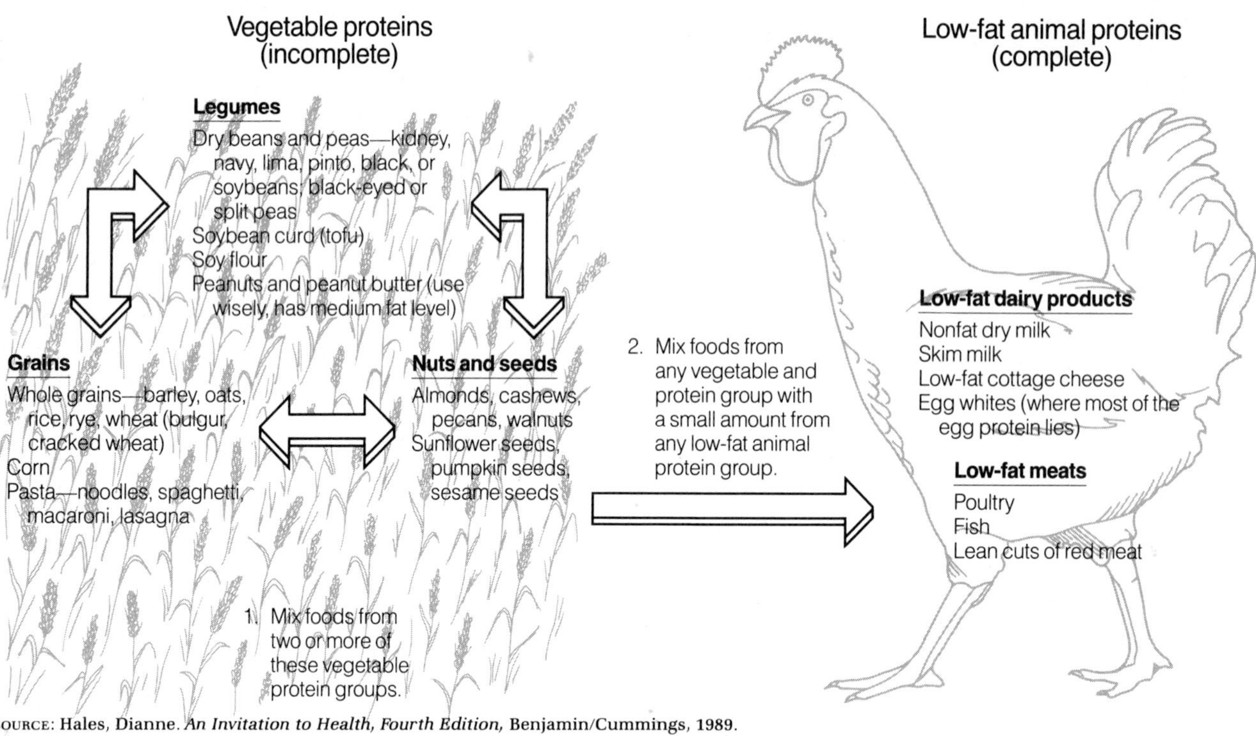


SOURCE: Hales, Dianne. *An Invitation to Health, Fourth Edition*, Benjamin/Cummings, 1989.

**FIGURE 4-1** By incorporating complementary protein sources in your diet, you can be sure your body has the complete protein it needs.

calories per gram. Sugars provide little more than a quick spurt of energy, whereas starches are rich in vitamins, minerals, and other nutrients.

Most nutrition experts recommend that at least 50 to 60 percent of daily calories come from complex carbohydrates. Carbohydrates include cereals; root vegetables such as potatoes and yams; legumes; dark-green leafy vegetables; yellow fruits and vegetables (winter squash, carrots); citrus fruits; and vegetables from the plant family that includes broccoli, cabbage, kohlrabi, and cauliflower (a family of vegetables called crucifers).

Many complex carbohydrates also supply a substance that our bodies can't digest but need nonetheless: fiber. (Animal products provide *no* fiber.) As fiber passes through our bodies, it creates a feeling of fullness, aids digestion, prevents constipation, and may protect us from cancer of the colon and other organs. High-fiber foods include fresh fruits with peels, berries, prunes, beans of all kinds, beet greens, broccoli, brussels sprouts, chick-peas, lentils, parsnips, peas, winter squash, bran cereals, bran flakes, and whole-grain cereals and breads. (See "Fiber: The Right Stuff?" later in this chapter for further discussion of fiber.)

**STRATEGY FOR CHANGE**

- Buy a big shaker like the ones pizza parlors use for cheese and oregano; fill the shaker with bran to shake on cereal or salads.
- Pack a salad bar for lunch. Include small bags of canned chick-peas, frozen peas, corn, fresh green peppers, or carrots, and so on.
- Reach for the darker greens, such as romaine lettuce, instead of iceberg. They provide more vitamins, plus beta-carotene, which may help prevent cancer.
- Go for pasta power: Pasta has 210 calories per cooked cup—only 9 calories from fat—and pasta is full of vitamins, plus some protein and iron (if enriched).

## Fats

A single teaspoonful of vegetable oil every day provides all the fat we need to store vitamins A, D, E, and K; keep skin healthy; give us stamina; and insulate us from shock and temperature extremes. Fat accounts for 42 percent of the daily calories in a typical American diet. There is no RDA for fat, and the American

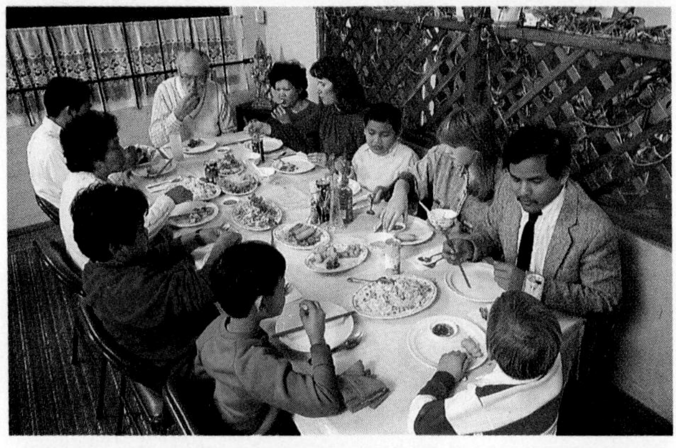

Americans are changing the way they eat to improve their nutrition and health.

Heart Association advises cutting back to 30 percent.[1] Some health experts believe 20 percent would be better.

Saturated fats, which come primarily from animal sources such as meat and dairy products, are dangerous to the heart and should account for no more than 10 percent of your daily calories. They are the number one culprit in increasing the amount of dangerous cholesterol, a type of fat, in the blood.

Unsaturated fats, which come from plants and include most vegetable oils (but not coconut), can actually benefit the heart. They include both polyunsaturated fats, such as those in safflower and sunflower oil, and monounsaturated fats, such as those in olive and canola oil. Polyunsaturates can lower cholesterol, but they lower beneficial types of cholesterol as well as harmful cholesterol. The monounsaturated fats lower only the harmful form of cholesterol. According to a 1990 study of almost 5,000 Italian men and women 20 to 59 years of age, in the *Journal of the American Medical Association*, monounsaturated fats may also benefit the heart by reducing blood pressure and blood sugar.[2]

Triglycerides are fatty substances, or lipids, that can be made up of saturated or unsaturated fats. Those with mostly saturated fats are solid at room temperature and are generally found in animal products, such as lard, grease, or butter. Those with mostly unsaturated fats are liquid at room temperature and are found in vegetable products, such as corn oil or cottonseed oil. (See Chapter 13 for more information on dietary risk factors.)

## Water

Although we can live for several weeks without food, we would die after a few days without water. A loss of 5 percent of the body's water causes weakness; a 15 to 20 percent loss can be fatal. Water is an important element in the production of sweat, which evaporates from the skin to cool the body.

Your body normally contains 40 to 50 quarts of water, which it uses to digest food and to transport nutrients to, and waste products from, cells. To make up for water lost through evaporation and elimination, drink at least six to eight glasses of liquids a day.

## Vitamins

A **vitamin** is an organic compound that is essential in very small amounts in our daily diet. Vitamins A, D, and E are **fat-soluble,** absorbed through the intestinal membranes and stored in the body. The B vitamins and vitamin C are **water-soluble** and are used up or washed out of the body in urine and sweat. They must be replaced daily. Recently the National Academy of Sciences began publishing an RDA for vitamin K, a water-soluble vitamin that helps regulate blood clotting and is found primarily in leafy green vegetables. (Men need 80 micrograms of vitamin K daily; women need 65 micrograms.)

The vitamins help put proteins, fats, and carbohydrates to use and help the body to produce the right chemical reactions at the right times. They're also involved in the manufacture of blood cells as well as hormones and other compounds.

The best vitamin sources are real foods, not tablets. If you rely on vitamin pills and fortified foods to make up for poor nutrition, you're kidding yourself—and you may be shortchanging your body. The only way of making sure your body gets what it needs is by eating a wide variety of nutritious foods.

Because vitamins are good for us, you might think that the more you get, the better you'll feel. It's not that simple. There are no proven benefits—and there are some serious risks—associated with huge amounts of any vitamin. The fat-soluble vitamins, primarily A and D, can build up in our bodies, and excess amounts can cause serious complications, such as damage to the kidneys, liver, or bones. Large doses of water-soluble vitamins, including C and the B vitamins, may also be harmful. Excessive $B_6$ (pyridoxine), a vitamin many women take to relieve premenstrual bloating, can cause neurological damage (an excessive amount is 1,000 or more times the recommended dose).

**vitamin** An organic substance needed by the body in a very small amount; carries out a variety of functions in metabolism and nutrition.

**fat-soluble vitamin** A vitamin absorbed, with the aid of fats in the diet or bile from the liver, through the intestinal membrane and stored in the body.

**water-soluble vitamin** A vitamin used up or excreted in urine and sweat; must be replaced daily.

## Minerals

Carbon, oxygen, hydrogen, and nitrogen make up 96 percent of your body weight. The other 4 percent consists of nearly 30 **minerals,** which help build bones and teeth, operate your muscles, and transmit messages along your nervous system. You need daily about 1/10 gram (or 100 mg) of each of the macrominerals: sodium, potassium, chlorine, calcium, phosphorus, and magnesium. You need also about 1/100 gram (10 mg) or less daily of each of the microminerals: iron, zinc, selenium, molybdenum, iodine, cobalt, copper, manganese, fluorine, and chromium.

Two of the most important minerals—and two you might not be getting enough of—are iron and calcium.

### Iron

Iron is an essential ingredient of **hemoglobin,** the protein that makes the blood red and carries oxygen to all our tissues. Because oxygen is needed to convert food into energy, too little iron—and thus hemoglobin—can trigger an internal energy crisis.

Getting enough iron is a big problem for women, whose iron stores are drained by menstruation, pregnancy, and nursing. Half of all women of childbearing age get less than the RDA of 15 mg, and 5 percent suffer from iron-deficiency anemia.

The symptoms of iron deficiency are chronic fatigue, edginess, depression, sleeplessness, and susceptibility to colds and infections. To boost your iron, include more iron-rich foods in your diet. Don't take iron supplements unless you've had a blood test; excess iron can cause severe constipation and other complications.

**STRATEGY FOR CHANGE**

**Put More Iron in Your Diet**

Use these guidelines to add more iron to your diet the natural way:

- Eat vegetables and starches high in iron: legumes, fresh fruits, whole-grain cereals, and broccoli.
- To increase the amount of iron your body absorbs from these vegetables, eat foods high in vitamin C at the same meal.
- Eat lean red meats, which are richest in the form of iron that your body utilizes best, two or three times a week.
- Eat iron-rich organ meats, like liver, once or twice a month.
- Don't drink tea with your meal—the tannin in it may interfere with iron absorption.

### Calcium

Calcium, the most abundant mineral in the body, builds strong bones and teeth, not just in children, but also in adults. The ongoing need for calcium is critical because our bodies keep breaking down and rebuilding bone tissue. In fact, every single cell in the body requires calcium. Without it, nerve cells cannot conduct impulses, the heart cannot beat, and the brain cannot function. Adequate calcium is especially important for pregnant or nursing women, who need it to meet the needs of the baby's body (see Chapter 8 for more on diet and pregnancy).

For both sexes the RDA of calcium is 1,200 mg from ages 11 to 24. Adequate calcium during this time period may be crucial to prevent osteoporosis, the bone-weakening disease that strikes one out of every four women over the age of 60 (see Chapters 5 and 17). The RDA for adults over age 24 is 800 mg, but some researchers believe that women should try to consume 1,000 to 1,500 mg of calcium a day.

**STRATEGY FOR CHANGE**

**Adding Calcium to Your Diet**

Use these guidelines to add more calcium to your diet:

- Dairy products are the best calcium sources, but be sure you choose those low in fat.
- Choose other calcium-rich alternatives, such as sardines (drained of oil), other canned fishes, tofu, and turnip or mustard greens.
- To boost absorption of calcium, eat foods rich in vitamin C (which helps iron absorption too) at the same time.
- Use an acidic dressing, made with citrus juices or vinegar, to enhance calcium absorption from salad greens.
- If you can't get enough calcium from food, supplements may be the only answer. But beware of those made with dolomite or bonemeal; they may be contaminated with lead.

## EATING RIGHT: THE BASIC FOUR FOOD GROUPS

Many foods are nutritious, but none provides all the nutrients, vitamins, and proteins your body needs.

**mineral** A naturally occurring inorganic substance; a small amount is essential to life.
**hemoglobin** The oxygen-transporting component of red blood cells.

**TABLE 4-2** Four Basic Food Groups and Their Major Nutrients

| | | Major Nutrients Supplied in Significant Amounts | |
|---|---|---|---|
| GROUP | EXAMPLE FOODS | BY ALL IN GROUP | BY ONLY SOME FOODS |
| Fruits and vegetables | Apples, bananas, dates, oranges, tomatoes, broccoli, cabbage, green beans, lettuce, potatoes | Carbohydrate, water | Vitamins: A, C, folacin; minerals: iron, calcium; fiber |
| Grain products (preferably whole grain; otherwise, enriched or fortified) | Breads, rolls, bagels, cereals (dry and cooked), pasta, rice, other grains, tortillas, pancakes, waffles, crackers, popcorn | Carbohydrate; protein; vitamins: thiamin, niacin; mineral: iron | Water, fiber |
| Milk and milk products | Milk, yogurt, cheese, ice cream, ice milk, frozen yogurt | Protein; fat; vitamins: A, riboflavin, $B_{12}$; minerals: calcium, phosphorus; water | Carbohydrate, vitamin D |
| Meats and meat alternatives | Meat, fish, poultry, eggs, seeds, nuts, nut butters, soybeans, tofu, other legumes (peas and beans) | Protein; vitamins: niacin, $B_6$; minerals: iron, zinc | Carbohydrate, fat, vitamin $B_{12}$, water, fiber |

SOURCE: Christian, Janet L. and Janet L. Greger. *Nutrition for Living, Second Edition*, Benjamin/Cummings, 1988.

That's why it's important to include items from the four basic food groups (see Table 4-2) in your daily diet.

## Vegetable and Fruit Group

Vegetables and fruits contribute vitamins A and C, are low in fat, and are high in fiber. Dark green vegetables are also good sources of riboflavin, folacin, iron, and magnesium; certain greens—collards, kale, turnip, and mustard—provide calcium. A serving consists of 1/2 cup or a typical portion, such as one potato, one-half grapefruit, or a bowl of salad.

## Bread and Cereal Group

Whole-grain and enriched breads and cereals are important sources of B vitamins, iron, and protein. This group includes bread, biscuits, cooked or ready-to-eat cereals, noodles, rice, rolled oats, barley, and bulgur. Count as one serving one slice of bread; 1/2 to 3/4 cup of cooked cereal, cornmeal, grits, macaroni, noodles, rice, or spaghetti; or 1 ounce of ready-to-eat cereal.

## Milk and Cheese Group

Most milk products are high in calcium and contribute riboflavin, protein, and vitamins A, $B_6$, and $B_{12}$. This group includes whole, skim, low-fat, evaporated, and nonfat dry milk; buttermilk; yogurt; ice cream; cottage cheese; and cheeses of all sorts. A serving consists of an 8-ounce cup of milk, 1 cup of plain yogurt, 2 cups of cottage cheese, 1 1/2 ounces of hard cheese, or 1 tablespoon of cheese spread. An 8-ounce glass of skim milk, with no fat, is a more nutritious choice than a tablespoon of a high-fat cheese spread.

## Meat, Poultry, Fish, and Bean Group

The foods in this group are good sources of protein, phosphorus, iron, zinc, vitamin $B_6$, niacin, and other vitamins and minerals. In addition to beef, veal, lamb, pork, poultry, and shellfish, this group includes dry beans, dry peas, soybeans, lentils, eggs, seeds, nuts, and peanuts. One egg, 1/2 to 3/4 cup of beans, 1/4 to 1/2 cup of nuts, or 2 tablespoons of peanut butter is the nutritional equivalent of 1 ounce of lean meat.

## Nonnutritive Foods: A Fifth Group

Some nutritionists classify fats, sweets, and alcohol in a separate, fifth food group. These foods provide relatively few nutrients in proportion to the calories in them. These "empty" calories provide no benefits and can contribute to weight problems.

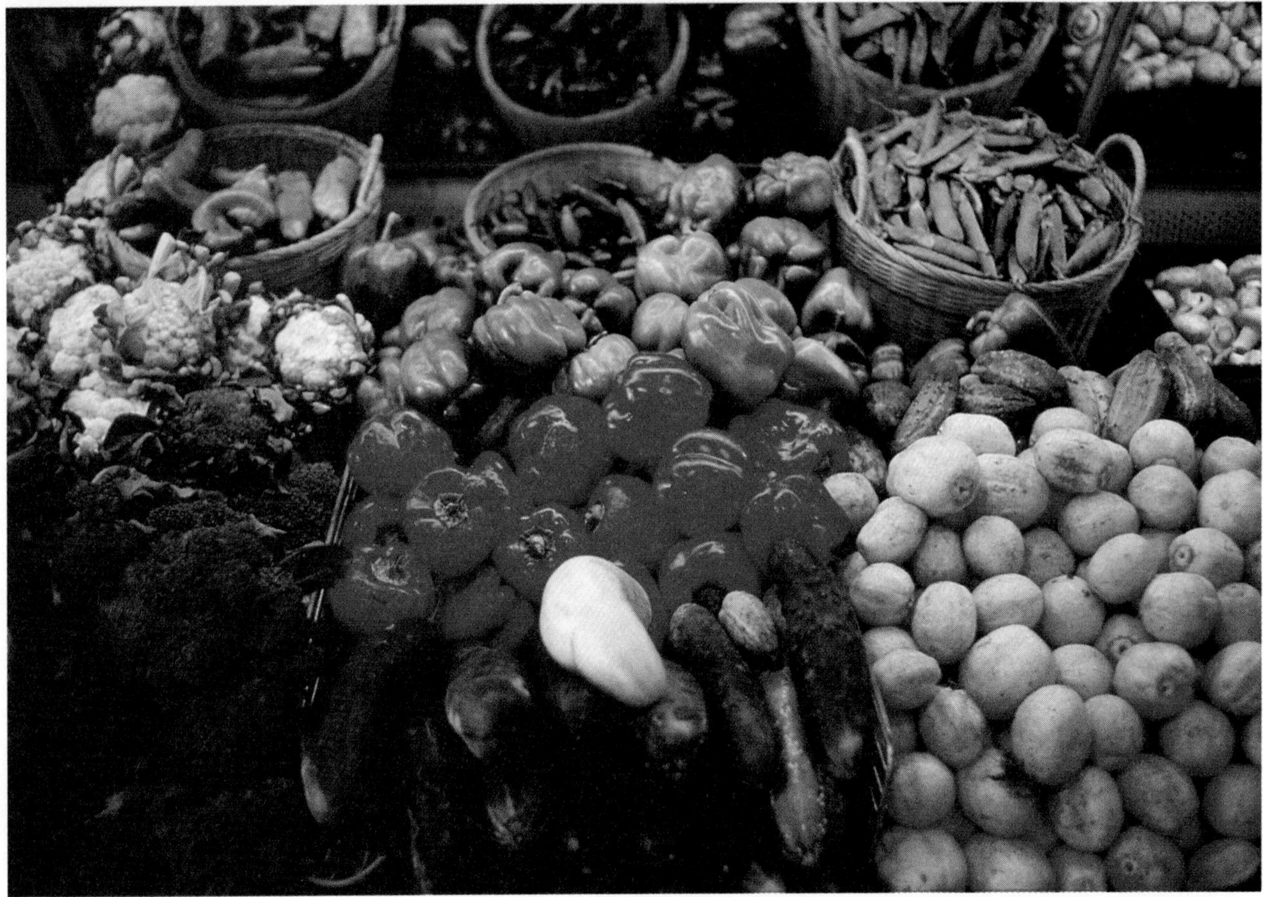

Fresh vegetables are an excellent source of fiber, vitamins and minerals.

## EATING TO PREVENT HEART DISEASE AND CANCER

The foods we eat can increase or decrease our risk of developing many illnesses, including the two most deadly diseases in the United States: heart disease and cancer. (See Chapters 13 and 14 for information on other risk factors.)

### Feeding the Healthy Heart

According to a report by the American Medical Association's Council on Scientific Affairs, Americans consume almost twice the maximum amount of saturated fat recommended to reduce heart disease.[3] If all Americans over age 2 were to cut cholesterol by 10 percent, there would be a 20 percent reduction in heart disease.

**STRATEGY FOR CHANGE**

**Heart-Saving Tips**

The American Heart Association's dietary recommendations for reducing the risk of heart disease are:

- Cut total fat to less than 30 percent of daily calories.
- Keep saturated fat below 10 percent, lower if possible. Keep polyunsaturated fats to less than 10 percent. You don't have to limit monounsaturated fats, as long as total fat is less than 30 percent.[4]
- Keep daily cholesterol intake to no more than 300 mg per day.
- Have no more than 55 ml of alcohol (2 drinks) a day.
- Limit sodium to no more than 1,000 mg per 1,000 calories, or 3,000 mg a day.

### Cholesterol: A Survival Guide

The body produces a substance called cholesterol that is a necessary component of various body cells.

**TABLE 4-3** Percentage of Fat Calories in Foods*

| FOOD TYPE | BELOW 20% | 20%–30% | 30%–40% | 40%–50% | 50%–60% | ABOVE 70% |
|---|---|---|---|---|---|---|
| Meat and fish | Turkey (light meat, no skin), cod, crab, flounder, scallops, sole, tuna in water | Chicken (light meat, no skin) | Lean sirloin, turkey (dark meat, no skin), catfish | Chicken (dark meat, no skin), lamb chops, veal roast | Ground beef, fish sticks | Bacon, Spam®, T-bone steak |
| Dairy products | Low-fat cottage cheese, skim milk | Buttermilk, milk (1% fat), low-fat yogurt (plain) | Milk (2% fat) | Whole milk | Eggs, part-skim ricotta | Cheddar cheese, cream cheese |
| Vegetables and grain-based foods | Most raw vegetables, bread (white and whole wheat), oatmeal, pasta, rice | Corn bread, wheat germ | Granola | Croissants, taco shells | Corn chips, tofu | |
| Desserts and snacks | Most raw and dried fruit, gelatin, sherbet | Graham crackers | Apple pie, chocolate-chip cookies | Carrot cake with icing, pound cake | Cream cheese cake, dough-nuts, ice cream (chocolate and vanilla), cashews, peanuts | Coconut, peanut butter |

*Chart based on nutrition information from the Center for Science in the Public Interest, Washington, D.C.

SOURCE: Copyright © 1987 by *New York Times Company*, Reprinted by permission. March 29, 1987.

But too much can be dangerous, especially to the heart. Foods high in saturated fat raise the level of cholesterol already in the blood and clog the arteries, adding to the risk of heart disease (see Chapter 13). The number one way of reducing blood cholesterol is cutting back on fats (see Table 4-3).

Everyone with moderate- to high-risk cholesterol levels should change their eating habits. Since cholesterol is found primarily in animal products, a reduction in the consumption of these products is an obvious place to start. The Step One diet calls for reducing fat to less than 30 percent of daily calories, limiting saturated fats to 10 percent or less of daily calories, and keeping cholesterol intake at less than 300 mg a day.

**STRATEGY FOR CHANGE**

### Two Steps to Lower Cholesterol

Begin by following the Step One diet to reduce your cholesterol level:

- Eat more fish and poultry; remove the skin.
- Choose lean red meats only. Avoid fatty cuts of beef, lamb, or pork (especially spareribs); sausage; cold cuts; hot dogs; and bacon.
- Drink skim or milk with 1 percent fat instead of whole milk or milk with 2 percent fat. Do not use cream, half-and-half, nondairy creamers (which can contain saturated fats), or whipped toppings. Substitute sherbet or sorbet for ice cream.
- Cut down on high-fat cheeses, like cheddar, Swiss, Camembert, and blue. Look for cheeses such as skim-milk mozzarella.
- Eat no more than three egg yolks a week. (Egg whites are cholesterol- and fat-free.)
- Eat more vegetables and fruits, but don't add any high-fat butter or cream sauces.
- Choose unsaturated vegetable oils (corn, olive, canola, safflower, or peanut) rather than butter, lard, chicken, or bacon fat. Don't use tropical oils, such as coconut and palm.
- Use baking cocoa instead of chocolate.
- Avoid commercially prepared baked goods, such as pies, cakes, doughnuts, and pastries.
- Choose rice or pasta over egg noodles.
- Eat whole-grain breads and cereals that do not have eggs or saturated fats as ingredients.

**HALES INDEX**

Number of Americans who've improved their eating habits in the last two years: 3 in 5

Amount Americans spend on vitamin and mineral supplements each year: $2.4 billion

Pounds of broccoli each American eats annually: 3

Pounds of ice cream: 29

Pounds of sugar: 140

Percentage of Americans who've increased the fiber they eat: 40

Percentage of Americans who would cut back on milk and meat before giving up dessert: 32

Percentage of adults between the ages of 25 and 74 who are on a diet: 25

Percentage of women who are overweight: 27

Percentage of women who think they're overweight: 78

Amount Americans spend for weight-loss programs each year: $10 billion

Odds that a person who's lost weight on a diet will gain it back: 9 to 1

SOURCES: **1** Gurin, Joel. "Eating Goes Back to Basics," *American Health,* March 1990. **2** Gilman, Margot. "Fiber Mania," *Psychology Today,* December 1989. **3, 4, 5** U.S. Department of Agriculture. **6** Long, Patricia. "What America Eats," *Hippocrates,* May/June 1989. **7** "Would You Take Advice from an Overweight Expert?" *Hippocrates,* May/June 1989. **8** "Goodbye Diet, Hello Diet Food," *Psychology Today,* November 1989. **9, 10** Jacoby, Susan. "The Body Image Blues," *Family Circle,* February 1, 1990. **11** O'Neill, Molly. "Congressional Hearings on Diet Industry," *New York Times,* March 28, 1990. **12** Simon, Cheryl. "The Triumphant Dieter," *Psychology Today,* June 1989.

After three months on this plan, have your cholesterol level rechecked. If your level has dropped, continue this diet, with regular retests four times the first year and two times each year thereafter.

If the Step One diet fails to reduce your cholesterol level, doctors advise following the more stringent Step Two diet:

- Cut saturated fats to 7 percent of your daily calories.
- Avoid all fried foods, and most red or fatty meats.
- Have no more than two egg yolks a week.

If this dietary program fails to sufficiently reduce your cholesterol level, doctors may recommend other approaches. (See Chapter 13 for more on preventing heart disease.)

### Meaty Matters

Much of our dietary cholesterol comes from red meat, particularly beef. The average American consumes more than 100 pounds of red meat a year; every bite contains 3 to 4 times more fat than protein. But the meat industry has put America's cows, sheep, and hogs on a diet. Today's hogs are 15 percent leaner than those of the 1950s; cattle and lamb are 10 percent leaner. Many nutritionists now feel that the way you prepare and eat meat matters just as much as the meat itself.[5]

**STRATEGY FOR CHANGE**

**Making the Most of Meat**

- Limit red meat (trimmed of all visible fat) to two or three servings a week, and keep portions between 2 and 3 ounces.
- When you buy meat, look for "lite" meats, as designated by the U.S. Department of Agriculture, which have 25 percent less fat than standard cuts.
- Cook stews, boiled meat, or soup stock ahead of time; refrigerate; and remove hardened fat.
- Baste meat with wine, tomato juice, or lemon juice instead of drippings, or rub raw meat with herbs and spices before cooking.
- Broil or roast meat instead of frying it.
- Don't oversalt. Salt delays browning and draws out moisture.

# Your Body

## An Owner's Manual

Your body is a marvelous machine. Moment-to-moment, hour-to-hour, year-to-year, it must respond to a myriad of signals and changes in your environment. Like any other precision machine, your body performs best and longest when well maintained by its owner—you. This manual supplies you with some unusual views of the body to help you understand the most fascinating and complex machine you'll ever own.

The image you see in your mirror each day is only the surface of an interconnected collection of organ systems. Each system functions in ways that are crucial to your every activity. In turn, your activities influence the operation of your body's systems.

In this "Owner's Manual," we invite you to take a tour of your body. You'll also pick up some tips for outward health behaviors that will help maintain your inner self.

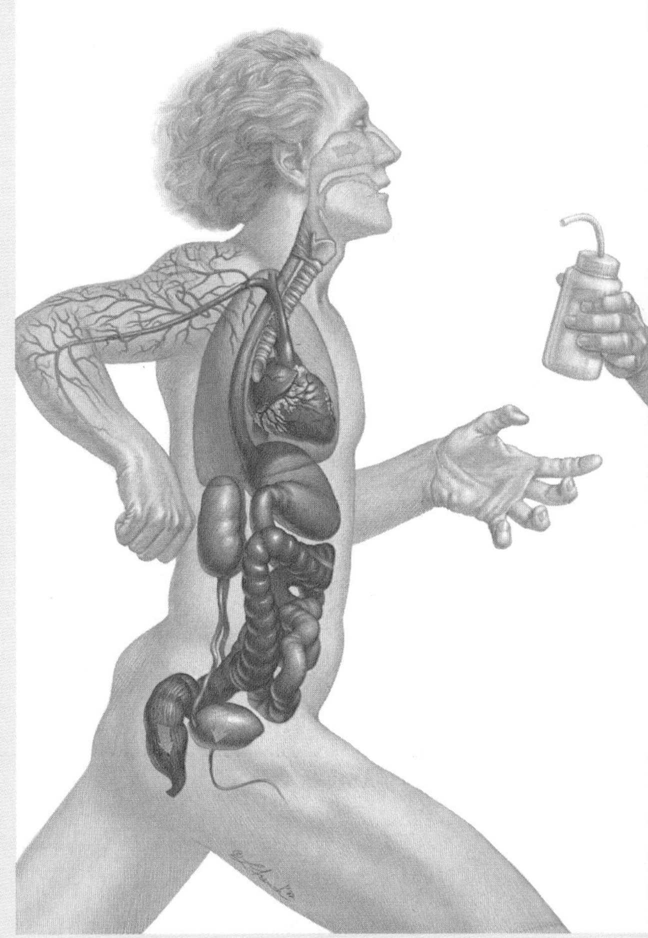

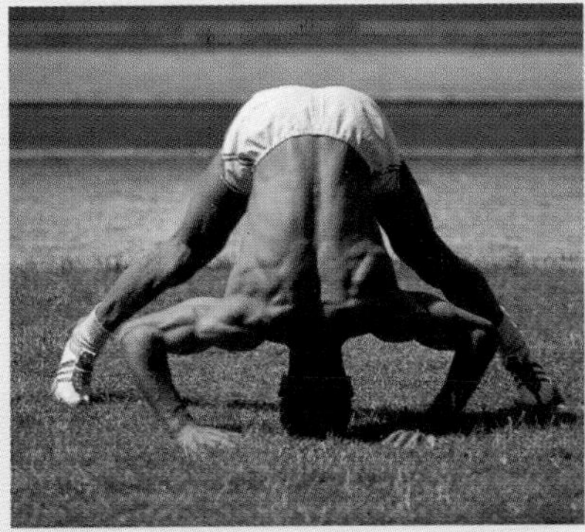

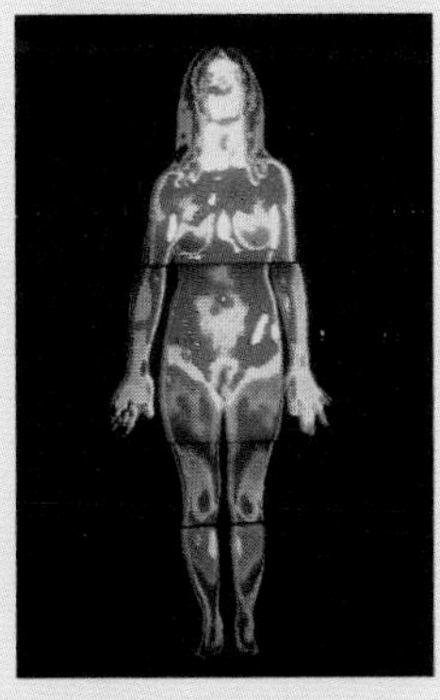

## Your Skeletal System

Your body's shape and mobility are provided by the skeletal system, a network of bones connected and cushioned by ligaments, joints, and cartilage. Accounting for nearly 20 percent of your body weight, the skeletal system is a framework that both supports and protects the other organs of your body. It also serves as a supply depot for minerals required elsewhere in your body.

Bones come in many sizes, from the thigh bone (femur), about 20 inches long and over 1 inch in diameter, to small sesamoid bones the size of sesame seeds, embedded in tendons of thumbs and toes. Although we usually think of bones as being long and narrow, their shape varies greatly, as in the lovely shell-shape of the inner ear bone (the cochlea). The secret of a bone's remarkable strength and resiliency is its internal structure, a meshwork of pliable protein strands embedded

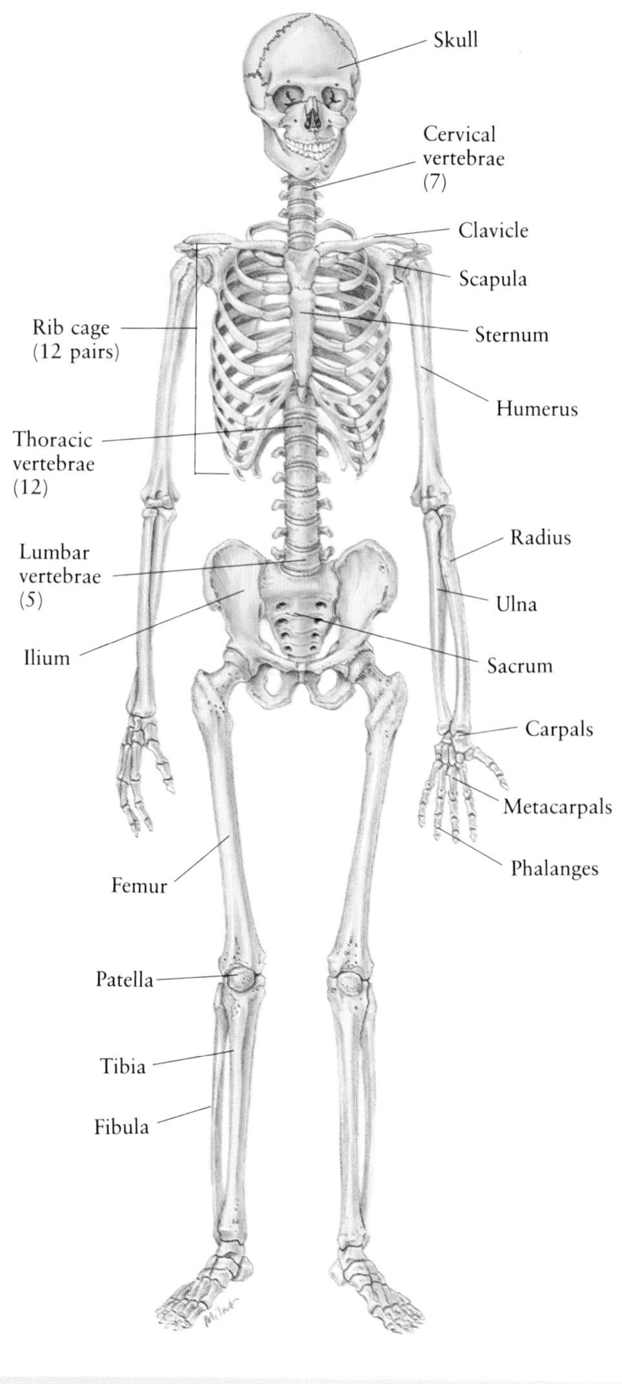


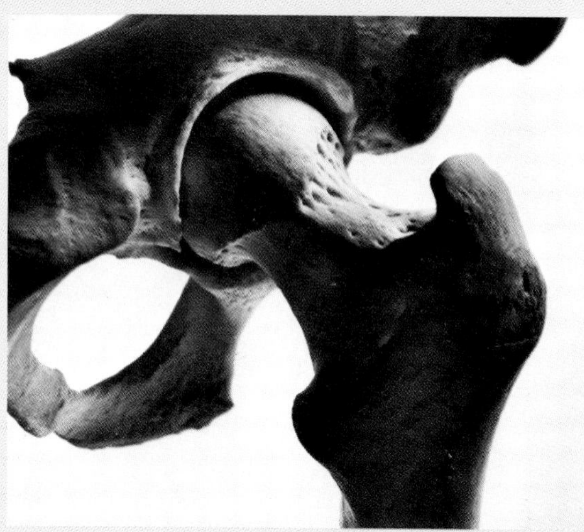

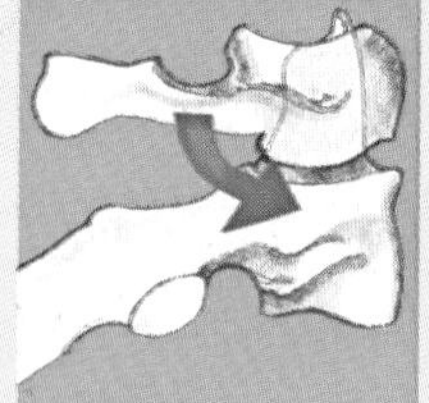
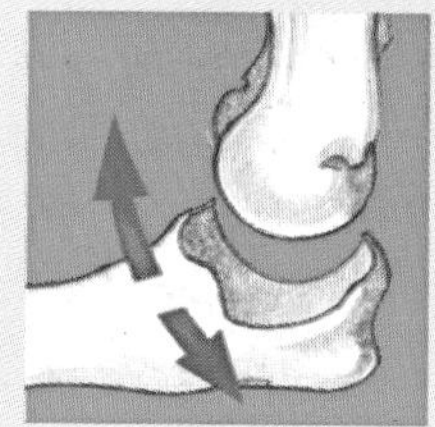
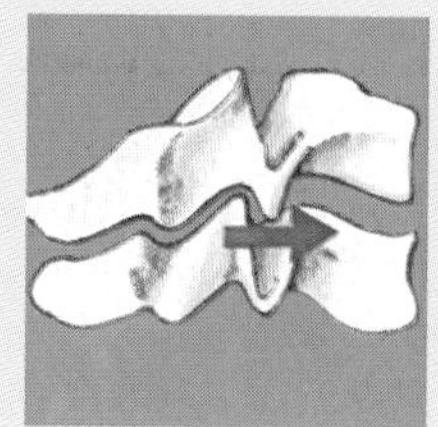
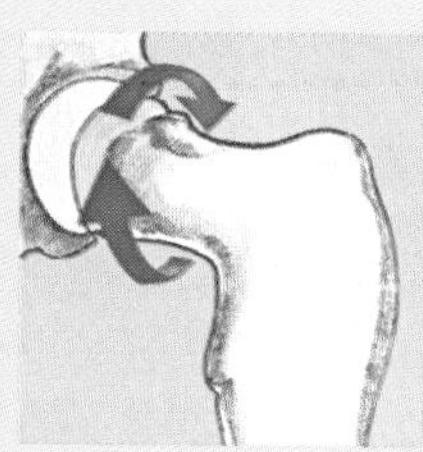

***Some Types of Joints*** *From left to right:* pivot (neck), hinge (elbow), sliding (ribs, vertebrae), ball-and-socket (shoulder).

with minerals, especially calcium. Bones must be strong. We subject some of them to between 12,000 and 15,000 pounds of pressure per square inch—just from walking! Bones are indeed alive. Marrow, a substance in the center of many bones, is the factory for production of blood cells, and bone itself contains many blood vessels.

Some bones are fused. Your skull, for example, is an assembly of 26 bones, fixed so they don't move. Other bones are connected by joints, which allow for some movement. A list of joint types may remind you of items in a hardware store; each type of joint allows connecting bones a specific range and degree of movement (see illustration on opposite page). For example, the pivot joint in the neck allows you to turn your head from side to side.

Sinewy connective tissues called ligaments help stabilize bone connections, whereas cartilage (a spongelike substance) both connects and cushions such bones as knees and vertebrae.

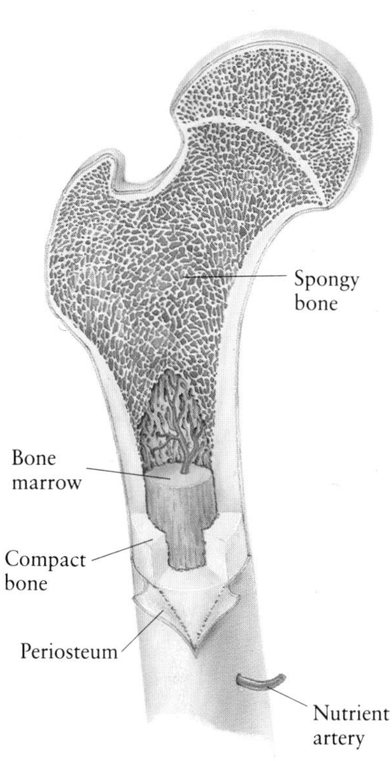


***Cross Section of Bone*** Spongy bone encases bone marrow. The outside layer of bone is the periosteum.

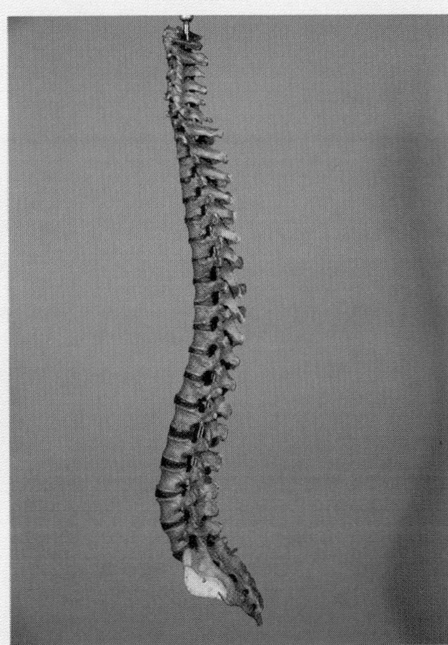

***The Spinal Column*** An S-shaped arrangement of vertebrae cushioned by cartilage, the spinal column not only affords our bodies their unique structure but houses and protects the spinal cord, the most critical path of nerves in our bodies.

## Maintenance Tips

- *Nutrition* Dairy products in your diet supply calcium, a critical component of bone.
- *Exercise* Inactivity can cause your bones to lose calcium, which makes them more susceptible to damage.
- *Safety* "Buckling up" and other safety precautions will prevent damage to your skeletal system from unfortunate impacts.

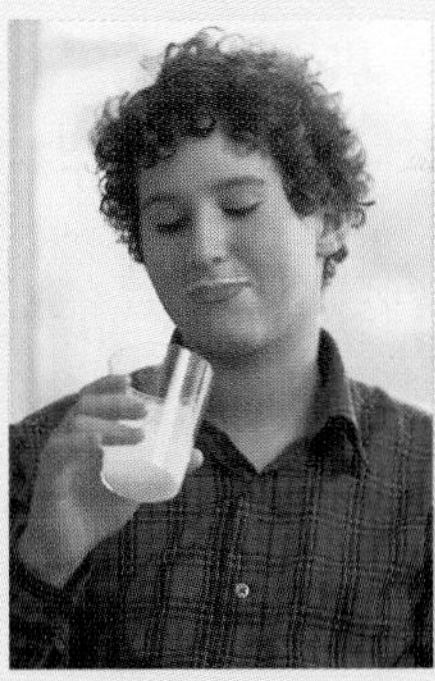

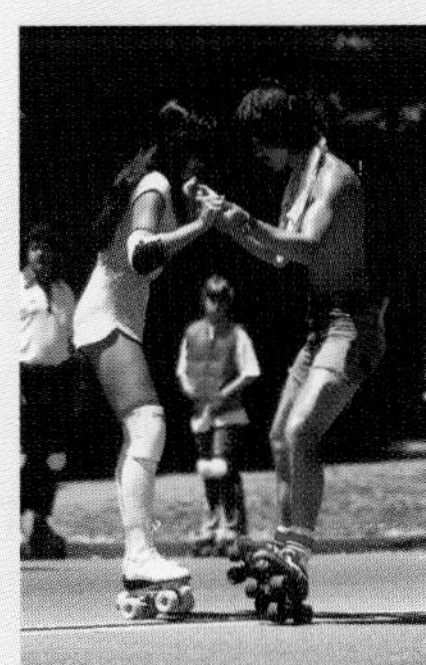

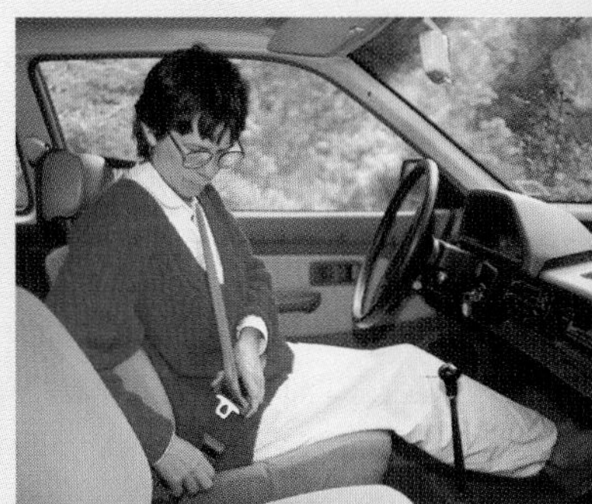

# Your Muscles

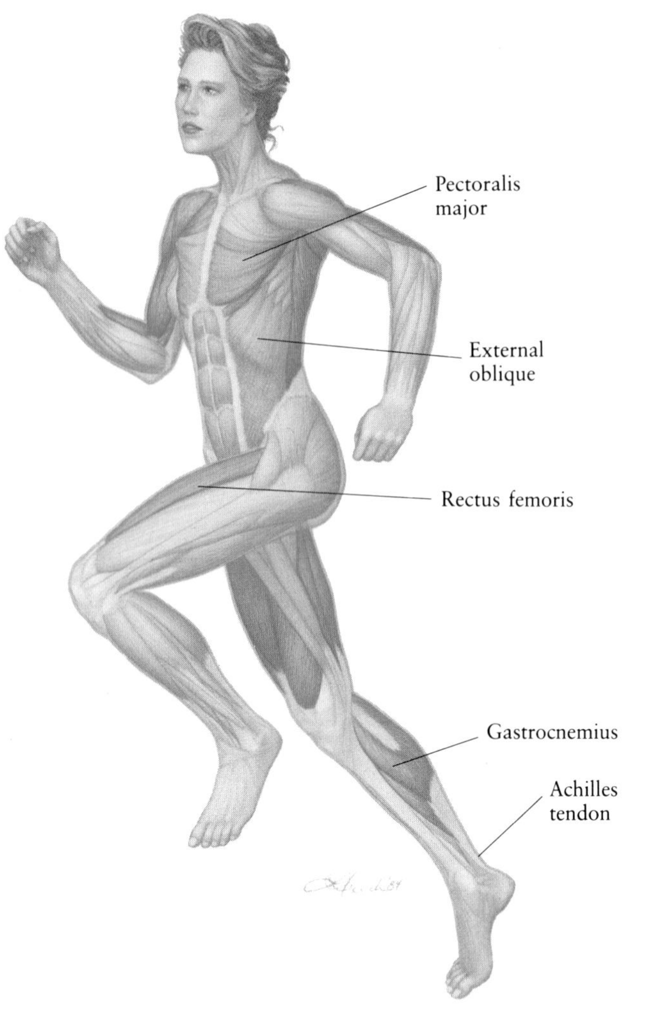


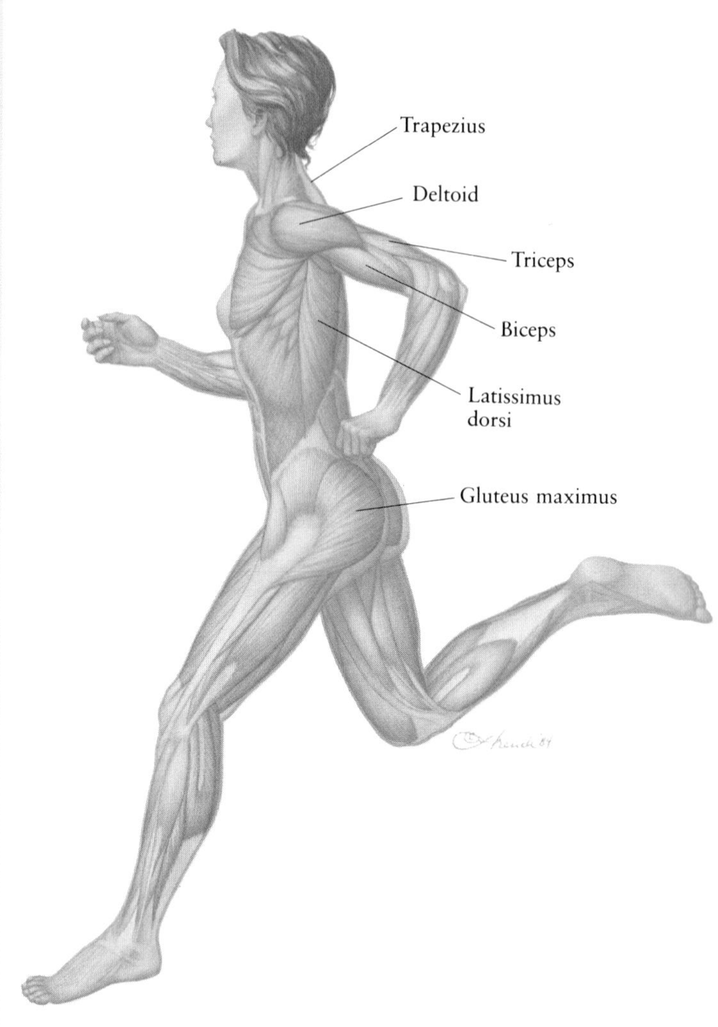


Muscles, muscles everywhere! Although muscles are most apparent in our arms and legs we have muscles located throughout our bodies. In fact, we have about 600 muscles. Altogether they compose 35 to 45 percent of one's body weight. Your heart is a muscle. Transportation of the food you eat and the oxygen you breathe is aided by the action of muscles in the stomach, intestines, and diaphragm. Facial muscles supply you with a large collection of expressions.

Muscles come in three basic varieties: skeletal, cardiac, and smooth. Skeletal muscle (sometimes called voluntary muscle) teams up with bones to produce the movements of our bodies. For example, in the flex of an arm, opposing muscle groups alternately contract and relax, pulling the attached bones up and down. Found only in the heart, cardiac muscle faithfully contracts and relaxes at a normal rate of seventy times per minute, 100,000 times per day, 2,500,000,000 times per lifetime. Smooth muscle, which is found in many of our internal organs, produces movements that are largely imperceptible, but crucial to respiration, digestion, elimination, and circulation. Nonvoluntary smooth muscles are constantly controlled by signals from a portion of the brainstem called the medulla.

All muscles are composed of fibers, each controlled by a nerve ending. Chemical signals from the brain cause muscle proteins in each fiber to slide, causing the fiber to contract. The coordinated contraction of millions of fibers produces noticeable movements like the flash of a smile or the tap of a foot.

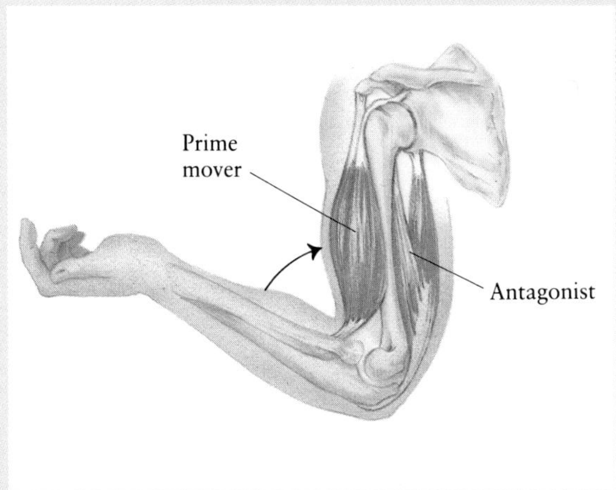


***Muscle Action*** Strong fibrous tissues (tendons) are continuous with bone and muscle as well as connect them.

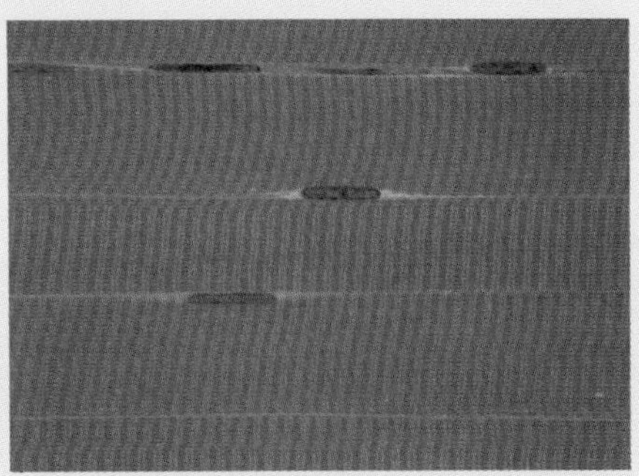

***Skeletal Muscle*** Long cells grouped into bundles give skeletal muscles their striped appearance.

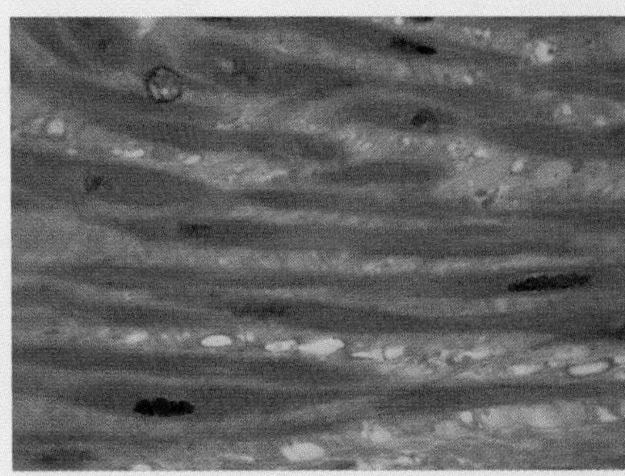

***Smooth Muscle*** These cells are smaller and not bunched into distinct arrangements.

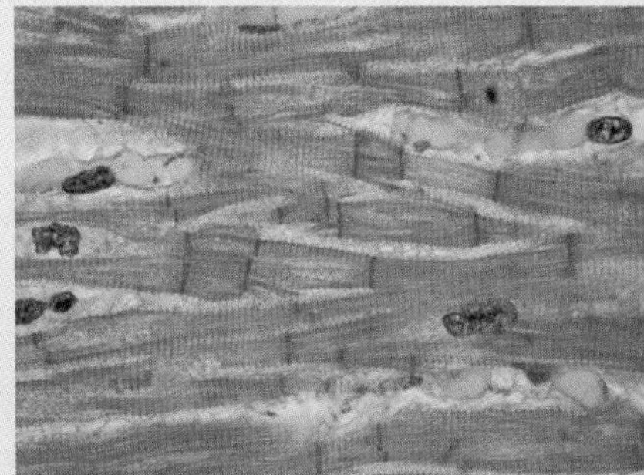

***Cardiac Muscle*** Cells of cardiac muscle branch and interweave to form thick bands.

## *Maintenance Tips*

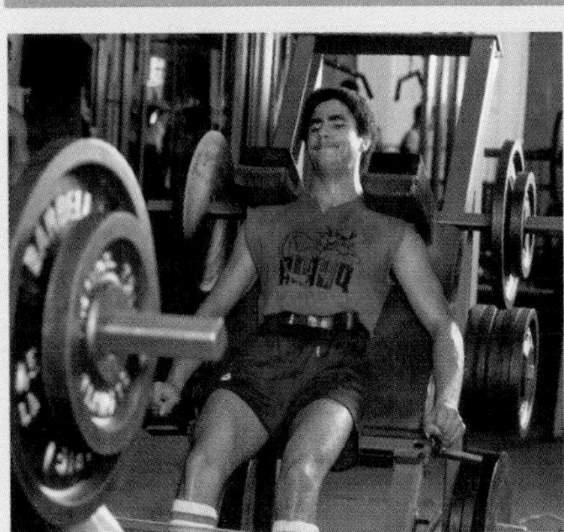

- *Exercise* Strengthening exercises help muscles bear heavy loads. Flexibility exercises increase the muscle's ability to stretch. Aerobic exercise ensures the muscle's oxygen supply.

- *Stress Management* Mental tension causes muscles to tighten involuntarily, creating everything from backaches to digestive disorders. Take time to relax.

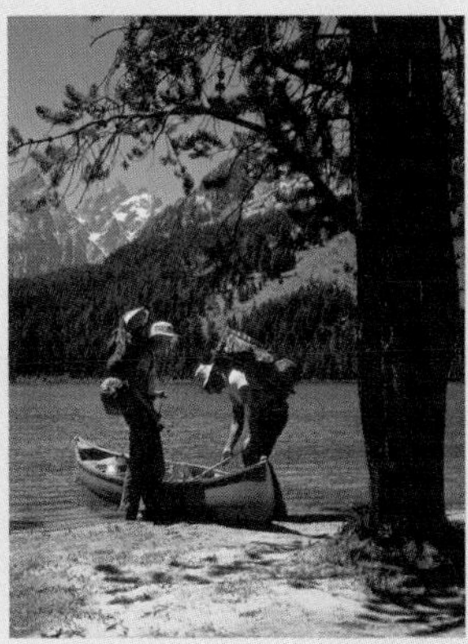

# Your Nervous System

Imagine a mission control room where one million gauges, buttons, and switches are receiving, processing, and transmitting information along a network of ten billion outside signal transmittors. Your nervous system, even more complex, is the "mission control" of your body. Playing a musical instrument, answering an exam question, flushing with sexual excitement, secreting digestive juices during a meal, quickening a heartbeat—these and millions of other behaviors are directed throughout your lifetime by your nervous system. Its billions of nerve cells receive, process, and transmit countless signals flowing through it.

The control room of your body, the central nervous system, consists of your brain and spinal cord. About 3 pounds and the consistency of an overripe avocado, the brain is composed of some ten billion nerve cells. It is divided into three parts: the cerebrum, your center for thinking and sensation; the cerebellum, primarily concerned with balance; and the medulla, which regulates essential internal activities of our bodies. The spinal cord, ½ inch in diameter and 18 inches long, is a central communication cable connecting the brain to the peripheral nervous system, a vast network of nerves running throughout the body.

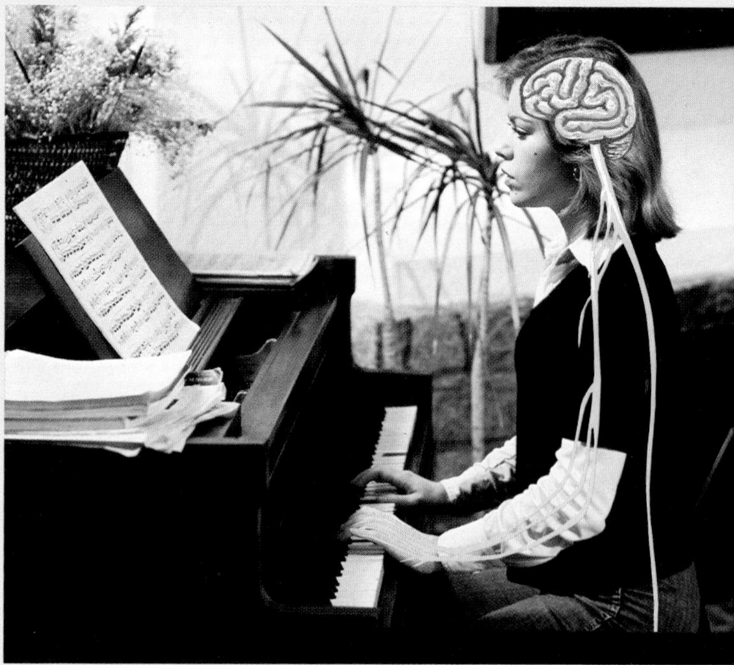

***Processing Information*** Sensory neurons carry images of musical notes from this piano player's eyes to her brain. In the cerebrum this information is processed then transmitted through the spinal column to the peripheral nerves in her arms, hands, and fingers.

The nerves of the peripheral nervous system are long cells, called neurons, that have specialized functions. *Sensory neurons* carry information to the brain. *Motor neurons* transmit information from the brain to skeletal muscles and internal organs. The information transported by neurons is actually a series of electrical signals—nerve impulses that jump from one nerve to the next. A mere blink of our eyes involves many thousands of these nerve impulses.

This body system is evidence that there is an awesome universe within us as well as around us.

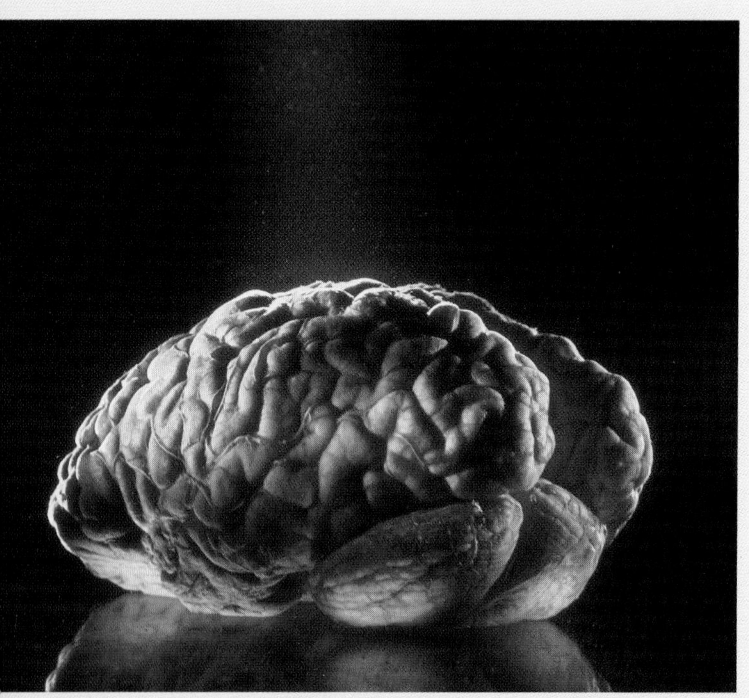

***The Human Brain*** Thinking, memory, and sensation occur in the large cerebrum. The small section at the lower right is the cerebellum.

**The Nerve Cell** This picture of a neuron shows its long extensions (dendrites), which convey electrical impulses to the main body of the cell.

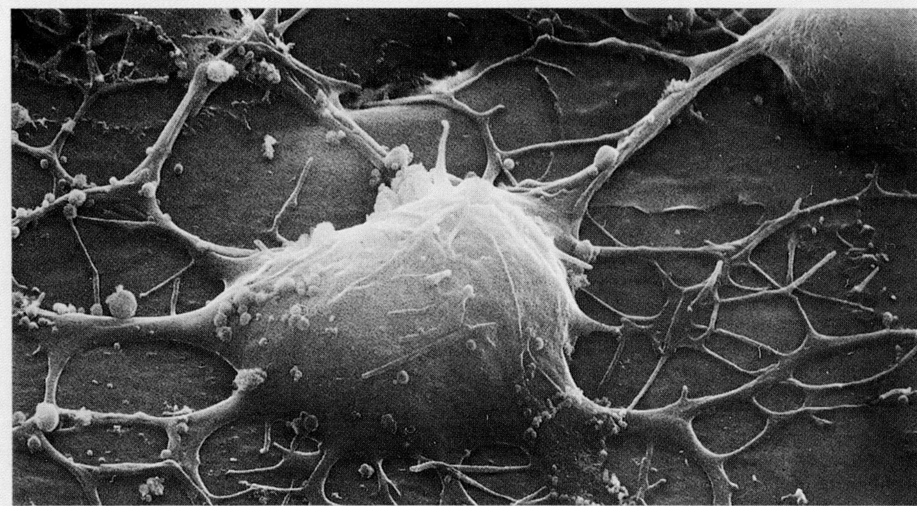

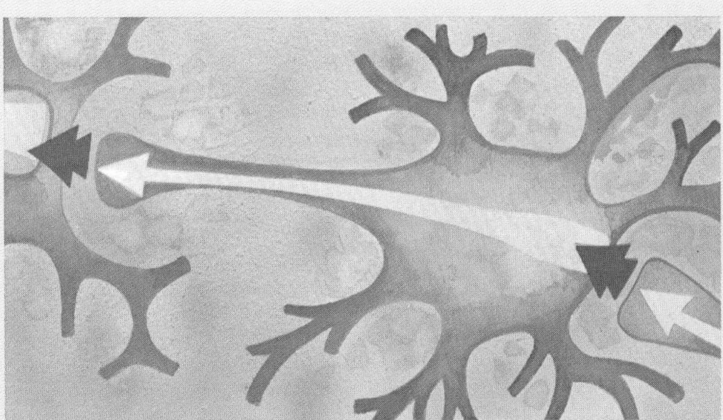

**Synapse** Nerve impulses, produced by small chemical transformations, travel across a bridge between nerve cells.

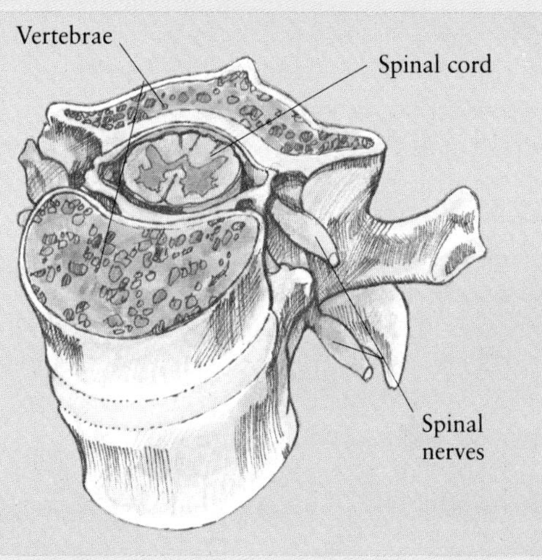


**The Spinal Cord** This cord is housed in a protective sheath formed by our vertebrae. Thirty-one pairs of spinal nerves, such as those pictured here, connect the central nervous system to the peripheral nervous system.

## Maintenance Tips

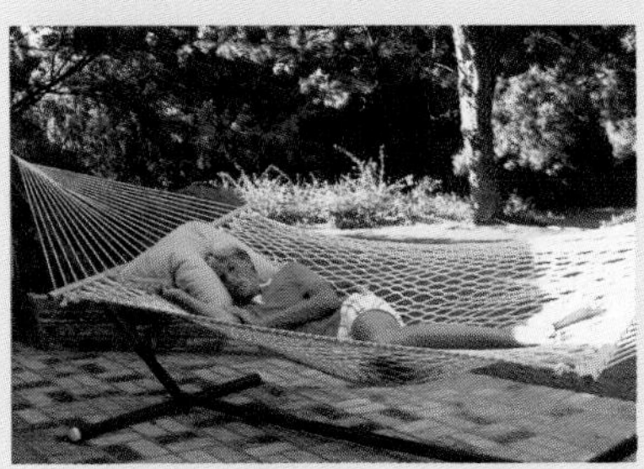

- *Rest* Although your nervous system never turns off, sleep and relaxation allow it to slow down and recharge for the busy day ahead.

- *Drugs* Drugs alter the chemical processes in your nervous system. Knowledgeable and responsible use of drugs will help preserve this vital system.

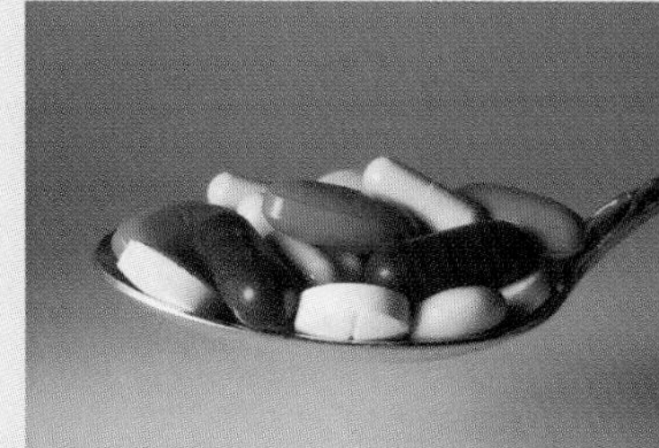

## Your Endocrine System

Major control stations, called endocrine glands, help the nervous system to regulate your body's many vital functions. Scattered about in strategic spots, these glands secrete hormones—chemicals that stimulate other body processes.

Located beneath the brain, the tiny pituitary is a powerful multipurpose gland that controls your body's growth and helps regulate the function of your kidneys. In females it also plays a role in pregnancy and lactation. Deep inside the brain is your smallest and most mysterious endocrine gland, the pineal body. Its exact function is still unknown. The thyroid gland in your neck oversees the rate of metabolism (production of heat and energy) in your body's cells. Strategically perched atop your kidneys, the adrenal glands help them to regulate the amount of water and salts in your system. These glands have other duties as well. They control protein building and breakdown and play a part in the formation of infection-fighting antibodies. In moments of alarm, the adrenal gland releases adrenalin, which stimulates your body's "fight-or-flight" response. In your pancreas, specialized endocrine cell clusters, called the islets of Langerhans, produce sugar-regulating hormones—insulin and glucagon. Two organs of the reproductive system, the ovaries and testes, are also endocrine glands; they produce progesterone and testosterone, respectively.

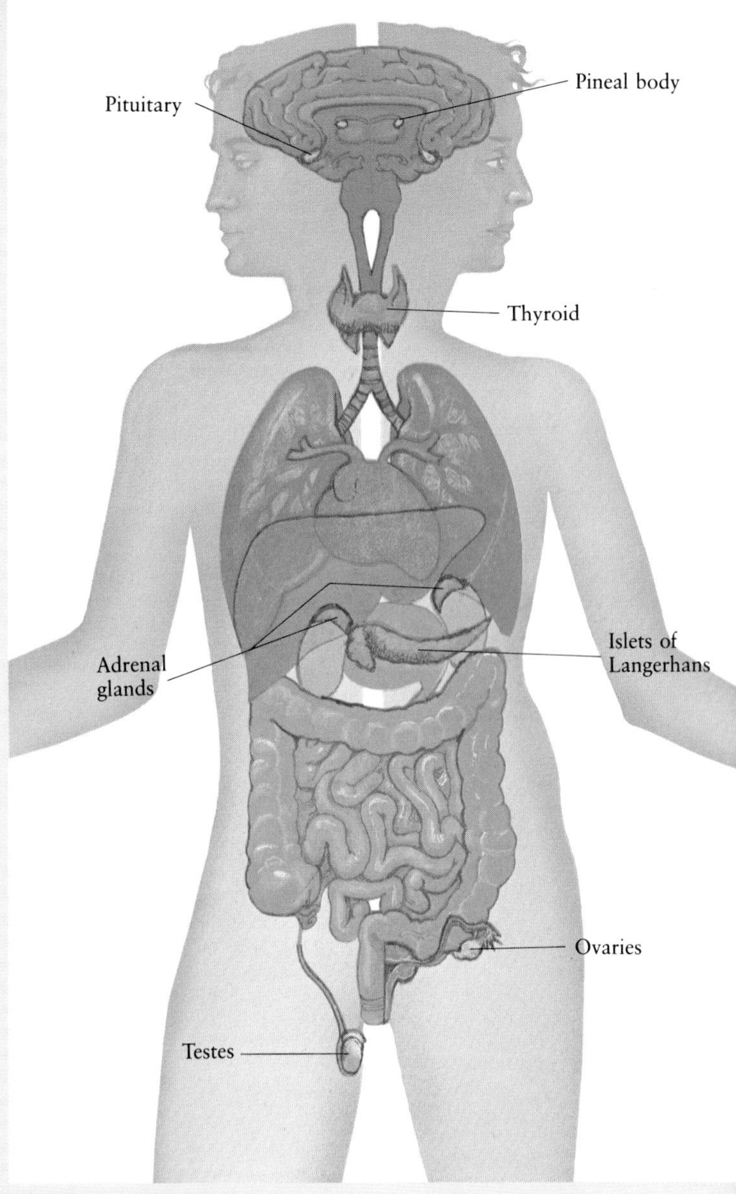


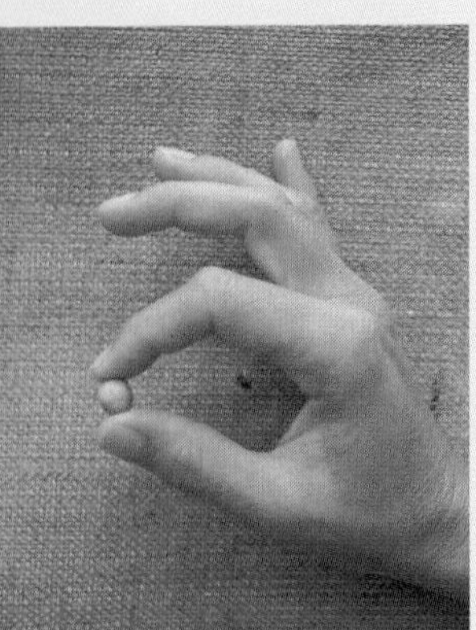

***Mighty Glands*** Endocrine glands are small, but powerful. The pineal body is the size of a pea; the pituitary, the size of an acorn. The total weight of all your endocrine glands does not add up to even one pound!

***The Hormone Testosterone*** Crystals of the hormone testosterone. The male hormone regulates growth, development, and sexual activity.

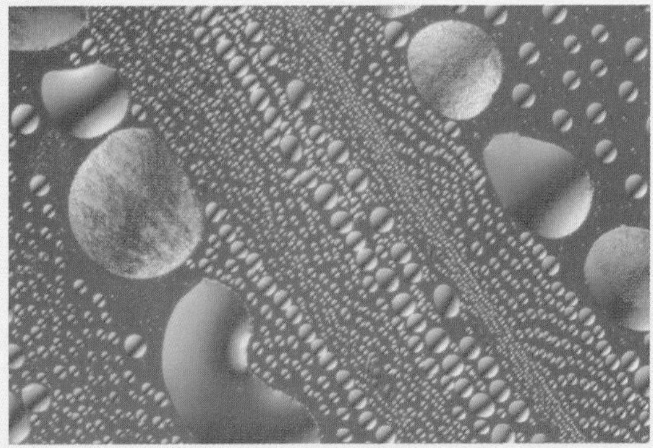

# Your Special Senses

Images of the outside world pour into your nervous system through your eyes, ears, nose, mouth, and skin. Your eyes can be compared to a camera; outside images flow through its lens. Like a shutter, the pupil controls the amount of light entering the eye. Unlike a camera, the eye simultaneously takes pictures of the outside world in both black and white and color. Rod cells in the retina register black and white images; cone cells are responsible for color perception. The combined image is then transmitted by the optic nerve to the brain.

Hearing is the function of perceiving and distinguishing sounds, which are really vibrations of varying frequencies that are processed and transmitted inside the ear by tiny bones with amazing shapes. Consider some of their names—drum, hammer, anvil, stirrup, cochlea (shell). The translated sound message is then sent on to the brain. Your ear can perceive sound in the range of 20 to 20,000 vibrations per second.

Smell and taste are closely connected. Odors can stream into your head through not only your nasal passage but also your mouth and throat, which has an open passage to your nasal cavity.



Tiny receptors high inside the nose transmit information on odor to the brain; taste buds are linked to the brain by a system of nerve fibers.

Your skin is also a sense organ. Distributed through it are millions of nerve endings that register contact, pressure, cold, heat, and pain. Sensation is just one of four vital functions of your skin. This crucial membrane also encloses the body's contents, helps regulate body temperature, and acts as a barrier to infection.

***Using the Senses*** Eating, nearly always a pleasurable activity, employs almost the full range of our special senses—taste, touch, sight, and smell.

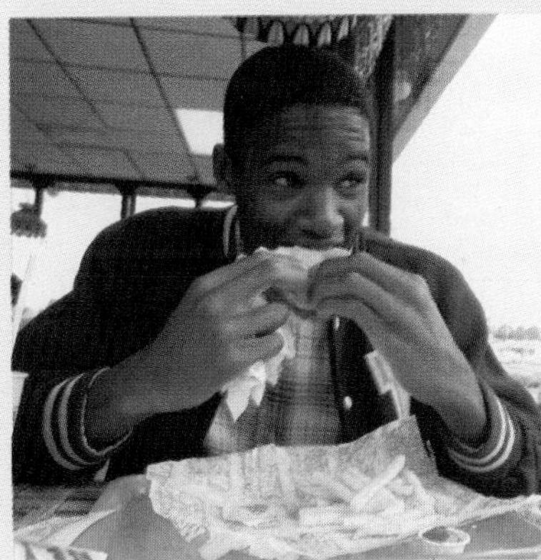

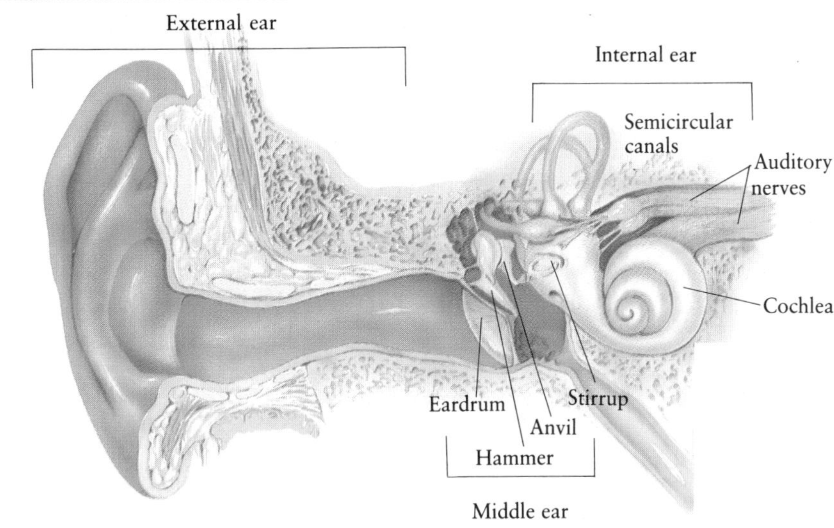

# Your Digestive System

Food that you eat at mealtime has been prepared in a kitchen. But, the cooking doesn't end there. Your digestive system can be thought of as a second kitchen where meals are prepared for your cells. Your body's kitchen is a 27 to 30 foot long corridor where food is mechanically and chemically processed into simple molecules.

Digestion begins in your mouth where teeth begin the mechanical breakdown of food, and saliva starts the chemical breakdown of starches. The act of swallowing pushes food into your esophagus, whose muscles move in a wave-like fashion to transport the food to your stomach. This next workstation is a 1½ quart pouch that processes your food for between 2 and 6 hours, depending on its composition. During this time the stomach's churning motion further softens your food, and acid gastric juices go to work to break down proteins. Food material, now called chyme, then moves through the pylorus (from the latin word for "gatekeeper") into your small intestine where progressive stages of chemical processing occur. First, al-

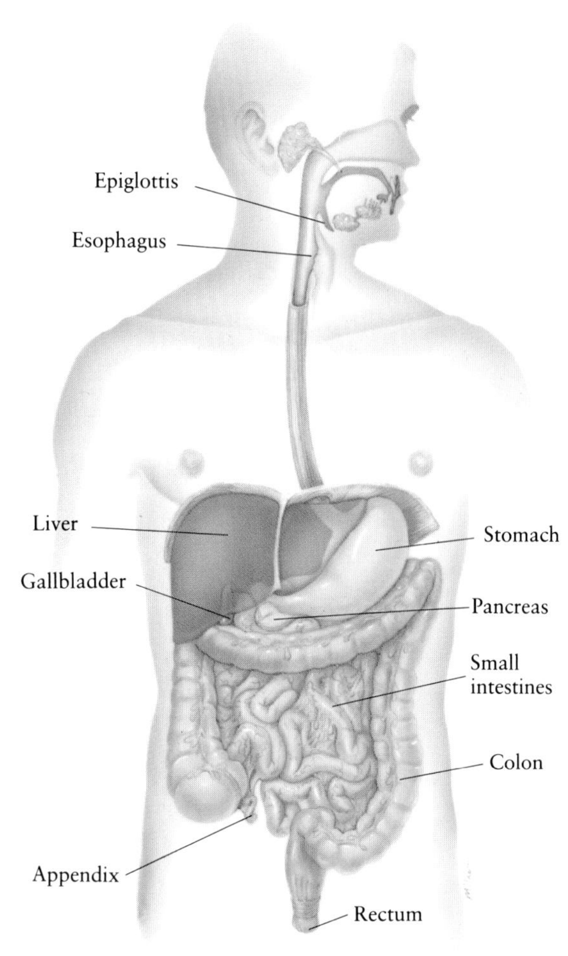


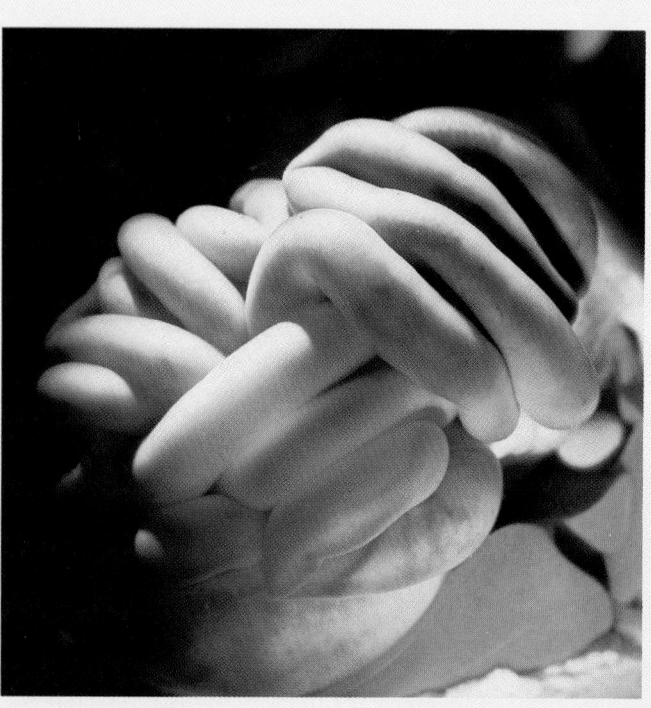

***Digestive Organs in an Infant*** The liver (red) manufactures bile, which is stored in the gallbladder (green). The liver also stores nutrients that have been processed by the small intestine, which is seen here in the foreground. The stomach can be seen in the lower right-hand portion.

kaline digestive juices from the pancreas neutralize the acidic chyme, and bile from the liver begins the process of breaking down fats. Next, proteins are broken down into amino acids, carbohydrates into sugars, fats into fatty acids and glycerol. Tiny fingerlike projections, called villi, in your small intestine then begin to absorb nutrients from chyme. Capillaries in the villi launch the nutrients into the bloodstream and on their way to the liver for storage. Finally, waste materials from digestion pass from the small intestine to the large intestine (colon), which absorbs water from the waste and prepares it for excretion through the rectum.

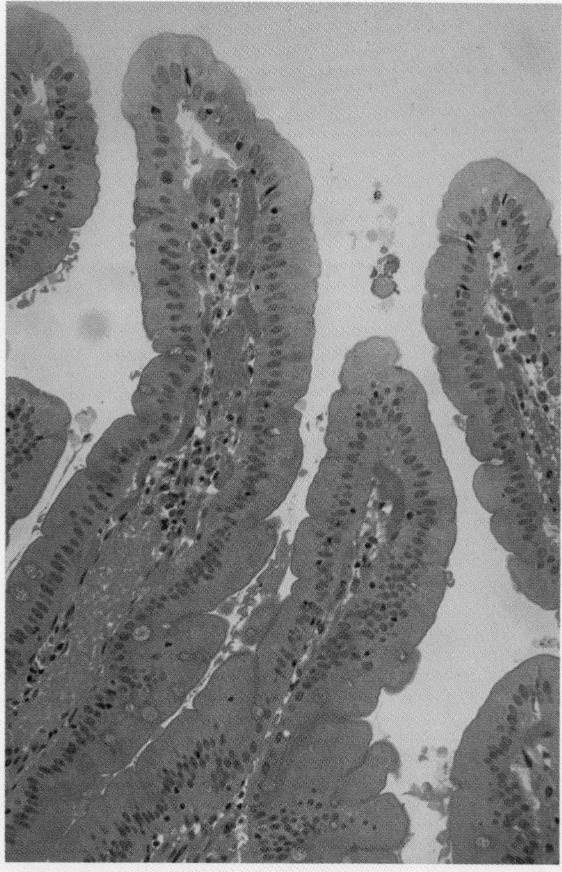

***Intestinal Villi*** Millions of these tiny structures line your intestinal walls.

## *Maintenance Tips*

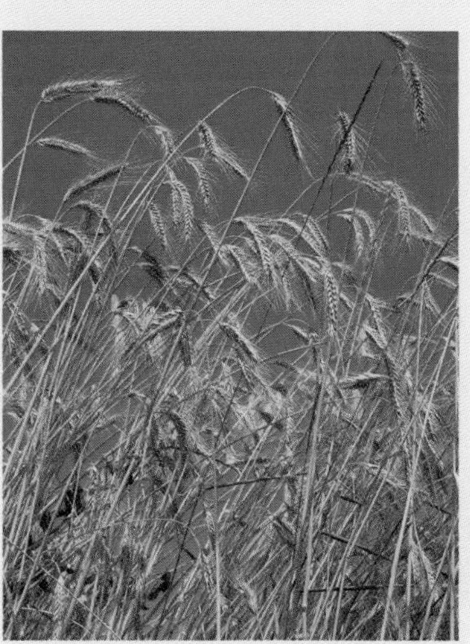

- *Diet* A high fiber diet aids the process of elimination and is thought to help guard against colon and rectal cancer.

- *Stress* Stress is commonly associated with digestive diseases such as ulcers, ileitus, and colitus. Finding healthy outlets for life's daily frustrations will help keep your digestive system free from disease.

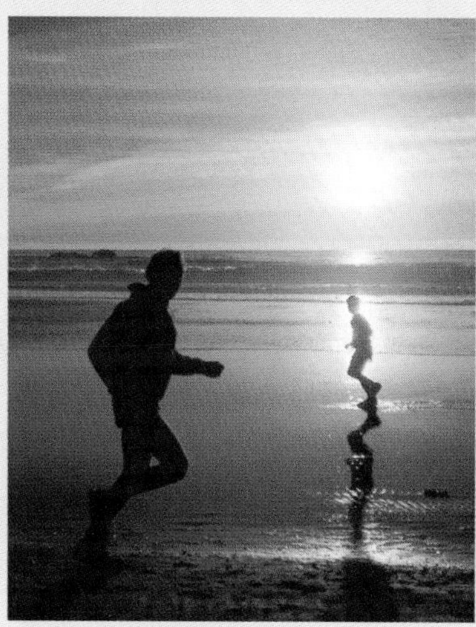

## *Your Respiratory System*

**M**oving, thinking, feeling—in other words, being alive—takes a flow of energy. From where does it arise?

Each of your body's trillions of cells is a tiny power plant, using nutrients and oxygen to produce energy and releasing byproducts, such as carbon dioxide and water. This process is called *cellular respiration.* Your body's respiratory system teams up with the cardiovascular system to supply oxygen to the cells and to carry away carbon dioxide.

During inspiration you take in approximately 2 gallons of air per minute in an average of 14 breaths. This air flows through the trachea and the bronchi—large channels leading into the lungs. Along the way, the air is cleansed of dust,

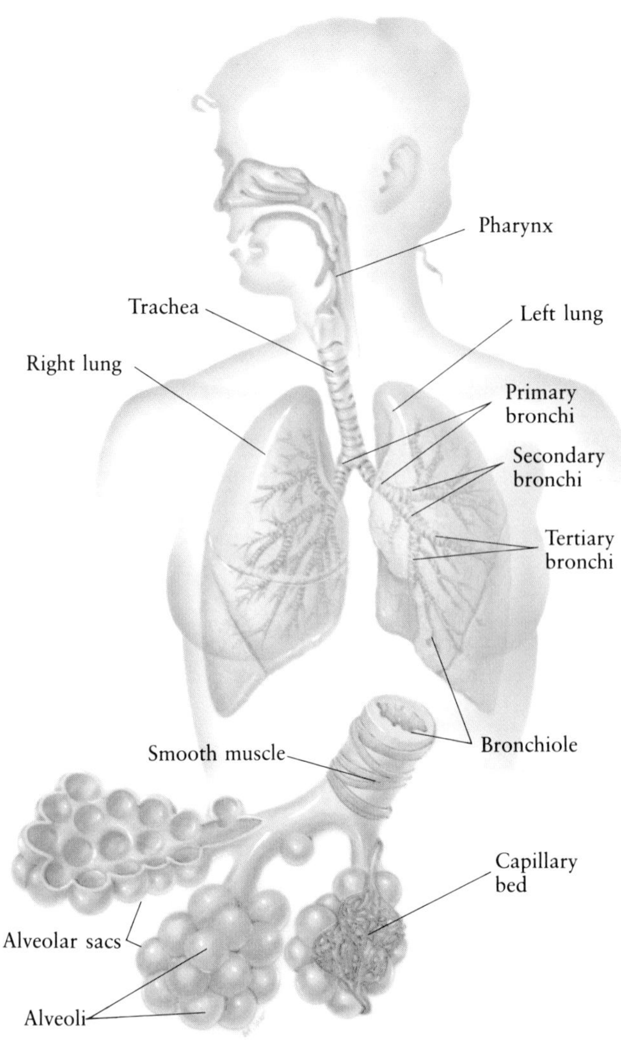


**The Lungs** These organs are infused with a dense system of blood vessels.

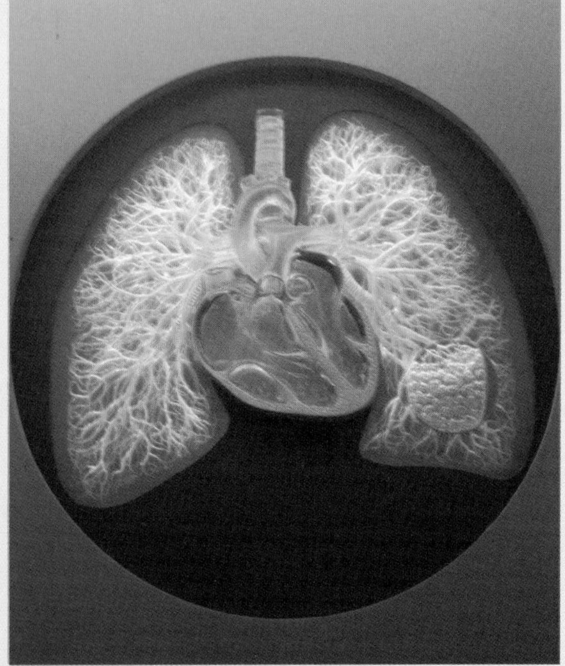

**Alveoli** These air cells are tiny round sacs that look something like a cluster of grapes.

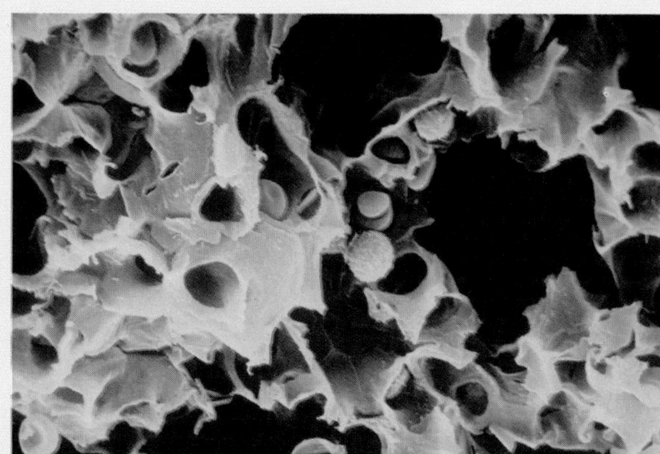

bacteria, and other harmful particles by mucus and *cilia*—tiny hairs lining the passageways. Continuing its journey inside the lung, the air moves from the bronchi through smaller branch-like *bronchioles* and finally into clusters of tiny sacs, called *alveoli*. Each of your lungs contains over 300 million alveoli which, if all laid out flat, would cover an area almost the size of a tennis court. In the alveoli, oxygen is picked up from the air by tiny capillaries interwoven with the alveolar tissue. It is then transported out of the lung and to your cells via a branching network of blood vessels.

Blood entering the lungs to pick up oxygen brings with it a cellular waste product, carbon dioxide. While picking up oxygen, blood also transfers carbon dioxide to air inside the alveoli. This transformed air is expelled from the lungs into the environment during expiration.

**Healthy Pink Lungs** These lungs are free to exchange oxygen and carbon dioxide at top capacity.

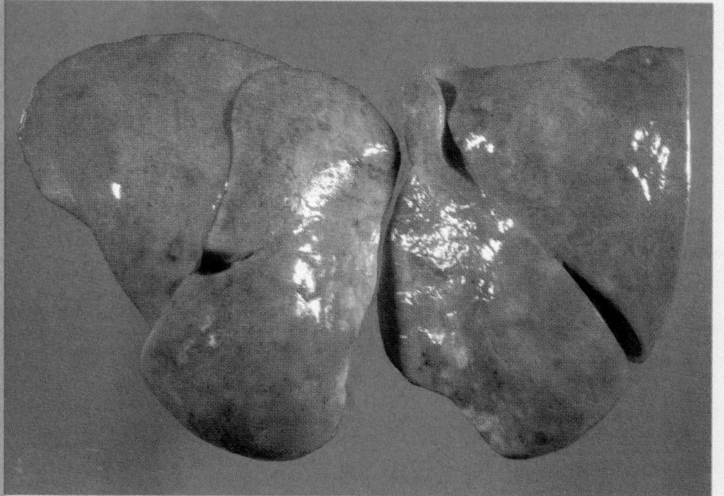

**A Smoker's Lung** The dark, mottled areas reveal that tar from cigarettes has settled into the bronchiole tubes of the lung. These tar deposits not only block the passage of air, but also damage the mucus and cilia and are furthermore associated with cancerous changes.

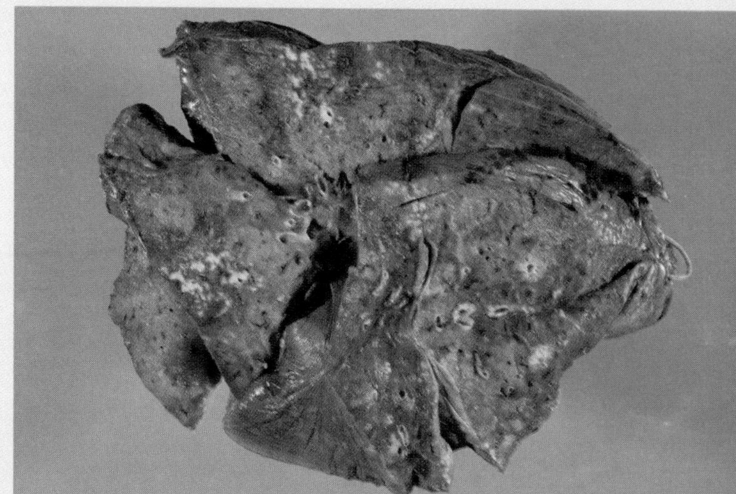

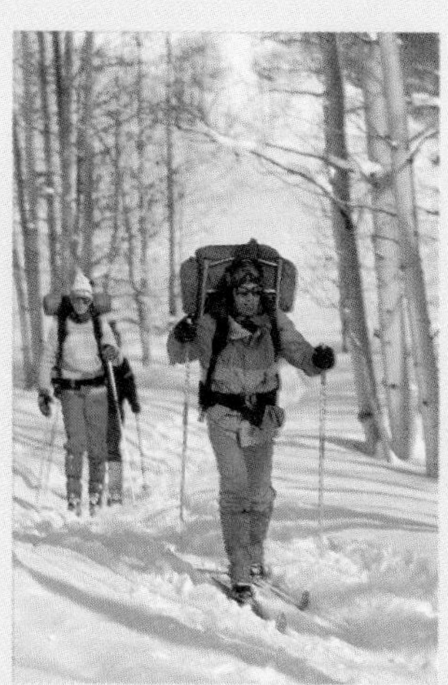

## Maintenance Tips

- *Exercise* Aerobic exercise enhances oxygen capacity in your respiratory and cardiovascular systems.
- *Environment* Clean air, unlike that above this city, helps to ensure healthy lungs.

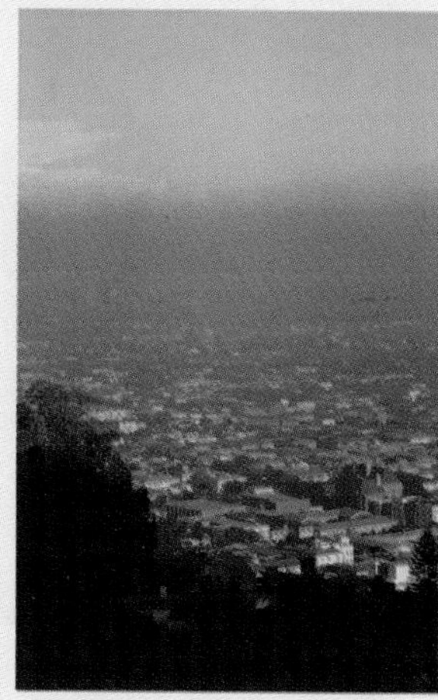

# Your Cardiovascular System

Sit completely still, hold your breath, and concentrate on your body. You should be able to sense the regular pulsing of your cardiovascular system as it nourishes and cleanses every cell in your body. No matter how still you manage to sit, inside, your cardiovascular system is a relentless maze of activity. Your heart is busy pumping 5 or 6 quarts of blood per minute through a complex system of blood vessels that ultimately extend to every cell.

This marvelous transport system distributes nutrients and oxygen to your active cells and carries off waste products—heat, water, carbon dioxide, urea, and other chemical compounds. But that's not all. It also disburses regulatory hormones and infection-fighting substances to strategic locations.

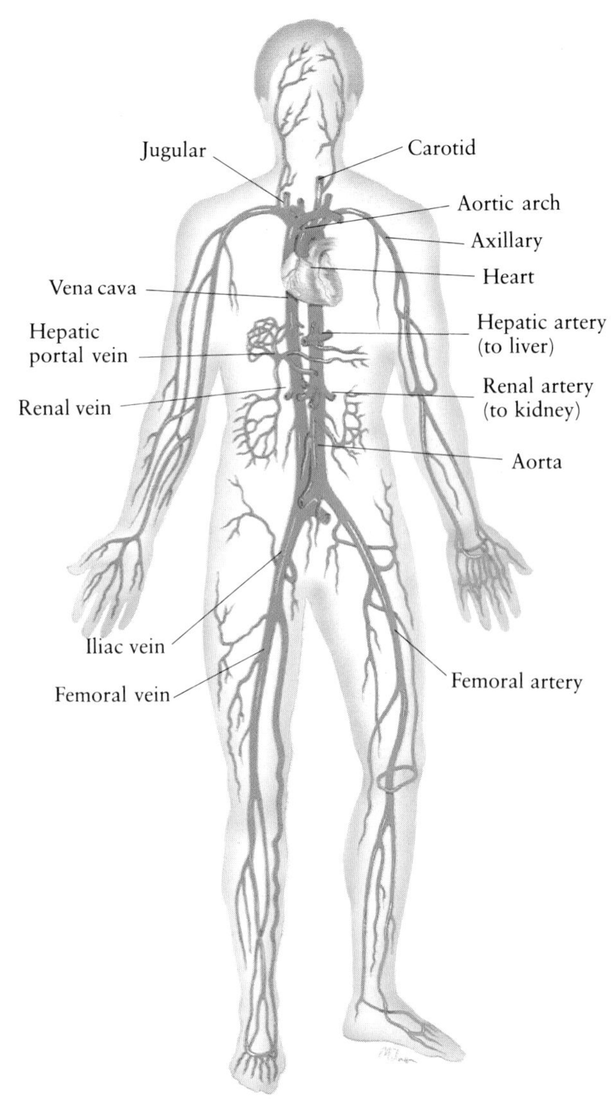


***The Circulatory Cycle*** Oxygenated blood is pumped through the left side of the heart to the body's cells. The right side of the heart receives blood containing carbon dioxide instead of oxygen. It sends this blood to the lungs where the carbon dioxide is expelled and new oxygen is picked up and sent to the left side of the heart.

***Red and White Blood Cells*** Red cells (flat) carry oxygen. White cells (round) defend the body from infection by foreign microorganisms. They are suspended in plasma, the liquid portion of the blood, which transports nutrients, hormones, and wastes.

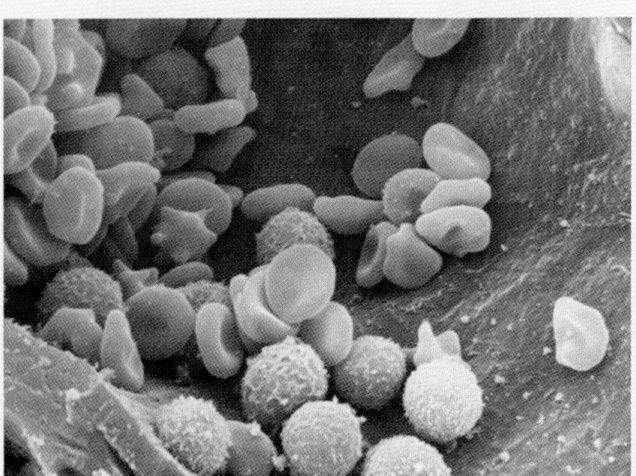

***Capillary Exchange*** As it moves through the capillary, a red blood cell will give up oxygen and take on carbon dioxide from neighboring cells.

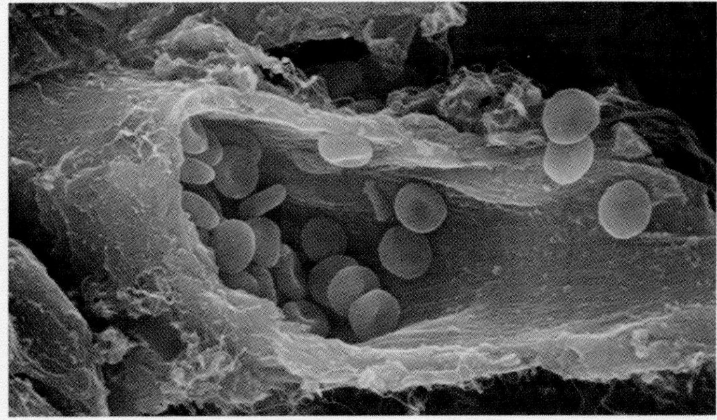

Your cardiovascular system is composed of a fist-sized heart, about 10 pints of blood, and a network of blood vessels so vast that it would extend 60,000 miles if laid out in a single line. This system is a closed loop through which your blood is recycled approximately 1000 times per day. Your heart is a powerful four-chambered pump. Its left and right atrial chambers receive blood: the right atrium accepts oxygen-depleted blood from the body while the left atrium takes in oxygen-rich blood from the lungs. These events occur during the brief time between heartbeats. Then, on an electrical cue from your nervous system, both atrial chambers contract to squeeze blood into corresponding left and right ventricles. Instantaneously thereafter, the ventricles contract

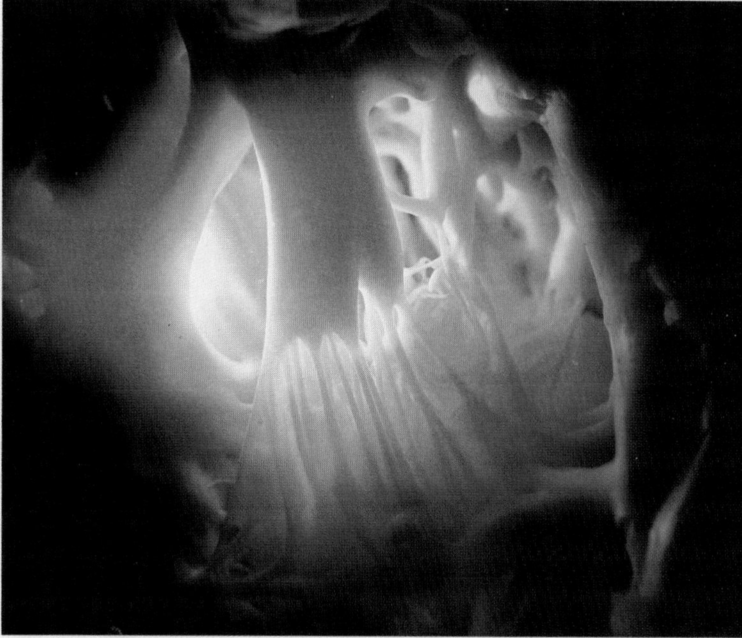

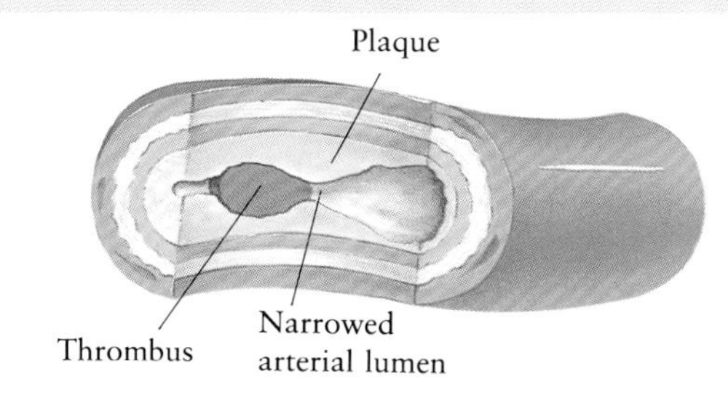


***Inside the Heart*** This bottom-to-top view begins in the right ventricle and looks toward the right atrium.

***Atherosclerosis*** Build-up of plaque in the blood vessels can seriously restrict blood flow, causing this life-threatening disease.

## *Maintenance Tips*

■ *Diet* Avoid foods that are high in fats and salts. A healthy diet consists of lots of grains and vegetables.

■ *Stress* Try not to let life's challenges turn into worry and stress. Worry and stress can turn into high blood pressure and heart disease.

■ *Exercise* Responsible exercise can help prevent or limit stress, excess weight, high blood pressure, and blood vessel disease—all major threats to the circulatory system.

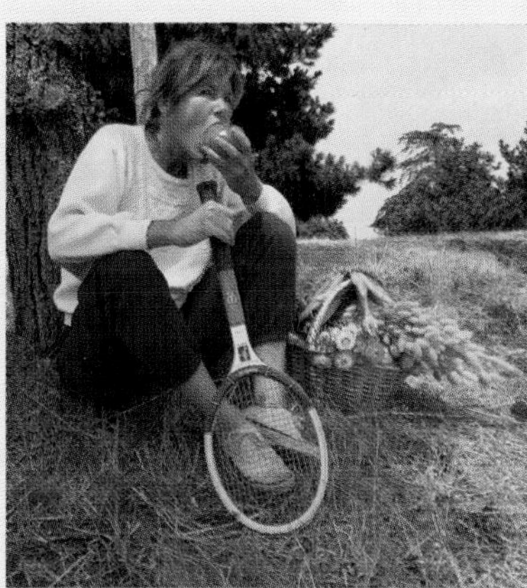

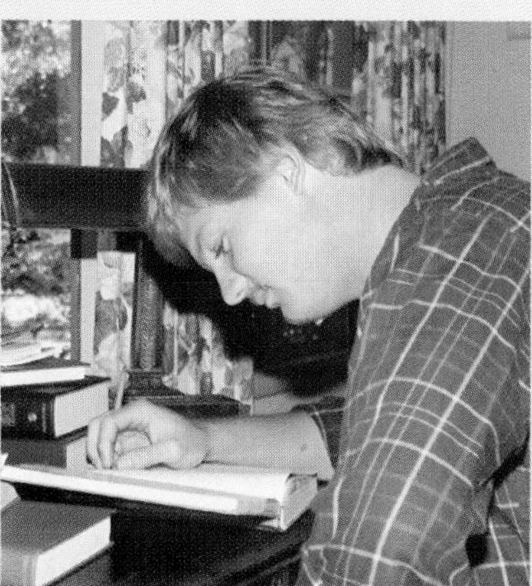

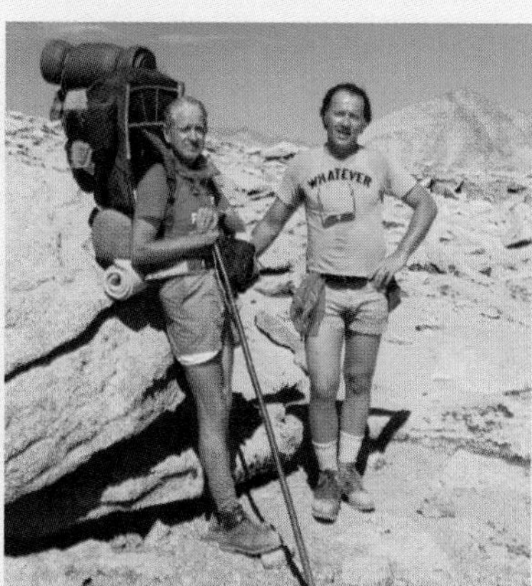

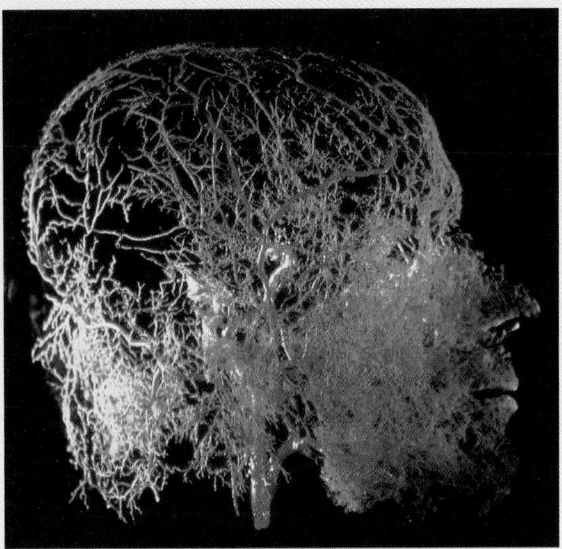

***Inside the Head*** Your body organs are penetrated by a complex network of arteries and veins. The model pictured here depicts arteries and veins penetrating the neck and brain.

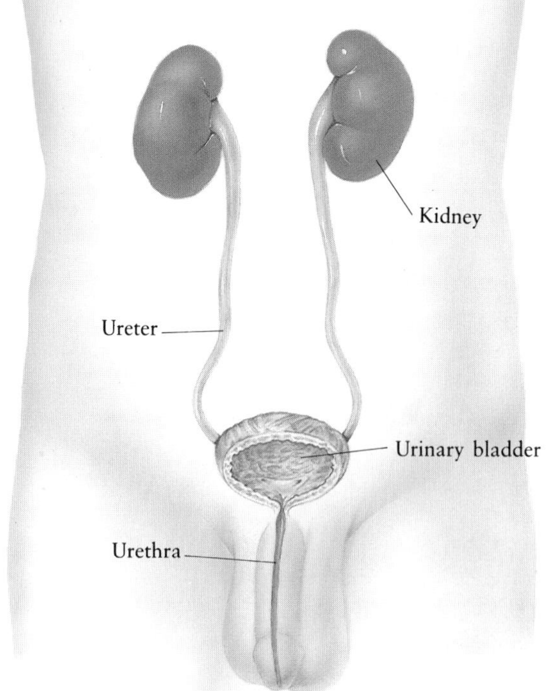


***The Urinary System***

and push this blood out of your heart. The right ventricle sends its oxygen-depleted blood through the pulmonary artery to your lungs to collect oxygen. The left ventricle pushes its oxygen-rich blood to the rest of your body where it will collect nutrients, then deliver its precious cargo to your body cells. See Chapter 17 for more information about your heart.

Arteries move blood away from the heart. They branch into smaller arterioles and then to tiny capillaries, which exchange substances with other cells. Capillaries widen into small venules and then to a system of larger and larger veins, which eventually return blood to the heart.

Your urinary system is an important substation of the circulatory system. Located in the small of your back, two bean-shaped kidneys process about one-fourth of the blood volume from every heartbeat. Their function is to rid the blood of various chemical waste products. Inside each kidney's one million nephrons, tiny sacs of capillaries, called glomeruli, absorb urea from the blood. The urea, then mixed with other kidney secretions, passes into the bladder as urine and is excreted.

***Glomeruli*** These tiny tiny sacs serve as a filtering device in the formation of urine.

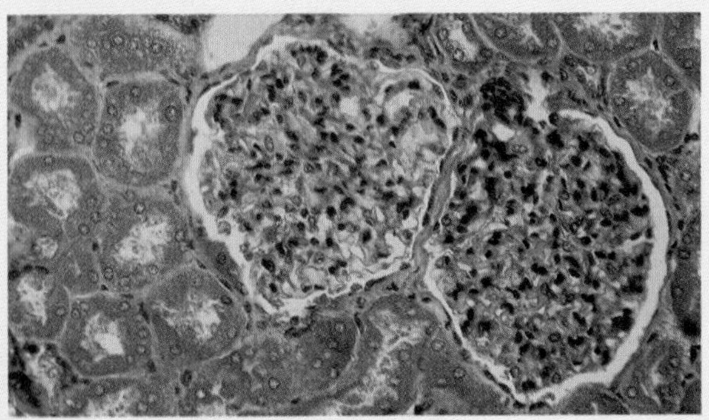

## Maintenance Tip

■ *Weight Control* Excess weight is hard on your entire circulatory system. Try to maintain a proper weight for your size and frame.

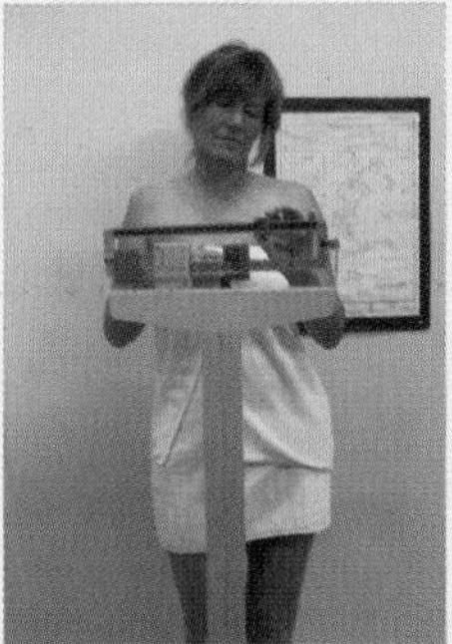

- Drain fat from ground beef after cooking.
- Stir-fry, slicing meat thin and cooking it over high heat.

### A Fish Story

Fish is low in calories, high in protein, and packed with vitamins and minerals—but that's not why fish has become a health food. Special unsaturated fats called omega-3 fatty acids, found in fish oils, have proven to be such powerful protectors of the heart that doctors are urging Americans to switch to fish.

According to one large-scale study, just two fish meals a week can reduce the risk of heart attack by 50 percent. The omega-3 fatty acids in fish oils change the chemistry of the blood to lower the likelihood of heart disease. They may also help prevent or treat a wide range of other ailments, including migraine headaches and rheumatoid arthritis.[6] Choose the real thing, not the fish-oil supplements sold in health-food stores. Their long-term risks are unknown, and no one has set minimum or maximum dosages.

**STRATEGY FOR CHANGE**

**Go Fishing**

- Substitute fish for meat two or three times a week.
- Fish that swim in cold ocean waters—such as salmon, mackerel, tuna, and sardines—are higher in omega-3 fatty acids.
- Even crab, shrimp, lobster, and other shellfish, though high in cholesterol, pack plenty of healthful omega-3s—and less cholesterol per serving than in a single egg.
- Nutritionists recommend steaming, grilling, baking, or poaching, Frying adds other fats and dilutes the beneficial effects.
- Don't reach for fast-food fish dishes. Processing and frying remove almost all their omega-3 fatty acids.

### Sodium

Too much sodium can aggravate high blood pressure, or hypertension, a major risk factor in heart disease.[7] The Food and Nutrition Board of the National Academy of Sciences recommends that daily intake of sodium be limited to 2,400 milligrams a day. But many Americans consume much more sodium than they need, mostly from salt. Many doctors advise people with a history of hypertension to cut back on salt; some experts believe everyone should.

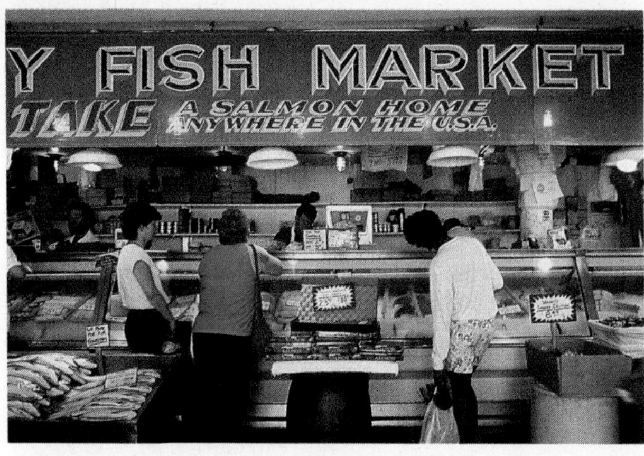


Fish is a smart buy because it's low in calories, high in protein and packed with vitamins and minerals.

**STRATEGY FOR CHANGE**

**How to Give Up Salt Without Suffering**

The best way to cut back on salt intake is to do so gradually and try substitute seasonings. Here are some ideas:

- Stop salting food automatically and avoid salty snacks.
- Steer clear of high-sodium processed foods, such as lunch meats, sausages, prepared sauces, gravies, salad dressings, and fast foods.
- Watch out for salt or sodium "hidden" in catsup, mustard, soy and steak sauces, and pickled foods.
- Experiment with different herbs and spices. Instead of salt, add lemon juice or vinegar to vegetables. To add flavor to meat and fish, rub or sprinkle seasonings like pepper, curry powder, dry mustard, or minced onion on the surface of the meat or fish before roasting or broiling.

## Fighting Cancer

We may be able to cut our cancer risk by a least 35 percent by changing the way we eat.[8] Medical scientists believe that a balanced, moderate diet may be best for preventing cancer. The greatest dietary risk factor for cancer may be fats, which have been linked to colon and breast cancer.

Whereas fat may be dangerous, fiber may protect us—but its role is controversial. Certain types of fiber, particularly the insoluble form found in wheat bran and many vegetables, seem most likely to protect against colon cancer.

Other cancer-fighting agents include vitamins C and E, beta-carotene (a precursor of vitamin A), and the mineral selenium. The best food source of these

**TABLE 4-4** Eating to Avoid Cancer

| CANCER FIGHTERS | FOOD SOURCES |
|---|---|
| Vitamin A | Liver, eggs, dairy products |
| Beta-carotene | Broccoli, dark-green leafy vegetables (such as kale, romaine, endive, spinach, chicory, escarole, watercress, collard, mustard, beet, and dandelion greens), asparagus, green and red peppers, cauliflower, cabbages, brussels sprouts, bean sprouts, mushrooms, green beans, onions, okra, tomatoes, yellow-orange vegetables (such as carrots, sweet potatoes, pumpkins, and winter squash) |
| Vitamin C | Oranges, grapefruit, broccoli, brussels sprouts, mustard greens, parsley, green peppers, lemons, limes, tangerines, juices made from citrus fruits |
| Vitamin E | Vegetable oils, eggs, whole-grain cereals |
| Fiber | Whole-grain products, such as bran muffins; breads made with brown, rye, oatmeal, or pumpernickel flour; whole-wheat cereals; barley; buckwheat groats; bulgur; fruits (with skins), including apples, pears, apricots, and berries; dry peas and beans, such as lentils, garbanzo beans, and black-eyed peas; vegetables, such as carrots, broccoli, potatoes, corn, cauliflower, brussels sprouts, cabbage, celery, green beans, summer squash, green peas, parsnips, kale, spinach, other greens, yams, sweet potatoes, and turnips |
| Folic acid (folate) | Liver, kidney, dark-green vegetables, fruits, wheat germ, peas |
| Natural anticancer chemicals | Brussels sprouts, cabbage, broccoli, cauliflower, rutabagas, turnips, soybeans, lima beans |
| Selenium | Seafoods, organ meats (kidney, liver), grains from selenium-rich areas |

desirable ingredients may be cruciferous vegetables, such as broccoli, cauliflower, cabbage, and brussels sprouts.

Other nutrients also protect us against cancer. For instance, both calcium and vitamin D (which is formed in skin in reaction with sunlight) ward off colon cancer. Calcium may bind with, or attach itself to, cancer-causing substances in the digestive tract and render them harmless compounds; vitamin D boosts calcium's effectiveness. (See Table 4-4 for a list of possible nutritional cancer fighters.)

**STRATEGY FOR CHANGE**

## An Anticancer Diet

The following recommendations, based on the latest research findings, show what you can do to protect yourself from cancer:

- Cut fats to no more than 30 percent of your total calories.
- Increase your fiber intake. The National Cancer Institute recommends your diet include 20 to 35 grams of fiber each day, the equivalent of five or six servings of high-fiber foods such as whole-grain cereals and fruits.
- Drink two to four glasses of low-fat milk each day. Milk drinkers have lower rates of colon and rectum cancer than those who don't drink milk.
- Choose fish two or three times a week. Hailed as a lifesaver because it lowers the risk of heart attacks, fish may also protect you from certain cancers.
- Eat two or three vegetables a day. In addition to providing dietary fiber, many vegetables contain natural chemicals that block the development and growth of cancer-promoting compounds.
- Eat cruciferous vegetables several times a week. Broccoli, cauliflower, brussels sprouts, kohlrabi, and other members of the mustard family help prevent the development of cancer.
- Make sure you're eating foods that supply vitamin A, which may help prevent various cancers.
- Have a carrot a day. Vegetables that contain beta-carotene—such as carrots, other yellow-orange vegetables, and dark greens (spinach, chicory, kale)—may reduce the risk of some cancers.
- Eat citrus fruits and other foods rich in vitamin C daily. Vitamin C may block the formation of cancer-causing chemicals, such as the nitrosamines produced when preserva-

tives like nitrite (used in bacon and hot dogs) are broken down in the body.

- Get more vitamin E in your daily diet. Like vitamin C, vitamin E prevents the formation of harmful compounds.
- Increase the amount of selenium-rich foods you eat. This trace metal, found in seafood, liver, kidney, and grains grown in selenium-rich soil, may help prevent certain cancers, perhaps by boosting the action of vitamin E.
- Get enough folate (folic acid). This B vitamin may help your body's repair system function better.
- Eat your hamburgers rare or medium-rare. Well-done hamburger meat contains at least six chemicals that cause changes in a cell's genetic blueprint, and these changes may increase the likelihood of cancer.
- Don't fry or grill often. Frying or grilling meat and fish can produce agents that induce cancer in animals. Safer cooking methods are baking, boiling, steaming, microwaving, poaching, and roasting.
- Don't have more than two alcoholic drinks a day. The deadliest duo is the combination of alcohol and cigarettes. Drinkers who smoke have higher rates of oral cancers than drinkers who don't smoke and than smokers who don't drink.

## HEALTH HEADLINE

### Future Fad: Fake Food

You may be able to savor more of the treats you once hated to love—such as high-fat, high-calorie cakes and ice cream—without guilt. In 1990 the Food and Drug Administration (FDA) approved Simplesse, the first low-calorie substitute for fat, and paved the way for a new generation of fat-free treats. Several companies have developed natural no-fat desserts by using nonfat milk and egg whites instead of whole eggs. But nutritionists warn that none of these "light" desserts has high nutritional value. They may be better than most junk food—but not as good as real, healthful foods.

SOURCES: "How to Pig Out but Avoid Fat," *Time*, February 5, 1990. O'Neill, Molly. "First Low-Calorie Substitute for Fats is Approved by U.S.," *New York Times*, February 23, 1990.

## EATING FOR GOOD HEALTH

Oat bran. Beta-carotene. Vitamin C. In recent years, substances like these have made headlines because of what they could, should, or would do to make us healthier. Almost always "superfoods" containing these nutrients haven't lived up to their claims. The following section can help you understand what is known and not known about some nutrition controversies; then you can decide for yourself which foods are best for your health.

### Fiber: The Right Stuff?

Fiber is rough stuff—the indigestible leaves, stems, skins, seeds, and hulls of grain and plants. Fiber helps prevent diverticulosis, a painful bowel inflammation that afflicts an estimated 40 percent of middle-aged Americans, and fiber may help lower the risk of colon cancer. Because it has few calories and may reduce the level of harmful blood fats, fiber also helps keep weight down and may lessen the risk of diabetes by keeping blood sugar down.

As with other nutrients, too much fiber can create problems. Some types of fiber interfere with absorption of minerals such as zinc, iron, and calcium. Nutritionists don't know exactly how much fiber is enough; but if half the foods you eat are complex carbohydrates, you should be getting all the fiber you need. (See Table 4-5.)

### Oat Bran

Oat bran, the hottest food fad of the late 1980s, fizzled in 1990. After studies suggested that the soluble fiber in oat bran might lower cholesterol levels, oat bran popped up in products ranging from pretzels to pasta. Then, in *The New England Journal of Medicine*, Harvard Medical School researchers reported that oat bran did not produce any greater reduction of cholesterol than low-fiber refined wheat.[9] The scientists did not say that oat bran was bad, just that it may not be as good as some (especially makers of oat bran products) would like us to believe. The bottom line from nutritionists: Continue to add a variety of fibers to your diet, rather than relying on any one.

**TABLE 4-5** Sources of Fiber

| RICH SOURCES OF DIETARY FIBER (4 OR MORE GRAMS OF FIBER PER SERVING) | MODERATELY RICH SOURCES OF DIETARY FIBER (1–3.9 G OF FIBER PER SERVING) | LOW SOURCES OF DIETARY FIBER (LESS THAN 1 G OF FIBER PER SERVING) |
|---|---|---|
| Cereals: All Bran-Extra Fiber®,* Fiber-One®,* All Bran Fruit & Almonds®,* 100% Bran®,* Bran Buds®,* Corn Bran®, Bran Chex®, Cracklin' Oat Bran®, Bran Flakes®, Raisin Bran®<br>Legumes: kidney beans, navy beans, lima beans<br>Fruits: dried prunes | Breads, grains, cereals and pasta: whole-wheat spaghetti, Most®, wheat germ, Shredded Wheat®, Wheat Chex®, Total®, Wheaties®, cooked oatmeal, Grapenuts®, whole-wheat bread, Cheerios®, regular spaghetti, brown rice, air-popped popcorn<br>Legumes (cooked) and nuts: lentils, peanuts, almonds<br>Vegetables: green peas, corn, parsnips, potatoes, brussels sprouts, carrots, broccoli, cooked spinach, sweet potatoes, string beans, turnips, bean sprouts, tomatoes, kale, red and white cabbages, summer squash, raw spinach, cauliflower, celery, asparagus<br>Fruits: apples, pears, raisins, strawberries, oranges, bananas, blueberries, dried dates, peaches, fresh apricots, grapefruits, dried apricots, cherries, pineapples, cantaloupes | Breads and cereals: white bread, cornflakes, white rice, Rice Krispies®<br>Vegetables: lettuce, mushrooms, onions, green peppers<br>Fruits: grapes, watermelons<br>Fruit juices: papaya, grape, grapefruit, orange, apple |

*This food has 6 g or more of fiber per serving.
SOURCE: National Cancer Institute, Bethesda, MD.

### Future Fibers

Will a new substance take oat bran's place as first among fibers? Psyllium, a grain high in soluble fiber and found in some breakfast cereals, has proven effective in lowering cholesterol but is mainly used as the active ingredient in the laxative Metamucil. Other candidates include rice bran and fiber-packed beans, which are gaining in popularity. According to the U.S. Department of Agriculture, each American is eating 3 pounds of beans more than in 1984. But while health experts expect fiber fads to continue to come and go, they urge consumers to take a commonsense approach to fiber as well as other foods.

**STRATEGY FOR CHANGE**

**Getting More Fiber**

- Try to include a high-fiber starch at every meal—for example, fruit instead of juice at breakfast, along with a whole-grain cereal or bran muffin (see Table 4-5).
- Add brown rice or barley to soups.
- Substitute whole-wheat rolls and bread for products made from white refined flour.
- Cultivate a love of vegetables.
- Eat fruit instead of pudding or cake for dessert.
- Don't add too much fiber too soon; it may cause intestinal distress.

## Sugar: A Villain in Search of a Crime?

Sugar accounts for more than 20 percent of average daily calories, mostly hidden in favorites such as soda (10 teaspoons per can), low-fat fruit yogurt (8 teaspoons per carton), and catsup (a teaspoon in every tablespoon).

Sugar has been blamed for obesity, heart problems, and metabolic disorders, but scientists have found no correlation between sugar intake and disease or behavior disorders.[10] Although sugar may do little harm, it does little, if any, good. And it's definitely a menace in the mouth. According to the American Dental Association, bacteria convert sugar, honey, candy, and other sweets into acids that attack protective tooth enamel. A sugary snack does provide a short-lived high as it rushes into your bloodstream. However, 15 minutes after munching a candy bar, your blood sugar plummets, and you're feeling down again.

In people with a relatively rare condition called **hypoglycemia,** or low blood sugar, the body consistently maintains low blood sugar. As a result, people with hypoglycemia may become weak, confused, ir-

**hypoglycemia** An abnormal decrease of sugar in the blood, which results in feelings of weakness, confusion, irratation, and forgetfulness.

ritable, and forgetful. They can prevent these symptoms by eating small, high-protein meals all day long.

Some people develop an uncontrollable craving (sometimes called an addiction) if they overindulge in sweets. The more sugar these people eat, the more they want. Some "sugarholics" go on cookie and candy binges, usually at times of emotional stress.

**STRATEGY FOR CHANGE**

**Giving Up the Sweet Life**

The average American's daily diet contains 500 calories of sugar, much more than any of us needs. Here are some practical and painless suggestions for learning to live with less sugar:

- Avoid temptation by not buying "for guests" treats such as boxes of elegant cookies or an assortment of ice cream flavors.
- Put a small, child-sized spoon in the sugar bowl.
- Try a drop of vanilla instead of sugar in your coffee.
- When you crave a sweet, reach for "nature's candy": fruit.
- If you want a daily sweet, have it as dessert, when you'll eat less of it, and when beverages and other foods will interfere with cavity-causing bacteria.
- Drink fruit juices and water instead of soft drinks.

## Artificial Sweeteners

Aspartame (NutraSweet), a combination of two natural amino acids that are broken down in the body just like protein, is 200 times sweeter than sugar and leaves no aftertaste. Individuals with the rare metabolic disorder called phenylketonuria should not use aspartame because it could affect, and potentially damage, their brain chemistry. Some scientists believe that, at high temperatures, aspartame in liquid form may decompose into toxic methyl alcohol. They have argued for a ban on aspartame in diet sodas and other drinks. The FDA has reported no evidence of "potential public harm."[11] Until we know more, the safest course is to use aspartame in moderate doses only (one or two aspartame-sweetened drinks or foods a day).

Saccharin, another widely used sugar substitute, is 300 times sweeter than sugar but leaves a metallic aftertaste that some users dislike. Although scientists consider saccharin relatively safe in low to moderate doses, there is evidence linking this sweetener to a higher incidence of bladder cancer, particularly in smokers.[12] The risk seems to increase with the amount of saccharin used.

## Vitamin C: What It Can and Can't Do

Vitamin C is essential for the formation of collagen (the all-important fibrous material that literally holds cells and tissues together); the production of nervous system chemicals; and the maintenance of blood vessels, bones, and teeth. Also, it protects other vitamins and certain chemicals in the body from being broken down by oxygen. Vitamin C may also:

- Reduce the length of a cold, but not the number of colds a person gets. An extra cup of orange juice (which provides 80 mg of vitamin C) in the morning provides the same benefits as a tablet.
- Help prevent iron deficiency in women. According the U.S. Department of Agriculture researchers, foods rich in vitamin C enhance absorption of iron from breads, cereals, and other plant foods.
- May help protect against heart disease. Some vitamin C supporters have claimed that massive doses (2 grams or higher) can prevent or reverse the

**HEALTH HEADLINE**

**Social Eating**

People eat less when they eat alone, according to Georgia State University psychologists. And the more individuals they eat with, the more they eat.

When 63 healthy adults between ages 19 and 54 kept a detailed diary of their daily food intake, their meal sizes increased by as much as 44 percent when others were around. They also tended to eat less fat and fewer calories when they dined by themselves. When others are around, people eat regardless of whether they're hungry and spend more time at the table. The greater the number of diners, the greater the number of calories each consumes.

SOURCE: Newman, Jennifer. "The Joys of Eating Alone," *American Health*, December 1989.

SELF-SURVEY

## What Kind of Eater Are You?

Your childhood experiences, way of life, and tastes all determine your personal eating style. This questionnaire will help you understand your eating patterns—and problems. Answer as accurately and honestly as possible.

| | NEVER | RARELY | SOME-TIMES | USUALLY | ALWAYS |
|---|---|---|---|---|---|
| 1. I have a snack or nibble when preparing meals. | N | R | S | U | A |
| 2. I overeat when I am happy. | N | R | S | U | A |
| 3. I have gone on eating binges that are hard to stop. | N | R | S | U | A |
| 4. I eat more than I should in restaurants or as a guest. | N | R | S | U | A |
| 5. As I overeat, I feel guilty but keep on eating. | N | R | S | U | A |
| 6. I eat more than usual when I am on vacation. | N | R | S | U | A |
| 7. The smell of good food is an irresistible temptation to eat. | N | R | S | U | A |
| 8. Food makes me feel better even when it isn't tasty. | N | R | S | U | A |
| 9. Once I begin to overeat, I eat more and more as the day goes on. | N | R | S | U | A |
| 10. I eat not when I'm really hungry, but just because food is around. | N | R | S | U | A |
| 11. I overeat when I'm angry or depressed. | N | R | S | U | A |
| 12. If I don't consciously restrain my eating, I overeat. | N | R | S | U | A |
| 13. I finish whatever is put in front of me. | N | R | S | U | A |
| 14. When I am bored, I eat for something to do. | N | R | S | U | A |
| 15. I overeat when I drink alcohol. | N | R | S | U | A |
| 16. When I'm served a small meal, I feel satisfied without seconds. | N | R | S | U | A |
| 17. Food is one of my major satisfactions. | N | R | S | U | A |
| 18. I think about food when I am not actually eating or preparing it. | N | R | S | U | A |
| 19. Seeing and thinking about food makes me hungry and likely to eat. | N | R | S | U | A |
| 20. Eating controls parts of my life. | N | R | S | U | A |
| 21. I do best on diets that tell me exactly what and how much to eat. | N | R | S | U | A |

***How to Rate Your Eating Pattern***

Below, cross out the number corresponding to each question to which you answered "usually" or "always." Then count the crossed-out numbers in each row to get your scores for three different types of eating:

| | | | | | | | | |
|---|---|---|---|---|---|---|---|---|
| 1 | 4 | 7 | 10 | 13 | 16 | 19 | Total Hyperresponsive: | ______ |
| 2 | 5 | 8 | 11 | 14 | 17 | 20 | Total Emotional: | ______ |
| 3 | 6 | 9 | 12 | 15 | 18 | 21 | Total Consciously Restrained: | ______ |

***Hyperresponsive to the Environment***
A score of 4 or more out of a possible 7 shows that the hyperresponsive pattern is common for you. When people are triggered to eat by environmental cues, they aren't eating to meet their body's physical needs. They may be hyperresponders—people who experience a rush of insulin, and a pang of hunger, at the sight, smell, or thought of a good meal (questions 7 and 19).

People in this category tend to eat whenever food is around, and to clean their plates—though if they're only served small meals, they'll be satisfied with those too (questions 10, 13, and 16). They can be hungrier when they see a lavish spread in a restaurant or a friend's home (question 4). Environmentally cued eaters are also likely to snack while cooking (question 1). It can be helpful for them to treat every snack as if it were a *real* meal and to eat only when sitting at the table, paying attention to the food and to the act of eating.

***Emotional Eating***
A score of 4 or more shows that you tend to eat for emotional reasons. Many such people overeat when they're happy, angry, depressed, or bored (questions 2, 11, and 14). Food may keep you feeling better and may even become a major source of satisfaction (question 17). The problem, though, is that food can become an emotional crutch and can come to control your life in various ways (questions 5 and 20).

One sign of this pattern is eating food that doesn't even taste good (question 8). You may use eating as a substitute for other pleasures or reward yourself with food. Unless you find new ways of rewarding yourself, a diet may make you feel nervous, anxious, and deprived.

***Consciously Restrained Eating***
If you score at least 4 here, you may be using sheer willpower to keep from eating as much as you'd like. Hyperresponders who stay thin, despite constant stimulation from the food around them, have to restrain themselves consciously. Many fat and formerly fat people control their weight this way (question 12). As a result, they can become obsessive about food, thinking about it quite a bit between meals (question 18).

It's hard to keep up the continuous, focused attention required to rein in the appetite. Any number of things—a drink of alcohol, the relaxed schedule of a vacation, the distractions of conversation or TV—can disrupt this concentration and lead a restrained eater to overeat (questions 6 and 15). And overeating can lead to still more overeating, in a vicious cycle (question 9). Having gone a bit out of control, restrained eaters may then really let go. This can lead to a pattern of private, secret binging, followed by guilt (question 3).

Restrained eaters often find it easier to eat in a restaurant than at home; portions are rationed and second helpings are usually unavailable. Because a constant diet of eating out is impractical, most restrained eaters choose diet plans that allow them next to no choice of what to eat from day to day (question 21). Although these diets may seem the easiest, plans that involve more choice and decision making are often more successful in the long term. They're closer to real life, and so they tend to be less easily broken.

SOURCE: Rodin. *American Health.*

**TABLE 4-6** What's in Fast Food*

| FAST FOOD | CALORIES | FAT % | SODIUM, MG |
|---|---|---|---|
| *Arby's* | | | |
| Chicken breast, roasted | 254 | 24 | 930 |
| Junior roast beef | 218 | 33 | 345 |
| Regular roast beef | 353 | 38 | 590 |
| Baked potato, plain | 290 | 2 | 12 |
| *Burger King* | | | |
| Chicken Tenders®, 6 pieces | 204 | 44 | 636 |
| Hamburger | 275 | 39 | 509 |
| Cheeseburger | 317 | 43 | 651 |
| *Domino's Pizza* | | | |
| 12-in. cheese pizza, 2 slices | 340 | 16 | 660 |
| *Hardee's* | | | |
| Hamburger | 276 | 50 | 589 |
| Cheeseburger | 309 | 37 | 825 |
| Roast beef sandwich | 312 | 36 | 826 |
| Side salad | 21 | 4 | 42 |
| *Kentucky Fried Chicken* | | | |
| Original recipe drumstick | 147 | 54 | 269 |
| Coleslaw | 105 | 50 | 171 |
| Corn on the cob | 176 | 16 | 10 |
| Mashed potatoes | 59 | 9 | 228 |
| *Long John Silver's* | | | |
| Kitchen-breaded fish, 1 piece | 122 | 44 | 374 |
| Chicken plank, 1 piece | 152 | 47 | 515 |
| Ocean chef salad (where available) | 229 | 31 | 986 |
| Coleslaw, drained on fork | 182 | 74 | 367 |
| Corn on the cob | 176 | 28 | — |
| *McDonald's* | | | |
| English muffin with butter | 186 | 26 | 310 |
| Hamburger | 263 | 39 | 506 |
| Scrambled eggs | 180 | 65 | 205 |
| *Roy Rogers* | | | |
| Roast beef sandwich | 317 | 29 | 785 |
| Chicken leg | 117 | 52 | 162 |
| Baked potato, plain | 211 | 1 | trace |
| Coleslaw | 110 | 56 | 261 |
| Potato salad | 107 | 51 | 696 |
| *Wendy's* | | | |
| Chicken sandwich, multigrain bun | 320 | 28 | 500 |
| Hamburger, kids' meal | 200 | 36 | 265 |
| Baked potato with chicken a la king | 350 | 15 | 820 |
| Baked potato, plain | 250 | 7 | trace |
| Omelet (mushroom, onion, and green pepper) | 210 | 64 | 200 |
| Pick-up window side salad | 110 | 49 | 540 |

*Note: Data supplied by individual food chains.

SOURCE: The Center for Science in the Public Interest. 

buildup of atherosclerotic plaque and lower heart-harming fats in the bloodstream. This has not been proven.

- Boost male fertility. A daily gram of vitamin C each day helps sperm swim freely to fertilize an egg.
- Help keep gums and teeth healthy. Monkeys given extra vitamin C were able to successfully fend off bacteria injected into their mouths. Without the supplements, they developed gum disease.

There is no proof that Vitamin C can cure cancer or other serious illnesses.

## What's Wrong with Fast Food?

Not all fast foods are junk foods—that is, high in calories, sugar, salt, and fat, and low in nutrients. Pizza, for example, provides reasonable amounts of protein, fat, and carbohydrates. Hamburgers, french fries, and shakes can also be nutritious, provided they aren't the only foods you eat. Table 4-6 shows the contents of a variety of popular fast foods. Some states require fast-food restaurants to post a nutrition analysis of the items they serve.

Though it's not all bad, fast food has definite disadvantages:[13] A meal in a fast-food restaurant may cost twice as much as the same meal prepared at home and easily provide half your daily allotment of calories. The fat content of many items is extremely high. A Burger King double-beef Whopper with cheese contains 709 calories and 45 grams of fat, 18 from saturated fat. A McDonald's sausage McMuffin with egg has 517 calories and 33 grams of fat, 13 saturated.

**STRATEGY FOR CHANGE**

**A Fast-Food Guide**

The major fast-food chains are offering lighter menu items. Here are guidelines you can follow to make the best fast-food selections:

- For breakfast, avoid croissants or muffins stuffed with eggs or meat; they pack as many as 700 calories. Better options include plain scrambled eggs (150 to 180 calories), hot cakes without butter or syrup (400 calories), and English muffins (185 calories each).
- Go for plain burgers, which average 275 to 350 calories. An even better choice is roast beef, which is lower in fat and calories.
- Order child-sized portions. They're lower in size, calories, and cost.
- Be wary of "fast" fish. With frying oil trapped in the breading and creamy tartar sauce on top, fried-fish sandwiches supply more calories (425 to 500) and fat than regular burgers.
- Avoid fried chicken. The coatings tend to retain grease. If you want bite-sized chicken, select "bites" made of chicken breasts, not processed chicken (which contains fatty ground-up skin).
- Ask for unsalted items; they are available. (Many chains have also reduced the amount of sodium used in cooking.)
- If you sample the salad bar, steer clear of mayonnaise, oily vegetable salads, and rich dressings.
- Choose milk (2 percent is now available at many chains) instead of a shake.

## Organic and Health Foods

In nutrition, the term **organic** refers to foods produced without the intentional use of commercial chemicals at any stage (though the residues from fertilizers, pesticides, and herbicides have been found in practically all agricultural soils and irrigation waters). Organic foods are a great deal more expensive than supermarket foods. However, since such well-publicized scares as the use of Alar (a potentially

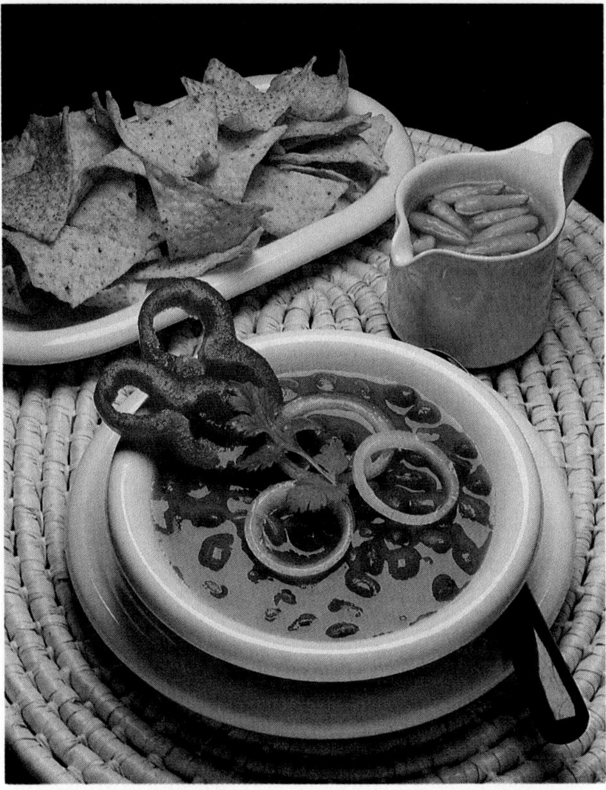

Cooking that features beans rice and corn is low in fat and high in nutrients.

cancer-causing pesticide) on apples, organic foods have become more popular.

Just because a product is sold in a health-food store doesn't mean it's healthful. To find out what you're really getting, read the product label carefully. Unfortunately, labels won't help when you're choosing produce. Even the so-called fresh vegetables in supermarkets have lost 50 percent of their vitamin C, health-food advocates say; they claim that overplanting and soil depletion have made conventional foods less nutritious than in the past.

## Vegetarian Diets

All vegetarians avoid meat. Some, called **lacto-vegetarians,** eat dairy products as well as fruits and vegetables; **ovo-lacto-vegetarians** eat eggs and dairy products in addition to fruits and vegetables. Pure vegetarians, called **vegans,** eat plant foods only; often

**organic** A term designating food produced with, or based on, fertilizer originating from plants or animals but without pesticides or chemically formulated fertilizers.
**lacto-vegetarian** A person whose diet consists of dairy products and vegetables only.
**ovo-lacto-vegetarian** A vegetarian who eats eggs as well as dairy products and vegetables.
**vegan** A vegetarian who eats only vegetables—no dairy products, eggs, or other animal-derived foods.

they take vitamin $B_{12}$ supplements, because that vitamin is normally found in animal products only. If they select their food with care, vegetarians can get sufficient amounts of protein, vitamin $B_{12}$, iron, and calcium.

Vegetarians' cholesterol levels are low, and vegetarians are seldom overweight. As a result, they're less apt to be candidates for heart disease than those who consume large quantities of meat. Also, vegetarians have lower incidences of breast and colon cancer and of osteoporosis.

## Additives: Risks Versus Benefits

**Additives** are substances added to food to lengthen the time it can be stored, change the taste in a way the manufacturer thinks is better, alter the color, or otherwise modify it to make it more appealing. The average American takes in more than 5 pounds of chemical food additives a year, and there are good reasons to worry about what these might do.

For example, nitrites—which are found in bacon, sausages, and lunch meats—inhibit spoilage; prevent botulism (an often lethal form of food poisoning), enhance flavor, and add color. But high heat from cooking—and even our own digestive systems—can convert nitrites to potent cancer-causing agents. Alternatives to nitrites—thermal processing, freeze-drying, irradiating, and freezing—would require new equipment and thus more money. Unfortunately, in a society that uses as many nitrites and other chemicals as ours does, there are no easy answers or substitutions.

### STRATEGY FOR CHANGE

### How to Read a Food Label

The U.S. government has ordered food manufacturers to include on product labels clearer, more accurate nutrition information about what is actually in products (see Figure 4-2). Here are some points to keep in mind as you read labels:

- Don't be misled by what the manufacturer says on other parts of the product. "Reduced fat" doesn't mean no or even low fat.
- Just because a product label says "no preservatives" doesn't mean other chemicals haven't been used in the product's processing.
- When comparing products, make sure to check serving size. A 7-ounce serving can be higher in nutrients simply because it's larger than a 3-ounce serving of another brand.

**FIGURE 4-2** New reading for the supermarket aisle.

☐ *To be omitted* (boxed items) ■ *To be added* (shaded items)

| PRESENT LABEL NUTRITION INFORMATION | | PROPOSED LABEL NUTRITION INFORMATION | |
|---|---|---|---|
| Serving Size | 1/4 Pizza | Serving Size | 1/4 Pizza |
| Servings Per Container | 4 | Servings Per Container | 4 |
| Calories | 240 | Calories | 240 |
| Protein | 9g | Calories from Fat | 63 |
| Carbohydrate | 35g | Protein | 9g |
| Fat | 7g | Carbohydrate | 35g |
| Sodium | 640g | Dietary Fiber | 2g |
| | | Fat | 7g |
| Percent of U.S. Recommended Daily Allowances | | Saturated Fat | 4g |
| | | Cholesterol | 15mg |
| Protein | 20 | Sodium | 640mg |
| Vitamin A | 15 | | |
| Vitamin C | 8 | Percent of U.S. Recommended Daily Allowances | |
| Thiamine | 8 | | |
| Riboflavin | 10 | Vitamin A | 15 |
| Niacin | 10 | Vitamin C | 8 |
| Calcium | 10 | Calcium | 10 |
| Iron | 6 | Iron | 6 |

SOURCE: U.S. Food and Drug Administration. Copyright 1990 by the New York Times Company. Reprinted by permission.

## Food Allergies

**Food allergies** are particularly common in babies, whose digestive systems haven't fully developed. However, older children and adults also can suffer violent reactions to ordinary foods. Cow's milk, eggs, seafood, wheat, soybeans, nuts, seeds, and chocolate have all been identified as triggers of allergic reactions.

The symptoms of food allergies vary. One person might sneeze if exposed to an irritating food; another might vomit or develop diarrhea; others might suffer headaches, dizziness, hives, or a rapid heartbeat. Symptoms may not develop for up to 72 hours, making it hard to pinpoint which food was responsible for the reaction. If you suspect that you have a food allergy, see a physician with specialized training in allergy diagnosis. Once you've identified the culprit, the wisest and simplest course is simply to avoid it.

**additive** A substance added to food to enhance certain qualities, such as appearance, taste, or freshness.
**food allergy** A hypersensitivity to particular foods.

## WEIGHT CONTROL

Do you watch your weight? Are you on a diet? If so, you're hardly alone. According to recent estimates, one of every four Americans is dieting. Yet, on the average, we weigh 6 pounds more than men and women did in 1960.

U.S. culture places such a high premium on thinness that dieting (restricting food intake for the sake of weight loss) has become a way of life for some people. In one study 75 percent of college women reported that they had dieted to control their weight.[14]

Although not all dieters develop eating disorders (see Chapter 2 for a discussion of anorexia nervosa, bulimia, and bulimarexia), they are at high risk. Thousands of young people starve, binge, purge, or combine all three behaviors at least occasionally. Recent surveys have found serious vitamin and mineral deficiencies in teenage girls and college women because of their constant dieting.[15]

Regardless of what you weigh, chances are that in your mind's eye you're fatter than you really are and than you want to be. Before you can manage your weight, you have to have realistic goals and expectations.

### What Should You Weigh?

Many factors determine what you weigh: heredity, eating behavior, food selection, amount of daily exercise. And there is a range of healthy weights for any height. Just as it is possible to be too heavy for your own good, it is also possible to be too thin. Some researchers believe that optimal weight rises with age and that the healthiest older people weigh more than they did in their twenties.[16]

**STRATEGY FOR CHANGE**

**Rethinking Your Weight Goals**

Stop looking at your scale or in your mirror, and look inside. Answer these questions as honestly as you can:

- If you could choose your weight, what would it be? Why? At what weight do you have

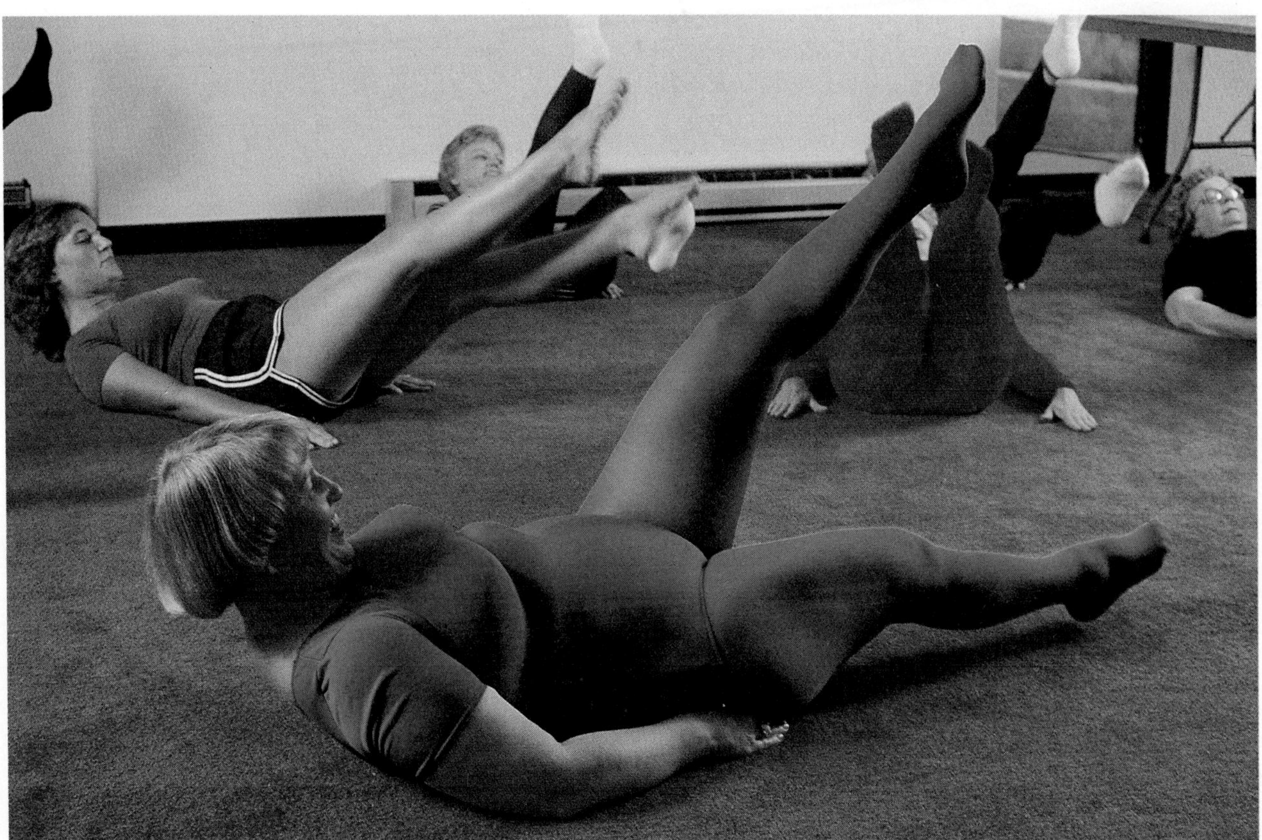

Exercise helps dieters lose fat rather than muscle and keep excess pounds off.

enough energy to make it through the day, yet not feel hungry all the time?
- What is the range of weight that's best for your height? How does this compare with what you consider your ideal weight?
- What do you think is a realistic weight? Have you ever gotten to, and stayed at, this weight? If you had to choose between the weight that was best for your health and the one you thought most attractive, which would you choose? Why?
- Is there a middle weight for which you could strive?

The most popular yardsticks for determining ideal weight ranges are the tables prepared by the insurance industry. (Table 4-7 is an example of such a table.) These tables relate weight and height with how long policyholders lived, not with their overall health, vitality, or appearance.

Another critical number is the percentage of fat in your body. In general, a range of 15 percent to 19 percent fat for men and 22 percent to 26 percent fat for women is considered good. Physicians and fitness experts rely on **hydrostatic immersion testing,** weighing a person in water to distinguish buoyant fat from denser muscle. **Skin calipers,** which pinch skin folds at the arms, waist, and back, are less accurate but more practical.

There are other simple methods for measuring body fat. One, a do-it-yourself technique developed by exercise physiologist Jack Wilmore at the University of Texas at Austin, requires only a tape measure and the charts in Figure 4-3.

Even simpler—and more revealing—is the **pinch test.** Stand naked before a full-length mirror and look at yourself objectively. Are there bulges at your waist or on your hips? Extend one arm out to the side. Using the thumb and index finger of your other hand, can you pinch more than an inch of skin at any point along the underside of your upper arm? If so, you need to firm up your muscles through exercise or to shed some pounds, or both.

The body has two different fat stores: one at the hips and one in the abdominal. Fat at the hips, which is more common in women and is more difficult to lose than abdomen fat, is stored primarily for special purposes, like extra energy needs during pregnancy

**hydrostatic immersion testing** The weighing of a person in water to distinguish buoyant fat from denser muscle.
**skin caliper** An instrument used to pinch skin folds at the arms, waist, and back to determine percentage of body fat.
**pinch test** A simple method of checking for excess body fat by using the thumb and index finger to pinch the loose skin on the underside of the upper arm; more than an inch of loose skin indicates a need for exercise or weight loss.

**TABLE 4-7** 1983 Metropolitan Life Insurance Company Height and Weight Tables*

| Men | | | | Women | | | |
|---|---|---|---|---|---|---|---|
| **Height** | **Weight, lb** | | | **Height** | **Weight, lb** | | |
| FT., IN. | SMALL FRAME | MEDIUM FRAME | LARGE FRAME | FT., IN. | SMALL FRAME | MEDIUM FRAME | LARGE FRAME |
| 5 1 | 123–129 | 126–136 | 133–145 | 4 9 | 98–108 | 106–118 | 115–128 |
| 5 2 | 125–131 | 128–138 | 135–148 | 4 10 | 100–110 | 108–120 | 117–131 |
| 5 3 | 127–133 | 130–140 | 137–151 | 4 11 | 101–112 | 110–123 | 119–134 |
| 5 4 | 129–135 | 132–143 | 139–155 | 5 0 | 103–115 | 112–126 | 122–137 |
| 5 5 | 131–137 | 134–146 | 141–159 | 5 1 | 105–118 | 115–129 | 125–140 |
| 5 6 | 133–140 | 137–149 | 144–163 | 5 2 | 108–121 | 118–132 | 128–144 |
| 5 7 | 135–143 | 140–152 | 147–167 | 5 3 | 111–124 | 121–135 | 131–148 |
| 5 8 | 137–146 | 143–155 | 150–171 | 5 4 | 114–127 | 124–138 | 134–152 |
| 5 9 | 139–149 | 146–158 | 153–175 | 5 5 | 117–130 | 127–141 | 137–156 |
| 5 10 | 141–152 | 149–161 | 156–179 | 5 6 | 120–133 | 130–144 | 140–160 |
| 5 11 | 144–155 | 152–165 | 159–183 | 5 7 | 123–136 | 133–147 | 143–164 |
| 6 0 | 147–159 | 155–169 | 163–187 | 5 8 | 126–139 | 136–150 | 146–167 |
| 6 1 | 150–163 | 159–173 | 167–192 | 5 9 | 129–142 | 139–153 | 149–170 |
| 6 2 | 153–167 | 162–177 | 171–197 | 5 10 | 132–145 | 142–156 | 152–173 |
| 6 3 | 157–171 | 166–182 | 176–202 | 5 11 | 135–148 | 145–159 | 155–176 |

*These weight ranges show weights in pounds at ages 25 to 29 based on lowest mortality. The tables have been adjusted to represent weights without clothes and heights without shoes.

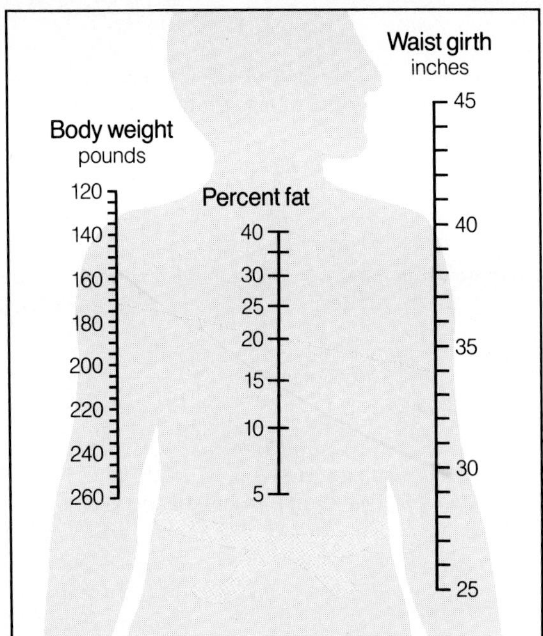


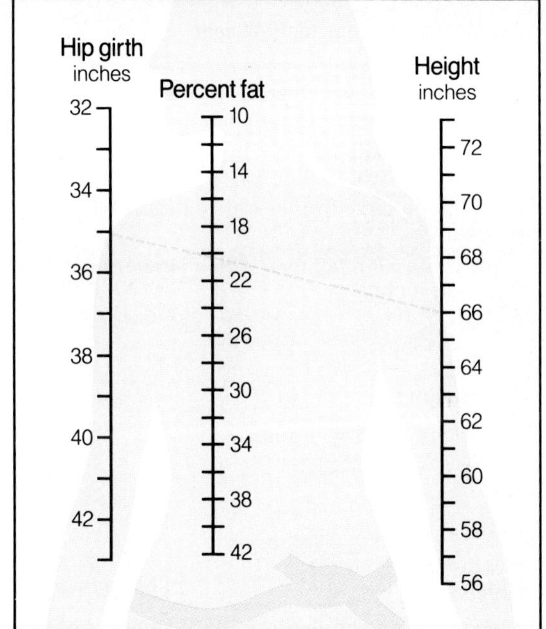


SOURCE: Wilmore, Jack H. *Sensible Fitness, Second Edition,* Champaign, IL: Leisure Press, 1986. Reprinted by permisssion.

**FIGURE 4-3** Estimating percentage of body fat.
**Men:** Body-fat percentage can be estimated from body weight, and abdominal or waist circumference. Measure the circumference of the waist at the exact level of the belly button, making sure to keep the tape perfectly horizontal. Using a straightedge and the chart, align this measurement and your body weight. Your body-fat percentage is indicated at the point the straightedge crosses the percent-fat line. Fit men should measure between 12 and 17 percent body fat.

**Women:** Body-fat percentage can be estimated from height and hip circumference. The circumference of the hips is measured at its widest point. Using a straightedge and the chart, align this measurement and your height. Your body-fat percentage is indicated at the point the straightedge crosses the percent-fat line. Fit women should measure between 19 and 24 percent body fat.

and nursing. Abdominal fat seems more dangerous, in that there is a correlation between it and increases in risk for diabetes, heart disease, and stroke.[17] Use Table 4-8 to calculate your ideal weight.

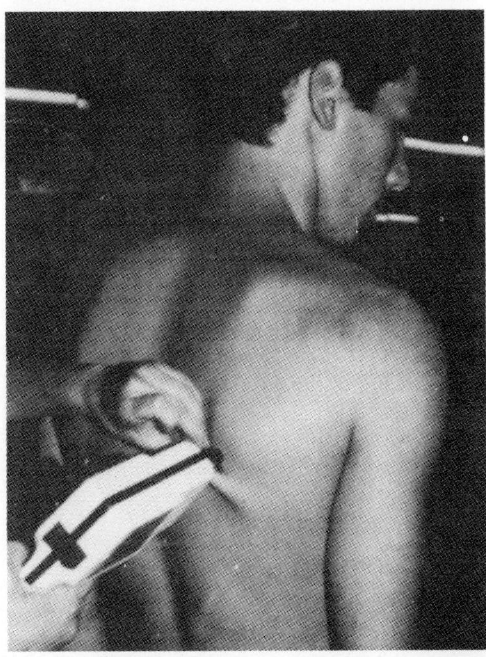

One way to determine body fat is to measure the fat that has accumulated under the skin with a skin caliper.

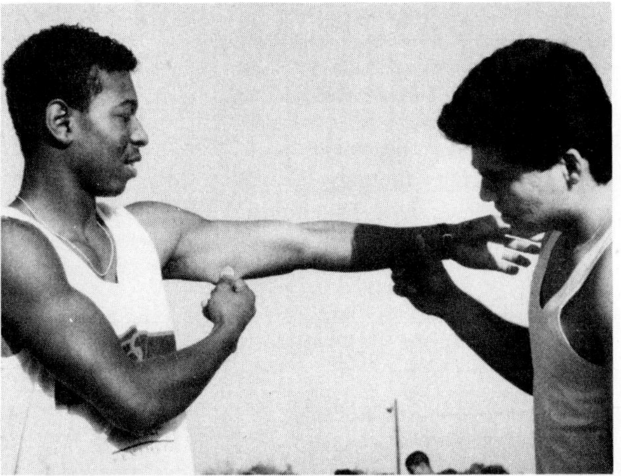

The pinch test is an easy way to tell if you have too much body fat.

**TABLE 4-8** Calculating Your Ideal Weight

Here are two widely used formulas for ideal weight, based on body-fat percentages of less than 20 percent for men and less than 26 percent for women. Use Table 4-9 to determine body-frame size.

**For men the formula is:**
height (in inches) × 4 − 128 = ideal weight

If you have a large frame, add 10 percent (0.10) to the total.

**Example using a 6-ft tall man with a large frame:**

| | |
|---|---|
| height (in inches) | 72 |
| multiply | × 4 |
| | 288 |
| | −128 |
| ideal weight | 160 lb |
| adjustment for large frame | 160 |
| | × .10 |
| add | 16 lb |
| | 160 |
| | + 16 |
| adjusted ideal weight | 176 lb |

The second, even simpler formula for men is to allow 106 lb, for the first 5 ft of height and add 6 lb for each additional inch of height thereafter.

**For a 6-FT man, the calculations are:**

| | |
|---|---|
| weight allowance for first 5 ft | 106 lb |
| add 6 lb for each additional inch | + 72 (12 × 6) |
| ideal weight | 178 lb |

**For women the formula is:**
height (in inches) × 3.5 − 108 = ideal weight

**Example using a 5-ft 4-in. woman with a medium frame:**

| | |
|---|---|
| height (in inches) | 64 |
| multiply | × 3.5 |
| | 224 |
| | −108 |
| ideal weight | 116 lb |

In applying the second formula, women should allow 100 lb for the first 5 ft of height and add 5 lb for each additional inch of height thereafter.

**For a 5-ft 4-in. woman, the calculations are:**

| | |
|---|---|
| weight allowance for first 5 ft | 100 lb |
| add 5 lb for each additional inch | + 20 (4 × 5) |
| ideal weight | 120 lb |

The fact that the numbers from the two formulas don't jibe perfectly underscores a key point about determining your ideal weight: Rather than aiming for one magic number, you should realize that there's a 5- to 10-lb range of ideal weight for every height.

### Calories: How Many Do You Need?

Calories are the measure of the amount of energy that can be derived from food. Science defines the **calorie** as the amount of energy required to raise the temperature of 1 gram of water by 1 degree Celsius. In the laboratory, the caloric content of food is measured in 1,000-calorie units called kilocalories. The calorie referred to in everyday usage is actually the equivalent of the laboratory kilocalorie.

The RDA for total calories for women 25 and older (with a median height of 5 feet 4 inches and a weight of 138 pounds) is 1,900 to 2,200 calories. For men (with a median height of 5 feet 10 inches and weight of 174 pounds), daily intake should be 2,300 to 2,900 calories. How many calories you need depends on your sex; age; body frame (see Table 4-9); weight; percentage of body fat; and **basal metabolic rate,** the number of calories needed to sustain your body at rest.

Your activity level also affects your calorie requirements (see Table 4-10). Regardless of whether you take food in as fat, protein, or carbohydrate, if you take in more calories than required to maintain your size and don't work them your body will convert the excess to fat. The average American consumes 3,300 calories a day—more than is required for anyone except an active 190-pound (or heavier) person.

## OBESITY

**Obesity** is a condition characterized by excessive accumulation of fat in the body, generally 20 percent or more above "desirable" weight, as determined by averaging the figures in Table 4-8. By this standard, 19 percent of men and 28 percent of women in the United States are obese. Obesity increases steadily from childhood to age 50, with a two- to threefold increase between the ages of 20 and 64.

Mild obesity refers to a body weight 20 percent to 40 percent above ideal weight; moderate, to a body weight 41 percent to 100 percent above ideal weight; and severe, to a body weight 100 percent or more above ideal weight. An estimated 11 million Americans are moderately obese. Some 200,000 adults are severely obese.[18]

**calorie** The amount of heat required to raise the temperature of 1 gram of water by 1 degree Celsius (the calorie of popular usage is actually 1,000 times larger than the calorie of science).
**basal metabolic rate** The number of calories required to maintain life-sustaining activities for a specified period of time.
**obesity** The excessive accumulation of fat in the body; a condition of being 20 percent or more above ideal weight.

**TABLE 4-9** How to Determine Your Body-Frame Size by Elbow Breadth

To make a simple approximation of your frame size, extend your arm and bend the forearm upwards at a 90° angle. Keep the fingers straight and turn the inside of your wrist away from your body. Place the thumb and index finger of your other hand on the two prominent bones on either side of your elbow. Measure the space between your fingers against a ruler or a tape measure.* Compare the measurements with those given below.

The elbow measurements listed below are for medium-framed men and women of various heights. Measurements lower than those listed indicate that you have a small frame; higher measurements indicate a large frame.

| Men | | Women | |
|---|---|---|---|
| HEIGHT | ELBOW BREADTH, IN. | HEIGHT | ELBOW BREADTH, IN. |
| 5′1″–5′2″ | 2½–2⅞ | 4′9″–4′10″ | 2¼–2½ |
| 5′3″–5′6″ | 2⅝–2⅞ | 4′11″–5′2″ | 2¼–2½ |
| 5′7″–5′10″ | 2¾–3 | 5′3″–5′6″ | 2⅜–2⅝ |
| 5′11″–6′2″ | 2¾–3⅛ | 5′7″–5′10″ | 2⅜–2⅝ |
| 6′3″ | 2⅞–3¼ | 5′11″ | 2½–2¾ |

*For the most accurate measurement, have your physician measure your elbow breadth with a caliper.
SOURCE: Adapted from the 1983 Metropolitan Height and Weight Tables. Reprinted courtesy of the Metropolitan Life Insurance Company.

**TABLE 4-10** How Many Calories Do You Need Daily?

| DESIRABLE WEIGHT | HIGH ACTIVITY | MEDIUM ACTIVITY | LOW ACTIVITY |
|---|---|---|---|
| *Women* | | | |
| 99 | 1,700 | 1,500 | 1,300 |
| 110 | 1,850 | 1,650 | 1,400 |
| 121 | 2,000 | 1,750 | 1,550 |
| 128 | 2,100 | 1,900 | 1,600 |
| 132 | 2,150 | 1,950 | 1,650 |
| 143 | 2,300 | 2,050 | 1,800 |
| 154 | 2,400 | 2,150 | 1,850 |
| 165 | 2,550 | 2,300 | 1,950 |
| *Men* | | | |
| 110 | 2,200 | 1,950 | 1,650 |
| 121 | 2,400 | 2,150 | 1,850 |
| 132 | 2,550 | 2,300 | 1,950 |
| 143 | 2,700 | 2,400 | 2,050 |
| 154 | 2,900 | 2,600 | 2,200 |
| 165 | 3,100 | 2,800 | 2,400 |
| 176 | 3,250 | 2,950 | 2,500 |
| 187 | 3,300 | 3,100 | 2,600 |

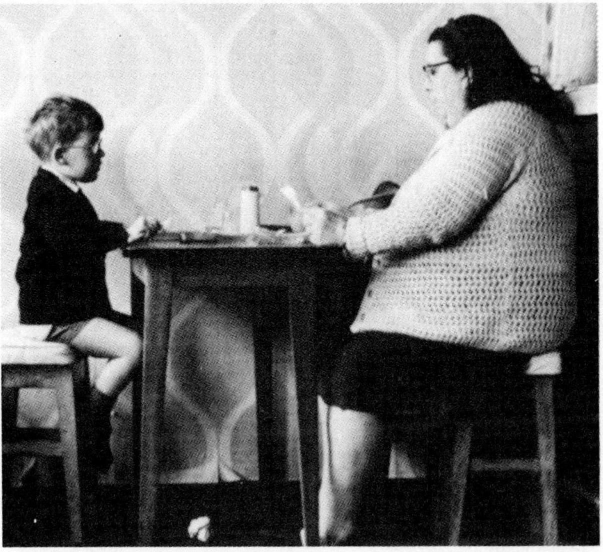

According to statistics, 80 percent of children with two obese parents, 40 percent of children with one obese parent, and only 10 percent of children with thin parents will become obese.

## The Causes of Obesity

According to statistics, 80 percent of children with two obese parents, 40 percent of children with one obese parent, and only 10 percent of children with thin parents will become obese.[19] However, people aren't "born to be fat." They might inherit a tendency to like high-fat foods; but if they're active and restrict those foods, they won't become obese.

Some obese people have a high number of fat cells, others have large fat cells, and the most severely obese have both more *and* larger fat cells. Whereas the size of fat cells can increase at any time in life, the number is set very early, possibly as the result of genetics and overfeeding early in life. Once formed, fat cells do not disappear. When obese people lose weight, they still have the same number of fat cells, which become smaller.

People who do not exercise regularly are more likely to become obese. Physical activity prevents obesity by increasing caloric use, decreasing food intake, and boosting metabolic rate.

In affluent countries, people in lower socioeconomic classes tend to be obese and those in the upper classes, who can afford as much food as they want, tend to be leaner. Education may be one factor; another is the price of nonfattening food. Often a healthy, nonfattening diet with plenty of fresh fruits and vegetables is more expensive.

Obese people are neither more nor less psychologically troubled than others. Psychological problems—such as irritability, depression and anxiety—are more likely to be the result of obesity than the cause.

## The Dangers of Obesity

Excess weight contributes to the death of many Americans, according to a panel of doctors and nutritionists assembled by the National Institutes of Health (NIH).[20] Obese people have 3 times the normal incidence of high blood pressure and diabetes; an increased risk of heart disease; a shorter life span; and a much greater risk of developing respiratory problems, arthritis, and certain types of cancer. Obese women are more likely to develop cancer of the uterus, cervical cancer, and breast cancer. Obese men have an increased chance of developing cancer of the colon, rectum, and prostate.

To put these risks into perspective, consider these estimates: In a group of 100 people of normal weight, 90 can expect to live to be age 60, 50 will survive to age 70, and 30 will live to age 80 and beyond. However, only 60 of every 100 obese individuals will make it to age 60, half of these 60 will live another decade, and no more than 10 will live to age 80.

Fat adults are far more susceptible to gout, blood clots, varicose veins, hemorrhoids, gall bladder and liver disease, and intestinal disorders. If fat adults have surgery, they're more likely to develop complications. Even relatively small amounts of excess fat—as little as 5 pounds—can be dangerous in those already at risk for hypertension and diabetes.

**STRATEGY FOR CHANGE**

### Psyching Yourself Up to Slim Down

One of the best ways to build motivation so that you can lose weight sensibly and safely is to build a better body image. Here are some suggestions to help:

- Act as if you're already slim. Don't put off special plans until you reach a certain magical weight.
- Start being the person you want to be; your body will catch up with you.
- Focus on the parts of your body you like. Maybe you have beautiful brown eyes or powerful shoulders.
- Don't put yourself down. Lots of fat people make jokes about their weight so others won't.
- Treat yourself with the respect you'd like from others.
- Create the body you want in your imagination. See yourself slimming down, and feeling lithe and thin.
- Try new activities. Don't let your weight-loss program be the center of your life. Take up folk-dancing, sailing, gardening, or some such hobby. The more active your new interest, the better.

## Treating Obesity

The best approach to overcoming obesity depends on how overweight a person is.

### Severe Obesity

Severe obesity (a body weight more than 100 percent over desirable weight) is life-threatening. Because of the medical dangers of their condition, such men and women, as a last resort, may undergo surgery to reduce the volume of their stomachs and to tighten the passageway from the stomach to the intestine. Others opt for a "gastric bubble," a soft, polyurethane sac placed in the stomach to make the person feel full while following a low-calorie diet. Obesity experts do not yet know whether people who lose weight with the bubble will be able to keep it off.

### Moderate Obesity

For those 41 percent to 100 percent over their ideal weight, doctors recommend a supervised diet and behavior modification. In addition to cutting down on daily calories, patients keep careful records of when, what, and why they eat; learn good nutrition; increase their physical activity; and work with therapists to overcome self-defeating attitudes.

### Mild Obesity

Rather than going on low-calorie diets, people 20 percent to 40 percent over ideal weight should cut back moderately on their food intake and concentrate on developing healthy lifelong eating habits. Many moderately to mildly overweight people turn to national organizations, such as TOPS (Take Off Pounds Sensibly, the largest nonprofit organization), Weight Watchers, and other commercial groups. Most offer behavior modification techniques, inspirational lectures, and carefully designed nutrition programs—but drop-out rates are high. In one study, 50 percent of the members dropped out within six weeks and 70 percent within twelve weeks.[21]

# BEYOND DIETING

What would you do if your weight crept up 10 or 20 pounds above what it should be? If your answer is "Go on a diet," think again. Diet aids—such as diuretics and laxatives, which speed up elimination of

HEALTH SPOTLIGHT

## A Nutritional Guide to Ethnic Foods

America, land of immigrants, has imported a wide variety of ethnic cuisines. Each has its own nutritional benefits—and potential drawbacks.

**Italian** The cuisine of southern Italy may be one of the world's healthiest because it consists mainly of pasta, vegetables, fruit, and fish. Olive oil, another essential in southern Italy, is also healthful because it's rich in monounsaturated fats. The cooking of northern Italy features much more beef, butter, and cream, and residents of this region have a greater incidence of heart disease than their southern neighbors.

**Chinese** The average diet in mainland China consists of 69 percent carbohydrates, 10 percent proteins, and only 21 percent fats—a healthy balance of nutrients. Chinese restaurants here serve more meat and sauces than are generally eaten in China, but their dishes remain relatively low in fat, with plenty of vegetables. Stir-frying—cooking very quickly in a lightly oiled, very hot wok—helps foods retain their vitamins. One drawback, at least for those prone to high blood pressure, is the high sodium content of soy and other sauces, and of a seasoner called MSG (monosodium glutamate). Most restaurants offer MSG-free dishes or leave out MSG on request.

**Japanese** The Japanese diet is very low in fat, which may be why the incidence of heart disease is low in Japan. Dietary staples include soybean products (like tofu), fish, vegetables, noodles, and rice. However, Japanese cuisine is high in salted, smoked, or pickled foods, which may play a role in the country's high incidence of stomach cancer.

**Mexican** The cuisine served in Mexico features rice, corn, and beans, which are low in fat and high in nutrients. However, the dishes Americans think of as Mexican are far less healthful. Burritos, for example, especially when topped with cheese and sour cream, are very high in fat.

**Indian** Many Indian dishes highlight healthful ingredients like vegetables and legumes (beans and peas). However, many also use ghee (clarified butter) or coconut oil, which is rich in harmful saturated fats. The best advice would be to ask how each dish is prepared when ordering at an Indian restaurant.

SOURCES: The Center for Science in the Public Interest, Washington, D.C. Saltman, Paul; Joel Gurin; and Ira Mothner. *The California Nutrition Book.* Boston: Little, Brown, 1987.

fluids and wastes—produce temporary weight loss only.

Diets, particularly very low-calorie diets, simply don't work. According to University of Pennsylvania researchers, crash dieting can be less than half as effective in the long run as the combination of behavioral modification and gradual weight loss.[22] Many diets not only fail to deliver on their promises, but also cause serious health problems.

### The Dangers of Fad Diets

Any diet that promises to take pounds off fast can be dangerous. The most risky are very low-calorie diets that provide fewer than 800 calories a day. According to a 1990 report in the *Journal of the American Medical Association* the drastic reduction in protein can weaken the heart and lead to heart failure and sudden death.[23] As much as 50 percent of the weight you lose may be muscle (so you look flabbier as well)—and because your heart is a muscle, it can become so weak that it can't pump blood through your body.

On a very low-calorie diet, your blood pressure may plummet, causing dizziness, lightheadedness, and fatigue. You may develop nausea and abdominal pain. You may lose hair. If you're a woman, your menstrual cycle may become irregular or you may stop menstruating altogether. As you lose more water, you lose essential vitamins too.

Semistarvation diets can backfire. When you cut way back on calories, your metabolism slows down. You might eat as few as 700 calories a day and not lose weight. Once you go off the diet—as you inevitably must—your metabolism remains slow. Your body continues to burn fewer calories, even though you're no longer restricting your intake. You gain back the pounds you just lost and often end up eating less and weighing more.

Liquid diet programs—such as Optifast, Medifast, and others—supply 420 to 800 calories a day and do include sufficient protein to preserve muscle tissue. For several months, dieters on these plans eat no solid food, consuming only the special liquid formula and water. This extreme diet, generally reserved for those at least 40 pounds overweight, does result in rapid weight loss.

Side-effects include dry skin, hair loss, constipation, gum disease, sensitivity to cold, and mood swings. In one study, 25 percent of dieters dropped out within the first three weeks.[24] And only 10 to 20 percent of those who enrolled managed to stay within 10 pounds of their target weight a year and a half after entering the program.

**STRATEGY FOR CHANGE**

**Evaluating a Diet**

If you hear about a new diet that promises to melt away fat, don't try it until you get answers to the following questions:

- Does it include a selection of nutritious foods?
- Does it emphasize moderate portions?
- Does it use foods that are easy to find and prepare?
- Does it give you enough variety?
- Can you use it wherever you eat—at home, work, restaurants, or parties?
- Is its cost reasonable?

If the answer to any of these questions is no, don't try the diet—and ask yourself one more question: Is losing weight worth losing your well-being?

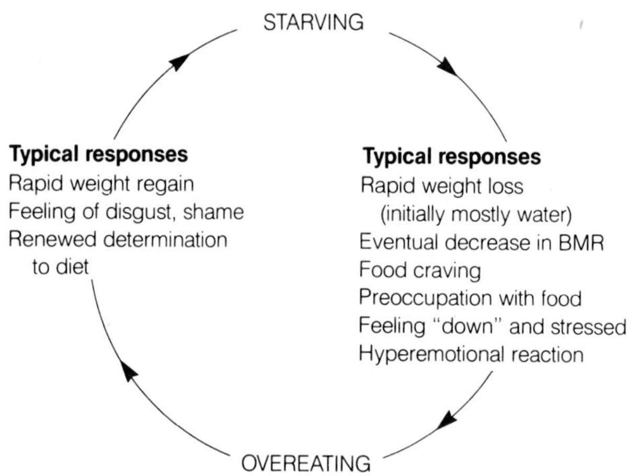


SOURCE: Christian, Janet L. and Janet L. Greger. *Nutrition for Living, Second Edition*, Benjamin/Cummings, 1988.

**FIGURE 4-4** The vicious cycle of chronic dieting and overeating. If a person uses a weight-loss diet that is very low in calories, the body and mind react against the severe deprivation; rebound eating is likely to occur. This results in weight regain and, often, self-criticism, which may lead to another and yet another trip around the circle.

## The Yo-Yo Syndrome

If you try to lose more than 1 or 2 pounds of fat a week, your body will try to find ways to resist. Here is what typically happens:

At first, you lose weight quickly. One-fourth of this initial loss is fat; most is water. Your basal metabolic rate may slow down by as much as 20 to 25 percent. Your pulse becomes slower; you feel chilly even in warm temperatures. Your body burns less fuel. Even if you force yourself to exercise, you won't lift your legs as high when you run or kick as vigorously when you swim.

Psychologically, you also feel the effects of dieting. You start to crave food. You may become so preoccupied with food that you can't concentrate. Your mood slumps, and you feel "down in the dumps." You're more irritable. You feel hassled and stressed.

As a result of such negative reactions, you're likely to go off your diet—and chances are that when you do, you'll overeat, possibly gaining more weight than you lost (see Figure 4-4). Ultimately, you'll feel helpless, miserable, weak-willed, and doomed to live in a body you've come to hate. You'll also forget how to eat normally.

## The Forever Diet

*Diet* is becoming a four-letter word. Increasingly, Americans have realized that quick fixes don't produce lasting results.[25] The number of people who say they are dieting has dropped, and more men and women are following "healthy eating plans" or "nutrition" programs. They're cutting back on fat; choos-

**TABLE 4-11** The Most Popular Ways to Lose Weight

| | PERCENTAGE OF AMERICANS TRYING TO LOSE WEIGHT |
|---|---|
| Just cut out snacks and desserts | 42 |
| Just eat less of everything | 37 |
| Start to exercise more | 32 |
| Cut down on fat | 32 |
| Stop eating at night | 29 |
| Eat more fruits and vegetables | 20 |
| Start counting calories | 19 |
| Eat less red meat | 17 |
| Use low-calorie foods and drinks | 12 |
| Follow a diet plan from a doctor | 11 |
| Eat more filling, low-calorie foods | 10 |
| Join a weight-loss group | 9 |
| Use a special diet food (e.g., protein powder) | 3 |
| Follow a diet book | 1 |

SOURCE: Gurin, Joel. "Eating Goes Back to Basics," *American Health,* March 1990.

ing more high-fiber, low-calorie foods; and exercising to stay in shape (see Table 4-11). Along the way they're learning a sensible approach to eating—an approach they can use, not just while they're trying to slim down, but for the rest of their lives.

**STRATEGY FOR CHANGE**

### Eating Light and Right

- Eat at a moderate pace. Your brain may not realize you're full for 20 minutes.
- Be sure not to neglect breakfast—but don't rely too much on all-American favorites like bacon and eggs (high in saturated fat and cholesterol) or presweetened cereals (some of which are more than 50 percent sugar).
- Preplan low-calorie, low-fat meals so moods, weekends, holidays, or schedules don't interfere with your goals.
- Remove all visible fat from meat and all skin from poultry. If you buy oil-packed tuna, rinse it thoroughly to eliminate fat.
- Use a vegetable-oil spray instead of shortening when frying eggs, hash browns, or meats.
- Gradually switch from whole milk to 2 percent; to 1 percent; to skim, or nonfat, milk. Substitute low-fat plain yogurt for sour cream.
- Put tempting high-calorie foods at the back of your freezer and cupboards. Don't leave any fattening foods in sight.
- Place baskets of washed, ready-to-munch fruits in the kitchen, family room, or dining room.
- Keep "bouquets" of celery and carrot sticks in the refrigerator.
- Begin your meals with a salad or soup.
- Use only low-calorie sweeteners and low-calorie salad dressing.
- Serve at least two vegetables, preferably fresh or frozen (without a sauce), at each meal.
- In seasoning foods, switch from sugar to a spice, such as cinnamon or vanilla.
- Gradually reduce the amount of sugar you put in custards, puddings, toppings, muffins, and cookies.
- Grate a carrot and add it in place of some of the sugar in tomato sauces, cakes, and cookies.
- Serve heavy desserts only as a rare treat. Substitute puddings, gelatins, and fruit.

## Changing Your Eating Habits

If you really want to lose your extra pounds, you've got to change the way you eat, as well as what you eat. A simple way to evaluate your diet is by keeping a food diary in which you record everything you eat in a day (see Figure 4-5). At a glance, you should be able to determine whether the four food groups are represented and whether you're getting adequate amounts of essential nutrients. If you aren't, pinpoint the deficiencies in your diet, such as too much fat and too little calcium.

The key to permanent weight control is establishing a way of eating that you can stick to for the rest of your life. You need to learn to eat only when you are hungry, to recognize situations and stresses that lead to overeating, and to eliminate impulse eating. Changing the way you eat is the first step to becoming slim and staying slim for the rest of your life (see Table 4-12).

## Exercise: Your Best Ally

You may think that exercise will make you want to eat more. Actually, it has the opposite effect. In one study of women 10 to 60 percent above their desirable weights, walking at least half an hour a day for a year led to weight losses ranging from 10 to 38 pounds—without any change in their food intake. And exercise helps keep off the pounds you do lose[26] (see Table 4-13).

Exercise also helps dieters lose fat rather than muscle. As you cut back on calories, 20 to 50 percent of the weight loss resulting from dieting by itself is a

**TABLE 4-12** Changing Unhealthy Eating Patterns

| EATING PATTERN | STRATEGY FOR CHANGE |
|---|---|
| *"External" Eater:* You're sensitive to outside cues, so you eat when others around you do—when watching food commercials on TV; when the clock strikes a certain hour, such as noon; or whenever you sit down in your favorite chair. | ■ Learn to recognize what stimulates your desire for food.<br>■ Stop eating by the clock.<br>■ Keep all food out of sight.<br>■ Before taking a single bite, ask yourself why you want something to eat, and eat only when you're genuinely hungry.<br>■ When you eat, sit down, and don't do anything but savor every spoonful. Keep meals independent of all other activities. |
| *The Garbage-Disposal Mentality:* You don't want to waste food. | ■ Start preparing smaller amounts for each meal.<br>■ Always leave one bite on your plate.<br>■ Give leftovers to your dog, or start a compost pile in your backyard.<br>■ Immediately upon serving your allotted portion, store leftovers. If possible, put them in the freezer.<br>■ Once you've finished eating, put a piece of sugarless gum in your mouth.<br>■ Try to get family members to take over the cleanup so you don't sneak snacks from their plates. |
| *Speed Eating:* You snarf down every morsel in sight within minutes. | ■ Time every meal, and don't leave the table for 20 minutes.<br>■ Put down your fork or spoon after each bite.<br>■ Concentrate on chewing. Notice the texture, the taste, the seasonings in your food.<br>■ Work at making your dining room as pleasant as possible, and take time to appreciate it and the people with whom you're dining. |
| *Junk-Food Junkie:* You're addicted to fast foods. | ■ Plan ahead for one fast-food meal every other day, then one every 3 days, then one every week.<br>■ Have only one item, like a hamburger, rather than a complete meal.<br>■ Eat fruit before you go in.<br>■ Treat yourself with a low-calorie dessert if you don't order a shake or pie |
| *The Starve/Stuff Syndrome:* You skip meals, then "pig out" later. | ■ Exercise early in the day so your hunger peaks in the morning or early afternoon.<br>■ Try eating six small meals a day, getting the bulk of your calories at breakfast and lunch.<br>■ If you don't have time for breakfast at home, try a blenderized milk-and-banana shake, or take along an apple or a bran muffin to munch at mid-morning.<br>■ Eat lunch early, and always start with a salad.<br>■ If you must have dinner late, eat lightly and plan a hearty breakfast for the morning. |
| *Boredom:* You eat to pass the time. | ■ Don't keep convenient snacks.<br>■ Follow a snack list, starting with low-calorie items like fresh fruit.<br>■ Do something physical.<br>■ Call up a friend.<br>■ On the brightest-colored paper you can find, make up a list of things to do—some chores, some fun—and post it on the refrigerator or cupboard door or wherever you store goodies.<br>■ Take up a hobby; read one of the books you've always meant to—just don't do it in the kitchen. |
| *Emotional Eater:* You eat because you feel bad or nervous. | ■ Recognize that food is not a cure or a comfort for your problems. Try other outlets; a hot bath, a new record, a quiet walk at sunset.<br>■ If stress drives you to eat, try deep breathing, regular exercise, or relaxation techniques.<br>■ Stay out of the kitchen when you're upset. |

SOURCE: U.S. Department of Agriculture

**TABLE 4-13** Exercise Away Your Calories*

| FOOD | CALORIES | RUNNING, MIN AT 7.5 MPH | SWIMMING, MIN AT 2 MPH | BICYCLING, MIN AT 9.4 MPH | WALKING, MIN AT 3 MPH | AEROBIC DANCING, MIN |
|---|---|---|---|---|---|---|
| **Breakfast Items** | | | | | | |
| Bagel with cream cheese | 265 | 20 | 33 | 42 | 70 | 40 |
| Cereal, dry (¾ cup) | 70 | 5 | 9 | 11 | 18 | 11 |
| English muffin, buttered | 186 | 14 | 23 | 29 | 49 | 28 |
| Fried egg | 115 | 9 | 14 | 18 | 30 | 17 |
| Oatmeal (⅔ cup) | 87 | 7 | 11 | 14 | 23 | 13 |
| Omelette, cheese (6 oz) | 340 | 26 | 42 | 54 | 89 | 52 |
| Pancakes (3) | 180 | 14 | 22 | 28 | 47 | 27 |
| Sweet roll, buttered | 260 | 20 | 32 | 41 | 68 | 39 |
| Waffles (1) | 210 | 16 | 26 | 33 | 55 | 32 |
| **Lunch Foods** | | | | | | |
| Bologna sandwich | 313 | 24 | 39 | 49 | 82 | 47 |
| Cheeseburger (¼ lb) | 518 | 39 | 64 | 82 | 136 | 78 |
| Chili with beans (¾ cup) | 250 | 19 | 31 | 39 | 66 | 38 |
| Club sandwich | 670 | 51 | 83 | 106 | 176 | 102 |
| Grilled cheese sandwich | 350 | 26 | 43 | 55 | 92 | 53 |
| Hamburger (¼ lb) | 418 | 32 | 52 | 66 | 110 | 63 |
| Ham sandwich | 350 | 27 | 43 | 55 | 92 | 53 |
| Pizza (1 slice) | 145 | 11 | 18 | 23 | 38 | 22 |
| Roast beef sandwich | 429 | 33 | 53 | 68 | 113 | 65 |
| **Dinner Foods** | | | | | | |
| Beef Stroganoff (1 cup) | 500 | 38 | 62 | 79 | 132 | 76 |
| Bluefish (3 oz) | 135 | 10 | 17 | 21 | 36 | 20 |
| Burrito, beef | 466 | 35 | 58 | 73 | 123 | 71 |
| Chicken wing, fried | 151 | 11 | 19 | 24 | 40 | 23 |
| Fried shrimp (3 oz) | 190 | 14 | 23 | 30 | 50 | 29 |
| Lamb chop | 360 | 27 | 44 | 57 | 95 | 55 |
| Macaroni and cheese (1 cup) | 430 | 33 | 53 | 68 | 113 | 65 |
| Pork chop | 305 | 23 | 38 | 48 | 80 | 46 |
| Pot roast | 140 | 11 | 17 | 22 | 37 | 21 |
| Spaghetti with sauce (1 cup) | 260 | 20 | 32 | 41 | 69 | 39 |
| **Desserts** | | | | | | |
| Banana split | 540 | 41 | 67 | 85 | 143 | 82 |
| Ice cream, hard (1 cup) | 270 | 20 | 33 | 43 | 71 | 41 |
| Gelatin (1 cup) | 140 | 11 | 17 | 22 | 37 | 21 |
| Pudding, chocolate (1 cup) | 385 | 29 | 48 | 61 | 101 | 58 |
| Sherbet, 2 percent fat (1 cup) | 270 | 20 | 33 | 43 | 71 | 41 |
| **Pies and Cakes** | | | | | | |
| Brownie with nuts | 95 | 7 | 12 | 15 | 25 | 14 |
| Cheesecake (5⁷⁄₁₀ oz) | 400 | 30 | 49 | 63 | 105 | 61 |
| Chocolate cake, iced (1 slice) | 250 | 19 | 31 | 39 | 66 | 38 |
| Cookies (4) | 200 | 15 | 25 | 31 | 53 | 30 |
| Pecan pie (1 slice) | 495 | 38 | 61 | 78 | 130 | 75 |
| Fruit pie | 345 | 26 | 43 | 54 | 91 | 52 |
| **Snacks and Sweets** | | | | | | |
| Candy, hard (1 oz) | 110 | 8 | 14 | 17 | 29 | 17 |
| Chocolate bar (1 oz) | 145 | 11 | 18 | 23 | 38 | 22 |
| French fries (10) | 135 | 10 | 17 | 21 | 36 | 20 |
| Mixed nuts (1 oz) | 180 | 14 | 22 | 28 | 47 | 27 |
| Popcorn, unbuttered (1 cup) | 25 | 2 | 3 | 4 | 7 | 4 |
| Potato chips (1 oz) | 150 | 11 | 19 | 24 | 39 | 23 |

*These calculations are based on a 150-lb individual who burns up 13.2 calories/min running, 8.1 calories/min swimming, 6.35 calories/min bicycling, 3.8 calories/min walking, and 6.6 calories/min dancing.

SOURCE: *Eater's Almanac.*

| Time | Minutes Spent Eating | M or S* | H** | Activity While Eating | Place of Eating | Food and Quantity | Others Present | Feeling Before Eating |
|---|---|---|---|---|---|---|---|---|
| 8:10 a.m. | 17 | M | 1 | standing, fixing lunch | kitchen | 1 c. O.J. 1 c. corn flakes | — | sleepy |
| | | | | | | 1/2 c. whole milk 2 t. sugar | | |
| | | | | | | black coffee | | |
| 10:30 a.m. | 10 | S | 1 | sitting, taking notes | classroom | 12 oz. cola | class | busy |
| 11:45 a.m. | 20 | M | 2 | sitting, talking | union | 1 sandwich 1 apple | friends | good |
| | | | | | | | | |
| 2:30 p.m. | 15 | S | 1 | sitting, studying | library | 12 oz. cola | friend | bored |
| 5:30 p.m. | 15 | M | 3 | sitting, talking | kitchen | 1 chicken leg 1 baked potato | roommate | good |
| | | | | | | 2 T. butter lettuce | | |
| | | | | | | 1 oz. dressing 1 c. whole milk | | |
| | | | | | | 4 cookies | | |
| 8:15 p.m. | 10 | S | 0 | sitting, studying | living room | 12 oz. cola | — | tired |
| | | | | | | | | |

SOURCE: Christian, Janet L. and Janet L. Greger. *Nutrition for Living, Second Edition*, Benjamin/Cummings, 1988.

**FIGURE 4-5** An example of a food diary, showing a day's worth of food intake.

loss of lean muscle tissue, not fat. Exercising builds up muscle tissue and burns off fat stores. You may not lose pounds, because muscle tissue weighs more than fat, but you will lose inches. Exercise also may reprogram your metabolism so that you burn up more calories during *and* after a workout (see Chapter 5).

## MAKING THIS CHAPTER WORK FOR YOU

### Feeding Yourself for a Healthy Future

**You truly are what you eat. Nutrition is the science that explores the connection between food and your health. The basic nutrients required for good health are proteins, carbohydrates, fats, water, vitamins, and**

## WHAT DO YOU THINK?

Luis is a junk-food junkie. His favorite breakfast is an Egg McMuffin, and he grabs a burger, burrito, or pizza for lunch and dinner. Between meals, he snacks on cupcakes and candy bars. He knows he's not eating well, but he says he doesn't have the time or skill to prepare more nutritious meals. What could Luis do to improve his daily diet? What is your worst eating or food habit? Do you want to change it? Why? How could you go about it?

In one study, fat college applicants were less likely to be accepted by top-ranked colleges than thinner students, even when everything else—grades, test scores, and activities—were equal. Do you think there is a bias against obese people? How do you feel when you see an extremely overweight man or women at the beach or at a restaurant? Why do you think you react the way you do?

For Mariette, dieting is a way of life. Ever since her early teens, she's tried every fad diet that's appeared. She always loses weight—and always gains it back. Now she's finding it harder than ever to stay at her ideal weight. What do you think she's doing wrong? What can she do to make sure she loses excess pounds and keeps them off?

minerals. To make sure that you get all the nutrients your body needs, you should include items from the four basic food groups in your daily diet.

By eating with care, you can reduce your risk of developing heart disease and cancer. The key to protecting your heart is eating less fat, particularly saturated fat, and reducing the levels of cholesterol in your blood. One of the best ways to begin eating a "heart smart" diet is to eat more fish, especially in place of red meat. To decrease your chances of developing cancer, limit your fat intake; make sure you get enough fiber; and eat foods that contain vitamins A, C, D, and E.

Some aspects of nutrition have become so controversial that it can be hard to sort out what you should and shouldn't eat. Fiber, the indigestible material in complex carbohydrates, aids digestion and elimination; prevents diverticulosis; is low in calories; and may lessen the risks of certain diseases, such as heart disease, bowel cancer, and diabetes. Sugar, high in calories and low in nutrients, can cause tooth decay. Artificial sweeteners, no- or low-calorie sugar substitutes, may have health risks. Vitamin C may have an effect on cold symptoms, atherosclerosis, male infertility, gum disease, and iron-deficiency anemia. Fast foods do supply nutrients but often are high in calories, fat, and sodium. The best way to become a smart nutrition consumer is to use common sense. Don't believe everything you hear or read about new products and never rely on fad foods to keep you healthy.

Many Americans, concerned with the safety of their foods, are choosing organic foods grown without chemicals and produced without additives—substances added to foods to increase their storage time or to alter their taste or appearance. Lacto-vegetarians avoid all meat but do eat dairy products. Ovo-lacto-vegetarians eat eggs as well as dairy products. Vegans eat only plant foods.

Many Americans worry as much about what they weigh as about what they eat. A person's ideal weight depends on his or her genetic makeup, height, age, eating habits, and amount of exercise. Although the most popular method of determining ideal weight is simply to refer to the weight charts published by the insurance industry, a more useful method is by measuring body fat.

When more calories are taken in than are used, the body converts the extra calories to fat. Mild obesity occurs when an individual is 20 to 40 percent above his or her ideal weight. An individual who is 41 to 100 percent above ideal weight is moderately obese, and a person who is more than 100 percent above ideal weight is severely obese.

Obese people are at risk for developing high blood pressure, diabetes, heart disease, certain kinds of cancer, and other life-threatening conditions. Severely obese people can be treated by stomach-reduction surgery; moderately and mildly obese individuals do best with diet and behavioral modification. Increasingly, Americans are turning away from fad diets and changing the way they eat. A lifelong change in unhealthy eating patterns and an increase in physical activity can control weight and enhance health.

If you decide to lose weight, set a realistic goal. Subtract your target weight from your actual weight and calculate how long it will take you to lose the difference, based on a weekly loss of 1 1/2 pounds. You didn't put those pounds on overnight, and you shouldn't expect to lose them overnight. Rather than looking for a crash diet, develop a plan, following these steps:

- *Make the commitment.* Join a group, such as Weight Watchers or Overeaters Anonymous, or sign up with a well-supervised health club or gym.
- *Keep a diary.* Keeping a diary for a week or two enables you to identify your eating and exercising patterns. Include in your diary all meals; snacks; and drinks; and all types of exercise, such as walking to class, climbing three flights of stairs, or bicycling.
- *Establish your goals.* Work at changing your eating habits along the lines given in this chapter, so that you have the right balance of protein, fat, and carbohydrates. But remember: Unless you change your eating habits *and* enjoy the food you eat, this program will not be any better than any other fad diet.
- *Watch your progress.* Continue your food diary and note any particular problems that need attention. Weigh yourself once a week, and be sure to reward yourself at the end of every week for the progress you have achieved.
- *Set a "danger" range—a weight 3 or 4 pounds above your desired weight.* Once you've reached your desired weight, don't let your weight climb above your danger range. If you hit your upper weight limit, take action immediately. If you let your weight continue to creep up, it may not stop until you have a serious weight problem—again.

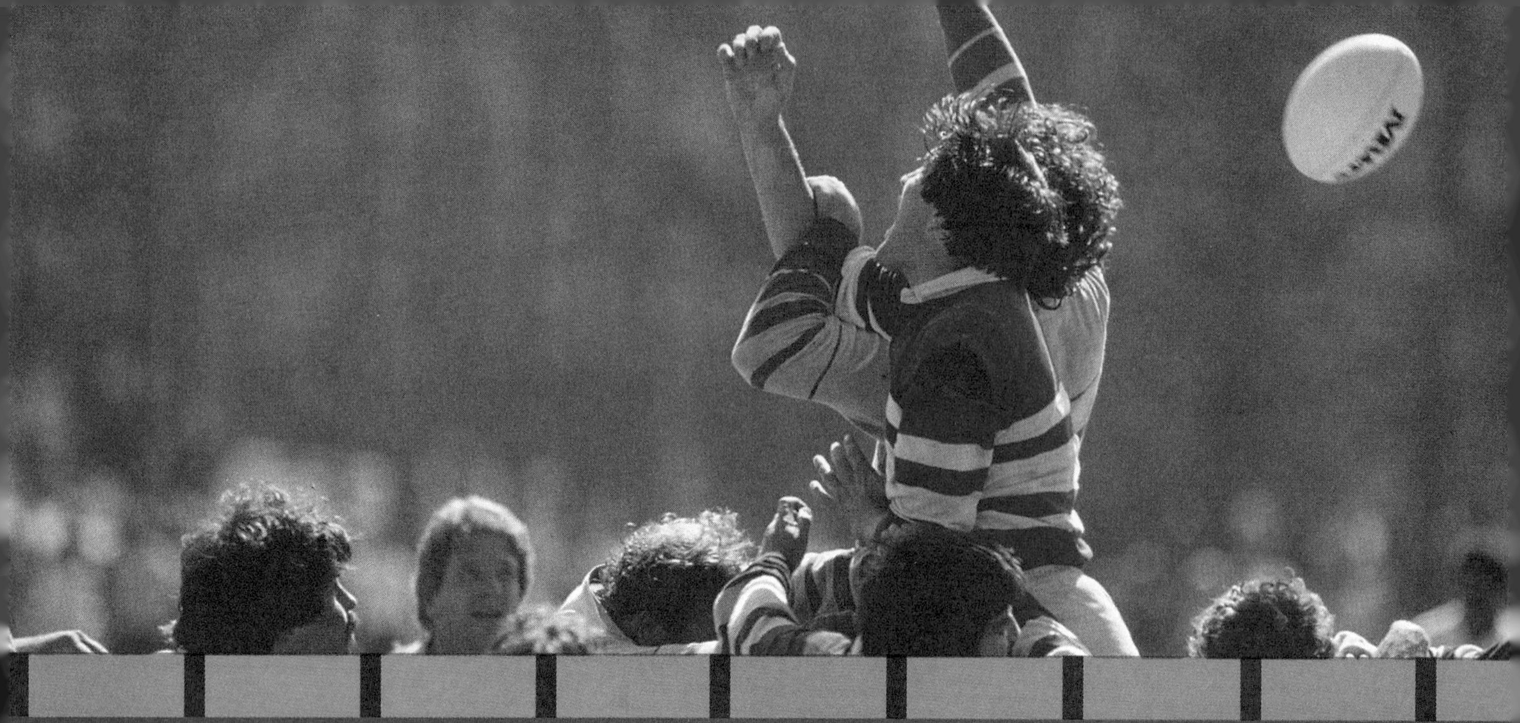

# 5 THE JOY OF FITNESS

In this chapter

What is physical fitness?

Flexibility

Cardiovascular or aerobic fitness

Muscular strength and endurance

Why exercise?

Men, women, and exercise

Nutrition for exercisers

Preventing problems

Making this chapter work for you: Shaping up

*Fitness means living in a body that's firm, flexible, strong, and responsive.* The payoffs of fitness include more energy, a hardier heart, a brighter outlook, and a trimmer torso. You don't have to exercise to the point of exhaustion or obsession to become fit. In fact, exercise should be enjoyable. This chapter describes various types of exercise, provides guidelines for getting into shape, and explains the benefits of different ways of working out.

## WHAT IS PHYSICAL FITNESS?

**Physical fitness** is the ability to meet routine physical demands, with enough extra energy to meet a sudden challenge. Fitness means your body will operate at maximum capacity for as many years as you live.[1]

Although every individual may think of fitness differently, there are three basic components: flexibility; cardiovascular, or aerobic, fitness; and muscular strength and endurance.

**Flexibility** is the range of motion that your joints allow—for example, the stretching you do to touch your toes. Flexibility depends on your age, sex, and posture; bone spurs; and how fat or muscular you are. Both muscles and connective tissue, such as tendons and ligaments, shorten with age. If they are not used at all or not used through their full range of motion, they can reduce flexibility. Women tend to be more flexible than men because of differences in their skeletons, muscle mass, and body composition, and because they tend to do more flexibility exercises.

**Cardiovascular fitness**—the ability of the heart to pump blood through the body efficiently—improves with **aerobic exercise** (any activity, such as brisk walking or swimming, in which the amount of oxygen taken into the body is slightly more than, or equal to, the amount of oxygen used by the body). In aerobic exercise, you work hard but avoid pushing to the point of breathlessness. **Anaerobic exercise** is activity in which the amount of oxygen taken in cannot meet the requirement of the work, and you literally run out of breath. An example is sprinting the quarter mile, which leaves even the best-trained athletes gasping for air. **Nonaerobic exercise** is a term used for sports with frequent rest periods—sports such as golf, bowling, softball, and doubles tennis. The body easily takes in all the oxygen needed for these activities, so the heart and lungs don't get a workout.

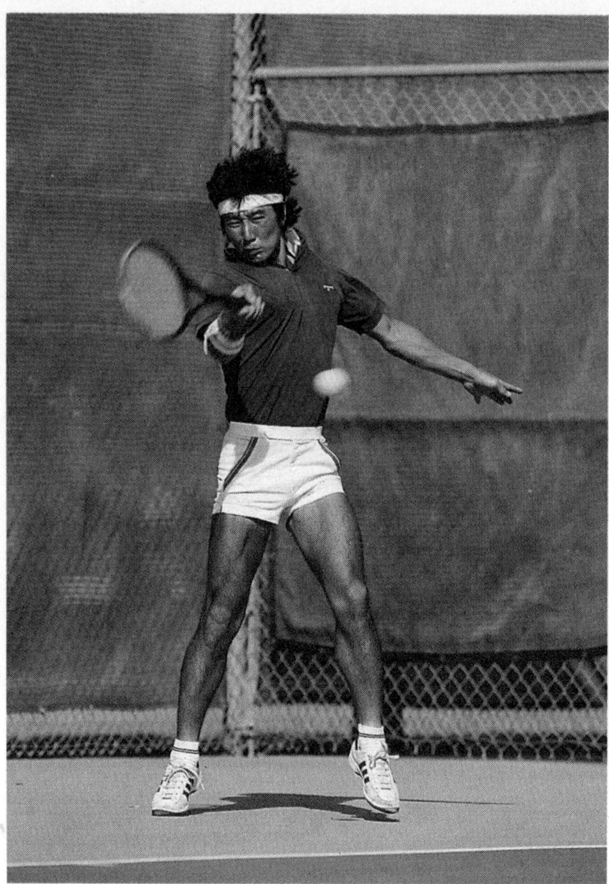

Tennis and other popular sports can be part of a total fitness program.

Most of us equate muscular fitness with **strength**—that is, with the absolute maximum weight that we can lift, push, or press in one effort. However, **endurance**—the ability to keep lifting, pushing, or

**physical fitness** A state of well-being in which a person has enough energy to meet daily needs as well as unexpected challenges.
**flexibility** The range of motion allowed by one's joints; determined by the length of muscles, tendons, and ligaments attached to the joints.
**cardiovascular fitness** The ability of the heart and blood vessels to work efficiently.
**aerobic exercise** Exercise requiring oxygen; exercise in which sufficient or excess oxygen is continually supplied to the body.
**anaerobic exercise** Exercise not using oxygen for energy production; exercise in which the body develops an oxygen deficit.
**nonaerobic exercise** Exercise in which the activity does not require extra effort by the heart and lungs to take in more oxygen.
**strength** Physical power; the maximum weight one can lift, push, or press in one effort.
**endurance** The ability to withstand the stress of physical exertion.

pressing—is just as important. You not only have to be strong enough to hoist a shovelful of snow, you've got to keep shoveling until the entire driveway is clear. Physical **conditioning,** or **training,** refers to the gradual building up of the body to enhance any aspect of fitness.

## FLEXIBILITY

Flexibility can protect you from injuries during exercise or daily activities. The key is stretching. But you have to start slow and keep at it, day by day.

Like a body yawn, stretching will loosen you up, and soothe and relax you. As part of your total fitness program, it can lengthen your muscles and help your coordination by increasing the range of motion of your joints.

Although stretching is one of the safest activities, it's important that you do it right so you don't end up hurting instead of helping yourself. **Static stretching,** or **passive stretching**—the safest way to stretch—consists of a relaxed, gradual stretch that you hold for a short time (6 to 60 seconds). To feel an example of such a stretch, let your hands slowly slide down the front of your straightened legs until you reach your toes; hold this final position for several seconds before straightening up.

**Ballistic stretching,** by comparison, uses rapid bouncing or jerking movements, such as the series of up-and-down bobs as you try again and again to touch your toes with your hands. These bounces can stretch muscle fibers too far; this causes the muscle to tighten rather than stretch.

When you stretch, you should never feel pain, though you should feel some discomfort as you extend your stretch. Reach to the point of discomfort and then back off slightly, relaxing and allowing your muscles to adjust for 20 to 30 seconds. You should hold this stretch until the feeling of tension diminishes. Concentrate on the feeling of the stretch itself, not on the flexibility you want to attain. (See Figure 5-1 for simple, effective stretches.)

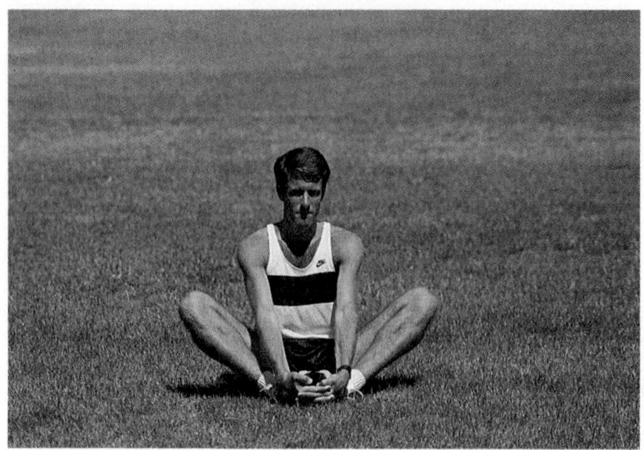

a

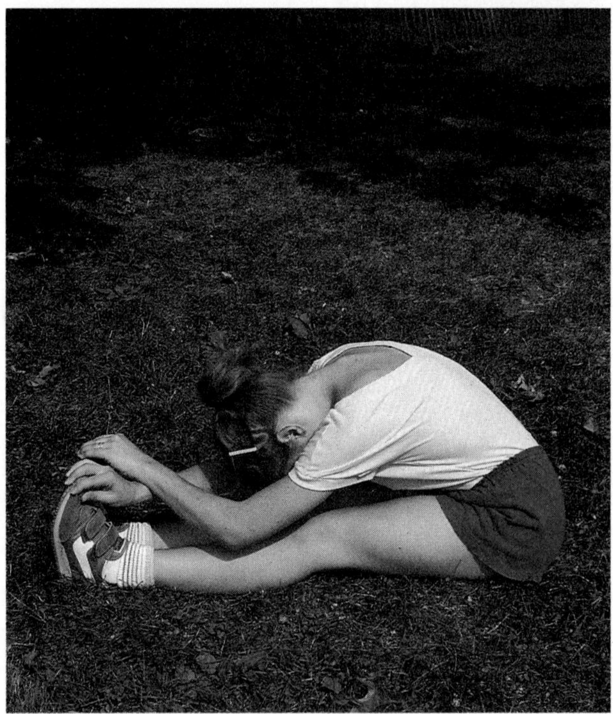

b

**FIGURE 5-1** These exercises will increase your flexibility **(a) Foot pull** (groin muscles and thighs)—Sit on the floor. Bend your legs so that the soles of your feet touch. Pull on your feet while pressing your knees down with your elbows. Hold for 10 seconds; repeat. **(b) Seated toe touch** (back and hamstring muscles)—Sit on the floor with your legs stretched out in front of you. Point your toes, and slide your hands down your legs until you feel the stretch. Holding this position, slowly lean forward and try to touch your toes. Hold for 10 seconds; repeat.

**conditioning** In sports, to bring one's body to a state of physical fitness.
**training** See *conditioning.*
**static stretching** A relaxed slow stretch held for 6 to 60 seconds.
**passive stretching** See *static stretching.*
**ballistic stretching** A potentially hazardous form of stretching that involves bouncing or jerking; can cause the muscles to contract rather than stretch.

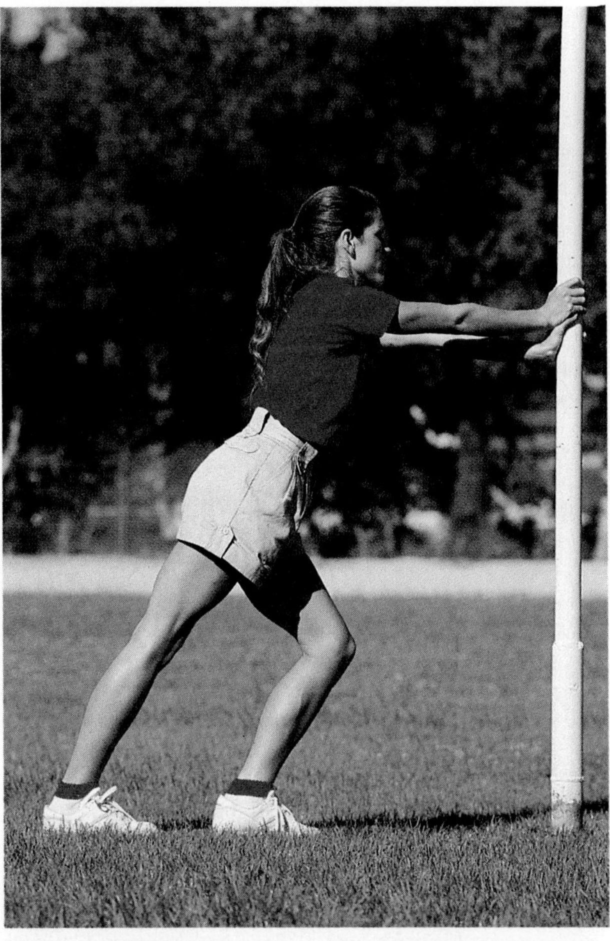

c

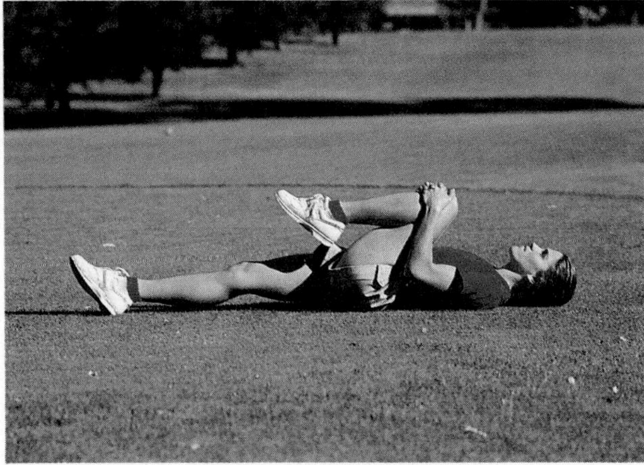

d

**(c) Wall stretch** (Achilles tendon)—Stand 3 feet from a wall with your feet slightly apart; put your hands flat on the wall. Keeping your heels on the ground, slowly lean forward. Hold for 10 seconds; repeat. **(d) Knee-chest pull** (lower back muscles)—While lying on your back, clasp one knee and pull it to your chest. Hold for 15 to 30 seconds; repeat with other knee.

**STRATEGY FOR CHANGE**

**Safe Stretching**

- Before you begin stretching, increase your body temperature by slowly running in place. Cold muscles are vulnerable to injury. Sweat signals that you're ready to start stretching.
- Don't force body parts to the point of pain or shaking.
- Do a minimum of five repetitions of each exercise.
- Continue breathing slowly and rhythmically throughout your stretch routines.
- To increase or maintain overall flexibility, stretch every muscle group or joint.
- Remember that exercises that don't create "stretch demand" (muscle lengthening beyond normal resting length) won't help.
- Perform stretching exercises regularly. "Use it or lose it" is the motto to keep in mind.
- Don't do any stretches that require deep knee bends or full squats. These positions can harm your knees and lower back.

## CARDIOVASCULAR OR AEROBIC FITNESS

Aerobics—regular exercise that strengthens the heart and lungs by boosting the body's consumption of oxygen—has brought the entire country to its feet. Millions of Americans of all sizes and ages are running, cycling, swimming, and sweating as if their lives depend on it—and to a remarkable extent, they do.

To get the full benefits of aerobic activity, you have to exercise hard, long, and often enough. How hard depends on the shape you're in. If you haven't been exercising regularly, even mild forms of exertion, such as a brisk walk, can seem rigorous. As you get in shape, your body will be able to handle much greater challenges.

### Your Target Heart Rate

The best way of making sure that you're working hard enough to condition your heart and lungs but not overdoing it is to use your pulse, or heart rate, as a guide. One of the easiest places to feel your pulse is in the carotid artery in the neck (see Figure 5-2). Tilt your head back slightly and to one side. Use your middle finger or forefinger or both to feel for your pulse. (Don't use your thumb, because it has a beat of its own.) To determine your heart rate, count the number of pulses for 10 seconds and multiply that number by 6 or count for 30 seconds and multiply by 2. Learn to recognize the pulsing of your heart when you are lying or sitting down. On your fitness record, make note of your **resting heart rate**—that is, the number of heartbeats per minute during inactivity.

Start taking your pulse during, or immediately after, exercise, when it is much more pronounced than when at rest. Three minutes after heavy exercise, take your pulse again. The closer that reading is to your resting pulse rate, the better your condition. If it takes a long time for your recovery pulse to return to resting level, your body's ability to handle physical stress is poor. As you continue working out, your pulse will return to normal much more quickly.

You don't want to push yourself to your maximum heart rate; yet you must exercise at about 60 to 85 percent of the maximum to get the benefits of training. This range is called your **target heart rate.** If you don't exercise intensely enough to raise your pulse at least to your target heart rate, your heart and lungs won't benefit from the workout. If you push too hard and aim for your absolute maximum, you run the risk of placing too great a burden on your heart. Table 5-1 lists target and maximum heart rates for various ages. You can also use the formulas in Table 5-2.

In the initial stages of training, aim for the lower part of your target zone (60 percent of your maximum), and gradually build up to 75 percent of your maximum heart rate. After six months or more of regular exercise, you can push up to 85 percent if you wish, though you don't have to work that hard just to stay in condition. As long as you use your target heart rate as your guide, your exercise intensity should be just right.

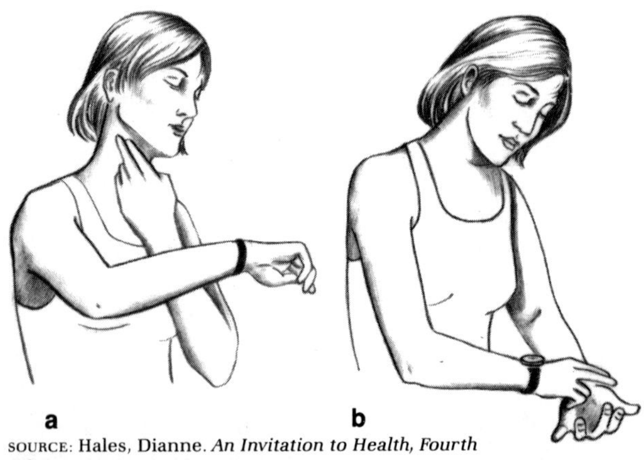


SOURCE: Hales, Dianne. *An Invitation to Health, Fourth Edition,* Benjamin/Cummings, 1989.

**FIGURE 5-2** You can take your pulse **(a)** at one of the carotid arteries in your neck (on either side of your Adam's apple) or **(b)** at your wrist.

**TABLE 5-1** Target Heart Rate

| | Beats per Minute | |
|---|---|---|
| AGE | AVERAGE MAXIMUM RATE (100%) | TARGET RATE (60%–75%) |
| 20 | 200 | 120–150 |
| 25 | 195 | 117–146 |
| 30 | 190 | 114–142 |
| 35 | 185 | 111–138 |
| 40 | 180 | 108–135 |
| 45 | 175 | 105–131 |
| 50 | 170 | 102–127 |
| 55 | 165 | 99–123 |
| 60 | 160 | 96–120 |
| 65 | 155 | 93–116 |
| 70 | 150 | 90–113 |

**TABLE 5-2** Calculation of Target Heart Rate per Minute

| **MEN:** | |
|---|---|
| **EXAMPLE FOR A 20-YEAR-OLD** | |
| All men start here | 220 |
| Subtract your age | − 20 |
| Maximum heart rate | 200 |
| Target rate for beginners | × .60 |
| Target heart rate | 120 |
| **WOMEN:** | |
| **EXAMPLE FOR A 20-YEAR-OLD** | |
| All women start here | 225 |
| Subtract your age | − 20 |
| Maximum heart rate | 205 |
| Target rate for beginners | × .60 |
| Target heart rate | 123 |

## How Much Is Enough?

Once you're working hard enough, you have to keep it up. Dr. Kenneth Cooper—the father of aerobics, who did some of the initial research on cardiovascular fitness—found that you need to work out at your target heart rate for at least 15 to 20 minutes a session to produce real benefits for your heart.[2]

If you exercise just once or twice a week, you can increase your aerobic capacity (your body's ability to use oxygen) by about 8 percent. If you work out three times a week—the minimum recommended by the American College of Sports Medicine—your aerobic capacity should improve by 15 percent. Four weekly workouts should produce a 25 percent improvement.

**resting heart rate** The number of heartbeats per minute during inactivity.
**target heart rate** A rate 60 to 85 percent of the maximum heart rate; the heart rate at which one derives maximum benefit from aerobic exercise.

Beyond a certain point, risks outdistance benefits. The primary hazard is injury. Exercising more than five times a week triples the injury rate in amateur athletes, and increasing exercise sessions from 30 to 45 minutes doubles the risk.

**STRATEGY FOR CHANGE**

### Designing Your Aerobic Workout

To some people, aerobics is running. To others, it's dancing. To yet others, it's a fast game of racquetball. These activities and many more (see Table 5-3) can be aerobic, as long as you follow the guidelines for exercising hard, long, and often enough. Whichever exercise you choose, your aerobic workout should follow this pattern:

- *For 5 minutes.* Warm up to elevate body temperature and prepare your body for more vigorous exercise. Jogging in place is an ideal warm-up.
- *For 5 to 10 minutes.* Stretch to loosen your muscles and prevent injuries.
- *For at least 20 minutes.* Exercise at your target heart rate.
- *For 5 minutes.* Cool down by moving more slowly.
- *For 5 to 10 minutes.* Stretch to prevent soreness the day after you exercise.

Figure 5-3 shows how the heart rate should change in a well-designed aerobic exercise program. Whatever you do, start slowly.

## Fitness Walking

If you do it fast and often enough, walking can do more than get you from one place to another. The American College of Sports Medicine suggests a 35-mile-a-week minimum, the equivalent of 3,500 calories, for walkers.[3]

How fast you go is as important as how far. Three or four times a week, you should walk at least 20 to 30 minutes at a pace that pushes your heart rate up to your target range. If you want more of a challenge, go farther, faster, or uphill.

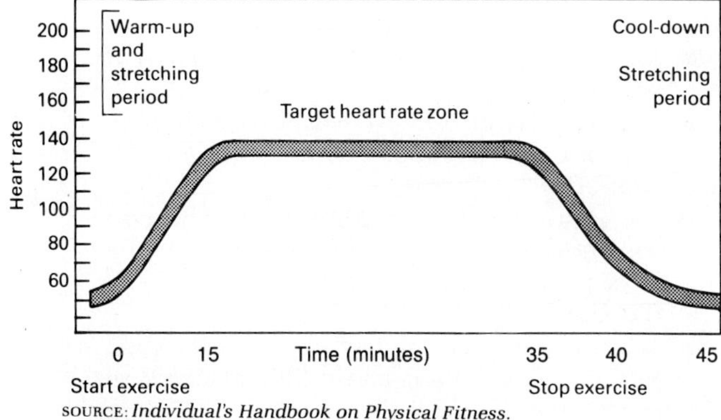


SOURCE: *Individual's Handbook on Physical Fitness.*

**FIGURE 5-3** This graph shows the changes in heart rate during an aerobic workout.

**TABLE 5-3** Aerobic Equivalents

| ACTIVITY | CALORIES PER MINUTE | EXERCISE EQUIVALENTS, MINUTES |
|---|---|---|
| Handball/squash | 16.7 | 22 |
| Skiing, cross-country | 16.7 | 22 |
| Running | 12.0 | 30 |
| Skating, ice or roller | 10.7 | 34 |
| Skiing, downhill | 9.0 | 40 |
| Swimming | 8.3 | 43 |
| Tennis | 8.3 | 43 |
| Dancing, aerobic | 8.3 | 43 |
| Cycling | 6.7 | 54 |
| Golf | 5.0 | 72 |
| Softball | 4.7 | 77 |
| Walking | 4.0 | 90 |
| Bowling | 2.5 | 144 |

SOURCE: President's Council on Physical Fitness.

**STRATEGY FOR CHANGE**

### Putting Your Best Foot Forward

- To avoid strain, always begin with a warm-up to limber your muscles.
- Walk very slowly for 5 minutes. Then do some simple stretches, such as the hamstring stretch (see Figure 5-1).
- Wear walking shoes that provide adequate support and cushioning.
- Maintain good posture. Focus your eyes ahead of you, stand erect, and pull in your stomach.
- Use the heel-and-toe method of walking. The heel of your leading foot should touch the ground before the ball of the foot or the toes. When you push off with the trailing foot, bend your knee as you raise your heel. You should be able to feel the action in the calf muscles.
- Pump your arms back and forth to burn up more calories.
- Walk at a comfortable pace. A good rule of thumb is making sure you can talk as you walk.
- End your walk the way you started it—slowly. Let your pace become more leisurely for the last 5 minutes.

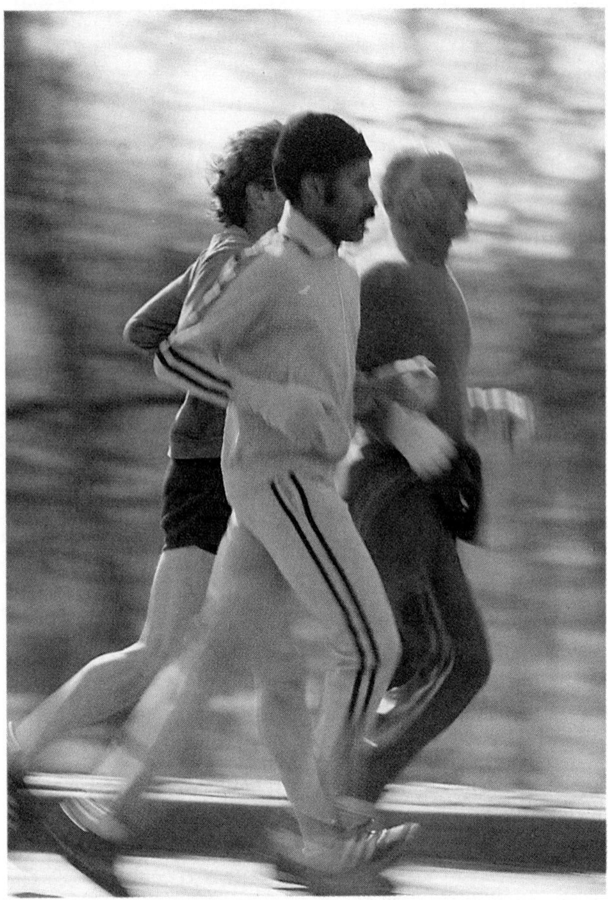

Jogging helps strengthen the heart and lungs, boost stamina and improve circulation.

## Jogging and Running

If you can walk, you can probably jog; if you can jog, you can run. (The difference between jogging and running is speed. If you move at a pace slower than 9 minutes a mile, you're a jogger. If you go faster, you're a runner.) However, there are different forms of jogging or running.

**Long, slow distance (LSD) running** is noncompetitive running over fairly long distances. It can be a training method or an end in itself. **Interval training** consists of repeated hard runs or sprints over a certain distance, with intervals of relaxed jogging in between. Depending on what suits you, you can vary the distance, duration, and number of fast runs, as well as the time and activity between them. According to recent studies, interval training can dramatically improve cardiovascular endurance and overall fitness.[4]

**long, slow distance (LSD) running** Noncompetitive running at a slow pace over fairly long distances.
**interval training** An aerobic conditioning method that involves repeated hard runs over a certain distance, with intervals of relaxed jogging in between.

If you've never run regularly before, start by walking for 15 to 20 minutes, three times a week. Walk at a comfortable pace, but don't overdo it. Continue at the same level until you don't feel sore or unduly fatigued the day after exercising. Then increase your walking time to 20 to 25 minutes, speeding up your pace too. When you can handle a brisk 25-minute walk, alternate fast walking with slow jogging. Begin each session walking, and gradually increase the amount of time you spend jogging. If you feel breathless while jogging, slow down and walk. Continue to alternate until you can jog for 10 minutes without stopping.

Conditioning expands the physical capacity of your heart and lungs. The following general guidelines can help you get the most out of your efforts:

- Gradually increase your jogging time by 1 or 2 minutes with each workout, until you build up from 10 to 20 or 25 minutes.
- Make sure you jog at least three times a week.
- Gradually increase your speed: Aim for 2.5 miles in 25 to 30 minutes.
- If you run out of breath, slow down; you're training too hard.
- If you feel tired and sore the day after exercising, you're going too fast or too far; cut back on your exercise work load.
- To maintain your aerobic fitness, don't let three days pass without exercising.[5]

**STRATEGY FOR CHANGE**

### Running Right

- As you run, keep your back straight and your head up. Run tall, with your buttocks tucked in.
- Look straight ahead. Hold your arms slightly away from your body. Your elbows should be bent slightly so that your forearms are almost parallel to the ground.
- Move your arms rhythmically to propel yourself along.
- Cup your hands loosely, with fingers touching your running shorts as they swing with your stride.
- Have your heel hit the ground first. Land on your heel, rock forward, and push off the ball of your foot. If this is difficult, try a more flat-footed style.
- Avoid running on the ball of your foot; this produces soreness because the muscles must contract for a longer time.
- To avoid shinsplints (a dull ache in the lower shins), stretch regularly to strengthen the

shin muscles and to develop greater flexibility in your ankle.
- Avoid running on hard surfaces and making sudden stops or turns.
- Breathe through your nose and mouth to get more volume. Learn to "belly breathe": When you breathe in, your belly should expand; when you breathe out, it should flatten. If your breathing becomes labored, try exhaling with resistance through pursed lips so that your body utilizes more oxygen per breath.
- When you approach a hill, shorten your stride. Lift your knees higher; pump your arms more. If the hill is really steep, lean forward. When you start downhill, lean forward, and run as if you were on a flat surface. Don't lean back, because this can strain your knees and the muscles in your legs.

## Swimming

More than 100 million Americans dive into the water every year. What matters for their heart's health is getting a workout, not just getting wet. Swimming is an excellent exercise for cardiovascular fitness and rates fairly high for weight control, muscular function, and flexibility.

For aerobic conditioning, you have to swim laps, using a crawl, butterfly, breast-, or backstroke. (The sidestroke is too easy.) You need to be a good enough swimmer to keep churning through the water for at least 20 minutes. Your heart will beat more slowly in water than on land, so your heart rate is not an accurate guide to exercise intensity. Try to keep up a steady pace that's fast enough to make you feel pleasantly tired, but not completely exhausted, by the time you get out of the pool.

**STRATEGY FOR CHANGE**

**Smart Swimming**

- Start by swimming 50 yards and rest when you feel breathless.
- Try to swim 100 yards, rest for a minute, and then swim another 100 yards.
- Increase your weekly yardage slowly, and work up to 700 yards in 18 minutes.
- Stick to the crawl, the butterfly, the back-, or breaststroke.

## Cycling

Bicycling, indoors and out, can be an excellent cardiovascular conditioner, as well as an effective way to control weight—if you aren't just along for the ride. A 10-speed bike or a mountain bike can make pedaling too easy, unless you choose gears carefully. If you often coast down hills, you'll have to ride longer on level ground for effective results.

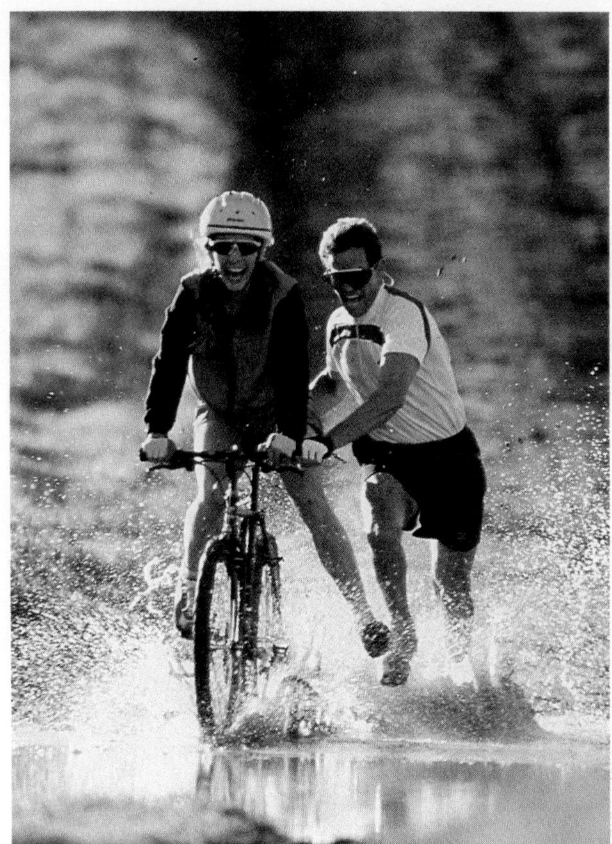

Cycling is a way of staying fit and having fun.

With a one-wheel stationary cycle with a tension-control knob, you can adjust the amount of effort required. Start with low resistance, and increase it until you're working at your target heart rate.[6] You can put the cycle in front of a television set if you feel the need for some "scenery."

**STRATEGY FOR CHANGE**

**Smart Cycling**

- If you're not used to cycling, start slowly. Limit your rides to 20 to 30 minutes for the first week.
- Increase your time and speed gradually so that you avoid sore thigh muscles. Rest when you feel breathless.
- Work up from 5 minutes of steady pedaling (interrupted by rest periods if necessary) to 10, 15, 20, and 25 minutes.
- Keep your elbows slightly bent to allow for a more relaxed upper body. Change your hand position periodically to avoid numbness.
- Monitor your heart rate to make sure you're working within your target range.

## HALES INDEX

Percentage of Americans aware of the value of regular exercise: 66

Percentage of U.S. population exercising moderately for 20 minutes three or more days a week: 50

Percentage of people who drop out of an exercise program within six months: 50

Percentage of people who cannot do at least ten sit-ups: 56

Primary reason why college students exercise: To improve appearance

Number of companies with an employee exercise area: 1 in 4

Number of Americans who do low-impact aerobics: 13.9 million

Fastest-growing form of aerobic exercise in 1990s: Stair-climbing

Minutes of running at 7.5 mph needed to burn off the calories in one slice of pizza: 11

Number of minutes of walking at 3 mph: 38

Number of minutes of aerobic dancing: 22

Value of black-market steroids sold by drug dealers each year: $100 million

Amount Americans spend on home-exercise equipment each year: $1.4 billion

SOURCES: **1, 2** "New Rules of Exercise," *U.S. News and World Report Health & Nutrition,* 1989. **3** "Shaping Up," *U.S. News and World Report,* May 29, 1989. **4** "The Non-Census," *USA Weekend,* March 16–18, 1990. **5** University of Alabama poll of 300 students. **6** Freudenheim, Milt. "Assessing the Corporate Fitness Craze," *New York Times,* March 14, 1990. **7** American Sports Data Institute, 1989 survey. Morain, Claudia. "The Future of Fitness," *San Francisco Chronicle,* January 29, 1990. **8** Williams, Linda. "America Goes Stair Crazy," *Time,* December 18, 1989. **9, 10, 11** *Eaters' Almanac,* U.S. Department of Agriculture. **12** Kashkin, K. B. and H. D. Kleber. "Hooked on Hormones?," *Journal of the American Medical Association,* January 11, 1990. **13** "The Great Home-Fitness Craze," *New York Times Magazine,* October 8, 1989.

## Skipping Rope

Skipping rope is excellent both as a heart conditioner and as a way of losing weight.[7] As with jogging and running, you should monitor your pulse rate, particularly when you first take up the activity. You should also warm up well and then stretch before you begin skipping. Try skipping to music, and vary the steps. Skip with both feet together, alternate your left and right feet, or jump up and down on one leg.

### STRATEGY FOR CHANGE

#### Jump with Joy

- Don't jump rope if you're more than 25 pounds overweight or if you have heart, circulatory, back, or joint problems.
- Vary your jumping style every few jumps to reduce stress on your ankle joints: Jump on your right foot, left foot, then both.
- Jump on cushioned surfaces, such as a hardwood floor or padded carpet, not on concrete or tiled floors.
- Wear athletic shoes that provide shock absorption and good arch support.

## Aerobic Dancing

Almost any kind of dancing is good exercise, but to shape up, consider a form of aerobic dance. You can choose from dozens of books, records, and videotapes; group classes are available on most campuses and in most communities across the country.

Aerobic dance combines music and kicking, bending, and jumping, to deliver the same benefits as running, bicycling, or swimming. A typical hour class (you can also dance at home) may consist of stretching exercises and sit-ups, followed by aerobic dances and cool-down exercises. Beginners start at exercise levels comparable to walking and progress to more vigorous levels resembling running or cycling. Aerobic classes usually emphasize safe and constant movement rather than dance skill. And most aerobic dancers enjoy the sound and stimulation of the music.

The American College of Sports Medicine recommends that, to get the most benefit from workouts, aerobic dancers follow these guidelines:

- Train 3 to 5 days a week.
- Work at 60 to 90 percent of maximum heart rate.
- Keep moving for 20 to 60 minutes at a time.
- Move all the large muscle groups—arms, legs, and back.

Aerobics can be good for the heart but hard on the body, particularly the joints and feet. Fitness experts have developed a safer approach, called low-impact aerobics. Low-impact aerobics replaces jogging and jumping with steps that don't jeopardize the joints. As long as exercisers work out at their target heart rates, they get all the benefits of high-impact aerobics.[8]

You can enroll in low-impact aerobics classes or use videotapes to exercise on your own. The routines call for rhythmic, continuous motion without bouncing. You'll do sidesteps, marches, and dance-walk combinations.

Even easier on muscles, joints, and bones is a new approach called "non-impact aerobics," that combines techniques of modern dance and martial arts in pain-free, cardiovascular workouts.

### Stair-climbing

An estimated 4 million Americans are stepping up to fitness, according to the American Sports Data Institute, and stair-climbing has become the hottest aerobic activity of the 1990s.[9] Men who climb more than five flights a day have 25 percent fewer heart attacks than those who rely on elevators or escalators to take them where they want to go.

The basic conditioning principles for any aerobic workout apply to stair-climbing. The session should include a warm-up, continuous activity for at least 20 minutes, and a cool-down. You could run up the stairs in an office building or dormitory, but most people use step-climbing machines in gyms and health clubs. (Versions of the machines are also available for the home.) On most, exercisers push a pair of pedals up and down while a computerized screen translates their efforts into "flights" climbed. A major advantage of stair-climbing is that it's easier on the feet and legs than many other aerobic activities.

**STRATEGY FOR CHANGE**

**Psyching Yourself Up to Get in Shape**

- Get a buddy. If you can't find a partner, join a group or class.
- Choose an activity you genuinely enjoy, such as aerobic dancing or bicycling. (See Table 5-4 for America's favorites.)
- Sign up for fun runs or charity walks—events that add extra enjoyment to working out.
- Set realistic goals. If you try to swim 30 laps the first time you jump into the pool, you may get too discouraged to dive in again.
- Aim for a small goal, reward yourself when you achieve it, and then set your sights a little higher.
- Find the best time in the day for a workout. Some people like to start the day with exercise; others prefer to exercise later to work off tension. Try both and see which you prefer.
- Vary your exercise routine. If you get tired of one activity, switch to another—at least temporarily.
- Keep track of your progress. In a diary or on your calendar, make notes on each session. Look back every 2 weeks to see how far you've come.
- Line up some cheerleaders. Let your friends and family know what you're trying to accomplish and why.
- Commit yourself to sticking to your new exercise routine for a minimum of eight weeks. By then, you may have the exercise "habit" and won't want to stop.

## MUSCULAR STRENGTH AND ENDURANCE

Aerobic workouts don't exercise many of the muscles that provide power when you need it—and muscular strength and endurance are critical for handling everyday burdens, like pulling a 40-pound stereo speaker from the back of a car.

**TABLE 5-4** Americans' Favorite Sports

| | PARTICIPANTS OLDER THAN 6 YEARS (IN MILLIONS) |
|---|---|
| Volleyball | 37.2 |
| Basketball | 36.1 |
| Stationary cycling | 36.0 |
| Running | 33.0 |
| Fitness walking | 29.7 |
| Fitness cycling | 27.9 |
| Free weights | 27.2 |
| Swimming | 24.7 |
| Golf | 22.4 |
| Tennis | 21.0 |
| Resistance machines | 16.8 |
| Downhill skiing | 15.8 |
| Low-impact aerobics | 13.9 |
| High-impact aerobics | 13.2 |
| Cross-country skiing | 7.4 |
| Treadmill machines | 6.1 |
| Stair-climbing | 2.8 |
| Mountain biking | 2.0 |

SOURCE: American Sports Data Institute, 1989 survey.

SELF-SURVEY

## How Fit Are You?

This self-survey is based on the National Fitness Test developed by the President's Council on Physical Fitness and Sports. You can determine your fitness level by doing the exercises described here.

For this test, you will need a partner to assist or time you. Keep track of your results; then see the accompanying table to find out how you rate.

***Push-ups***

*Women:* Place your hands on the floor, directly under your shoulders, and bend your knees. Keep your shoulders, back, and buttocks straight. Bend your elbows until your chest touches the floor.

*Men:* Position yourself the same as for women but keep your legs straight. Lower yourself until your chest touches your partner's upright fist.

Do as many push-ups as you can, without stopping, for a maximum of 90 seconds or until you reach the top number for your age group (see the accompanying table).

***Curls***

Lie on your back with your knees bent. Place your hands on your thighs or on the floor. Raise your head, followed by your shoulders and then upper trunk. At the same time, lift your hands until your fingertips touch the middle of your kneecap; then return your upper trunk, shoulders, and head to the floor. Do as many as you can for a maximum of 90 seconds or until you reach the top number for your age group.

***Sit and Reach***

Place a piece of tape on the floor. Sit with your legs extended and your heels about 5 inches apart. Make sure that your soles are touching the near edge of the tape. Place a yardstick between your legs; make sure that the 15-inch mark is on the near edge of the tape. Keeping your knees straight, slowly reach forward with both hands as far as you can. Have your partner read the yardstick to see how far you reach.

***Three-Minute Step Test***

Step up onto a 12-inch block or bench by bringing up one foot, then the other. Then step down by bringing one foot down, then the other. You *must* do 24 full steps a minute for 3 minutes. Sit down immediately after finishing. Five seconds after you finish the exercise, have your partner count your heart rate for 1 minute.

***Arm Hang***

With your legs straight and feet clearing the ground, grasp the bar with your palms facing forward. Hang as long as you can or until you reach the top time for your age group.

***Your Results***

The following scorecard will help you find what you're best at and which parts of your fitness routine need work. Very few people will get a gold rating across the board; most can stand to do better in some area. Runners, for example, are likely to rate silver or gold on the 3-minute step test, but may score a low bronze in push-ups.

Try the test, thinking of it as a way to check out your body's different capabilities. If you have any health conditions that might make exercise a problem, check with your doctor first.

Exercise enables muscles to work efficiently and reliably. Conditioned muscles function more smoothly and contract somewhat more vigorously, and with less effort, than unconditioned muscles. With exercise, muscle tissue becomes firmer and can withstand much more strain.

Prolonged exercise prepares the muscles for sustained work by improving the circulation of blood in

**Your Strengths and Weaknesses**

| Push-ups, *Number Completed* | | | | | | | | | | |
|---|---|---|---|---|---|---|---|---|---|---|
| Age | 18–29 | | 30–39 | | 40–49 | | 50–59 | | 60+ | |
| | F | M | F | M | F | M | F | M | F | M |
| Gold | 46+ | 51+ | 41+ | 46+ | 36+ | 41+ | 31+ | 36+ | 26+ | 31+ |
| Silver | 17–45 | 25–50 | 12–40 | 22–45 | 8–35 | 19–40 | 6–30 | 15–35 | 5–25 | 10–30 |
| Bronze | 0–16 | 0–24 | 0–11 | 0–21 | 0–7 | 0–18 | 0–5 | 0–14 | 0–4 | 0–9 |

| Curls, *Number Completed* | | | | | | | | | | |
|---|---|---|---|---|---|---|---|---|---|---|
| Age | 18–29 | | 30–39 | | 40–49 | | 50–59 | | 60+ | |
| | F | M | F | M | F | M | F | M | F | M |
| Gold | 46+ | 51+ | 41+ | 46+ | 36+ | 41+ | 31+ | 36+ | 26+ | 31+ |
| Silver | 25–45 | 30–50 | 20–40 | 22–45 | 16–35 | 21–40 | 12–30 | 18–35 | 11–25 | 15–30 |
| Bronze | 0–24 | 0–29 | 0–19 | 0–21 | 0–15 | 0–20 | 0–11 | 0–17 | 0–10 | 0–14 |

| Sit and Reach, *Inches* | | | | | | | | | | |
|---|---|---|---|---|---|---|---|---|---|---|
| Age | 18–29 | | 30–39 | | 40–49 | | 50–59 | | 60+ | |
| | F | M | F | M | F | M | F | M | F | M |
| Gold | 23+ | 22+ | 23+ | 22+ | 22+ | 21+ | 21+ | 20+ | 21+ | 20+ |
| Silver | 17–22 | 13–21 | 17–22 | 13–21 | 15–21 | 13–20 | 14–20 | 12–19 | 14–20 | 12–19 |
| Bronze | 0–16 | 0–12 | 0–16 | 0–12 | 0–14 | 0–12 | 0–13 | 0–11 | 0–13 | 0–11 |

| 3-Minute Step Test (Heart Rate), *Beats per Minute* | | | | | | | | | | |
|---|---|---|---|---|---|---|---|---|---|---|
| Age | 18–29 | | 30–39 | | 40–49 | | 50–59 | | 60+ | |
| | F | M | F | M | F | M | F | M | F | M |
| Gold | to 79 | to 74 | to 83 | to 77 | to 87 | to 79 | to 91 | to 84 | to 94 | to 89 |
| Silver | 80–110 | 75–100 | 84–115 | 78–109 | 88–118 | 80–112 | 92–123 | 85–115 | 95–127 | 90–118 |
| Bronze | 111+ | 101+ | 116+ | 110+ | 119+ | 113+ | 124+ | 116+ | 128+ | 119+ |

| Arm Hang, *Minute* | | | | | |
|---|---|---|---|---|---|
| Age | 18–29 | 30–39 | 40–49 | 50–59 | 60+ |
| | F/M | F/M | F/M | F/M | F/M |
| Gold | 1:31+<br>2:01+ | 1:21+<br>1:51+ | 1:11+<br>1:36+ | 1:01+<br>1:21+ | 0:51+<br>1:11+ |
| Silver | 0:46–1:30<br>1:00–2:00 | 0:40–1:20<br>0:50–1:50 | 0:30–1:10<br>0:45–1:35 | 0:30–1:00<br>0:35–1:20 | 0:21–0:50<br>0:30–1:10 |
| Bronze | 0–0:45<br>0–0:59 | 0–0:39<br>0–0:49 | 0–0:29<br>0–0:44 | 0–0:29<br>0–0:34 | 0–0:20<br>0–0:29 |

SOURCE: *American Health* 1984.

the tissue. Tiny blood vessels called **capillaries** increase by as much as 50 percent in regularly exercised muscles; existing capillaries open wider so total circulation increases by as much as 400 percent, thus

**capillary** A network of minute blood vessels connecting tiny arteries to tiny veins.

providing the muscles with a much greater supply of nutrients. This increase takes about 8 to 12 weeks in young persons and longer in older individuals. Inactivity reverses the process and shuts down extra capillaries.

### Exercise and Muscles

Your muscles never stay the same. If you don't use them, they **atrophy,** or break down. If you use them rigorously and regularly, they grow stronger. Such growth, or **hypertrophy,** is the normal response of muscle cells when they're challenged by weight lifting.

The only way to develop muscles is by demanding more of them than you usually do. This is called overloading. As you train, you have to increase the number of repetitions or the amount of resistance gradually and work the muscle to temporary fatigue. That's why it's important not to quit when your muscles start to tire. Some exercise enthusiasts believe that the experience of pain—the "burn"—signals that exercise is paying off; others contend that it means you're pushing too hard and risking injury.

You exercise differently to develop strength than to extend your endurance. To develop strength, do a few repetitions with heavy loads. As you increase the weight your muscles must move, you increase your strength. To increase endurance, do many more repetitions with lighter loads. If your muscles are weak and you need to gain strength in your upper body, you may have to work for weeks to do a half dozen regular push-ups. Then you can start building endurance by doing as many push-ups as you can before exhaustion. (Later in this chapter see the Self-survey entitled "How Fit Are You?")

**Isometric** exercises are those in which you push or pull against an immovable object, hold each muscle contraction for 5 to 8 seconds, and repeat these steps 5 to 10 times daily. Isometric exercises seem to raise blood pressure in some people, and this can be dangerous. Isometrics are not generally used to develop muscle strength.

**Isotonic** exercises are those in which the muscle moves a moderate load several times, as in weight lifting or calisthenics. The best isotonic exercises for muscular strength combine high resistance and a low number of repetitions. You can develop the greatest flexibility, coordination, and endurance with low resistance and frequent repetitions.

For isotonic exercise, you can use free weights, like barbells and dumbbells, or Nautilus or Universal equipment, which is found in most gyms and health clubs. Nautilus and Universal weight-training machines use the principle of progressive resistance. The Universal equipment is a system of cables, pulleys, and weights. Nautilus machines have a special cam—a pulley with an off-center axis—that adjusts the resistance automatically for exercise in all positions.

**Isokinetic** exercises use special machines that provide resistance to overload muscles throughout the entire range of motion. These exercises are highly effective in strengthening specific muscle groups, but the sophisticated mechanical devices are generally available only at commercial fitness clubs.

Muscular training is specific, which means that you have to exercise certain muscles for certain re-

**atrophy** To waste away.
**hypertrophy** To enlarge, as muscles do when lifting heavy weights.
**isometric** An increase in muscular tension without the muscle shortening in length, as when pushing an immovable object.
**isotonic** The repetition of an action to create muscular tension, as occurs in calisthenics.
**isokinetic** An exercise with specialized equipment that provides resistance through the whole range of motion.

## HEALTH HEADLINE

### Does Exercise Make You Sexy?

**According to behavior scientists at Bentley College, regular exercise doesn't just increase energy, improve health, and reduce stress; it also boosts sexual interest and activity.**

**In the study, master swimmers in their forties had intercourse as often as many people in their twenties (seven times a month); swimmers in their sixties were nearly as sexually active as those in their forties. Overall, 94 percent of the swimmers said they enjoyed sex "a lot." But more exercise didn't necessarily mean more sex. Extremely rigorous training dampened sexual desire among both men and women.**

SOURCE: Longstreet, Dana. "When Exercise is Sexercise," *American Health,* March 1989. Whitten, Phillip and Elizabeth Whiteside. "Can Exercise Make You Sexier?" *Psychology Today,* April 1989.

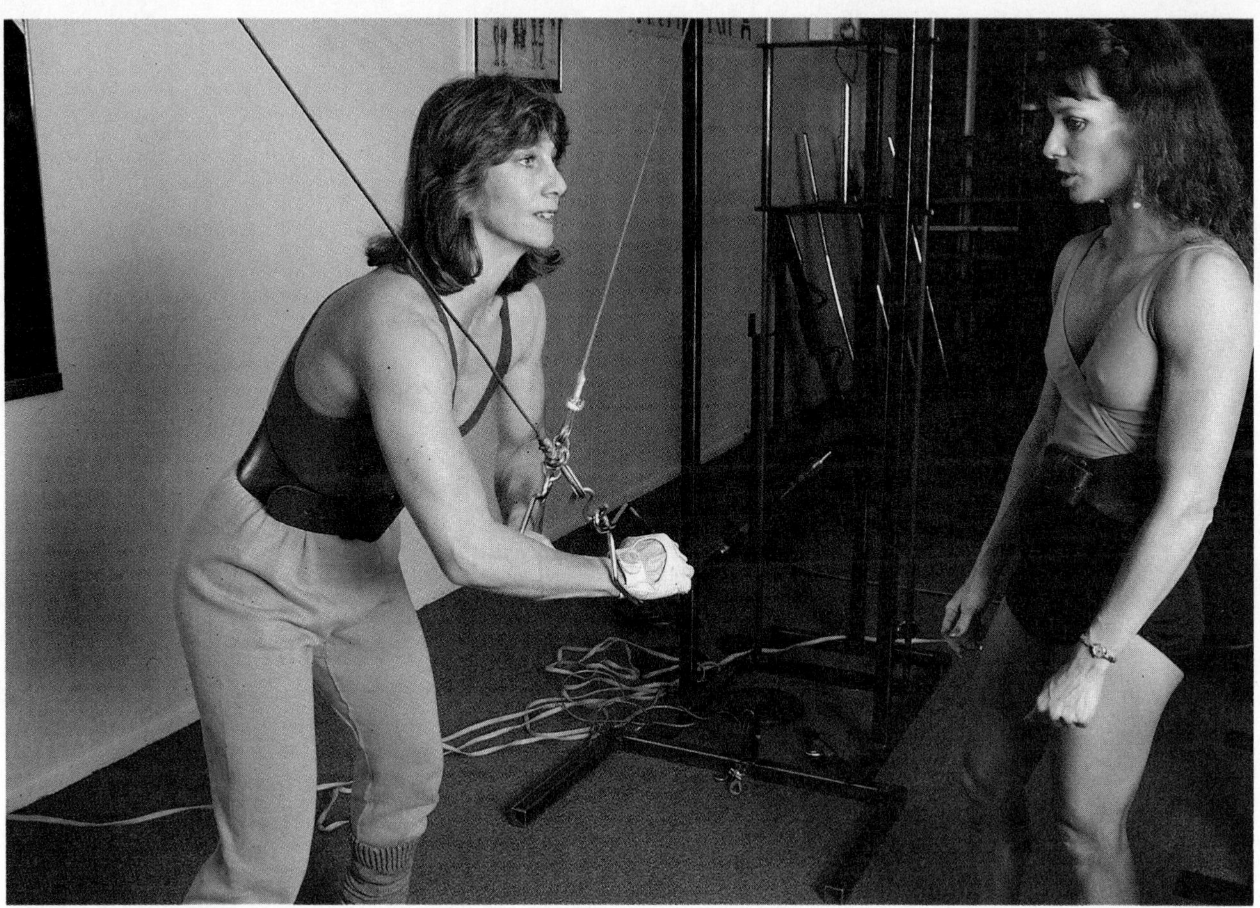

Conditioning enables muscles to work more efficiently and reliably.

sults. If you want to build up your leg muscles to run a marathon, push-ups won't help—just as running a marathon won't develop your upper body. If you're training for specific goals, you have to tailor your exercise program to make sure you meet them.

## Designing a Muscle Workout

A workout with weights should exercise your body's primary muscle groups: the deltoids (shoulders), pectorals (chest), triceps and biceps (back and front of upper arm), quadriceps (front thigh), gluteus maximus (buttocks), and abdomen. Various machines and free-weight routines focus on each muscle group, but the principle is always the same: Muscles contract as you raise and lower a weight, and you repeat the lift-and-lower routine until the muscle group is tired.

A weight-training program is made up of both **sets** (set numbers of the same movement) and **reps** (the single performance of an exercise, such as lifting 75 pounds once). You should allow your breath to return to normal before moving on to each new set or rep. Pushing yourself to the limit builds strength.

Maintaining proper breathing techniques is crucial. To breathe correctly, inhale when muscles are relaxed, and exhale when you push or lift. Don't hold your breath, because oxygen flow helps prevent muscle fatigue and injury.

Your muscles need 48 hours to recover from a training session. Two or three 30-minute sessions a week are sufficient for building strength and endurance. Figure 5-4 shows recovery patterns following six strength-building workouts in a 12-day period. For total fitness, you may want to schedule aerobic workouts for your days off from weight training.

**set** In conditioning, a specified number of repetitions of the same movement or exercise.
**rep** In exercise, a single repetition, or performance, of a movement.

**STRATEGY FOR CHANGE**

### Working with Weights

If you plan to work with free weights, here are some guidelines for using them safely and effectively:

- Don't train alone—for safety's sake as well as motivation.
- Work with a partner so you can serve as spotters for each other.

- Always warm up and stretch before weight training.
- Begin with relatively light weights (50 percent of your maximum), and increase the load slowly until you find the weight that will cause muscle failure at anywhere from 8 to 12 repetitions. (Muscle failure is the point during a workout at which you can no longer perform or complete a repetition through the entire range of motion.)
- In the beginning, don't work at maximum intensity. Increase your level of exertion gradually over 2 to 6 weeks to allow your body to adapt to new stress without soreness.
- Always use proper form. Unnecessary twisting, lurching, lunging, or arching can cause serious injury.
- Always train your entire body, starting with the larger muscle groups.
- Don't focus on specific areas only, although you may want to concentrate on your weakest muscles.
- In order for your body to recover from a workout and to avoid overtraining, allow no less than 48 hours, but no more than 96 hours, between training sessions. Workouts on consecutive days do more harm than good, because the body can't adapt that quickly. However, your muscles will begin to atrophy if you let more than three or four days pass without exercising them.
- Quality matters more than quantity. One properly performed set of lifts can produce a greater increase in strength and muscle mass than many sets of improperly performed lifts.

## Aerobic Circuit Training: Working Heart and Muscles

The state-of-the-art workout for the 1990s may be aerobic or interval circuit training, which combines aerobic and strength exercises to build both cardiovascular endurance and muscular strength.

Done individually or in a group at a gym or health club, aerobic circuit training generally involves weight training equipment (such as free weights or Nautilus or Universal machines) and aerobic stations (such as treadmills, stationary bikes, or cross-country ski machines). By alternating weight and aerobic stations and moving quickly from one station to the next, exercisers can get a total body workout. Some trainers have reported that interval training results in significant improvements in aerobic capacity as well as enhanced toning and shaping of muscles.[10]

## Pumping Steroids

Doctors use **anabolic steroids,** synthetic derivatives of the male hormone testosterone, in treating severe burns and injuries. For years, however, bodybuilders, weight lifters, football players, and other athletes have been using steroids, usually in dangerous forms and doses, to gain weight and strength. Some inject high doses of steroids intended only for horses. Others, in a practice called stacking, take several different steroids at the same time. Anabolic steroids have also

**anabolic steroid** A drug derived from testosterone and approved for medical use but often used by athletes to increase their musculature and weight.

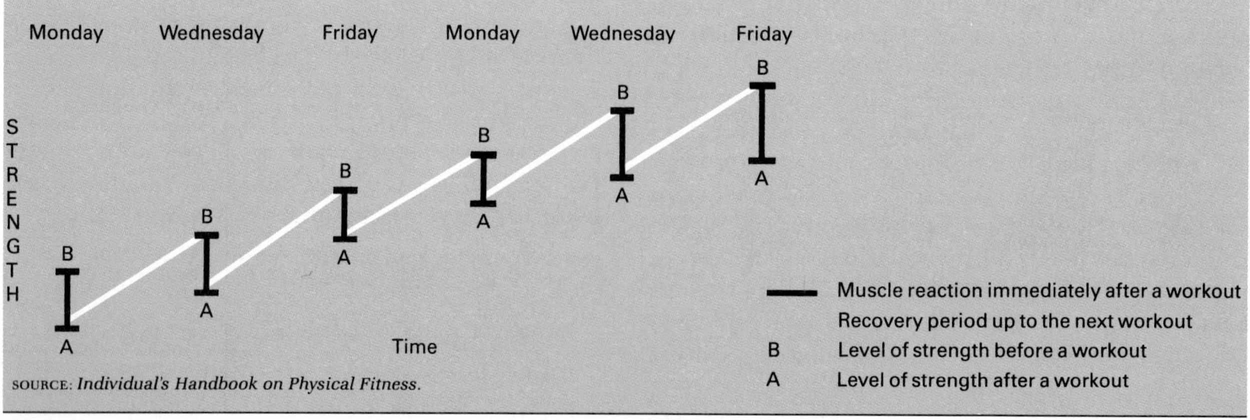


**FIGURE 5-4** This graph shows the muscle recovery patterns before and after alternate-day strength-building workouts. To avoid overtraining, no less than 48 hours and no more than 96 hours should pass between training sessions. Strength-building workouts on consecutive days do more harm than good, because the body can't recover that quickly.

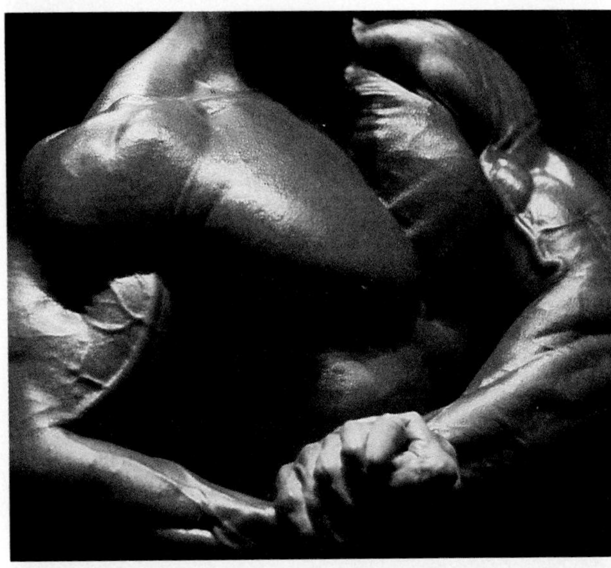

Men and women who use steroids in combination with heavy resistance training will increase their muscle and bone mass, but may also experience severe side effects, and in some cases, death.

become popular among nonathletes, particularly teenagers, who want to look muscular (see Chapter 9).

Steroids do increase weight and muscle strength, but they have dangerous side effects on the liver, the cardiovascular system, the reproductive organs, and the mind. The adverse effects in men include:

- breast enlargement
- atrophy of the testicles, with decreased sperm count, abnormal sperm shapes and movement, and possible infertility
- impotence
- enlarged prostate

In women, the adverse effects include:

- enlargement of the clitoris
- beard growth
- baldness
- deepened voice
- breast diminution

Both sexes can develop these side effects of steroids:

- increased risk of heart disease, stroke, or obstructed blood vessels
- increased aggression (known as "'roid rage")
- liver tumors and jaundice
- in preteens and teenagers, the growing plates in bones close prematurely, resulting in permanent shortness
- acne

In addition, the sharing of needles to inject steroids could result in transmission of the virus that causes AIDS from an infected person to others. (See Chapters 7 and 15 for more on AIDS transmission.)

According to a 1990 report in the *Journal of the American Medical Association,* anabolic steroids have profound psychological effects. Long-term, high-dose anabolic steroid use may lead to a preoccupation with drug use; difficulty stopping despite psychological side effects; drug craving; and withdrawal symptoms, including depression, when drug use stops.[11]

Despite their popularity, steroids do not give bodybuilders or athletes a competitive edge. In careful studies, researchers have concluded that prior and ongoing training, particularly when combined with an adequate diet, improves muscle strength and performance more significantly than does drug use, without the side effects and long-term risks associated with steroids.[12,13,14]

**STRATEGY FOR CHANGE**

### Evaluating Fitness Products

Just as you have to be a good health-care consumer (see Chapter 12), you should be a smart fitness consumer. Here are some guidelines:

- Don't buy any equipment without first trying it out. If you decide to buy a stationary bicycle, for instance, read all the product information. Ask someone in the physical education department for recommendations. Try out a bicycle at a gym.
- Make sure any equipment you purchase is safe and durable.
- Think about your fitness goals before you buy equipment. If you're primarily interested in aerobic stamina, try out stationary bicycles, rowing machines, treadmills, and cross-country skiing machines.
- Spend 5 to 10 minutes working at moderate intensity. How do the movements feel to you—awkward or fluid, extremely difficult or surprisingly easy?
- If you're considering strength-training equipment, remember that free weights are the cheapest option. The best resistance machines are also the most expensive, with prices soaring over $1,000. Would you use one often enough to justify its cost?
- Think about your exercise style. Are you going to find sitting at a stationary bicycle for 30 minutes too boring? Are you motivated enough to hoist free weights on your own several times a week? The best home equipment does no good unless it's used.

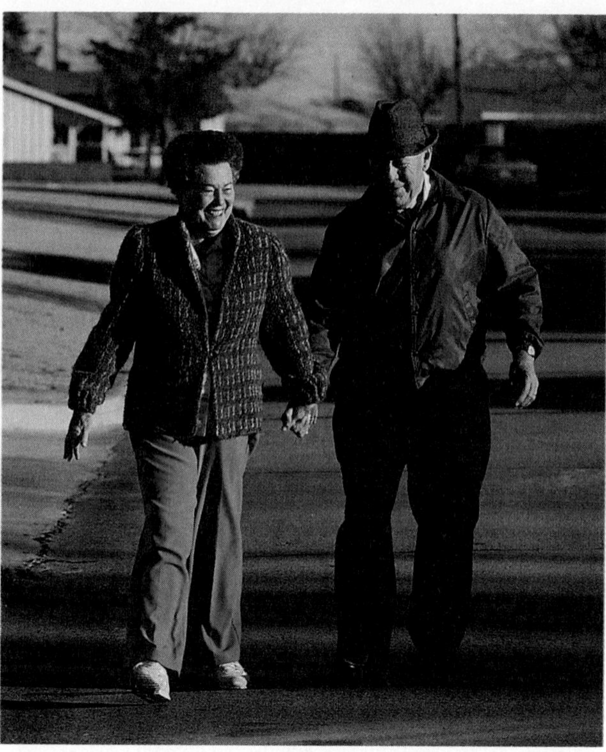

Regular aerobic exercise, such as brisk walking, can help older people feel younger than their years.

## WHY EXERCISE?

The primary benefit of exercise is that it extends your life span. In a major study of 10,224 men and 3,120 women by researchers at the Institute for Aerobics Research, published in the *Journal of the American Medical Association,* physical fitness greatly reduced the risk of dying of heart disease, cancer, and other illnesses.[15] Even modest levels of fitness improve survival, but the fitter you are, the longer you'll live. Each hour of exercise may add almost 2 hours to your life.

Exercise does far more than increase the quantity of life; it enhances the quality of life as well. As you get into shape, your heart muscles become stronger and thicker and pump blood more efficiently. Your heart rate and resting pulse slow down. Red blood cells may increase and blood pressure may drop slightly. Because exercise speeds up metabolism during and after workouts, it burns up calories and fat. As a result, your percentage of body fat decreases and you may trim inches from your torso.

There are yet other benefits of exercising: Conditioning thickens the bones, possibly preventing the slow loss of calcium with age. Exercise increases flexibility in the joints and improves digestion and elimination. It raises body temperature several degrees, killing potential pathogens (organisms that cause disease). It also heightens sensitivity to insulin (a great benefit for diabetics) and enhances clot-dissolving substances in the blood, helping to prevent strokes, heart attacks, and pulmonary embolisms (clots in the lungs).

### Turning Back the Clock

Getting in shape slows several age-associated processes: the loss of lean muscle tissue, the increase in body fat, and the decrease in work capacity. With regular exercise, a person in late middle age can match the physical capacity of someone 20 years younger.

### A Hardier Heart and Stronger Lungs

Over the long term, regular exercise can help protect you against heart disease, in part by lowering the cholesterol that can lead to heart attacks and strokes. (See Chapter 13 for more information on cholesterol and heart disease.)

Another beneficial effect of aerobic exercise is an increased ability to dissolve blood clots that can cause heart attacks and strokes. Jogging for about 30 minutes three times a week enhances the biochemical process that breaks down obstructions in the blood vessels. Vigorous exercisers have a lower risk of sudden death.[16,17]

In addition to its effects on the heart, exercise makes the lungs more efficient. They take in more oxygen, and their vital capacity (ability to take in and expel air) is increased. This not only provides greater energy, but may predict how long you'll live.

### Better Bones

Weak and brittle bones are common among people who do not exercise. **Osteoporosis** is the demineralizing of bones—a process that makes them frail and prone to injury. Osteoporosis affects a great many older people. Women, in particular, are vulnerable because their bones are less dense to begin with and because female hormones, particularly estrogen, can diminish bone minerals. Bone mass (or density) is at its peak between the ages of 30 and 40; after that it declines.

Exercise may stop or prevent osteoporosis—and the best way to work out to prevent it may be by combining weight lifting and aerobics. In a study at the University of California, San Francisco, 46 young

**osteoporosis** A condition common in older people, in which their bones become increasingly soft and porous, making them susceptible to injury.

men who participated about 6 hours a week in both aerobics and a weight program—with either free weights or Nautilus-type equipment—developed the densest bones (as determined by computerized X-rays of the spine).[18] (See Chapter 17 for an extensive discussion of osteoporosis.)

### Brighter Mood

In a variety of studies of people who were not under psychiatric care, the least physically fit were the most emotionally troubled.[19] When they began exercising, they improved more dramatically—in body and mind—than those who started off in better shape. According to a growing number of reports, exercise also increases energy, reduces hostility, improves concentration and alertness, and makes people less self-conscious and better able to handle stress.

### Protection from Certain Cancers and Diseases

Women who were varsity athletes in high school or college are less likely to develop cancer of the breast or reproductive organs than those who weren't competitive athletes.[20] Fitness, before and after graduation, pays off by lowering the risk, not only of cancer, but also of diabetes and bone fractures.

### Lower Weight

As you exercise, your body responds to the increased demand from your muscles for nutrients, and your metabolic rate rises. As a result, aerobic exercise burns off calories during your workout. This surge persists for several hours after exercise, so you continue to use up more calories than usual. In addition, aerobic exercise dampens appetite, so you aren't as tempted to eat. If you exercise while dieting, you lose more fat and less muscle. (See Chapter 4 for more information on weight control.)

## MEN, WOMEN, AND EXERCISE

The average man is 4 to 5 inches taller, is 25 to 40 pounds heavier, and has larger muscles and internal organs than the average woman. Because she has less testosterone, the average woman's muscles won't become as bulky as a man's, regardless of how much iron she pumps. However, when lean body mass is compared pound for pound, the differences aren't as dramatic, particularly in equally conditioned men and women.

Men and women respond to aerobic conditioning in much the same ways, but even after training, a woman's aerobic capacity remains about 27 percent lower than that of an equally fit man. With training, a woman's relative leg strength can equal or surpass a man's. Women still lag behind on upper body strength, but in other aspects of fitness—such as reaction time—women often outscore men. In many fitness categories, there are greater differences between individuals than between the two sexes, with some women outperforming almost all men.

Women's naturally higher percentage of body fat may have more of an effect on their physical performance than any other factor. Although women weigh approximately 25 pounds less than men, they have 10 to 15 pounds more fatty tissue. Even female athletes have roughly twice the percentage of body fat that male athletes have. This extra fat is essential for reproduction and a woman's health.

Because men have a 50 percent greater ratio of muscle mass to body weight, they're faster and more powerful than women. Simply because of this difference, women run slower, jump less far, and are able to do fewer push-ups and pull-ups. Although some experts have speculated that women's larger fat stores

## HEALTH HEADLINE

### Who Stays Fit?

**Outgoing, well-adjusted college students are more likely than their anxious or shy classmates to work out frequently when they reach their sixties, according to a long-term study of Harvard College graduates begun almost 50 years ago.**

**The key to predicting which men would remain active was not how fit or athletic they were in college, but what their personalities were like. The lifelong exercisers tended to be practical, outgoing, and interested in politics during their college days; those who rarely exercised in their sixties were more likely to have been loners with artistic or cultural interests as students.**

SOURCE: Stark, Ellen. "Who Stays Fit," *Psychology Today*, November 1989.

HEALTH SPOTLIGHT

## How to Buy Athletic Shoes

Here are some guidelines, developed by Dr. Lloyd Nesbitt of the Canadian Podiatric Sports Medicine Academy, that you can follow to put your best foot forward:

When buying shoes for exercise, have both feet measured in athletic socks. (One foot is generally larger than the other.) Shop for shoes in the late afternoon, when your feet are most likely to be somewhat swollen—just as they will be after a workout.

For walking shoes, look for a shoe that's lightweight, flexible, and roomy enough for your toes to wiggle. It should have a well-cushioned curved sole, good support at the heel, and an upper part made of a material that "breathes" (allows air in and out).

A running shoe should provide maximum cushioning, support, and stability while still being soft, flexible, and lightweight (see the accompanying illustration). The sole should be durable on the outside, with a moderately soft layer in the midsole. The midsole should be flexible enough to bend easily by hand. Without this flexibility, you may stress your Achilles tendon and calf muscles as you propel off the ball of your foot into your next step.

Look for adequate cushioning under the ball of your foot. The insole should be firm but provide adequate shock absorption. Running—particularly sprinting—exerts a great deal of pressure in this area. The shoe should have a solid, but not a snug, heel cup. The heel counter should be firm and well padded to prevent too much side-to-side motion. The heel itself has to absorb the shock of impact with the ground. A slightly elevated heel lessens the strain on the back of your legs. You should be able to wiggle your toes easily, but the front of your foot shouldn't slide from side to side, which could cause blisters.

Your toes shouldn't touch the end of the shoe, because your feet will swell with activity. Allow about 1/2 inch from the longest toe to the tip of the shoe. The tongue and upper sole should be well padded and fashioned to stay in place as you run. The shank area, under the arch of the shoe, needs to be rigid and lie flush with the ground. If it buckles at foot contact, it may cause heel and arch injuries. As a test, try bending the shoe in this area. If it flexes easily, it may not offer enough support.

For racquetball shoes, look for reinforcement at the toe for protection during foot drag. The sole should allow minimal slippage. There should be some heel elevation to lessen strain on the back of the leg and Achilles tendon. The shoe should have a long "throat" to ensure greater control by the laces.

For tennis shoes, look for reinforcement of the toe. The sole at the ball of the foot should be well padded, because that's where most pressure is exerted. The sides of the shoe should be sturdy, for stability during continuous side-to-side motions. The toe box should allow

might prove an advantage in endurance events like a marathon, the opposite seems true: The hormone estrogen blocks fat metabolism, so women's bodies release the energy stored in fat cells more slowly than do men's.

Contrary to many clichés, most women can perform consistently throughout their menstrual cycles. Researchers have found no significant differences in physical capabilities, such as oxygen intake, throughout a woman's cycle.[21]

ample room and some cushioning at the tip. A long throat ensures greater control by the laces. Don't wear wet shoes for training. Let them air-dry, because a heater will cause them to stiffen or shrink. Use powder in your shoes to absorb moisture, lessen friction, and prevent fungal infections. Break in new shoes for several days before wearing them for a long-distance run or a competition.

SOURCE: Canadian Podiatric Sports Medicine Academy.

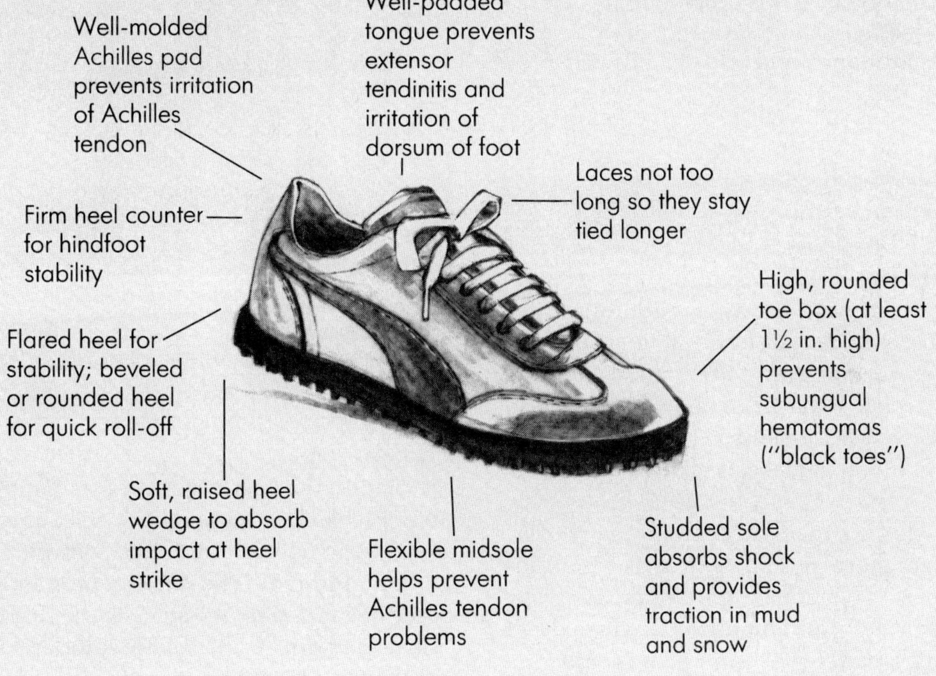


Moderate exercise thickens women's bones and helps prevent the slow loss of calcium that culminates in osteoporosis. But very vigorous exercise can actually increase the risk of bone deterioration by interfering with hormone balance. Women marathoners who train by running 50 miles a week are more likely to stop menstruating (possibly because of a drop in body fat) than those logging fewer miles. (See Chapter 7 for information on menstrual problems.)

**STRATEGY FOR CHANGE**

**Do's and Don'ts for Women Athletes**

Here are some guidelines for women who want to be both healthy *and* fit:

- If you're running or doing aerobics, make sure you have comfortable, sturdy shoes that provide the extra shock absorption most women need.
- Don't push yourself to exercise when you're feeling unusual pain or fatigue.
- Don't exercise so hard that your periods stop or become irregular. If you do stop menstruating, see a gynecologist.
- Don't go on a low-calorie diet while undertaking a strenuous exercise regimen. If you allow yourself to become too thin, both your athletic performance and your health will suffer.

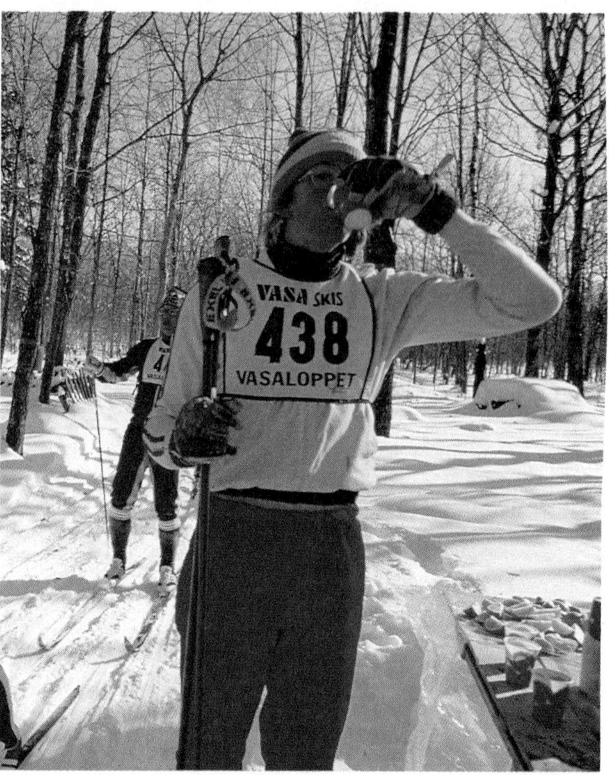

To prevent problems while exercising outdoors, drink plenty of fluids and dress appropriately for the weather.

## NUTRITION FOR EXERCISERS

A balanced diet can supply everything most exercisers need to perform well. However, endurance athletes whose workouts last an hour or more do best with a diet high in complex carbohydrates, which help keep the level of sugar in the blood steady and increase the body's fuel reserve. This diet prevents sudden drops in blood glucose, weakness, and lightheadedness.

Because muscles are made of protein, many exercisers think that more protein will make muscles stronger. Yet heavy workouts don't increase your body's need for protein, and high-protein diets don't lead to high performance. The American Dietetic Association has warned that too much protein can impair athletic performance by placing an excessive burden on the kidneys and liver.

If you're interested in "high-octane" nutrition to enhance your performance, you may be tempted to try "body-building" or "high-energy" foods, drugs, or dietary supplements, such as amino acids. Don't. You'll be wasting a lot of money, and you might end up feeling worse, rather than better, because of a nutrition imbalance.

What you *do* need before and during a workout is water. On a hot day, you can lose 1/2 pound of weight during your first hour of running. Some athletes lose 2 pounds during a summer training session; that amounts to a quart of sweat. As their bodies become dehydrated, their hearts find it more difficult to satisfy the demands of the muscles.

Water works best to prevent dehydration, because water is absorbed more quickly than any athletic drink or beverage containing sugar, sodium, potassium, or other ingredients. The American Dietetic Association describes "plain cool water" as the fluid of choice for "most persons undertaking moderate exercise in moderate temperature conditions."

Although you may have heard a great deal about salt tablets, stay away from them. They're unnecessary and potentially dangerous. Although you do lose some salt in sweat, the loss is minimal—and more than made up for by the huge amounts of sodium most Americans get in their daily diet.

## PREVENTING PROBLEMS

Shaping up takes time, sweat, and perseverance—and common sense. Some simple precautions can prevent problems before they happen. Should you need it, you can find information on the treatment and future prevention of common sports injuries in "Your Survival and Self-care Guide" in the appendix.

### Feet First

Your feet have 52 bones, one-fourth of all the bones in the body, plus 214 ligaments and 38 muscles. The comfort—and to some degree the safety—of all of them depends on the fit of the shoe. Well-fitting, supportive shoes are especially important for runners. Although the sole of the shoe may have 30 square inches of surface, only a small area touches the ground at any one time. (In this chapter see "Health Spotlight: How to Buy Athletic Shoes.")

### Handling Heat

Prevention is the wisest approach to heat problems. Always wear as little as possible when exercising in hot weather. Choose loose-fitting, lightweight, white or light-colored clothes. Cotton is a good choice because it absorbs perspiration. Never wear rubberized or plastic pants and jackets to sweat off pounds. These sauna suits cause only a loss in water, not fat, and they can be dangerous because they hold heat. On humid days carry a damp washcloth to wipe off perspiration and cool yourself down. Be sure to get plenty of fluids, and watch for the earliest signs of heat problems, including cramps, stress, exhaustion and heat stroke. (See "Your Survival and Self-care Guide" in the appendix.)

### Coping with Cold

Protect yourself by covering as much of your body as possible, but don't overdress. Wear one layer less than you would if you were outside but not exercising. Don't use warm-up clothes of waterproof material because they tend to trap heat and keep perspiration from evaporating. Make sure your clothes are loose enough to allow movement and exercise of the hands, feet, and other body parts, thereby maintaining proper circulation. Choose dark colors that absorb heat. Because 40 percent or more of body heat is lost through your head and neck, wear a hat, turtleneck, or scarf. Make sure you cover your hands and feet as well. (Mittens provide more warmth and protection than gloves.) In addition, watch for signs of frost nip, frostbite, and hypothermia (see "Your Survival and Self-care Guide").

## MAKING THIS CHAPTER WORK FOR YOU

### Shaping Up

**A physically fit person has enough energy to meet routine physical demands as well as any unexpected challenges. Fitness itself has three basic components: flexibility, cardiovascular fitness, and muscular strength and endurance. Stretching can improve flexibility. Aerobic exercise, which causes the heart and lungs to work harder and more efficiently, improves cardiovascular fitness. Building up strength and endurance ensures muscular fitness. A complete fitness program should include exercises for flexibility, stamina, and strength.**

## WHAT DO YOU THINK?

Mai Li hates to sweat, and she jokes that she gets her exercise by pushing the buttons on the TV's remote control. Although she knows that exercise is good for health, she figures that she can keep her weight down by dieting and worry about her heart and health when she gets older. "I look good. I feel okay. Why should I bother exercising?" she asks. What would you say in reply?

Manny, who felt that his thin arms and chest made him look like a wimp, started working out. At the gym he learned that some of the guys with the most impressive muscles took anabolic steroids. He decided to try them himself. Sure enough, his muscles got bigger. But his acne also got much worse, his breasts enlarged, and he's had bouts of unexplainable anger. He tried stopping steroids once, but found his cravings for the drug too hard to handle. What has happened to Manny? What do you think he should do?

When he started working out, Jeff simply wanted to stay in shape. But he felt so pleased with the way his body looked and responded that he kept doing more. Now he runs 10 miles a day (longer on weekends), lifts weights and works out on Nautilus equipment almost every day, and plays racquetball or squash whenever he gets a chance. Is Jeff getting too much of a good thing? Is there any danger in his fitness program? What would be a more reasonable approach?

Every aerobic workout should begin with a warm-up and stretching exercises, include 20 minutes of continuous aerobic activity, and end with a cool-down and more stretching exercises. Among the options for aerobic exercise are brisk walking, jogging or running, swimming, indoor and outdoor cycling, skipping rope, aerobic dancing (including low-impact aerobics), and stair-climbing. A weight-training program for muscular fitness should exercise the body's primary muscle groups.

The benefits of regular exercise include longer life, improved circulation, greater lung capacity, increased metabolism, stronger bones, greater flexibility, increased levels of high-density lipoproteins (HDLs), lower risk of heart disease and sudden death, less danger of osteoporosis, increased energy, less anxiety, and a more positive mood. Being fit may also provide some protection from cancer.

To get the most of physical activity, you need to eat a balanced diet; to use common sense to prevent injuries; to protect yourself from heat and cold; and to stay away from potential dangers, such as anabolic steroids. Although these powerful drugs can increase weight and muscle bulk, they can damage the cardiovascular system, the liver, the reproductive organs, and mental abilities.

Getting physical does *not* mean joining a health club, buying designer sportswear, or working out on expensive bodybuilding equipment. All you need, other than some good shoes for your feet, is a genuine commitment to making the most of your body.

If you stick to your exercise plan, you'll eventually notice how much trimmer, firmer, faster, and stronger you've become. You'll have more energy at the end of the day. You'll feel less stressed, despite daily pressures. And you'll discover for yourself the special joys of fitness: the thrill of feeling newly toughened muscles bend to your will; the satisfaction of a long, smooth stretch after a stressful day; the sweetness of the crisp morning air on an early run; and the pure pleasure of living in the body you deserve.

SECTION III

# YOUR SEXUALITY

Our most special relationships are those that bring us closer to others—friends, partners, spouses, parents, children. Such intimacy is the most rewarding and the most demanding of human involvements. The giving of ourselves to another—sharing thoughts, feelings, experiences, sexual pleasure—touches the essence of what it means to be a human being. This section provides a comprehensive view of both philosophical and practical matters of relating to others. Each of the chapters focuses on the unique form of personal responsibility involved in every close relationship: a responsibility that looks beyond the self and extends to those we care for and love.

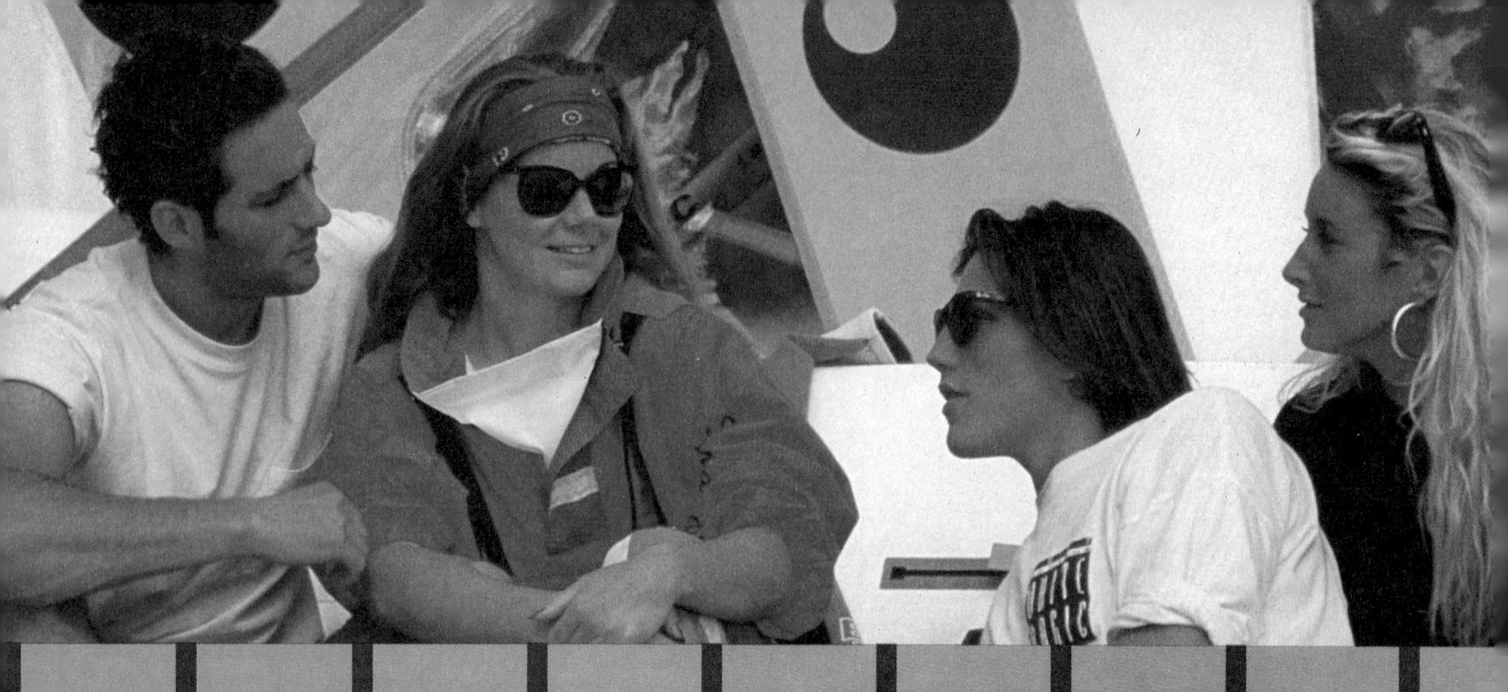

# 6 YOUR RELATIONSHIPS

In this chapter

Forming relationships

Life-style choices

Marriage

Parenthood

Family ties

Making this chapter work for you: Building better relationships

*All of us need people; all of us need each other.* Relating—caring and wanting to be cared about, feeling for others and wanting others to feel for us, sharing ideas and experiences—is essential to human life. We need each other to survive and to carry on the species.

This chapter discusses the needs we all share, the ways some of us respond to those needs, and the possibilities that exist for coming together from our solitude to warm ourselves in each other's glow of life.

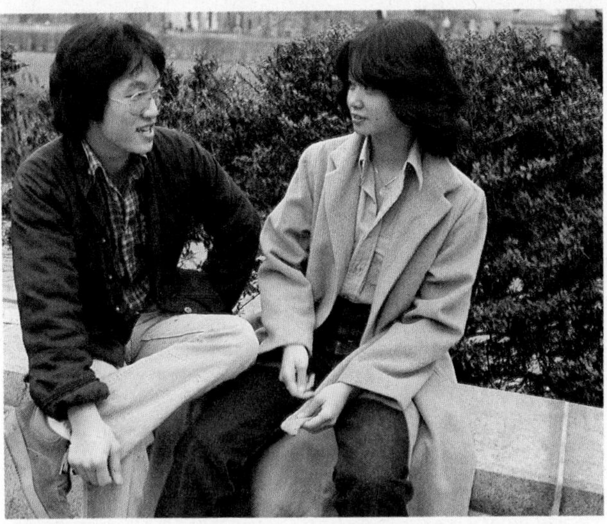

Sharing thoughts, feelings and experiences builds true intimacy between two people.

## FORMING RELATIONSHIPS

Throughout life, intimate relationships, tested and strengthened by time, allow us to explore the depths of our souls and the heights of our emotions.

### I, Myself, and Me

Self-esteem and self-love provide a positive foundation for our relationships with others. Self-love does not mean vanity or preoccupation with our own needs; rather, it is a genuine concern and respect for ourselves. We cannot love or accept others until we love and accept ourselves, however imperfect we may be.

### Communication

You are constantly sending messages to other people through your words, gestures, expressions, and behaviors. In your closest relationships, your messages must be clear and accurate. No one can read your mind. Only you can express what you really feel.

You choose the information about yourself that you want to share and that you want to hide. Some parts of yourself may remain mysterious even to you, until you form an intimate relationship. We all increase our self-knowledge by opening ourselves to others.

However, it can be very difficult to express certain emotions. Some people have difficulty saying "I appreciate you" or "I care about you," even though they are genuinely appreciative and caring. Others find it hard to know what to say in response.

Sometimes it seems easier not to use words—to convey our emotions with a kiss or a hug or with a slap. Such nonverbal messages are immediately effective, but they're not precise enough to communicate your exact thoughts. Stalking out of a room and slamming the door may be clear signs of anger, but they don't explain what caused the anger or suggest what to do about it. You must learn how to communicate your feelings, negative as well as positive, if you hope to achieve true intimacy.

Couples must sharpen their communication skills so they can discuss all the issues they may confront. They must learn how to communicate anger, frustration, and disappointment, as well as pleasure, satisfaction, and affection. And they must listen as carefully as they speak.

**STRATEGY FOR CHANGE**

**Effective Communication**

- Be sure of your own feelings. If you don't know what you're trying to say, no one else will be able to understand what you mean.
- When discussing something important, make and maintain eye contact. Holding or touching helps when you're talking about sensitive personal subjects.
- Remember that your point of view is not the only one. Try to see things through your partner's eyes too.
- When you're not sure you understand what your partner is saying, try paraphrasing it. Start with a phrase such as "So what you're saying is. . . ."
- Always try to say something positive, even when you're also raising negative points.
- Be specific about what you want and how strongly you want it.
- Only you know what's inside your head. Don't expect your partner to be a mind reader.
- Make your point and then be quiet. If you keep repeating yourself, your partner will tune you out.

## Friendship

A friend is one who knows you as you are,
Understands where you've been,
Accepts who you've become,
And still gently invites you to grow.

*Anonymous*

Friends can be a basic source of happiness, a connection to a larger world, a source of comfort in times of trouble. Although we have different friends throughout life, often the friendships of adolescence and young adulthood are the closest we ever form. These relationships ease the normal transition from childhood to independence.

Men and women may form different types of friendships with members of the same sex. Most women, allowed from childhood to be open with their feelings, find it easy to confide in and become close to other women. That's not usually the case with men, who have few role models for friendships. In school, sports, and business, the pressure to get ahead or win comes between men. They learn at an early age not to admit weaknesses, not to express fears, not to reveal too much.

However, both men and women are capable of loyalty, commitment, and trust. Men may find it harder initially to be open and receptive. But when they are, friendship can offer as many rewards for them as it does for women.

**STRATEGY FOR CHANGE**

### Maintaining Friendships

Like all relationships, friendships require attention and work to survive. Here are some behaviors that can keep you close to those you care about most:

- Be willing to open up. The more you share, the deeper the bond between you and your friend will become.
- Be sensitive to your friend's feelings. Keep in mind that, like you, your friend has unique needs, desires, and dreams.
- Express appreciation. Be generous with your compliments. Let your friends know you recognize their kindnesses.
- See friends clearly. Admitting their faults need not reduce your respect for them.
- Know that friends will disappoint you from time to time. They, too, are only human.
- Talk about your friendship. Evaluate the relationship periodically. If you have any gripes or frustrations, air them.

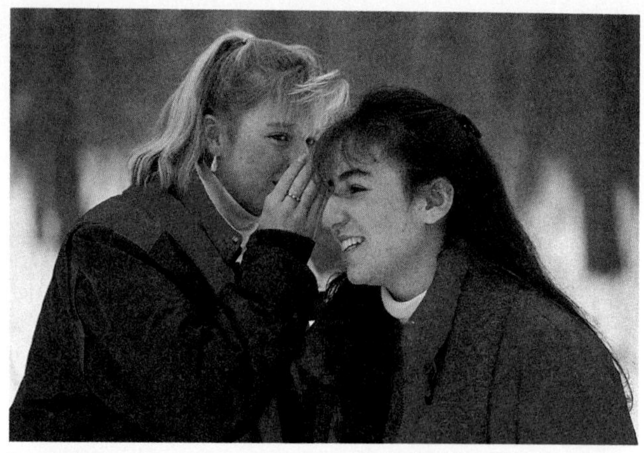

Often the friendships of adolescence and young adulthood are the closest we ever form.

## Dating

A date is any occasion during which people share their time: It can be a Friday night dance, a bicycle ride, a dinner for two, or a walk in the park. We talk about good dates and bad dates, hot dates and blind dates, steady dating and group dating. Friends and lovers go on dates. So do complete strangers. Some women date other women; some men date other men. We don't expect to love, or even like, everyone we date. Yet the people you date reveal something about the sort of person you are.

While in school, you may date people you meet in class or on campus. However, with more people remaining single longer, the search for a good date has become more complex. Singles bars have become less popular because of the dangers of drinking and casual sex. Personal ads have become a more popular way to meet other single people, with advertisements sometimes filling dozens of pages in some publications.

Personal ads allow you to define your ideal date, though that description may vary from one year to the next. However, dating can do more than help you meet a certain type of person. By dating, you can learn how to make conversation; get to know more about other people; and share feelings, opinions, and interests.

Dating is also an opportunity for exploring your sexual identity. It's not unusual for either men or women, particularly when young, to choose a date by appearance alone. Sexual curiosity and attraction bring many couples together. They may later discover common bonds, or they may break up after the attraction cools.

Some people date for months and never share more than a good-night kiss. Others may fall into bed together before they fall into love—or even "like." It's often puzzling to sort out your emotional feelings

## HALES INDEX

Percentage of teenage girls who have sex for the sake of love: 11

Percentage of teenage boys who have sex for the sake of love: 6

Percentage of American Jews who marry non-Jews: 33

Percentage of married people who would marry their spouses again: 80

Percentage of married people who say their spouses are their best friends: 75

Percentage of married couples who pray together: 61

Percentage of couples having serious problems in the first year of marriage: 49

Percentage of couples married less than seven years who say they make love often: 83

Percentage of couples married more than seven years who say they make love often: 69

Percentage of Americans who disapprove of extramarital sex: 91

Decline in divorce rate in 1989: 4

SOURCES: **1, 2** Stark, Ellen. "Teen Sex: Not for Love," *Psychology Today,* May 1989. **3** "Interfaith Anxiety," *Psychology Today,* December 1989. **4, 5, 6** Schmidt, William. "Valentine in a Survey: Fidelity Is Thriving," *New York Times,* February 12, 1990. **7** Burden, Dorian. "First Year of Marriage: Down to Real," *Psychology Today,* May 1989. **8, 9, 10** Greeley, Andrew. "Faithful Attraction," *Psychology Today,* March 1990. **11** "Staying Power," *Marin Independent Journal,* March 19, 1990.

from your sexual desires. The first step to making responsible sexual decisions is respecting your sexual values and those of your partner. If you care about the other person—not just his or her body—and the relationship you're creating, sex will be an important, but not the all-important, factor while you're dating.

### STRATEGY FOR CHANGE

#### How to Say No to Sex

Not every date or relationship has to end up in bed. Here are some ways to deal with what can be a very awkward situation:

- First of all, recognize your own values and feelings. If you feel that sex is something to be shared only by people who've already become close in other ways, be true to that belief.
- If you're feeling pressured, let your date know that you're uncomfortable. Be simple and direct.
- Avoid leading your date on. If you flirt throughout the evening, your date may feel that you're expecting sex.
- Think ahead so you can avoid getting trapped in a situation in which you feel you have no alternative. If your date's been drinking, arrange to go home on your own or with friends.
- Communicate your feelings to your date sooner rather than later. It's easier to say "I don't want to go to your apartment" than to fight off unwelcome advances once you're there.
- Watch out for emotional blackmail. If your date says "If you really liked me, you'd want to make love," point out that if he or she really liked you, he or she wouldn't try to force you to do something you don't want to do.
- Remember that if saying no to sex puts an end to a relationship, it wasn't much of a relationship.

## Falling in Love

Falling in love is an intense, dizzying experience. A person not only enters your life, but takes possession. You are intrigued, flattered, delighted—but is this love or a love of loving? At the time you're experiencing it, there is no difference between infatuation and lasting love. You feel the same giddy, wonderful way. However, infatuation refers only to falling in love. People genuinely in love with each other do more than

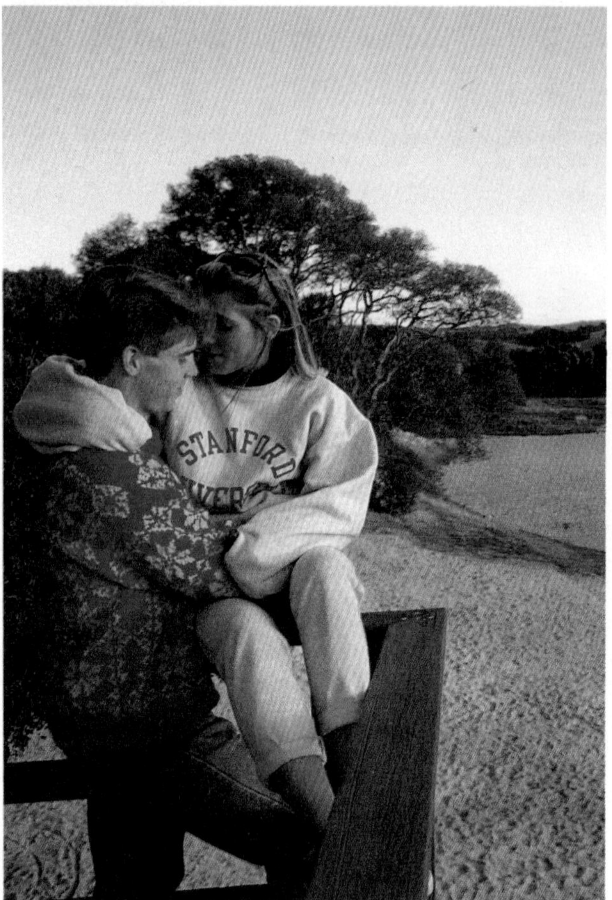

Falling in love can be an intense, dizzying experience that makes every moment together seem special.

fall: They start building a relationship together. Infatuation can be a disguise for something quite different: a strong sex drive, a fear of loneliness, loneliness itself, or a hunger for approval.

You've met someone, gone out a few times, and enjoyed yourself. Is it infatuation, "like," or love? Should you keep seeing each other? Here are some positive indications of a relationship worth continuing: you feel at ease with your new partner; you feel good about your new partner when you're together and when you're not; your partner is open with you about his or her life—past, present, and future; you can say no to each other without feeling guilty; you feel cared for, appreciated, and accepted as you are; your partner really listens to what you have to say.

### Love

All of our close relationships, whether they're with parents or friends, have a great deal in common. We feel we can count on these people in times of need. We feel that they understand us and we understand them. We give and receive emotional support. We care about their happiness and welfare. However, when we choose one person above all others to share a life with, there is something more—something deeper and richer—that we call love.

### Intimacy

The term **intimacy**—which implies the sharing of close, confidential communication—comes from the Latin word for within. Intimacy doesn't happen at first sight or in a day or a week or a number of weeks. Intimacy requires time and nurturing: It is a process of revealing rather than hiding; of wanting to know another and to be known by that other. Although intimacy doesn't require sex, an intimate relationship often includes a sexual relationship—heterosexual or homosexual.

For some people, intimacy is scary: To be intimate with someone means to be vulnerable. Some people fear rejection; others fear suffocation—and there is risk of both in any intimate relationship. Only experiences of closeness over time can replace that fear with trust and satisfaction.

## LIFE-STYLE CHOICES

Today's adults have many choices to explore: living alone, returning to one's primary family, living with a roommate or a group of friends, living in a long-term relationship with a lover of the same or opposite sex, and marriage.

### Living Alone

According to the Census Bureau, by 1990 there were more than 66 million single adult Americans.[1] In their young adult years, male singles outnumber women; after age 40, there are more single women than men (see Figure 6-1). More than one-fifth of the households in the nation are one-person homes, and approximately 10 percent of today's young men and women will never marry.

There is a difference in the quality of singles' lives today, as well as in their numbers. In the past, living alone was seen as a short, distinct period between living with parents and living with a spouse. College students were expected to be on their own for only a few years before entering into a long-term relationship. Today young people are postponing such commitments for a longer time—and more commitments are dissolving, creating a new population of

**intimacy** The state of closeness between people; characterized by the desire and ability to share innermost feelings with each other.

older, second-time-around singles. Being single no longer seems a transition phase, but an accepted, appealing life-style that can be as fulfilling as marriage or a commitment to any one person.

**STRATEGY FOR CHANGE**

**How to Be Alone Without Being Lonely**

- Fill your life with meaningful work, experiences, and people.
- Build a social support network of friends who care for you and about you.
- Try not to spend holidays alone.
- Be open to new experiences that can expand your feelings about yourself and your world.
- Don't miss out on a special event because you don't have someone to accompany you. Go alone.
- Volunteer to help others less fortunate, or become involved in church and social organizations.

## Living with Parents

According to the Census Bureau, in 1990 young adults between ages 18 and 24 were more likely to be living in their parents' homes than young people were in 1970.[2] Their reasons include the high cost of housing and the low incomes most men and women earn in their early twenties. Another reason is a delay in getting married. In 1960, the average first-time groom was 22.8 years old; his bride was likely to be just 20.3 years old. By 1990, the median age at first marriage had crept up to 25.9 years for men and 23.6 years for women (see Figure 6-2).

## Living Together

Couples have always lived together in informal relationships without any official ties; but "living together" has become more common. The number of people under age 25 living together outside marriage has increased more than eightfold in the last two decades. By 1990 more than 2,500,000 unmarried cou-

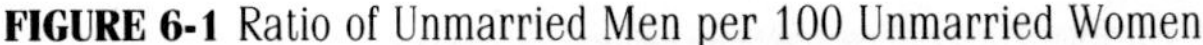

**FIGURE 6-1** Ratio of Unmarried Men per 100 Unmarried Women

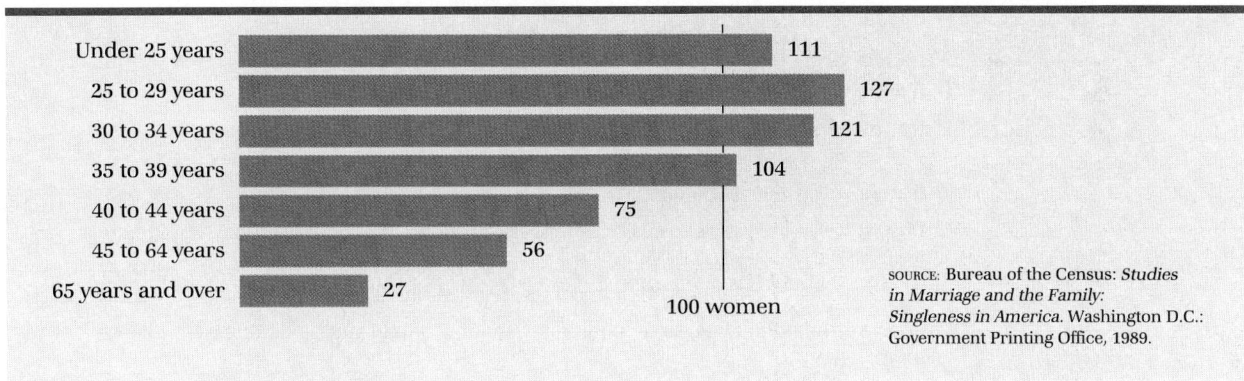


**FIGURE 6-2** Median Age at First Marriage, by Sex

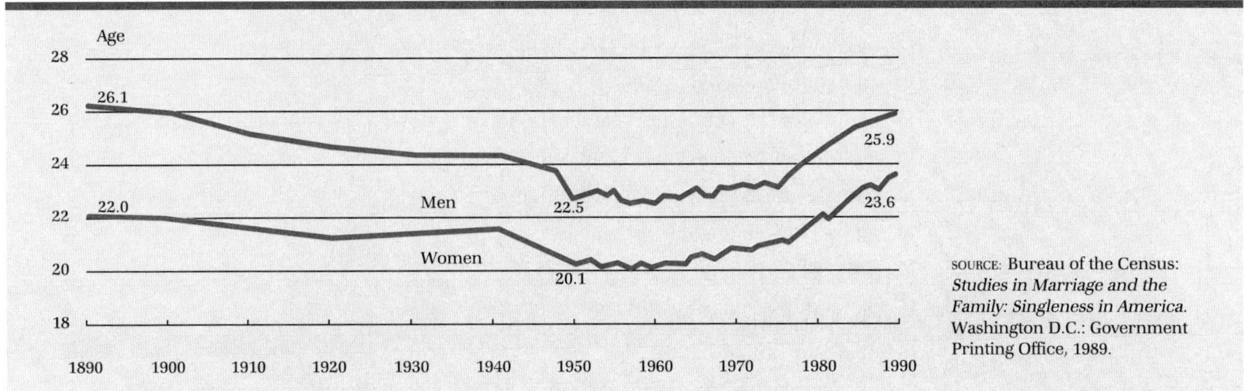

SELF-SURVEY

## How Close Can You Get?

This exercise is designed to measure your capacity for intimacy—how well you have fared in, and what you have learned from, your interpersonal relationships from infancy through adulthood. In a general way, it helps measure your sense of security and self-acceptance, which gives you the courage to risk the embarrassment of proffering love or friendship or respect, and getting no response. This exercise can provide insight and can alert you to weaknesses that may be reducing your performance in everything from meeting and interacting with potential mates to ordering food in a restaurant.

***Directions***

Read each question carefully. If your response is yes or mostly yes, place a plus (+) on the line preceding the question. If your response is no or mostly no, place a minus (−) on the line. If you honestly can't decide, place a zero (0) on the line; but try to enter as few zeros as possible. Even if a particular question doesn't apply to you, try to imagine yourself in the situation described and answer accordingly. Don't look for any significance in the number or the frequency of plus or minus answers. Simply be honest when answering the questions.

_______ 1. Do you have more than your share of colds?

_______ 2. Do you believe that emotions have very little to do with physical ills?

_______ 3. Do you often have indigestion?

_______ 4. Do you frequently worry about your health?

_______ 5. Would a nutritionist be appalled by your diet?

_______ 6. Do you usually watch sports rather than participate in them?

_______ 7. Do you often feel depressed or in a bad mood?

_______ 8. Are you irritable when things go wrong?

_______ 9. Were you happier in the past than you are right now?

_______ 10. Do you believe it possible that a person's character can be read, or one's future foretold, by means of astrology, I Ching, tarot cards, or the like?

_______ 11. Do you worry about the future?

_______ 12. Do you try to hold in your anger as long as possible and then sometimes explode in a rage?

_______ 13. Do people you care about often make you feel jealous?

_______ 14. If your intimate partner were unfaithful one time, would you be unable to forgive and forget?

_______ 15. Do you have difficulty making important decisions?

_______ 16. Would you abandon a goal rather than take risks to reach it?

_______ 17. When you go on a vacation, do you take some work along?

_______ 18. Do you usually wear clothes that are dark or neutral in color?

_______ 19. Do you usually do what you feel like doing, regardless of social pressures or criticism?

_______ 20. Does a beautiful speaking voice turn you on?

_______ 21. Do you always take an interest in where you are and what's happening around you?

_______ 22. Do you find most odors interesting rather than offensive?

_______ 23. Do you enjoy trying new and different foods?

_______ 24. Do you like to touch and be touched?

_______ 25. Are you easily amused?

_______ 26. Do you often do things spontaneously or impulsively?

_______ 27. Can you sit still through a long committee meeting or lecture without twiddling your thumbs or wriggling in your chair?

_______ 28. Can you usually fall asleep and stay asleep without the use of sleeping pills or tranquilizers?

_______ 29. Are you a moderate drinker rather than either a heavy drinker or a teetotaler?

_______ 30. Do you smoke not at all or very little?

_______ 31. Can you put yourself in another person's place and experience their emotions?

_______ 32. Are you seriously concerned about social problems even when they don't affect you personally?

_______ 33. Do you think most people can be trusted?

_______ 34. Can you talk to a celebrity or a stranger as easily as you talk to your neighbors?

_______ 35. Do you get along well with salesclerks, waiters, service-station attendants, and cabdrivers?

_______ 36. In mixed company, can you discuss sex easily and without feeling uncomfortable?

_______ 37. Can you express appreciation for a gift or a favor without feeling uneasy?

_______ 38. When you feel affection for someone, can you express it physically as well as verbally?

_______ 39. Do you sometimes feel that you have extrasensory perception?

_______ 40. Do you like yourself?

_______ 41. Do you like others of your own sex?

_______ 42. Do you enjoy an evening alone?

_______ 43. Do you vary your schedule to avoid doing the same things at the same times each day?

_______ 44. Is love more important to you than money or status?

_______ 45. Do you place a higher premium on kindness than on truthfulness?

_______ 46. Do you think it is possible to be too rational?

_______ 47. Have you attended, or would you like to attend, a sensitivity or encounter-group session?

_______ 48. Do you discourage friends from dropping in unannounced?

_______ 49. Would you feel it a sign of weakness to seek help for a sexual problem?

_______ 50. Are you upset when a homosexual seems attracted to you?

_______ 51. Do you have difficulty communicating with someone of the opposite sex?

_______ 52. Do you believe that men who write poetry are less masculine than men who drive trucks?

_______ 53. Do most women prefer men with well-developed muscles to men with well-developed emotions?

_______ 54. Are you generally indifferent to the kind of place in which you live?

_______ 55. Do you consider it a waste of money to buy flowers for yourself or for others?

_______ 56. When you see an art object you like, do you pass it up if the cost would mean cutting back on your food budget?

_______ 57. Do you think it pretentious and extravagant to have an elegant dinner when alone or with members of your immediate family?

_______ 58. Are you often bored?

_______ 59. Do Sundays depress you?
_______ 60. Do you frequently feel nervous?
_______ 61. Do you dislike the work you do to earn a living?
_______ 62. Do you think a carefree hippie life-style would have no delights for you?
_______ 63. Do you watch TV selectively rather than simply to kill time?
_______ 64. Have you read any good books recently?
_______ 65. Do you often daydream?
_______ 66. Do you like to fondle pets?
_______ 67. Do you like many different forms and styles of art?
_______ 68. Do you enjoy watching an attractive person of the opposite sex?
_______ 69. Can you describe how your date or mate looked the last time you went out together?
_______ 70. Do you find it easy to talk to new acquaintances?
_______ 71. Do you communicate with others through touch as well as through words?
_______ 72. Do you enjoy pleasing members of your family?
_______ 73. Do you avoid joining clubs or organizations?
_______ 74. Do you worry more about how you present yourself to prospective dates than about how you treat them?
_______ 75. Are you afraid that if people knew you too well they wouldn't like you?
_______ 76. Do you fall in love at first sight?
_______ 77. Do you always fall in love with someone who reminds you of your parent of the opposite sex?
_______ 78. Do you think love is all you currently need to be happy?
_______ 79. Do you feel a sense of rejection if a person you love tries to preserve his or her independence?
_______ 80. Can you accept your loved one's anger and still believe in his or her love?
_______ 81. Can you express your innermost thoughts and feelings to the person you love?
_______ 82. Do you talk over disagreements with your partner rather than silently worry about them?
_______ 83. Can you easily accept the fact that your partner has loved others before you and not worry about how you compare with them?
_______ 84. Can you accept a partner's disinterest in sex without feeling rejected?
_______ 85. Can you accept occasional sessions of unsatisfactory sex without blaming yourself or your partner?
_______ 86. Should unmarried adolescents be denied contraceptives?
_______ 87. Do you believe that even for adults in private there are some sexual acts that should remain illegal?
_______ 88. Do you think that hippie communes and Israeli kibbutzim have nothing useful to teach the average American?
_______ 89. Should a couple put up with an unhappy marriage for the sake of their children?
_______ 90. Do you think that mate swappers necessarily have unhappy marriages?
_______ 91. Should older men and women be content not to have sex?

_______ 92. Do you believe that pornography contributes to sex crimes?

_______ 93. Is sexual abstinence beneficial to a person's health, strength, wisdom, or character?

_______ 94. Can a truly loving wife or husband sometimes be sexually unreceptive?

_______ 95. Can intercourse during a woman's menstrual period be as appealing as at any other time?

_______ 96. Should a woman concentrate on her own sensual pleasure during intercourse rather than pretend enjoyment to increase her partner's pleasure?

_______ 97. Can a man's effort to bring his partner to orgasm reduce his own pleasure?

_______ 98. Should fun and sensual pleasure be the principal goals in sexual relations?

_______ 99. Is pressure to perform well a common cause of sexual incapacity?

_______ 100. Is sexual intercourse an uninhibited romp rather than a demonstration of sexual ability?

***Explanation of Scoring***

Questions 1–18, count your minuses: _______

Questions 19–47, count your pluses: _______

Questions 48–62, count your minuses: _______

Questions 63–72, count your pluses: _______

Questions 73–79, count your minuses: _______

Questions 80–85, count your pluses: _______

Questions 86–93, count your minuses: _______

Questions 94–100, count your pluses: _______

Total: _______

To obtain your corrected score, subtract from this total half the total number of zero answers.

If your corrected score is under 30, you have a shell like a tortoise and tend to draw your head in at the first sign of psychological danger. Probably life handed you some bad blows when you were too young to fight back; so you've erected strong defenses against the kind of intimacy that could leave you vulnerable.

If you scored between 30 and 60, you're about average, which shows you have potential. You've erected some strong defenses; but you've matured enough and have had enough good experiences that you're willing to take a few chances with other human beings, confident that you'll survive regardless.

Any score over 60 means you possess the self-confidence and sense of security not only to run the risks of intimacy, but also to enjoy it. This could be a little discomforting to another person who doesn't have your capacity or potential for close interpersonal relationships; but you're definitely ahead in the game, and you can make the right person extremely happy just by being yourself. If your score approaches 100, either you're an intimate superstar or you're worried too much about giving right answers.

If convenient, do this exercise with someone with whom you feel intimate. Afterward, compare and discuss your answers. The results may indicate how compatible you are, socially or sexually.

Capacity for intimacy is one aspect of interpersonal relationships in which opposites do not necessarily attract. A person of high intimacy capacity can intimidate someone of low capacity who is fearful to respond; but those of similar capacities will tend to make no excessive demands on each other and, for that reason, will find themselves capable of an increasingly intimate and mutually fulfilling relationship.

SOURCE: Adapted from *Go to Health*, copyright 1973 by Communications Research Machines, Inc. Used with permission of Delacorte Press.

ples were living together as domestic partners.

Young people often live together in a trial marriage, getting to know each other better to see whether they're compatible. People who've been married and divorced may be content just sharing their lives with another. Unmarried couples are not very different from married couples: They share, they talk, they quarrel. Marriage counselors in some cities say that more than half the couples they see are not married.

According to a 1989 report in the *Journal of Marriage and the Family,* which studied more than 14,000 couples, 40 percent of those who had lived together eventually got married.[3] And these "cohabitors" were 7.25 times more likely to stay married than the couples who had not shared a home before marriage. However, a Yale University sociologist reported in the *American Sociological Review* that Swedish women who lived with male partners were 80 percent more likely to separate or divorce than women who hadn't moved in with their would-be mates.[4]

## MARRIAGE

Contemporary marriage has been described as an institution that everyone on the outside wants to enter and everyone on the inside wants to leave. About 90 percent of all American adults marry—for as long as they both love, if not live. Ten percent of adults who ever marry get a divorce. By 1990, there were about 105 million Americans married and living with their spouses and 14 million divorced men and women. That means that about 133 of every 1,000 marriages to date have ended in divorce.

Yet 70 to 75 percent of Americans who divorce remarry—generally within two years. Even after their hopes for happiness with one spouse end, men and women still yearn for the challenges and rewards of meshing two personalities, two life histories, and two dreams into a marriage.

### HEALTH HEADLINE

**Where Does Living Together Lead?**

**Marriage isn't automatically the next step for couples who live together. In fact, equal numbers of men and women split up or marry after cohabitation. In a study of more than nine hundred 23-year-old men and women, University of Michigan researchers found that 40 percent of the men and 23 percent of the women separated from their domestic partners within two years. In that same time period, 23 percent of the men and 37 percent of the women married their live-in lovers.**

SOURCE: "Does Cohabitation Last?" *Psychology Today,* June 1989.

### Whom and Why We Marry

Not too long ago, marriage was often a business deal, a contract made by parents for economic or political reasons when the spouses-to-be were still very young. Today, some ethnic groups, such as Asians who've recently immigrated to the United States, still "arrange" marriages.

Generally today's men and women marry people from the geographical area that they grew up in and from the same social background. However, we don't simply choose the most convenient partners. We choose mates very much like ourselves—and couples with the same level of education, the same values, and the same economic status are more likely to stay married. Differences in religion and race add to the pressures on any marriage. Differences in age can create difficulties years after the ceremony.

Even in this day and age, partners often marry because they "have to"—one of every six brides is pregnant on her wedding day—and many young couples marry as a way to escape from their parents' homes and authority. But most people say they marry for love.

The best indicators of whether a marriage will succeed are not the reasons for the marriage, but the ages of the bride and groom.[5] Half of the marriages between people under age 20 break up within five years; another 25 percent dissolve later. People who marry in their late twenties tend to have more successful marriages than those who marry younger.

What keeps two people together? According to psychologist Robert Sternberg of Yale University, the crucial ingredients of commitment are the following:

- shared values
- a willingness to change in response to each other
- a willingness to tolerate flaws
- a match in religious beliefs
- the ability to communicate effectively

STRATEGY FOR CHANGE

**When to Think Twice About a Relationship**

Don't get married if:

- You or your partner is constantly asking the other questions like "Are you sure you love me?"
- You spend most of your time together disagreeing and quarreling.
- You are both still very young (under age 20).
- You are really looking for a "mother" or "father," not an equal.
- You frequently have thoughts like "He/she will change after we're married."
- Your boyfriend/girlfriend has behaviors (such as nonstop talking), traits (such as bossiness), or problems (such as drinking too much) that really bother you.
- Your partner wants you to stop seeing your friends, quit a job you enjoy, or change your life in a way that limits rather than enhances your satisfaction with your life.

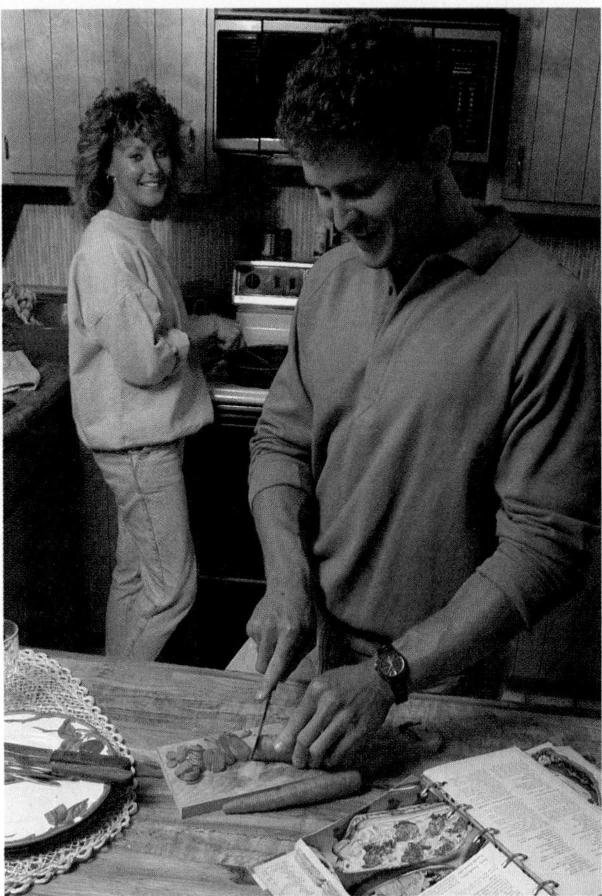

In any enduring relationship, couples have to learn to work together as partners.

## Building a Partnership

Studies of "couples development" have shown that most marriages go through four basic stages. In the first, the spouses are self-centered, interested in what the relationship can do for them. In the second stage, the couple starts negotiating, trading one service for another ("I'll do the dishes if you take the car to the garage for a tune-up," for example). During the third stage, the spouses begin to appreciate each other's individuality and to make accommodations for the good of the marriage. By the fourth stage, they have developed "rules of the relationship," by which they avoid or deal with problems.

No two people can live together in perfect harmony all the time. Among the issues that crop up in any long-term relationship are unrealistic expectations, communication problems, money, and sex.

### Unrealistic Expectations

Spouses may think their mates should always be as attractive, charming, and tolerant as when they were dating. They may assume that their partners will always agree with them or will automatically see their point of view. Or they may believe that their one true love will always be able to meet all their needs. Because no one could ever live up to such expectations, the partners are doomed to disappointment.

### Communication Problems

Some fighting can be a good thing, but too much isn't. If the two of you are always squabbling, take a deeper look at what sets off your quarrels. Are you fighting out of boredom? Or to convince yourselves that you still care about each other when you really don't? Are you secretly hoping for a fight so nasty that you'll be able to break up without feeling guilty? The art of arguing is a skill, like bicycle riding, that anyone can master with time, patience, and plenty of practice.

STRATEGY FOR CHANGE

**How to Fight Fairly**

- Start your sentences with "I," not "you." Instead of attacking with a statement like "You're jealous and immature," say "I feel hurt when you quiz me about my old relationships."
- Make sure you're arguing about the right issue. Are you angry simply because your partner's never on time? Or because you don't seem to be the top priority?

HEALTH SPOTLIGHT

## Lessons from Happy Marriages

Many long-running relationships not only survive but also thrive through the years. What's the secret? Here are some of the characteristics that researchers have found in happy couples:

- They're best friends. They share secrets, work, and play; they hang out together; and they laugh a lot.
- They listen to, and confide in, each other. They discuss and debate everything—and they reveal their innermost feelings and fears to each other.
- They're tuned in to each other's feelings. Unlike the stereotype of silent, cold men, the husbands in good marriages "are just as expressive as the women."
- They can deal with negative emotions and keep them from getting out of control.
- They know how to handle conflict. Happy couples focus on an issue; deal only with the current problem; and criticize the spouse's action, not the spouse.
- They're less than brutally honest. Although they express their feelings clearly, they know that hurtful words can leave scars.
- They trust each other. In a good marriage partners can show their weakest side and know they'll still be loved.
- They're committed to making the marriage work. Even in the roughest times, they choose to stick it out with each other.
- They share interests and values. And their common interests create a bond that keeps their relationship strong.
- They're flexible enough to change and tolerate change. In fact, their marriages endure and improve—not despite the changes and challenges, but because of them.

- Don't embarrass each other by fighting in front of others.
- Even if you're alone, don't attack each other so viciously that one of you is backed into a corner.
- Avoid generalizations, like "You always interrupt me."
- Be fair. Whenever there's a cheap shot, one of you should stop the fight by crying "Foul!"
- Focus on the issue at hand.
- Think before you open your mouth. Taking a few deep breaths will give you a chance to weigh your words.
- Learn to listen. Rather than thinking about what you're going to say next, tune in to your partner's words, gestures, or expression.
- If you can't come to terms on a particular issue, agree to disagree or to keep talking about your differences in the future.

### Money

Money, which makes the business world go around, has the opposite effect on marriages: It knocks them off their tracks, brings them to a halt, twists them upside down. However, even though almost all couples quarrel about money, they rarely fight over how much they have. What matters more—whether they make $10,000 or $100,000 a year—is what money means to both partners. How does each person use money to meet emotional needs? Who decides how the money is spent? Who keeps track? Until they resolve these issues, couples may quarrel over money as long as they're together.

STRATEGY FOR CHANGE

#### How to Stop Fighting About Money

Set a specific time to have a serious talk about money and what it means to you and your relationship.

- Try to understand that being different in money values or expectations doesn't make one of you right and the other wrong.
- Recognize the value of unpaid work. A spouse who's finishing school or taking care of the children is making an important contribution to the family and its future.
- Go over your finances together so you have a firm reality base for what you can and can't afford.
- Talk about the financial goals you hope to attain five years from now. Set priorities to meet them.
- Set aside money for each of you to spend without asking or answering to the other.

### Sex

According to a 1990 survey by the National Opinion Research Center at the University of Chicago, married couples have intercourse slightly more than once a week.[6] The happiest couples have sex most often. In the survey, the people reporting the happiest marriages said they had sex 74.8 times on average in the past year, compared with 42.9 times for those who said they were unhappy. The "pretty happy" couples had sex 57.7 times a year.

But when it comes to sex, numbers aren't what matter most. What is important is whether both partners are satisfied with both the quantity and quality of their sexual activity. (Chapter 7 presents guidelines for making sex better.)

## Two-Career Couples

Two-career couples now head 67 percent of families with children under age 18. More than 60 percent of women with children under age 18 work—a dramatic increase from the 1960s, when only 30 percent of mothers worked outside the home.[7]

Many wives work to help make financial ends meet, but work can also bring new challenges and satisfactions to their lives. In extensive studies on health and social roles, working wives and mothers are healthier and happier—though often more hassled—than women who don't work outside their homes.

Two careers can lead to additional pressures on a relationship. Partners pursuing individual careers sometimes face difficult choices. What happens, for example, if the husband is offered a promising job in another city? What if she's offered a promising job elsewhere? Does the spouse automatically pack up and go? Some couples resolve such dilemmas by working in different cities and spending weekends together.

**STRATEGY FOR CHANGE**

### Handling Dual-Career Stress

Marital therapists report that they are seeing more two-career couples struggling with the demands of their double lives. Here are some suggestions to help working couples cope:

- Plan your weekends. List your priorities, and take turns selecting what you'll do.
- Keep dating. Block out a time at least once a week to enjoy each other's company and to talk about your concerns and feelings.
- Spend a night—or, if possible, a weekend—alone once every three months.
- You both know what it's like to deal with office politics, angry bosses, and rush-hour traffic. Empathize and reassure each other.
- Accept help without imposing your standards. Whoever does the shopping or washes the car shouldn't have to do it your way. Just be grateful you didn't have to do it yourself.

## Can This Marriage Be Saved? Lessons from Marital Therapy

According to the Association of Family and Marital Therapists, at least one out of every five couples in this country needs professional counseling. However, there is good news for troubled partners: Marital therapy can and does help. According to recent research, the relationships of about two-thirds of those who get counseling do improve—both in the couples' own judgments and according to objective measures of marital satisfaction.

A well-trained counselor can spot destructive behavior patterns and help couples see their situations in a new light. Therapy often helps stop spouses from hurting each other so badly that they can't stay together. If nothing else, it can help both partners decide whether to continue or end the relationship.

## Extramarital Affairs

According to recent studies, most married partners don't cheat on each other. In sociologist Andrew Greeley's survey of 657 couples, reported in *Psychology Today* in 1990, 90 percent of husbands and wives have never been unfaithful to each other.[8] But when extramarital affairs do occur, they can be devastating. A husband or wife who learns about a spouse's affair typically feels an overwhelming sense of betrayal as well as deep feelings of guilt, shame, fear of abandonment, depression, and anger. Two crucial questions determine whether a marriage can survive: Do the spouses still feel a serious commitment toward each other? Do they love each other and want to grow old together?

**STRATEGY FOR CHANGE**

**How to Stay Married**

Focus on what's right with your spouse.

- Learn to negotiate for what you want. One effective approach is offering your mate what he or she wants in return.
- Look for the problem behind the problem. Often an affair or a lack of sexual interest is merely a symptom; the real question is why the problem developed.
- Keep your perspective. Uncapped toothpaste tubes or socks on the floor may be annoying, but are they worth a fight?
- Rather than thinking of all the things your partner is or isn't doing, focus on what you can do to make your marriage better.

### The Rewards of Marriage

Despite its problems, marriage endures because it's a fulfilling way for two people to live. Marriage can make people both happy and healthy. Married men and women live longer than the unmarried. Divorced, widowed, and single people—regardless of race or sex—are more likely to die of heart disease and other illnesses. Married men are much less prone to accidents, alcoholism, and illness than unmarried men. Married people may even get fewer colds. In a study comparing the immune system (the protective network that wards off health threats), University of Ohio researchers found that happily married women had the healthiest immune function.[9] Those in unhappy unions had the weakest immune systems.

Marriage's impact on the mind is just as profound. In surveys that assess which adults are most happy and satisfied with their lives, the highest scores consistently come from married persons, especially husbands. Marriage seems to serve as a protective barrier against life's stresses. Although it can't prevent economic and social upheavals, it buffers their impact so that married men and women are far less likely to be depressed or anxious than are divorced, separated, or single persons.

**HEALTH HEADLINE**

**Fidelity Becomes a Fad**

**Ninety percent of American husbands and wives have never been unfaithful to each other, according to a 1990 survey of 657 couples. Nearly two-thirds of the spouses said they were very happy in their marriages, and four of five said they would wed the same person again. Three out of four described their mates as physically attractive. According to the poll, the three key factors in making a marriage happy are communication, cooperation in child care and housework, and romance. Perhaps in a backlash to the sexual revolution, 51 percent of the women under 35 in the survey regretted having had a premarital affair; 16 percent of the men felt that way.**

SOURCE: Greeley, Andrew. "Faithful Attraction," *Psychology Today,* March 1990.

## PARENTHOOD

Parenting is a 24-hour-a-day, 7-day-a-week, 52-week-a-year job, with no sabbaticals or sick leaves and no opportunity to renegotiate the contract. Though caring for children is no easier than parenting ever was, today's parents have more options and greater flexibility in defining their roles, sharing their responsibilities, and asserting their own rights.

Styles of parenting are less important than the needs of the child. The greatest need is for love—the feeling of being wanted and cared for, of being special, and of realizing that the parents like the child for himself or herself. Children have other needs, too: security, protection, confidence, a feeling of belonging, a set of standards and human values, models to teach behavior, and clearly defined limits and controls.

### When Baby Makes Three

Experts in family development have been studying the changes a baby brings to a marriage. The bad news is that marital satisfaction invariably declines, if only slightly, while the number of separations and divorces rises. However, researchers have also found some unexpected good news: Couples who stick together as partners through the process of becoming parents can keep their marriages strong.

**STRATEGY FOR CHANGE**

**Staying Close as Partners and Parents**

- Make sure your expectations are realistic. Learn as much as you can—from books, friends, or your own parents—about the facts of life with a newborn.
- Express your negative feelings. It's not wrong to feel trapped, overwhelmed, or resentful at times; in fact, it's normal.
- Make time for just the two of you.
- Talk with other parents. You'll find comfort in comparing notes and sharing problems.
- Focus on the positives. The feel of a fuzzy little head against your cheek, the toothless grins, and the first big hugs put the hassles into perspective.

## New Roles for Fathers

Fathers contribute to a child's social and intellectual growth in unique ways. Whereas mothers tend to touch their infants for caretaking purposes—such as feeding, changing, and bathing—fathers spend more time than mothers playing games with infants. Fathers tend to be more tactile and less verbal. They swing the baby into the air; mothers play peekaboo. Babies who interact extensively with their fathers are more at ease with strangers.

**STRATEGY FOR CHANGE**

**How to Be a Better Parent**

Among the principles taught at parenting classes are the following:

- Give attention and praise for good behavior, not bad.
- To avoid misbehaviors, try to figure out what's causing the problem: boredom, insecurity, lack of attention, and so on.
- Learn how to listen to your children rather than rushing to explain, criticize, or comfort.
- When possible, offer your child two acceptable choices.
- Involve children in problem solving. Write down all possible solutions to a problem, without commenting on them. Add yours to the list. Then choose one you all can live with.

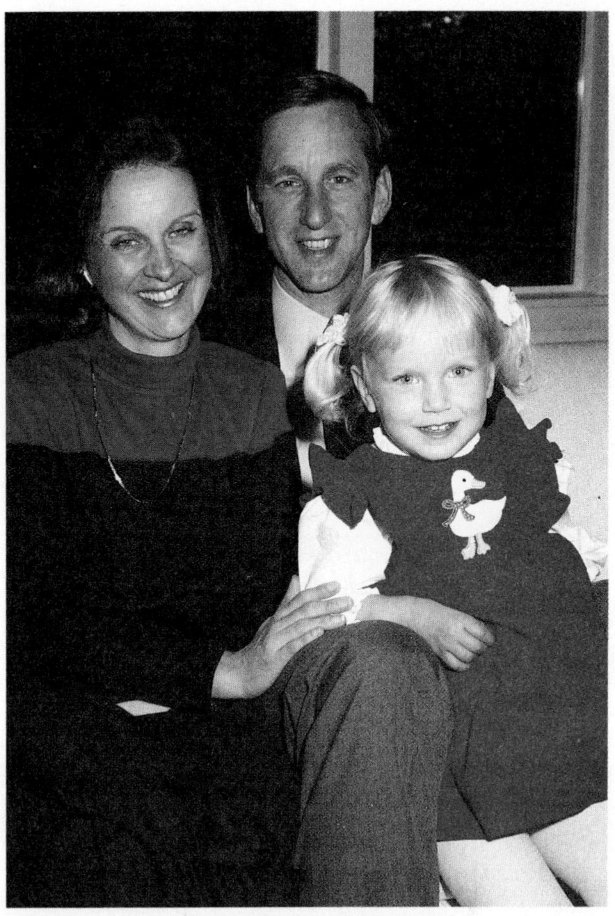

Whether large or small, the family serves as a training ground for living and for loving.

## New Responsibilities for Mothers

More than half of today's mothers work outside the home. In many ways these women are forging into new territory. Without any role models or rules for being a mother plus a doctor, banker, or carpenter, many working mothers feel anxious—even guilty—about their dual careers. Most experts say they shouldn't.

"There's no one right way to be a mother," says psychologist Helen Cleminshaw, director of the Center for Family Studies at the University of Akron.[10] "But women should know that they have options, that they can have a life outside the home and still meet their children's needs." Ultimately, the happiest children are those whose mothers are happy with their decision to work or not.

## STRATEGY FOR CHANGE

### Working and Caring

- Make your children your top priority when you're home. In addition to special activities, spend quiet times together.
- Set aside a few minutes for a one-to-one conversation with each child every night before bedtime.
- If you can't be home when your children get out of school, check in with them by telephone.
- Talk about your job with your children. Let them see where you work so they know what you're doing when you're not home.

## FAMILY TIES

Children who spend their entire childhood in a two-parent family will become a minority in the twenty-first century. The number of two-parent families is dropping, and the number of one-parent families is soaring. More than half of the children born this year will spend at least one year living in a single-parent household before they reach age 18.

### Divorce

More than 1.2 million marriages end in divorce every year. The divorce rate soared in the 1960s and 1970s but held steady in the 1980s.[11] Yet more than one in every five men and women who've ever been married has been divorced.

Legally, divorce has become easier. Many states have no-fault divorce laws in which both partners simply agree to separate without blaming one or the other. Throughout the country, alimony is no longer considered the "wronged" spouse's due. Often money is awarded only if one partner does not have job training and needs funds for education.

Emotionally, divorce remains as painful as ever. And divorce affects others besides the two adults who once vowed to love each other. Each year divorce separates more than a million children from their parents. For most children, divorce is a personal, familial, and social loss.

Divorce has an enormous impact on many aspects of a child's life, including his or her standard of living. A national survey has shown that the incomes of women who do not remarry after a divorce fall by 30 percent. Among black women, the decline is even greater.[12]

After divorce, very young children may become more babyish, irritable, and dependent. Preschool or young school-age children may blame themselves, feeling that "Daddy left because I was bad." The reactions of school-age children are more complex. Children in this age group may feel lonely, helpless, and depressed; they may develop illnesses or have problems in their friendships. Preteens may experiment with alcohol, drugs, and sex. For teenagers, divorce may make separating from the family and establishing an adult identity even harder.

According to various reports, 15 to 20 percent of all children whose parents divorce may require professional therapy.[13] The impact of divorce may be more

## WHAT DO YOU THINK?

Kevin and Hannah both enjoy windsurfing, long walks, and Thai food, and they look forward to spending more time together. But if they should get involved, they may face some serious issues. The reason: Kevin is black; Hannah is white. Though our society has become more tolerant, interracial couples still face special pressures. What are they? How do you feel about romances between people of different races? What about different religions? Why?

Priana, 21 years old and a junior in college, and Steve, 20 years old and a sophomore, have dated since high school. Both work part-time; their parents occasionally help them out financially. They've talked about getting married, but Steve thinks they should live together until they're financially secure. Priana feels the real reason is that Steve doesn't want to make a commitment. If they were your friends, what would you say?

Bethene and Michael, a married couple in their early thirties, have successful careers that involve long hours. Bethene is a high school principal and wants to run for a seat on her county school board. Michael hopes to become the chief physical therapist at the hospital. Both also want children. What issues should they address before having a baby? How would you juggle the demands of your job and those of children? Would your answer be different if you were the other-sex parent?

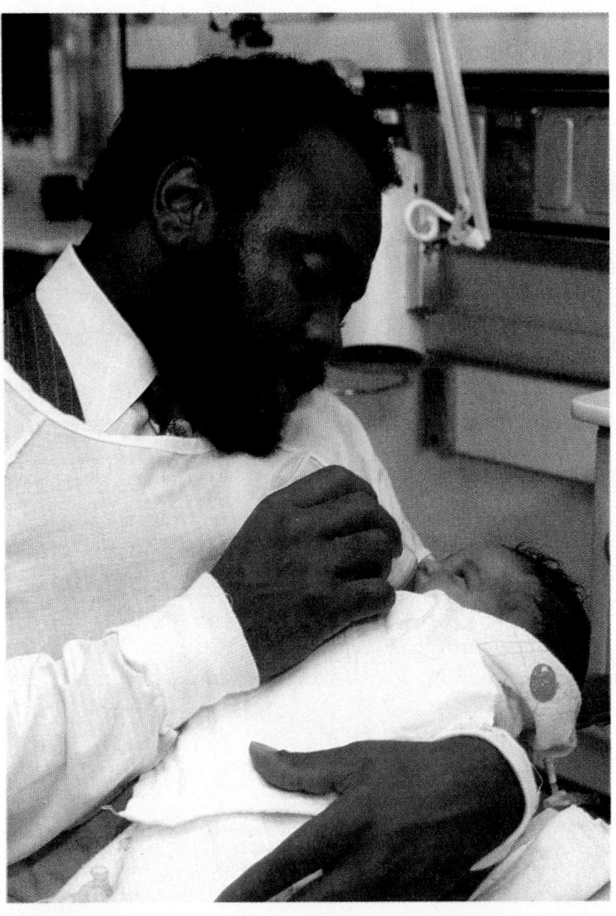

Involved, loving fathers contribute to a child's development in unique ways.

intense and enduring for boys than for girls. One long-term effect of divorce that affects girls more is a greater likelihood of divorce when they grow up and marry.

## Single-Parent Families

Single-parent families are all different, as are two-parent families. An educated divorced woman in her thirties with one school-age child has very different options and opportunities than a young, unskilled, never married woman with three preschoolers. However, at every economic level, the amount of time single parents spend with their children is not significantly different from that spent by parents in two-parent families—and psychologists have found no negative impact of a single-parent family on a child's intellectual or academic achievement.

## Blended Families

Each year about half a million children become part of a new "blended" family after their parents remarry. Stepfamilies are as successful as other families in adapting to change and solving problems. Children in blended families fare better economically than those in single-parent homes, but they have more behavior problems than those in families that have not experienced divorce. The recent growth in stepfamilies has occurred so quickly that individuals, families, and society have had little time to develop ways of coping with the problems that blending families can create.

## MAKING THIS CHAPTER WORK FOR YOU

### Building Better Relationships

We are born social. From our first days of life, we reach out to others. People make us smile, laugh, cry, hope, and pray. The fabric of our personalities and lives becomes richer as others weave through it the threads of their experiences.

Intimacy is essential to close, emotionally satisfying relationships. How we feel about ourselves affects how others feel about us. But we must also learn how to express our feelings and needs. Relationships begin with signals: yes, no, and maybe. From the first, we should try to make our signals clear. As we progress to messages, we should try to reach within and without: within to be sure we are responding honestly and naturally, without to express our feelings as precisely as we can.

Some people feel that relationships shouldn't require any effort, that there's no need to talk of responsibility between people who care about each other. Yet responsibility is implicit in our dealings with anyone or anything we value—and what is more valuable than the ways we share our lives?

Friends often become our extended family, providing acceptance, warmth, and loyalty. Dating provides opportunities to get to know other people, to practice social skills, and to explore one's sexuality. Love brings an extra dimension to heterosexual and homosexual relationships: commitment, tenderness, and passion.

Increasingly, young adults are spending longer periods of time living alone, with their parents or with a partner. If they decide to marry, many couples do so for love. The older and more similar two people are, the more likely they are to have a successful marriage.

Even happily married couples must contend with many complex issues, including two careers, money, sex, and communication problems. Conflict in a relationship can be constructive, as long as the partners are able to fight fairly. Marriage therapy can teach couples skills and behaviors that can improve their relationships. For all its challenges, marriage provides many rewards. Married people tend to be healthier, to live longer, and to cope with stress better than single people.

Parenthood is the most demanding, difficult, and gratifying job two people will ever have. The roles and responsibilities of parents today are not as rigidly defined as they were in the past; more fathers are actively involved with their children and more mothers have careers. Both parents must realize that, at each stage of their development, children have special needs and abilities.

Although divorce laws have become more fair and divorce is more socially acceptable, it is still painful for the couple as well as for their children. The response of children to the divorce of their parents depends on their age and on the amount of fighting before and after the divorce.

Throughout life, each of us is responsible for keeping up our end of many relationships, be they with friends, dates, partner, spouse, or children. Yet our words seldom fully express what we feel. This means that every relationship involves a healthy and vital struggle toward understanding. Here are some guidelines to help:

- Develop the habit of asking the other people in your life about their feelings, thoughts, interests, and desires. Never assume.
- With friends, partners, and families, function as a team. Work at making decisions and solving problems together.
- Give the people you care about daily doses of the four *As*: attention, acceptance, approval, and affection.
- Build common interests.
- Don't play games, such as trying to make a friend jealous, getting even, or proving someone wrong.
- Be polite. Politeness is a way of saying "I care about you," and it means more than an expensive gift.
- Give as much of yourself as you can. The more time you can give to the people who mean the most to you, the closer you'll become. You won't have to wonder what you're getting out of your relationships; you'll discover that the getting comes with the giving.

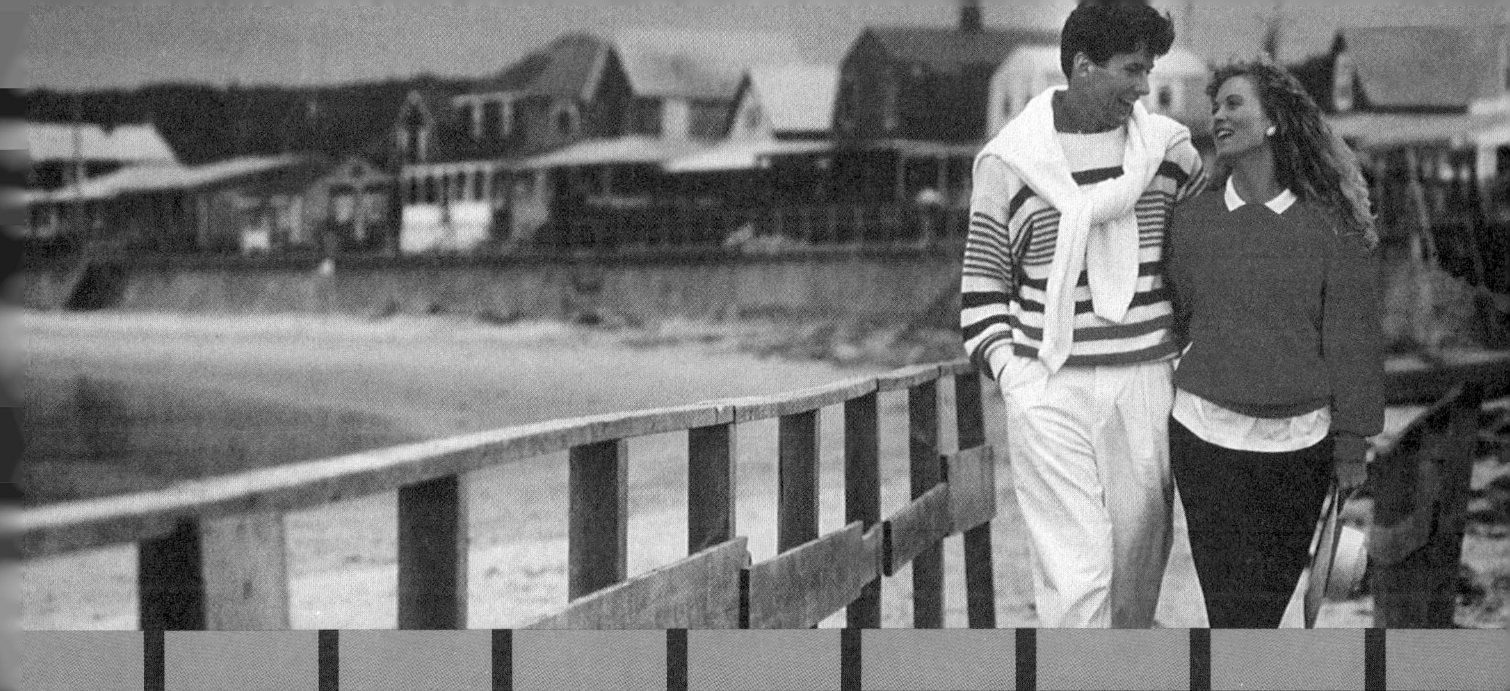

# 7 SEXUAL HEALTH AND BEHAVIOR

In this chapter

Women's sexual health

Men's sexual health

Sexual development

Sex and gender

Sexual preference

Sexual intimacy

Safer sex: Avoiding health risks

Sexual difficulty

Sexual assault

The business of sex

Making this chapter work for you: Responsible sexuality

*You are ultimately responsible for your sexual health and satisfaction.* You make decisions that affect how you express your sexuality, how you respond sexually, and how you give and get pleasure. Yet most sexual activity involves another person. Therefore, your decisions about sex—more so than those you make about nutrition, drugs, or exercise—have important effects on other people. Recognizing that fact is the key to responsible sexuality.

Sexual responsibility involves learning about your body, your partner's body, your sexual development and preference, and various sexual behaviors. It also means protecting yourself and your partner from sexually transmitted diseases, including common infections and the disease our society has come to dread most—acquired immune deficiency syndrome (AIDS). In today's world, you need to understand the risks of various sexual activities and to learn about safer sex practices for a simple reason: Your life may depend on it.

This chapter is an introduction to your sexual self and an exploration of sexual issues in today's world. It provides the information and insight you need to make decisions and to choose behaviors that are responsible for all concerned.

## WOMEN'S SEXUAL HEALTH

In part because more of women's sex organs are hidden from view than are men's, female sexuality has long seemed mysterious. Only recently has a realistic understanding of women's sexual health and problems emerged.

### Female Sex Organs

As illustrated in Figure 7-1(a), the **mons pubis** is the hair-covered area over the pubic bone. The folds of skin that form the outer lips of a woman's genital area are called the **labia majora.** They cover soft flaps of skin (inner lips) called the **labia minora.** The inner

**mons pubis** The rounded fleshy area over the junction of the pubic bones.
**labia majora** The fleshy outer folds that border the female genital area.
**labia minora** The fleshy inner folds that border the female genital area.

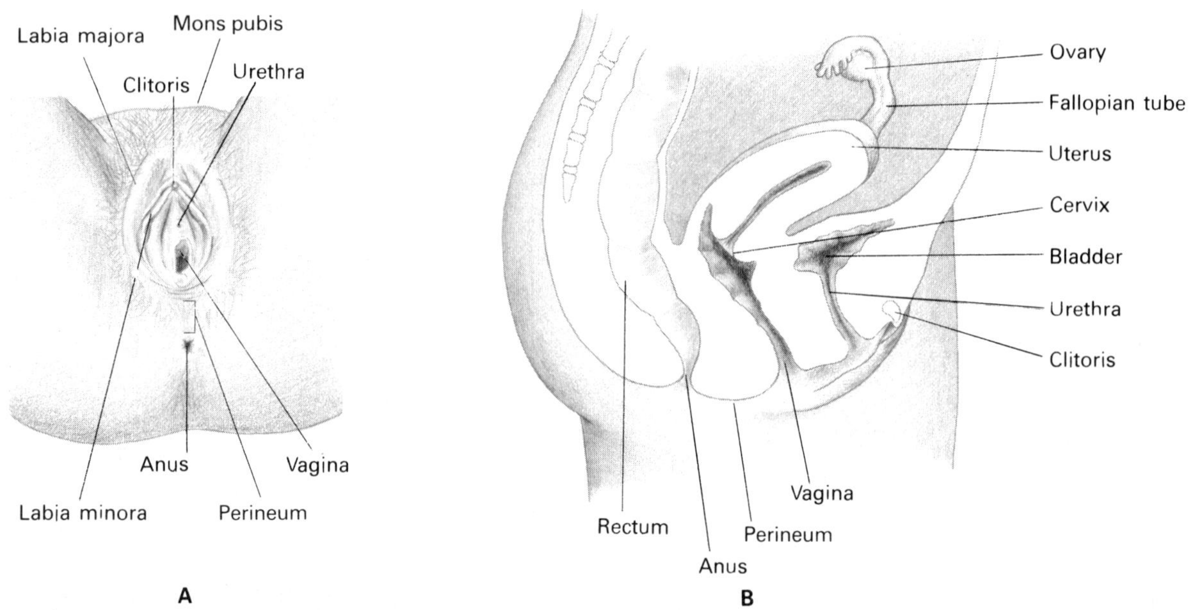


SOURCE: Hales, Dianne. *An Invitation to Health, Fourth Edition,* Benjamin/Cummings, 1989.

**FIGURE 7-1** Female sexual and reproductive anatomy. **(a)** External view of the female genitals; **(b)** cross section of the female organs.

lips join at the top to form a hood over the **clitoris,** the most sensitive spot in the entire genital area. Below the clitoris is the **urethra,** the outer opening of the thin tube that carries urine from the bladder. Below that is a larger opening, the mouth of the **vagina,** the canal that leads to the primary internal organs of reproduction. The **perineum** is the area between the vagina and the anus (the opening to the rectum and large intestine).

At the back of the vagina is the **cervix,** the opening to the womb, or **uterus** (Figure 7-1(b)). The **ovaries,** about the size and shape of almonds, are located on either side of the uterus and produce both **ova** (egg cells) and female sex hormones. Extending outward and back from the upper uterus are the **fallopian tubes,** the vessels that transport ova from the ovaries to the uterus. When an egg is released from an ovary, the fingerlike ends of the adjacent fallopian tube "catch" the egg and direct it into the tube.

## The Menstrual Cycle

As shown in Figure 7-2, the pituitary gland sets the menstrual cycle into motion by releasing **follicle-stimulating hormone (FSH)** and **luteinizing hormone (LH).** In the ovary, these hormones stimulate the growth of a few of the 400,000 to 500,000 egg-containing follicles stored in every woman's body. Usually only one follicle matures completely during each cycle. As it does, this follicle increases its production of the female sex hormone **estrogen,** which in turn causes the pituitary to release a larger surge of LH.

At mid-cycle, the increased hormones trigger ovulation, the release of the egg cell, or ovum. The cells of the follicle then enlarge, change character, and form the corpus luteum, or yellow body. In the second half of the menstrual cycle, the corpus luteum secretes both estrogen and **progesterone,** the hormone that prepares the uterus for implantation of a fertilized ovum and the breasts for nursing.

If the ovum is not fertilized, the corpus luteum disintegrates. Levels of the female sex hormones estrogen and progesterone drop, and the uterine lining is shed in a menstrual period. If the egg is fertilized, the cells that eventually develop into the placenta secrete human chorionic gonadotropin (HCG), a messenger hormone that signals the pituitary not to start a new menstrual cycle. The corpus luteum then steps up its hormone production.

Many women experience physical or psychological changes, or both, during their monthly cycles. Usually the changes are minor, but more serious problems can occur.

### Premenstrual Problems

Many women develop physical and psychological distress—including water retention, bloating, breast tenderness, fatigue, lethargy, irritability, crying spells, anxiety, constipation, acne, headaches, and a craving for sweet or salty foods, before their menstrual periods begin.

The majority of menstruating women notice at least one emotional, behavioral, or physical change in the week before menstruation. Some 3 to 10 percent suffer disabling symptoms and changes that may disrupt their lives for a week or more. **Premenstrual syndrome (PMS)** refers to the most severe symptoms; milder cases are described as premenstrual tension.

Once dismissed as a psychological problem, PMS has been recognized as a very real physiological disorder that may be caused by a hormonal deficiency; changes in brain chemicals; or social and environmental factors, particularly stress. For some women with PMS, treatment with diuretics (drugs that speed up fluid elimination) relieves the problem. Others use behavioral approaches, such as exercise, and chart their cycles to know when they're vulnerable. Researchers are hoping that promising research with a high-carbohydrate diet and with drugs that reduce some symptoms of PMS may provide more help for more women in the future.

---

**clitoris** A small erectile structure on the female, corresponding to the penis on the male.
**urethra** The canal through which urine from the bladder leaves the body; in the males, serves as the conduit for semen as well.
**vagina** The canal leading from the exterior opening in the female genital area to the uterus.
**perineum** The area between the anus and the vagina in the female and between the anus and the scrotum in the male.
**cervix** The opening between the vagina and the uterus.
**uterus** The female organ that houses the fetus until birth.
**ovary** The female sex organ in which ova are produced.
**ovum** (plural: *ova*) The female gamete (egg cell).
**fallopian tubes** The pair of tubes that transport ova from the ovaries to the uterus; the usual site of fertilization.
**follicle-stimulating hormone (FSH)** A hormone, produced by the pituitary gland, that stimulates the growth of ovarian follicles in females and sperm production in males.
**luteinizing hormone (LH)** A hormone, produced by the pituitary gland, that stimulates maturation of ovarian egg cells in the female and production of testosterone in males.
**estrogen** The female sex hormone that stimulates female secondary sex characteristics.
**progesterone** A hormone that stimulates the uterus, preparing it for the arrival of a fertilized egg.
**premenstrual syndrome (PMS)** A disorder that causes physical discomfort and psychological distress prior to a woman's menstrual period.

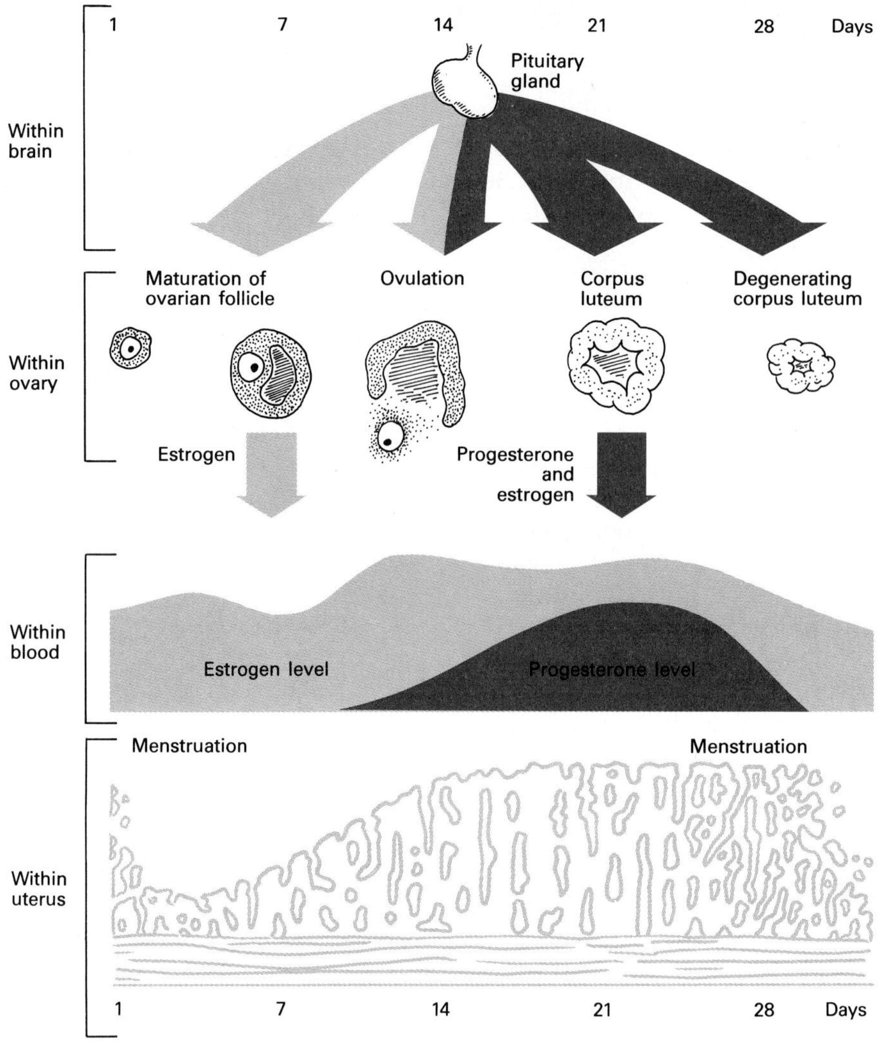


SOURCE: Hales, Dianne. *An Invitation to Health, Fourth Edition*, Benjamin/Cummings, 1989.

**FIGURE 7-2** The menstrual cycle. The pituitary gland secretes hormones that promote the maturation of an *ovarian follicle*, one of many tiny cavities in the ovary containing an ovum. The ovarian follicle matures rapidly until it ruptures, releasing the ovum into the fallopian tube. The remnant of the ovarian follicle then begins to secrete progesterone, which stimulates the growth of the uterine lining, preparing it for implantation of the fertilized egg. If the egg is not fertilized, progesterone production decreases, the uterine lining is shed in menstruation, and the cycle begins again.

STRATEGY FOR CHANGE

### Coping with Premenstrual Problems

- Get plenty of exercise. Physically fit women usually have fewer problems both before and during their periods.
- Eat often and nutritiously. In the week before your period, your body doesn't regulate the levels of sugar, or glucose, in your blood as well as it usually does.
- Get sufficient vitamins.
- Swear off salt. If you stop using salt at the table and while cooking, you may gain less weight premenstrually, feel less bloated, and suffer less from headaches and irritability.
- Cut back on caffeine. Coffee, colas, diet colas, chocolate, and tea can increase breast tenderness and other symptoms.
- Don't drink or smoke. Some women become so sensitive to alcohol's effects before their periods that a glass of wine hits with the impact of several stiff drinks. Nicotine worsens low-blood-sugar problems.

### Menstrual Cramps

About half of all menstruating women suffer from **dysmenorrhea,** the medical name for the discom-

**dysmenorrhea** Painful menstruation.

forts—abdominal cramps and pain, back and leg pain, diarrhea, tension, water retention, fatigue, and depression—that accompany menstruation. The cause seems to be an overproduction of bodily substances called prostaglandins, which typically rise during menstruation.

### Amenorrhea

Women may stop menstruating—a condition called **amenorrhea**—for a variety of reasons, including a hormonal disorder, drastic weight loss, or change in environment. "Boarding-school amenorrhea" is common among young women who leave home for school. Distance running and strenuous exercise can also lead to amenorrhea. The reason may be a drop in body fat from the normal 18 to 22 percent to 10 to 12 percent. Prolonged amenorrhea can have serious health consequences, including a loss of bone density that could lead to stress fractures and osteoporosis.

### Toxic Shock Syndrome

This rare, potentially deadly bacterial infection primarily strikes menstruating women under the age of 30 who use tampons. Symptoms include a high fever; a rash that leads to peeling of the skin on the fingers, toes, palms, and soles; dizziness; dangerously low blood pressure; and abnormalities in several organ systems (the digestive tract and the kidneys) and in the muscles and blood. (See Chapter 15 for a more extensive discussion of this disease.)

To reduce their risk of Toxic Shock Syndrome, menstruating women should use sanitary napkins instead of tampons. If they do use tampons, they should use regular instead of superabsorbent, change them three or four times during the day, and use napkins during the night or for some time during each day of menstrual flow.

### Menopause

The median age of **menopause,** the end of monthly menstrual cycles, among women in the United States is 51.4 years. Usually the "change of life" is a gradual process. By the time a woman reaches her forties, her ovaries do not respond as they once did to stimulation by the pituitary hormones. Her periods become irregular. Eventually the ovaries do not respond at all, and estrogen decreases rapidly.

For some women, menopause triggers psychological as well as physiological change. Yet most women today seem to take menopause in stride. In a survey of 2,500 healthy women between the ages of 45 and 55, National Institute on Aging researchers found that few experienced severe symptoms, and 75 percent expressed either relief or no particular feelings about having arrived at menopause.[1]

## MEN'S SEXUAL HEALTH

Because the male reproductive system is simpler in many ways, it's often ignored—especially by healthy young men. However, just like women, men should make regular self-exams (including the checks of their penises, testes, and breasts described in Chapter 12) part of their routine.

### Male Sex Organs

The visible parts of the male sexual system are the **penis** and the **scrotum,** the pouch that contains the **testes,** which manufacture testosterone and **sperm** cells (Figure 7-3(a)). Sperm are stored in the **epididymis,** a collection of coiled tubes adjacent to each testis (Figure 7-3(b)).

The penis contains three hollow cylinders loosely covered with skin. The two major cylinders, the corpora cavernosa, extend side by side through the length of the penis. The third cylinder, the corpus spongiosum, surrounds the urethra, the channel for both seminal fluid and urine.

When hanging down loosely, the average penis measures 3 3/4 inches in length. During erection, its internal cylinders fill with so much blood that they become rigid, and the penis stretches to an average length of 6 1/4 inches. About 90 percent of all men have erect penises measuring between 5 and 7 inches in length. There is no relation between penis size and female satisfaction; a woman's vagina naturally adjusts to the size of the penis.

---

**amenorrhea** The absence or suppression of menstruation.
**menopause** The period during which menstruation ceases and a woman's reproductive ability ends.
**penis** The organ of sex and urination in the male.
**scrotum** The sack of skin that holds the testes.
**testes** (singular: *testis*) The primary male sex organs that produce sperm.
**sperm** Cells produced in the seminiferous tubules of the male reproductive system and ejaculated through the penis.
**epididymis** A collection of coiled tubes adjacent to each testis, where sperm are stored.

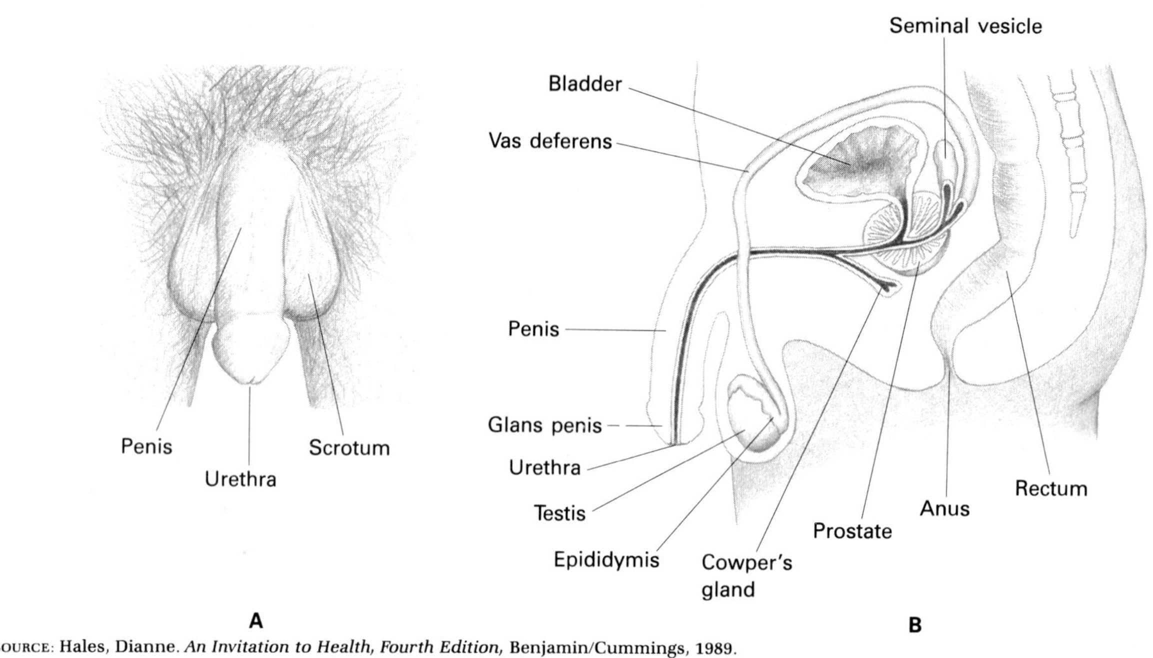


SOURCE: Hales, Dianne. *An Invitation to Health, Fourth Edition,* Benjamin/Cummings, 1989.

**FIGURE 7-3** Male sexual anatomy. **(a)** External view of the male genitals; **(b)** cross section of the male organs.

Inside the body are the **vas deferens,** two tubes that carry sperm from the testes to the urethra; the **prostate gland,** where sperm cells are mixed with seminal fluid, or **semen** (the liquid in which sperm cells are carried out of the body during **ejaculation**); and the **Cowper's glands,** two pea-sized structures located one to each side of the urethra (just below where it emerges from the prostate gland) and connected to it via tiny ducts.

When a man is sexually aroused, the Cowper's glands often secrete a fluid that appears as a droplet at the tip of the penis. This fluid is not semen, but it occasionally contains sperm. Also inside the body are the **seminal vesicles,** which make some of the seminal fluid, and the tubes linking different parts of the system.

**vas deferens** The two tubes that carry sperm from the testes to the urethra.
**prostate gland** A gland, wrapped around the male urethra, that provides a secretion that helps liquefy the semen from the testes.
**semen** The viscous whitish liquid that is the complete male ejaculate; a combination of secretions from the prostate gland, seminal vesicles, and other glands.
**ejaculation** The sudden ejection of semen from the penis at orgasm.
**Cowper's glands** The small glands that discharge into the male urethra.
**seminal vesicles** Glands in the male reproductive system that produce the major portion of the fluid of semen.
**circumcision** The surgical removal of the foreskin of the penis.

## Circumcision

In its natural state, the tip of the penis is covered by a fold of skin called the foreskin. In many societies, including our own, the foreskin is removed in a procedure called **circumcision.** The most common benefit of circumcision is that it prevents the accu-

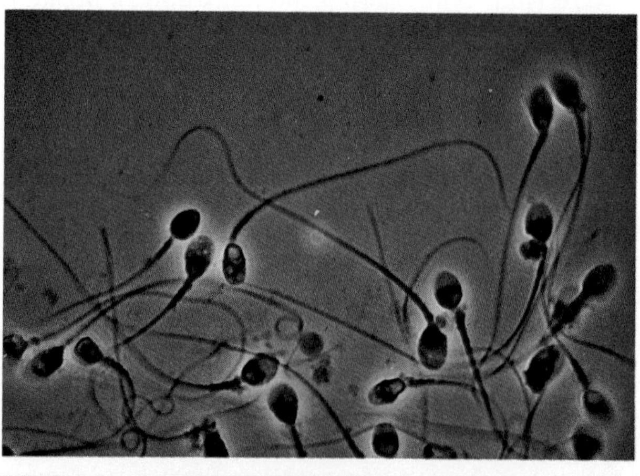

Sperm, as seen under a microscope.

mulation of oils and secretions under the foreskin, which could cause swelling or infection. Uncircumcised men can prevent problems by regular washing of the head of the penis beneath the foreskin.

For years, sex experts have debated whether circumcision enhances or diminishes sexual response. Sex therapists William Masters and Virginia Johnson could find no differences in sensitivity to stimulation between circumcised and uncircumcised men. Others claim that the membrane at the tip of the penis thickens by as much as 10 times after circumcision, and so the man loses a great deal of sensitivity.[2]

### Prostate Problems

The chestnut-sized prostate gland, wrapped around the urethra (urinary tube) at the base of the bladder, is a common source of concern. The most common problem in younger men is infection, or prostatitis, which can cause fever, pain during bowel movements, pain during a rectal exam, and pus in the urine. Infrequent sexual activity is one cause, and occasional bursts of sexual activity between long periods of abstinence are likely to produce this problem. Prostatitis is usually treated with antibiotics, such as sulfa.

After age 40, the prostate enlarges; this condition is called benign prostatic hypertrophy and occurs in every man. As it expands, the prostate tends to pinch the urethra, decreasing urinary flow and creating a sense of urinary urgency, particularly at night. Zinc-rich foods (whole grains, milk, nuts, fresh peas and carrots, and oysters) may help prevent such problems. In some cases, a surgical procedure called transurethral resection is necessary to scrape out the inner core of the prostate and relieve severe symptoms.

The older a man gets, the more likely he is to develop prostate cancer, which claims about 20,000 lives a year. Men over age 35 should have their prostates examined by a doctor annually. The doctor inserts a finger into the rectum and feels the prostate.

### "Man-o-pause"

Although men do not experience the dramatic hormonal upheaval that women do at mid-life, many do undergo significant personal changes, sometimes referred to as **male menopause.** The most visible is loss of hair on the head, which can be a major blow to self-esteem.

Production of the male sex hormone **testosterone** declines after age 40, but sexual ability and enjoyment do not. Men should expect some differences in sexual response as they grow older, including the following:

- a need for more time and arousal to achieve erection
- a longer time for ejaculation
- a briefer orgasm
- a decrease in the force of expulsion of the semen at orgasm
- a smaller volume of ejaculate
- a more rapid loss of erection after orgasm
- a lengthening of the time after ejaculation until the capability for intercourse and orgasm returns

## SEXUAL DEVELOPMENT

*Sex* refers to biological maleness or femaleness; *sexuality* refers to the quality of being sexual and includes psychological and social influences as well as physical drives.

### Childhood Sexuality

From birth, a warm physical relationship with the mother arouses an intense sensuality. The mouth is the principal source of sensual pleasure, but infants are also sensitive to genital and general body contact.

By the age of 3 or 4, children recognize the genital differences between males and females and may develop childhood romances. Curiosity about adults' and other children's genitals, about where babies come from, and about breasts on women and beards on men continues until age 8 or 9. At that time, interest in sex play is less common, but curiosity about sex remains high—especially regarding where babies come from.

### Adolescent Sexuality

At puberty, sexual curiosity explodes—along with everything else. Breasts grow, hair sprouts, skin erupts with pimples, voices drop. The process starts in the brain, which secretes a hormone called luteinizing hormone-releasing hormone (LHRH), which causes the pituitary gland to release hormones called **gonadotropins.** These, in turn, stimulate the **gonads,** the ovaries in girls and the testes in boys, to make sex hormones.

---

**male menopause** A period of change and possible crisis for men at mid-life.
**testosterone** The male sex hormone that stimulates male secondary sex characteristics.
**gonadotropins** The gonad-stimulating hormones produced by the pituitary gland.
**gonad** A sex organ: in women, the ovaries; in men, the testes.

The sex hormones change the growth pattern of childhood so that a boy or girl may spurt up 4 to 6 inches a year. The skeleton matures very rapidly until, at the end of puberty (usually around age 18), the growth centers at the ends of the bones close off. Estrogen causes the process to happen earlier in girls than in boys.

In females, the first menstrual period—the **menarche**—marks the "coming of age." The age of menarche has been dropping steadily in the past century. Physicians attribute this drop in age at menarche to improved nutrition. Most girls experience menarche when they reach a critical body weight—or, more precisely, a certain ratio of lean to fat tissue.

At that point, the pituitary gland manufactures hormones that travel to the ovary and stimulate the production of estrogen. As estrogen increases, a girl's breasts become fuller, her external genitals enlarge, and fat is deposited on her hips and buttocks. Estrogen keeps her hair thick and skin smooth. Most of all, it prepares her body to conceive and carry a baby.

In boys, testosterone triggers profound changes: Their voices deepen, hair grows on their faces and bodies, their penises become larger and longer, and their muscles become stronger. These effects are called the male secondary sex characteristics. It's not unusual for teenage boys to experience frequent erections during the day and night, including "wet dreams," during which ejaculation occurs.

According to a survey by the National Center for Health Statistics released in 1990, America's teenage girls are having sex earlier.[3] More than half—54 percent—of girls 15 to 19 had intercourse at least once.

### Adult Sexuality

Our sexual identities, needs, likes, and dislikes become clearer in adulthood, but we continue to change and evolve. As our lives become more complex and varied, sex becomes one among many needs and pleasures.

Sexual interest is most intense in men at age 18 and in women in their thirties. Although age brings changes in sexual responsiveness, we never outgrow our sexuality. Given the opportunity, men and women can continue to enjoy sex well into their eighties—and possibly beyond.

## SEX AND GENDER

**Sex** refers to physiological maleness or femaleness, including the sex chromosomes and genital anatomy. **Gender** includes the psychological and sociological, as well as the physical, aspects of being male or female. You are born with a certain sexual identity; you, your parents, and the society in which you mature mold your gender identity.

### Physical Differences

Biologically, only four absolute differences separate the sexes: Males alone can make sperm; females alone can menstruate, give birth, and breastfeed babies. These basic physiological capabilities are controlled by chemicals called hormones, which are manufactured in the body.

### Sex Hormones

In Greek, *hormon* means set into motion—and that's exactly what our hormones do. They arouse certain cells and organs to specific activities, influencing the way we look, feel, develop, and behave. The hormones most crucial to women are the sex hormones estrogen and progesterone, which are produced by the ovaries. For men, the primary sex hormone is testosterone, which is produced by the testes and the adrenal glands.

Hormones start their job before birth. About six weeks after conception, hormones begin the work of making the fetus into a boy or a girl (see Chapter 8 for a more complete discussion). Prenatal hormones may also create a predisposition to certain ways of thinking or acting; however, their impact is subtle. For instance, prenatal testosterone may somehow enhance "spatial" ability—the capacity of thinking in three dimensions. Girls exposed to male hormones before birth score higher on spatial ability tests than other girls, and boys born with severe testosterone deficiencies have much poorer spatial ability than other boys.

### Sex Differences

Are there other differences in male and female brains? The corpus callosum, a nerve cable connecting the brain's two halves, may be thicker in women and allow more "crosstalk" between the hemispheres. But the evidence for even this distinction is far from conclusive.

In just about every aspect of behavior or ability, the differences among individual men and among indi-

**menarche** The onset of menstruation at puberty.
**sex** Maleness or femaleness resulting from structural, functional, and genetic factors.
**gender** Maleness or femaleness as determined by a combination of anatomical, physiological, and psychological factors and learned behaviors.

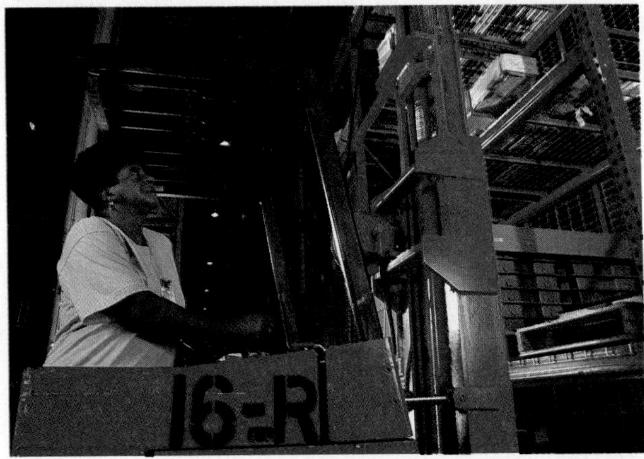


Today's men and women are challenging traditional notions about "men's work" and "women's work."

vidual women are as striking as those between them. Most men run faster than most women, but some women can outrun most men. Most women show more nurturing behaviors than most men, but some men show extraordinary tenderness. Though no one argues that boys and girls are—or should be—identical in ability and potential, the real issue may not be what makes them different, but what difference the differences make.

### Sexual Stereotypes

Being male is not the same as being masculine, and being female is not the same as being feminine. Today more men and women are breaking out of traditional stereotypes. Men are acknowledging their feelings and fears and taking on "feminine" jobs, becoming nurses and secretaries and acting as partners who shop for groceries and do the laundry. Although there still aren't any female linebackers in the National Football League, and no one expects that there will be, women have begun to take their places among truck drivers, engineers, architects, coal miners, physicians, and executives.

Many people are working toward the concept of **androgyny,** a word that literally translates as "man-woman." Androgynous individuals combine aspects of both masculinity and femininity into their personalities and life-styles. They act in ways that seem appropriate in a given situation, instead of responding in a way that seems appropriately masculine or feminine.

## SEXUAL PREFERENCE

Sigmund Freud argued that we all start off **bisexual,** or attracted to both sexes. But by the time they reach adulthood, most males prefer female sexual partners, and most females prefer male partners. **Heterosexual** is the term used for individuals whose primary orientation is toward members of the other sex. In virtually all cultures and eras, some men and women have been **homosexual** (preferring partners of their own sex).

### Sexual Orientation

Your **sexual orientation** (attraction to a certain sex) involves physiological, psychological, and social factors. In our society, we tend to view heterosexuality and homosexuality as very different. In reality, these orientations are opposite ends of a broad range of sexual preferences.

As Figure 7-4 illustrates, sex researcher Alfred Kinsey devised a seven-point continuum representing sexual orientation of men and women in American society. At one end are those exclusively attracted to members of the other sex; at the other end are those exclusively attracted to those of the same sex. In between are varying degrees of homosexual and heterosexual orientation.

According to recent studies, approximately 2 percent of men and 1 percent of women in America seem to be exclusively homosexual, about 75 percent of the men and 85 percent of the women are exclusively heterosexual, and roughly 23 percent of the men and 14 percent of the women have had both types of experience.[4]

Some individuals are **transsexuals** and consider themselves to be of the sex opposite their biological sex. Most are males who feel deeply that they are more truly females. More than 3,000 Americans have undergone complex medical procedures to change their genital and secondary sex characteristics.

### Bisexuality

Bisexuality—sexual attraction to, and interaction with, both males and females—can surface at any point in one's life. Some people identify themselves as bisex-

**androgyny** The expression of both masculine and feminine traits.
**bisexual** The sexual attraction to, and relationships with, people of either sex; a person who is attracted in such a way.
**heterosexual** The sexual attraction to, and relationships with, persons of the other sex; a person who is attracted in such a way.
**homosexual** The sexual attraction to, and relationships with, persons of the same sex; a person who is attracted in such a way.
**sexual orientation** One's preference in sexual partners; preference can be for the other sex, same sex, or both sexes.
**transsexual** One who undergoes complex medical treatment to change genitals and secondary sex characteristics.

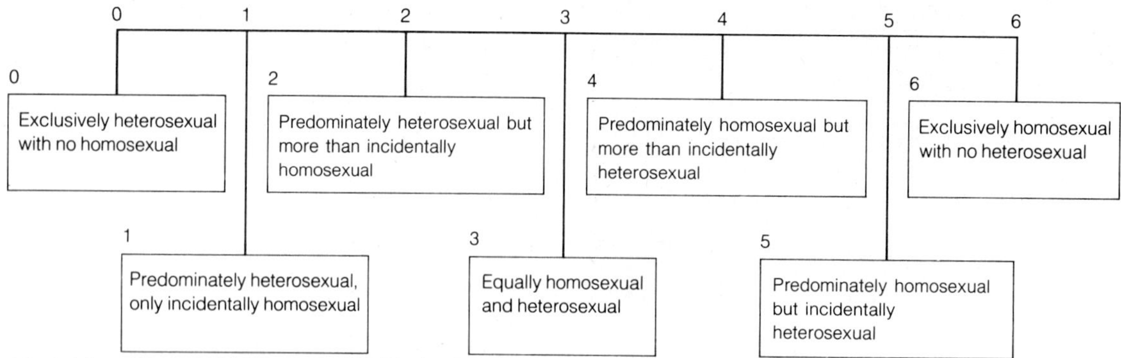


SOURCE: Adapted from Kinsey, A.; W. Pomeroy; and C. Martin. *Sexual Behavior in the Human Male.* Philadelphia: Saunders, 1948.

**FIGURE 7-4** Continuum of sexual orientation.

ual even if they do not participate in bisexual behavior. Some are "serial" bisexuals—that is, they are sexually involved with same-sex partners and then partners of the other sex or vice versa.

## HEALTH HEADLINE

### HIV in the Inner City

**In a study of 196 inner-city teenagers in New York City, 58 percent had engaged in sexual intercourse; 12 percent had never used contraception. Almost half—47 percent—"never" or "rarely" worried about AIDS. But 39 percent reported changing their sexual behavior because of concern about AIDS. Of those reporting changes, 66 percent (25 percent of the total study group) claimed to be using condoms currently, and 16 percent (6 percent of the total group) claimed to be abstaining from sex. Of sexually active girls, 73 percent had not insisted on condom use the last time they had sex, whereas 51 percent of the sexually active boys said they'd used condoms. Twenty-one percent said they'd commit suicide if they tested positive for HIV infection.**

SOURCE: Goodman, E. and A. T. Cohall. "Acquired Immunodeficiency Syndrome and Adolescents: Knowledge, Attitudes, Beliefs, and Behaviors in New York City Adolescent Minority Population," *Pediatrics,* July 1989.

An estimated 7 to 10 million men, about twice the number thought to be exclusively homosexual, could be described as bisexual during some extended period of their lives. The largest group are married, rarely have sexual relations with women other than their wives, and have secret sexual involvements with men.

The fear of AIDS, particularly among heterosexual women who worry about becoming involved with a bisexual man, has sparked concern about bisexuality. About 2 to 3 percent of people with AIDS are women infected by bisexual partners, and health officials fear that bisexual men who hide their homosexual affairs could transmit the virus to many more women.

## Homosexuality

Homosexuality—social, emotional, and sexual attraction to members of the same sex—exists in almost all cultures. Men and women homosexuals are commonly referred to as gay; women homosexuals are also called lesbians.

Homosexuality threatens and upsets many people, perhaps just because homosexuals are viewed as different, or perhaps because no one understands why some people are heterosexual and others homosexual. Since the emergence of AIDS as a major health problem, many people see homosexuals as a societal danger. **Homophobia,** a dislike and fear of homosexuals, has intensified in many communities.

### The Roots of Homosexuality

For decades, behavioral and medical specialists have debated whether homosexuality is biologically or socially determined. Some say a genetic defect is the

**homophobia** The fear and dislike of homosexuals.

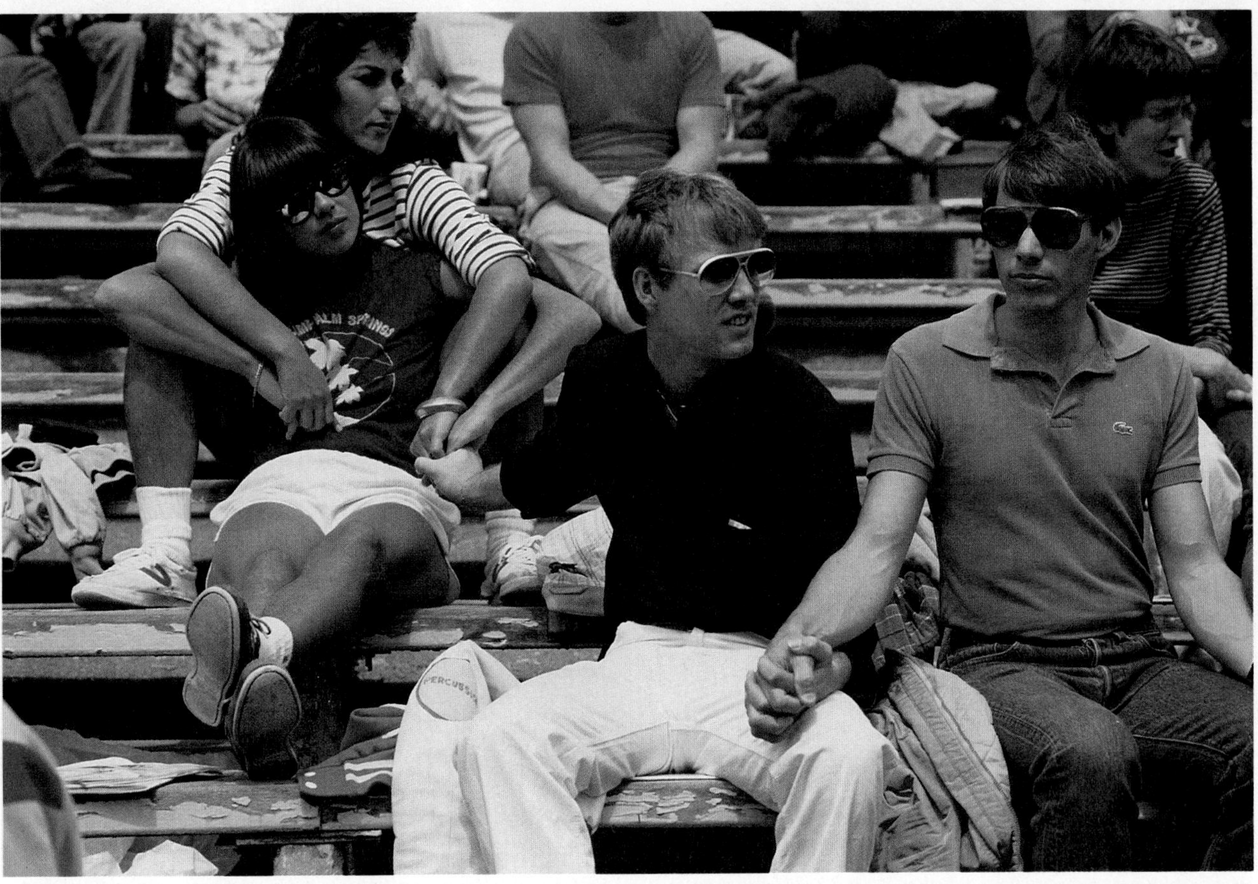

About two percent of men and one percent of women in America are exclusively homosexual.

cause. Others argue that prenatal hormones influence sexual preference. Some psychotherapists have argued that mothers foster homosexuality by loving their sons too much and their daughters too little. Others have traced homosexuality to broken homes, seductive friends, and failure at "dating and mating."

Which theory is right? After almost 1,500 interviews and 10 years of statistical analysis, researchers from the Alfred C. Kinsey Institute of Sex Research at Indiana University concluded that homosexuality "can *not* be traced back to a single social or psychological root."[5]

### Homosexual Life-styles

After a 10-year study of almost 10,000 male and female homosexuals, social scientists at the Institute for Sex Research concluded that "relatively large numbers of homosexual men manage their homosexuality with little difficulty, while a homosexual way of life is problematic for only a distinct minority."[6] Those who were happiest and best adjusted were those (about one-half of the men and three-fourths of the women) in "close-couple" relationships, the equivalent of stable heterosexual marriages.

For male homosexuals, the emergence of AIDS has had a profound impact. As of 1990, the Centers for Disease Control reported that more than half of people with AIDS have been homosexual or bisexual men, many of whom had had multiple sex partners. In the 1980s, many gay men changed their sexual habits because of a fear of AIDS and refrained from sexual activity or from "unsafe" sex practices.[7] However, a 1990 survey found that a third of gay men in San Francisco engaged in unsafe sex practices.[8] (You can find more information on safe sex, AIDS, and other sexually transmitted diseases later in this chapter and in Chapter 15.)

## SEXUAL INTIMACY

Like other forms of intimacy (see Chapter 6), sexual intimacy, or closeness and mutual sharing, should develop slowly, and both partners should think and talk about what each wants and expects. Many couples move slowly through various forms of sexual intimacy, including hugging, kissing, and touching. They don't necessarily say "no" to sexual intercourse, but "not yet."

## HALES INDEX

Percentage of adults who had no sex partners in previous year: 22

Percentage of singles who wonder if they've gotten a sexually transmitted disease after sex with a new partner: 62

Percentage of teenagers with a sexually transmitted disease: 17

Percentage of college students infected with the AIDS virus: 0.2

Percentage of college men who say they would lie to obtain sex: 33

Percentage of college women who say they would lie to obtain sex: 10

Percentage of college men who would lie about testing positive for the AIDS virus: 20

Percentage of college women who would lie about testing positive for the AIDS virus: 4

Percentage of acquaintance rapes that occur during a date: 50

Percentage of college women who've experienced sexual harassment: 20

Average number of sex partners for 18- to 29-year-old adults: 6.08

Number of times men and women under age 40 have intercourse in a year: 78

SOURCES: **1** National Opinion Research Center of the University of Chicago, report on sexual behavior, American Association for the Advancement of Science meeting, February 1990. **2** "Fear of Sleeping," *Psychology Today,* May 1989. **3** Byrd, Robert. "Teen Girls Having Sex Sooner," *San Francisco Chronicle,* February 6, 1990. **4** Leary, Warren. "AIDS Risk Among College Students Is Real but Not Rampant, Tests Find," *New York Times,* May 23, 1989. **5, 6, 7, 8** Cochran, Susan and Vickie Mays, letter, *New England Journal of Medicine,* March 15, 1990. **9** Goleman, Daniel. "When the Rapist Is Not a Stranger," *New York Times,* August 29, 1989. **10** Camody, Deirdre. "Sexual Harassment on Campus: A Growing Issue," *New York Times,* July 5, 1989. **11, 12** National Opinion Research Center of the University of Chicago, report on sexual behavior, American Association for the Advancement of Science meeting, February 1990.

As you consider a sexual relationship, you also have to think about the significance of your actions. "Having sex" refers to the motions two people go through to achieve sexual pleasure; "making love" is a profound sharing of emotion and experience. Which would you be doing in your relationship?

### STRATEGY FOR CHANGE

#### Are You Ready for Sex?

Before getting sexually involved, you should know what you want and expect of yourself, your partner, and your relationship. Here are some questions to consider:

- What role do I want relationships and sex to occupy in my life at this time?
- What are my values as they pertain to sexual relationships?
- Will a decision to engage in sex enhance my positive feelings about myself or my partner?
- Do I and my partner both want to have sex?
- Is my partner pressuring me in any way? Am I pressuring my partner?
- Have my partner and I discussed and taken precautions against unwanted pregnancy and sexually transmitted diseases?

## Sexual Activity

Part of learning about your own sexuality is having a clear understanding of human sexual behaviors. Understanding frees us from feelings of fear and anxiety so that we may accept ourselves and others as the natural sexual beings we all are.

### Celibacy

A celibate person does not engage in sexual activity. Complete **celibacy** means that the person does not masturbate (stimulate himself or herself sexually) or become involved in sexual activity with a partner. In partial celibacy, the person masturbates but doesn't have sexual contact with others.

Though we think of celibacy most often as the lifelong choice of priests and nuns, many people may decide to be celibate at certain times of their lives. In a 1990 survey presented at the American Association for the Advancement of Science, 22 percent of Americans said they had not had sex with a partner during the previous year.[9] Some worried about sexually transmitted diseases; others hadn't found suitable

**celibacy** Abstention from sexual activity.

partners. Many simply had other priorities, like finishing school or starting a career.

### Fantasy

The mind is the most powerful sex organ in the body. Fantasies that are erotic (those that are sexually stimulating) can accompany sexual activity or be pleasurable in themselves. A study of college students found that 60 percent of men and women fantasized during sexual intercourse.

Fantasies generally enhance sexual arousal, reduce anxiety, and boost sexual desire. They are also a way to anticipate and rehearse new sexual experiences and to bolster a person's self-image and feelings of desirability. Part of what makes fantasies exciting is that they provide an opportunity for expressing forbidden desires, such as sex with a different partner or with a past lover.

### Masturbation

Not everybody masturbates but most people do. Kinsey estimated that 7 out of 10 women and 19 out of 20 men masturbate (and admit they do). Their reason is simple: It feels good. **Masturbation** produces the same physical responses as sexual activity with a partner, but the psychological and emotional differences are great.

Masturbation has been described as immature; unsocial; tiring; frustrating; and a cause of hairy palms, warts, and blemishes. None of these myths is true. Even Freud felt that masturbation was normal for children. Yet many people associate masturbation with mental illness, perhaps because some severely ill psychiatric patients may masturbate in front of others.

### Kissing and Touching

A kiss is a universal sign of affection. A kiss can be just a kiss—a quick press of the lips—or it can lead to much more. Usually kissing is the first sexual activity that couples engage in; and even after years of sexual experimentation and sharing, it remains an enduring pleasure for partners.

Touching is a silent form of communication between parent and child, friends and lovers. Although a touch to any part of the body can be thrilling, some areas, such as the breasts and genitals, are especially sensitive. Stimulating these **erogenous** regions can lead to orgasm in both men and women. Though such forms of stimulation often accompany intercourse, more couples are gaining an appreciation of them as sources of sexual fulfillment in themselves—and as safer alternatives to intercourse.

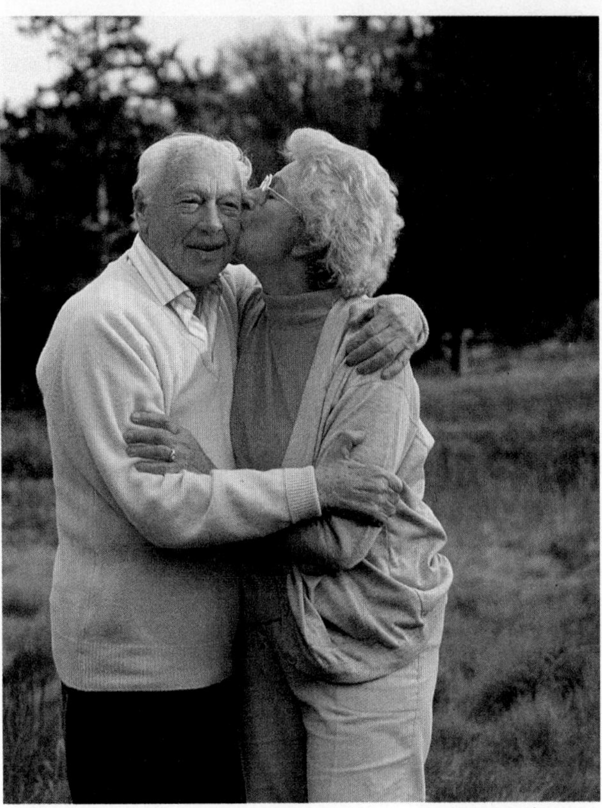

Neither men nor women ever outgrow their sexual feelings and needs.

### Intercourse

Sexual **intercourse,** or **coitus,** refers to the penetration of the vagina by the penis. This is the preferred form of sexual intimacy for most couples, who may use a wide variety of positions. The most familiar in our society is the so-called missionary position, with the man on top and facing the woman (Figure 7-5). In an alternative position the woman is on top, either lying down or sitting upright. Other positions include lying side-by-side and face-to-face or having the man's penis enter the woman's vagina from the rear. Many couples move into several different positions during a single episode of lovemaking; others may have a personal favorite or may choose different positions at different times.

### Oral-Genital Sex

Our mouths and genitals give us some of our most intense pleasures. Though it might therefore seem logical to combine the two, many people are horri-

**masturbation** Self-stimulation of the genitals, resulting in orgasm.
**erogenous** Sexually sensitive.
**intercourse** Sexual activity in which the penis repeatedly penetrates the vagina until orgasm and ejaculation occur.
**coitus** See *intercourse.*

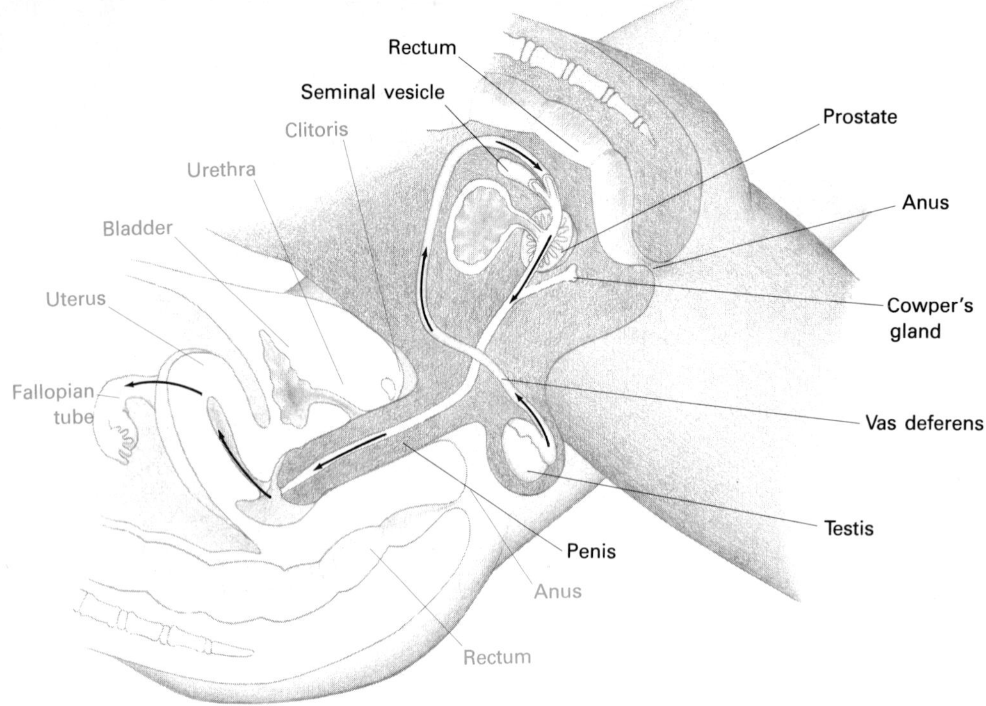


SOURCE: Hales, Dianne. *An Invitation to Health, Fourth Edition,* Benjamin/Cummings, 1989.

**FIGURE 7-5** Cross section of sexual intercourse. Sperm are formed in each testis and stored in the epididymis. When a man ejaculates, sperm, in semen, travel up the vas deferens. (The prostate gland, seminal vesicles, and Cowper's glands all contribute components of the semen.) The semen passes out of the penis through the urethra and is deposited in the vagina, near the cervix. During sexual excitement and orgasm in a woman, the upper end of the vagina enlarges, and the uterus elevates. During the resolution phase, these organs return to their normal states and positions, and the cervix descends into the pool of semen.

fied by that thought. Some people consider oral-genital sex a perversion; it is against the law in many states and a sin in some religions.

The formal terms for oral sex are cunnilingus, which refers to oral stimulation of the woman's genitals, and fellatio, which refers to oral stimulation of the male's genitals. For many couples, oral-genital sex is a regular part of lovemaking. For others, it is an occasional experiment. However, oral-genital sex with a partner infected with one of several venereal diseases, such as herpes, may lead to infection. (See "Safer Sex: Avoiding Health Risks" later in this chapter and further discussion in Chapter 15.)

### Anal Stimulation and Intercourse

Because the anus has many nerve endings, it can produce intense erotic responses. Both homosexual and heterosexual couples use stimulation of the anus by fingers or mouth as a source of sexual arousal and engage in penile penetration of the anus (anal intercourse). In one study, 25 percent of married couples under 35 reported that they occasionally engaged in anal intercourse.[10] However, anal sex involves important health risks, such as damage to sensitive tissues, and transmission of various intestinal infections, hepatitis, and sexually transmitted diseases, including AIDS.

**STRATEGY FOR CHANGE**

**Talking About Sex**

Some simple guidelines can make communication about sex—the key to any satisfying sexual relationship—more effective:

- Remember that your feelings are neither wrong nor right. They simply are.
- Use an "I" statement, such as "I really enjoy making love, but I'm so tired right now that I won't be a responsive partner. Why don't we get the kids to bed early tomorrow so we can enjoy ourselves a little earlier?"
- Remember that neither you nor your partner can always explain your feelings.
- When your partner is talking, don't dismiss his or her feelings as crazy or irrational or selfish.
- If your partner has temporarily lost interest in sex, express concern and ask what the two of you might do to make things better. Don't blame yourself.

- Speak up if something hurts during sex. Be specific.
- If you would like to try something different, say so. Practice saying the words if they embarrass you. If your partner feels uncomfortable, don't force the issue, but try talking it through.
- Set aside time for a weekly sex talk. Take turns bringing up topics. Mention special pleasures or particular problems.

## Sexual Response

Sexuality involves every part of you: mind and body, muscles and skin, glands and genitals. The pioneers in finding out exactly how human beings respond to sex were William Masters and Virginia Johnson, who first studied more than 800 individuals in their laboratory in the 1950s. They discovered that sexual response is a well-ordered sequence of events, so predictable it could be divided into four phases: excitement, plateau, orgasm, and resolution. In real life, individuals don't necessarily follow this well-ordered pattern. But the responses for both sexes are remarkably similar. And sexual response is always the same, whether the means of stimulation is masturbation, intercourse, or oral-genital sex.

### Excitement

Stimulation is the first step: a touch, a look, a fantasy. In men, sexual stimuli set off a rush of blood to the genitals. The penis fills with blood, and valves in the veins keep the blood from flowing out. Because these vessels are wrapped in a thick sheath of tissue, the penis becomes erect. The testes lift.

Women respond to stimulation with vaginal lubrication within 10 to 20 seconds of exposure to sexual stimuli. The clitoris becomes larger, as do the vaginal lips (the labia), the nipples, and later the breasts. The vagina lengthens, and its lower two-thirds increase in size. The uterus lifts, further increasing the free space in the vagina.

### Plateau

During this stage, the changes begun in the excitement stage continue and intensify. The penis further increases in both length and diameter. The outer one-third of the vagina swells. During intercourse, the vaginal muscles grasp the penis to increase stimulation for both partners. The upper two-thirds of the vagina become wider as the uterus moves up. Eventually the diameter of the vagina is 2 1/2 to 3 inches.

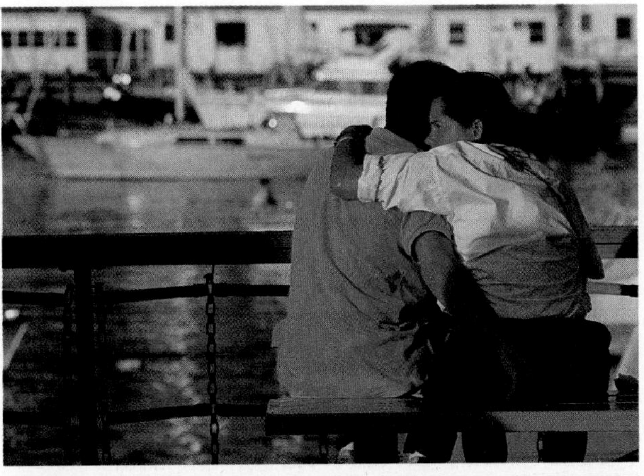

Like other forms of intimacy, sexual intimacy can develop at a pace that is comfortable for both partners.

### Orgasm

Orgasm is remarkably similar in men and women. Both experience three to twelve pelvic muscle contractions approximately 4/5 second apart and lasting up to 60 seconds. Both undergo other muscle contractions and spasms, as well as increases in breathing and pulse rates and blood pressure. Both can sometimes have orgasms with no involvement of the genitals—from kisses, stimulation of the breasts or other parts of the body, or fantasy alone. The major difference is that men ejaculate (discharge semen); women do not.

The process of ejaculation requires two separate events. First, the vas deferens, the seminal vesicles, the prostate, and the upper portion of the urethra contract. The man perceives these subtle contractions deep in his pelvis just before the point of no return, which therapists refer to as the point of ejaculatory inevitability. Then, seconds later, muscle contractions force semen out of the penis via the urethra.

Female orgasms follow several patterns. One pattern is almost the same as a man's. Another pattern of female orgasm—a series of miniorgasms—has been referred to as skimming. Another pattern consists of rapid excitement and plateau stages and then a prolonged orgasm. This is the most frequent response to stimulation by a vibrator.

Whatever the pattern, female orgasms are triggered by the clitoris, the primary sensory sexual organ in the female. When stimulation reaches an adequate level, the vagina responds by contracting. Although it sometimes seems that vaginal stimulation alone can set off an orgasm, the clitoris is almost always involved—at least indirectly during full penetration.

There is no evidence that there is a vaginal, as distinct from a clitoral, orgasm.

Researchers have identified what they call the Grafenberg area (or G area) just behind the front wall of the vagina, between the cervix and back of the pubic bone. When this region is stimulated during intercourse, women may experience a rush, or ejaculation, of fluid from the urethra at orgasm. There is considerable controversy over this area's possible role in sexual pleasure.

### Resolution

The sexual organs of men and women return to their normal, nonexcited state during this final phase of sexual response. Heightened skin color quickly fades after orgasm; the heart rate, blood pressure, and breathing rate soon return to normal. The clitoris also resumes its normal position and appearance very shortly thereafter, whereas the penis may remain somewhat erect for up to 30 minutes.

After orgasm, the male enters a **refractory period,** during which he is incapable of another orgasm. The duration of this period varies from minutes to days, depending on age and the frequency of previous sexual activity. If either partner does not have an orgasm after becoming highly aroused, resolution may be much slower and may be accompanied by a sense of discomfort.

**STRATEGY FOR CHANGE**

**How to Make Sex Better**

Sooner or later, sexual partners may want to request changes or make complaints. Here are some suggestions for how to tackle these touchy topics:

- Choose a good time. That usually means not immediately before, during, or after sex. Select a time when you're both relaxed and feeling close to each other.
- Start with positive statements. Instead of complaining that you don't make love often enough, let your partner know how much you enjoy having sex, and then express your desire to enjoy lovemaking more often or in different ways.
- Avoid questions that start with *why.* If you ask "Why don't you want to make love in different positions?" you sound as if you're accusing your partner.
- Encourage small changes. If you want your partner to be less inhibited, start slowly, perhaps by suggesting you occasionally leave the light on during sex.

## SAFER SEX: AVOIDING HEALTH RISKS

Sex has never been safe. For centuries, sexual diseases, such as gonorrhea and syphilis, caused great suffering and many deaths. Modern medicine has developed effective treatments for these health threats, but other sexually transmitted diseases (STDs), such as herpes and chlamydia, have become serious health problems. However, no STD in recent history has had the impact of **acquired immune deficiency syndrome (AIDS).** (Chapter 15 provides a complete discussion of the nature, history, symptoms, diagnosis, and treatment of AIDS; AIDS-related problems; and other STDs, including syphilis, gonorrhea, herpes, and chlamydia.)

Truly safe sex is 100 percent safe—and that means one of two things: abstinence or sex with a partner who has never been exposed to the AIDS virus or other sexually transmitted diseases.

### Abstinence

Abstinence is an increasingly popular choice among homosexuals and heterosexuals. Particularly for young people, abstinence may be wise; it protects them from the dangers of situations in which they may lose sexual control, and it guarantees that they will indeed have many years in the future for safe and fulfilling sex. For the sake of preventing STDs, you don't have to abstain from all sexual activity. Fantasizing, touching, and hugging are safe and pleasurable.

### A Safe Partner

Sex with a person who has never been exposed to the virus that causes AIDS or to other STDs is safe, regardless of what type of sexual activity you engage in. If you are lucky enough to have been in a mutually faithful relationship with one partner for the last ten years, you are both safe. However, if either of you has sex with another partner or uses IV drugs, you are no longer safe. The only way of being sure that a potential partner is safe is by blood tests for antibodies against the virus that causes AIDS and for other STDs.

**refractory period** The period, following sexual intercourse, during which the male cannot ejaculate again.

**acquired immune deficiency syndrome (AIDS)** A fatal disease caused by a virus that destroys the ability of the immune system to fight disease; transmitted primarily by sexual contact and the contaminated needles of drug users and, less commonly, through contaminated blood products.

**STRATEGY FOR CHANGE**

**Playing It Safe**

- Start any new relationship very slowly. Learn as much as possible about a potential lover.
- Limit your sexual relationships. By reducing your number of partners, you reduce the odds of exposure to someone with an STD.
- Avoid any sex practices that involve contact with semen or vaginal fluids. Think of what you can do rather than what you can't.
- The male should wear a condom from the beginning to the end of every sexual encounter. Latex condoms treated with a spermicide containing nonoxynol-9 offer more protection.
- For additional protection, the woman should use a diaphragm with a spermicide containing nonoxynol-9. Because the virus could still pass through the vaginal lining, a diaphragm alone is not sufficient to protect a woman. Her partner must still wear a condom.

## Acquired Immune Deficiency Syndrome (AIDS)

AIDS is the last stage of a disease process caused by a virus, known as HIV (human immunodeficiency virus), that cripples the body's protective immune system, leaving victims vulnerable to certain types of cancer and to serious infections that are rare or would otherwise produce only mild symptoms. The HIV virus came to the United States in the late 1970s. Throughout the 1980s, HIV spread primarily among homosexual men, intravenous drug users and their partners. By 1990, 4.4 percent of people with AIDS had been infected through heterosexual contacts.[11]

The rate of HIV infection among teenagers has begun to skyrocket. Not only are more teenagers becoming infected with the virus, but equal numbers of boys and girls are getting the disease through heterosexual intercourse. Teenagers are at high risk because many have multiple sex partners and very few use condoms.

On college campuses, researchers describe the threat of HIV infection and AIDS as real but not yet widespread.[12] Federal officials estimated in 1989 that 25,000 college students may be infected with HIV—an infection rate similar to that in other groups not considered at particularly high risk for the disease.

### Myths and Misconceptions About AIDS and HIV Infection

AIDS is such a frightening disease that some people have exaggerated its dangers, whereas others have understated them. Here is what you should know about HIV transmission:

- Casual contact does not spread HIV. Compared to other viruses, HIV is extremely difficult to get. In studies of family members sharing dishes, food, clothing, and frequent hugs with people with HIV infection or AIDS, no one has ever contracted the virus.

**HEALTH HEADLINE**

**HIV on Campus**

Health officials describe HIV infection as "an actual, active problem" on campuses, yet students have not greatly changed their sexual behavior. According to a study of 132 women students, today's students are just as willing as their counterparts in the pre-AIDS 1970s to engage in oral or anal sex or to have multiple sex partners. Some 41 percent said that they did use condoms during intercourse—an increase from in the past. Yet as the women became seriously involved with men, they tended to use less, rather than more, protection, which the researchers describe as "a potentially dangerous habit, since just knowing someone better doesn't make you more safe."

In a check of 16,861 blood samples from students at 19 colleges across the country, 0.2 percent were positive. If that infection rate applies to the nation's 12.5 million college students, some 25,000 may already carry HIV. The infection rate is about the same as in other groups that are not considered high risk.

SOURCE: Leary, Warren. "AIDS Risk Among College Students Is Real but Not Rampant, Tests Find," *New York Times*, May 23, 1989. Zinner, Stephen. *New England Journal of Medicine*, March 22, 1990.

- A person can be infected only by exposure, through any sexual act, to the semen of a man or to the vaginal fluids of a woman carrying HIV.
- During vaginal intercourse, the virus may invade tiny breaks in the surface of the vagina or the penis, or it may cross the soft tissues in the genital area.
- During anal intercourse, the virus may enter the bloodstream through tiny breaks in the lining of the rectum or through direct infection of cells.
- No cases of HIV transmission by deep kissing have been reported, but it could happen. In a study of fifty AIDS patients, one had HIV in his saliva. Social (dry) kissing is safe; only deep, very wet kissing may be at all risky.
- Oral sex jeopardizes a person—at least in theory—because the virus in any semen that enters the mouth could make its way to the bloodstream through tiny nicks or sores. The risk in performing oral sex on a woman is smaller because a woman's genital fluids have much lower concentrations of AIDS virus than does semen.
- The chance of HIV infection from a single sexual encounter with an infected partner is low but increases if the relationship continues. The risk of contracting HIV during one sexual encounter is less than 1 percent. With repeated sex with an infected person, the risk rises to between 10 and 45 percent for the uninfected partner—whether male or female.
- You cannot tell whether a partner is carrying HIV. Only a blood test can detect the antibodies the body produces to fight HIV.

**STRATEGY FOR CHANGE**

**HIV Infection and Dating**

How can you tell if someone you're dating or would like to date has been exposed to HIV? The bad news is, you can't. But the good news is, as long as sexual activity and sharing drug needles are avoided, it doesn't matter.

You are going to have to be careful about the person you become sexually involved with, making your own decision based on your own best judgment. That can be difficult. The questions you must keep in mind are:

- Has this person had any sexually transmitted diseases?
- How many people has he or she been to bed with?
- Has this person experimented with drugs?

You have a personal responsibility to find out the answers. Think of it this way. If you know someone well enough to have sex, then you should be able to talk about HIV infection and AIDS. If someone is unwilling to talk, you shouldn't have sex.

SOURCE: *Understanding AIDS: A Message From The Surgeon General*, Department of Health and Human Services, 1989.

## Who's at Risk?

When it comes to HIV infection, no one is immune, but HIV is a particularly serious threat to certain groups. Approximately half of the AIDS patients in the United States are white; almost 30 percent are black and 16.5 percent are Hispanic. Rates per 100,000 people are highest for blacks and Hispanics, who make up the majority of AIDS patients with a history of intravenous (IV) drug use. The majority of homosexuals and bisexuals with AIDS are white. The majority of women with AIDS in this country are young, poor, and black or Hispanic. Most used IV drugs or slept with men who did.

Your risk of HIV infection depends on what you do sexually and with whom you do it. If you abstain from sexual activity or you and your partner have not had sex with anyone else for at least 10 years, if you both have never used needles to inject drugs, and if neither of you had a blood transfusion between 1978 (when HIV entered the blood supply) and 1985 (when screening for HIV began), you are not in danger.

These factors increase chances of infection:

- IV drug use or sex with an IV drug user. Needle-sharing by IV drug users has been the number one source of AIDS in heterosexual men; sleeping with IV drug users has been the number one cause of AIDS in women. (Chapter 9 discusses IV drug use and its risks.)
- Sex with partners whose sexual histories you do not know. These days you don't go to bed with just one individual; you go to bed with all the people with whom your partner has had sex.
- Sex with people who received blood transfusions between 1978 and 1985. For unknown reasons, transfusion recipients are not as likely to pass HIV on to their partners as are other carriers. The infection rate among their spouses is 10 to 20 percent, compared to 45 percent among partners of IV drug users.
- The locale of your sexual activity. The highest-risk areas for contracting HIV are metropolitan New York, San Francisco, Los Angeles, Houston, Miami, Newark, Chicago, Dallas, Philadelphia, Atlanta,

HEALTH SPOTLIGHT

### A Letter from a Gay Man to His Parents

Dear Mom and Dad,

Hi! I hope that all is well with you.

Well, I was waiting to tell you about my sexuality—waiting for a time when it would be best for you to deal with it. But now that it is out in the open, I'm happy that I can share that part of my life with you. My relationship with Bob is a big part of what is positive in my life; so not being able to share that has really been difficult for me.

I would hope that my sharing this with you will bring us closer together. I would like to do anything I can to help you to understand me and to understand what it's like to be gay. Please realize that you are in no way responsible for my sexual preference. What you did or didn't do as parents is not what determined my sexuality. I want to be absolutely clear—you are not to "blame"; it is not your "fault"—it's just part of who I am, and it is a beautiful part of me. So do not feel guilty. Besides, accepting my feelings has made me truly happy for the first time in my life. My being gay is not a tragedy—it's just part of who I am.

I know that my preference to be in a relationship with a man is going to be difficult for you to understand and difficult to accept. There is a lot of social pressure and programming against it. For that reason, I had a hard time accepting it myself. I tried to deny it, in fact, for 29 years. I didn't want to disappoint you as parents, and I wanted to be "normal" and accepted by those around me. As I said, it was not easy to accept the social context; but I firmly believe, deep in my heart and soul, that being with another man is going to make me happy and fulfilled. (It has already.)

My feelings for a man are deeper, more beautiful, and more intense than anything I have felt with a woman. How can it be wrong if it fills me full of joy and happiness? How can it be wrong when being with a man is just so comfortable and easy?

How can it be wrong? . . . Because the Catholic Church says so? Because ignorant people who know nothing about it and are afraid of looking at their own sexuality say so? Who has the right to tell me that my feelings are wrong?

I hope you can accept my relationship, because it is the most important aspect of my life—that love and caring form a base for everything else that I do. I would very much like you to share my life, and I hope that you can see that I'm still the same person that you have always loved and cared about. I definitely do not want to be in the position of having to choose between your approval and my happiness—because from my perspective, the choice would be an obvious, but unfortunate one.

Also, please try to react out of love—not fear, guilt, or sadness. I tried to write this letter from my heart, and I hope that you will receive it in the same spirit in which it was written.

I love you very much,

Don

SOURCE: Crooks, Robert and Karla Baur. *Our Sexuality*, Fourth Edition, Benjamin/Cummings, 1990 (author's files).

Boston, and Washington, D.C. In these cities, as many as one in every 30 men carries the virus. Some mostly rural states, such as the Dakotas and Montana, have reported few cases of AIDS.

### HIV Infection and Homosexuals

More than half of all people with AIDS in the United States have been homosexual men. Several factors—including frequent sexual activity with multiple, anonymous partners and dangerous sexual practices, such as anal intercourse—may have caused the quick spread of the virus through the gay community. Though the spread of HIV among gays slowed in the late 1980s, a 1990 survey of 401 gay and bisexual men in San Francisco found that 30 percent were engaging in unsafe, unprotected sex. Young men age 18 to 29 were most likely to risk HIV infection.

HIV infection is not widespread among lesbians. However, there has been at least one documented case of HIV transmission from a bisexual woman, who contracted HIV infection from a male partner, to her lesbian lover.

**STRATEGY FOR CHANGE**

**Protecting Your Sexual Health If You're Homosexual**

- Don't have sexual contact (including prolonged open-mouth kissing) with anyone who is or might be infected with HIV.
- Avoid having multiple or anonymous sex partners.
- Avoid having sex with anyone who has multiple or anonymous sex partners or who has a sex partner infected with HIV.
- Avoid contact with your partner's blood, semen, urine, or feces.
- Use a latex condom during each sexual act, from start to finish.
- Don't have sexual contact with individuals who use IV drugs.
- Avoid receptive anal intercourse or insertion of your fingers or fist into the anus, because these acts could tear the rectal tissues, allowing direct access to the bloodstream.
- Do not use amyl nitrate (poppers), a sexual stimulant popular among homosexuals. The drug may be associated with the development of a cancer associated with AIDS.

### HIV Infection and Heterosexuals

Both men and women can transmit HIV to their sexual partners. HIV has been found in vaginal and cervical fluids and in menstrual blood. Women are more vulnerable than heterosexual men. The virus is much more highly concentrated in semen than in vaginal fluids, making male-to-female transmission more likely.

In heterosexuals, vaginal sex is just as risky as anal intercourse. Although most homosexuals transmitted the virus by anal intercourse, women are just as likely to be infected by what one researcher calls "plain old sex." Most women who got HIV from their sexual partners had only vaginal intercourse.

It's not the number, but the nature, of sex partners that adds to the risk. According to researchers, it seems more dangerous to have one moderately prolonged relationship with a man at risk (because of IV drug use or homosexual affairs) than 40 to 50 encounters with partners who live in low-risk areas.[13]

The risk of becoming infected with HIV does not depend simply on the number of times an individual has intercourse with an infected partner. A study of 80 couples in which one spouse had acquired the virus from a blood transfusion found that one woman contracted HIV after a single episode of sexual intercourse with her husband.[14] Eleven other women remained uninfected, although each had intercourse with her husband more than 200 times. Transmission was more likely from husbands to wives than vice versa. All but two of the couples engaged in vaginal intercourse only.

Bisexual partners are a potential source of infection for heterosexual women. A small—but dangerous—percentage of bisexual men have many male and female lovers.

Prostitutes or men who frequent prostitutes can infect their partners. Only a small number of AIDS cases in heterosexual men has been traced to prostitutes, but the risk may be growing. In big cities as many as half of the prostitutes tested have been exposed to HIV, almost all through IV drug use or sex with users.

Individuals may be at greater risk if they have an active sexual infection. Sexually transmitted diseases—such as herpes, gonorrhea, and syphilis—increase the risk of HIV transmission during sex with an infected partner.

Pregnancy can endanger the life of an HIV-infected woman and her unborn child. Possibly because it alters the immune system, AIDS often develops or worsens when a woman already infected with the virus becomes pregnant.

**STRATEGY FOR CHANGE**

**Protecting Your Sexual Health If You're Heterosexual**

- Avoid having multiple or anonymous sex partners.
- Don't have sexual contact with anyone who has symptoms of AIDS, is infected with HIV, or is at high risk of HIV infection because of his or her behavior.
- Avoid sexual contact with anyone who has had sex with people at risk of getting HIV infection.
- Don't have sex with prostitutes.

- Men should use a latex condom during each sexual act, from start to finish; women should use a diaphragm with a spermicide containing nonoxynol-9. One method alone may not be sufficient.
- Avoid prolonged, open-mouth kissing with partners you are not sure are HIV-free.

### The HIV Antibody Test

The HIV antibody test does not detect the HIV virus itself, but antibodies the body forms in response to exposure to the virus. Most county agencies offering free tests for the HIV antibody use the ELISA test, which is 95 to 98 percent accurate. (The Western Blot, which may cost up to $300 at a private physician's office, is even more precise.) Because false positives occur in about 2 percent of the tests, most centers repeat the test if the initial results are positive. Experienced counselors can then refer men and women with two positive readings (virtual certainty of infection) to physicians who specialize in AIDS-related problems. (See Chapter 15 for information on what to do if you test positive for the HIV antibody.) A negative result indicates no exposure to the HIV—at least as of 3 to 6 months prior to testing. (It can take that long for the body to produce the telltale antibodies.)

A positive result to an HIV antibody test indicates exposure to the virus, not active infection. An estimated 30 to 50 percent of HIV carriers eventually develop symptomatic HIV infection or AIDS. Whether or not symptoms develop, individuals remain infected for life and can transmit the virus to any sex partner and to anyone with whom they might share a needle. Because a woman can pass the virus to any children she conceives, she should consider taking the HIV test before getting pregnant. Infected men and women should notify all their partners, past and present (see Chapter 15).

**TABLE 7-1** What Makes Sex Safe

**Risky Behavior**

Sharing drug needles and syringes

Anal sex, with or without a condom

Vaginal or oral sex with someone who shoots drugs or engages in anal sex

Sex with someone you don't know well (a pickup or prostitute) or with someone you know has several sex partners

Unprotected sex (without a condom) with an infected person

**Safe Behavior**

Not having sex

Sex with one mutually faithful, uninfected partner

Not shooting drugs

SOURCE: *Surgeon General's Handbook on AIDS*. 1989.

**STRATEGY FOR CHANGE**

**Should You Be Tested?**

You should undergo testing for antibodies to HIV if any of the following is true for you:

- You are male and have had sex with a male in the last 10 years.
- You use IV drugs and have shared needles or had sex with someone who has done so.
- You have had sex with prostitutes in the last 10 years.
- You are female and have had sex with a bisexual male.
- You have had sex with someone from a country or region with a high incidence of AIDS (such as central Africa).
- You have had many sex partners you did not know well and are worried about being infected.

### Unsafe Sex

Although you can't always make sex safe, you can make it safer. Avoiding the most dangerous sexual practices (see Table 7-1) can help:

- *Anal Intercourse*—The risk is higher for the partner whose rectum is penetrated by a penis; this is called anal-receptive intercourse and has been the most common route of HIV transmission among homosexuals. Because there are many blood vessels in the anus and rectum, and particularly because anal intercourse results often in tiny tears in the lining of the rectum, the virus may pass easily into the bloodstream. HIV may also be able to infect cells of the rectum directly. The risk of HIV infection is lower for the person inserting his penis into a partner's rectum. In one study, the incidence of HIV infection was 2 to 3 percent in homosexual men in the invasive role, compared to 50 to 60 percent in those in the receptive role. Among heterosexuals, anal intercourse is as risky, but there is no evidence that it is more dangerous than vaginal intercourse.
- *Vaginal Intercourse*—This practice is particularly dangerous for women because semen carrying HIV

SELF-SURVEY

## How Do You Feel About Sex?

This exercise is designed for you to respond to a number of statements dealing with human sexuality in our culture, and then analyze your sexual attitudes on a liberal/conservative or accepting/nonaccepting continuum.

***Directions***
Read each statement carefully and indicate your reaction to each by placing SA = Strongly Agree, A = Agree, D = Disagree, or SD = Strongly Disagree in the space provided to the left of each statement.

***Response***

_______ 1. Homosexuals should be put in a place where the rest of society does not have to put up with them.

_______ 2. Masturbation by a married person is a sign of poor marital adjustment.

_______ 3. Oral-genital contact can provide a higher degree of effective erotic stimulation than can sexual intercourse.

_______ 4. Sex education should not be taught in school.

_______ 5. The practice of birth control is worthwhile.

_______ 6. Premarital intercourse between consenting adults is acceptable.

_______ 7. College marriages are usually doomed to failure.

_______ 8. Venereal disease is contracted only by people of lower socioeconomic status.

_______ 9. Rape is an easy crime to commit and never be convicted of.

_______ 10. Abortion should be prohibited under all circumstances.

_______ 11. Pornography has a detrimental impact on moral character and therefore is related to sex crimes.

_______ 12. Living together is practiced only by white middle-class youth.

_______ 13. Sexual intercourse is a kind of communication.

_______ 14. Homosexuals should not be employed in occupations where they might serve as role models.

_______ 15. Masturbation is acceptable when the objective is simply the attainment of sensory enjoyment.

_______ 16. Oral-genital contact should be regarded as an acceptable form of erotic play.

_______ 17. Sex education should be as common a school subject as math or English.

_______ 18. Birth control is as much a man's responsibility as a woman's.

_______ 19. Sexual intercourse should occur between married partners only.

_______ 20. College marriages are no different from any other marriages.

_______ 21. Masturbation is generally unhealthy.

_______ 22. Preserving the physical health of the mother should be the only basis for abortion.

_______ 23. Communication barriers are the key factors causing sexual problems.

_______ 24. Homosexuality should be regarded as an illness.

_______ 25. Relieving tension by masturbating is a healthy practice.

_______ 26. Women should be as willing as men to participate in oral-genital sex play.

_______ 27. Too much fuss is made over sex education.

_______ 28. The practice of birth control leads to increased sexual activity.

_______ 29. Women should experience sexual intercourse prior to marriage.

_______ 30. It takes a mature couple to make a college marriage work.

_______ 31. Venereal disease does not exist among upper- and middle-class people.

_______ 32. The ultimate goal of rape is sexual satisfaction.

_______ 33. Abortion is murder.

_______ 34. Pornography is not harmful to young children, and there is no need to be concerned about their coming in contact with it.

_______ 35. A couple's living together is often an indication of their strong sexual need for each other.

_______ 36. The basis of sexual communication is touching.

_______ 37. Homosexuality repulses me.

_______ 38. Oral-genital contact repulses me.

_______ 39. Sex education at the college level serves no purpose.

_______ 40. Birth control pills should be available at a college health service.

_______ 41. Men should experience sexual intercourse prior to marriage.

_______ 42. College marriages add but one more problem to an already frustrating time of life.

_______ 43. Rape usually occurs within a mile of the victim's home.

_______ 44. Abortion should be permitted whenever desired by the pregnant woman.

_______ 45. Masturbation should be encouraged under certain conditions.

_______ 46. Homosexuality is all right between two consenting adults.

***Explanation of Scoring***

After responding to these statements, compare your results with friends, classmates, and the person with whom you are in a relationship (if applicable). Discussion of these statements will help make clear that we all differ in our sexual values and that we bring these differences into a relationship. It will be helpful to group your responses by topic as follows:

- *Sexual Stereotypes*—Questions 4, 8, 9, 11, 17, 27, 31, 32, 34, 39, and 43 refer to sexual items that tend to be stereotypical in nature and exist prior to formal sex education at the college level.
- *Masturbation*—Questions 2, 15, 21, 25, and 45 refer to the sexual behavior of masturbation.
- *Premarital Intercourse*—Questions 6, 12, 19, 29, 35, and 41 deal with premarital intercourse in our society.
- *Homosexuality*—Questions 1, 14, 24, 37, and 46 indicate attitudes toward homosexuality.
- *Sexual Communication*—Questions 13, 23, and 36 deal with the process of sexual communication in a sexual situation and within a relationship.
- *College Marriages*—Questions 7, 20, 30, and 42 refer to getting married while still in college or while involved in any academic pursuit.
- *Abortion*—Questions 10, 22, 33, and 44 address the topic of abortion in our culture.
- *Oral-Genital Sex*—Questions 3, 16, 26, and 38 explore attitudes toward the practice of oral-genital sex in our society.
- *Birth Control*—Questions 5, 18, 28, and 40 refer to the practice of birth control and to responsibility for it.

SOURCE: "The Valois Sexual Attitude Questionnaire," reprinted by permission from Cox, Stafford et al., *Wellness R.S.V.P.*, Benjamin/Cummings, 1981.

can make its way into the bloodstream through sores or tiny openings in the vagina, cervix, or external genitals. The risk may be greater if the woman is menstruating or using tampons, or if the uninfected partner has another sexually transmitted disease.

- *Oral-Anal Stimulation*—Contact between the tongue and the anus is less likely to spread the HIV than is any form of intercourse, but it can happen. The virus has been found in saliva and in feces.
- *Oral-Genital Stimulation*—HIV in semen or vaginal fluids could enter the mouth and thence, through tiny openings, the bloodstream. The risk may be greater with semen, which contains a high concentration of HIV.

## SEXUAL DIFFICULTY

In general, sexual difficulties are classified as primary or secondary. Typically, in a primary difficulty, the man or woman has never experienced excitement or orgasm. In a secondary difficulty, the man or woman is not responding the way he or she used to or does in other circumstances.

**STRATEGY FOR CHANGE**

**When to Seek Help**

Almost everyone experiences a sexual problem at some time. You and your partner should consider consulting a sex therapist if any of the following is true for you:

- Sex is painful or physically uncomfortable.
- You are having sex less and less.
- You have a general fear of, or revulsion for, sex.
- Your sexual pleasure is declining.
- Your sexual desire is diminishing.
- Your sexual problems are increasing in frequency or persisting for longer periods.

### Common Sexual Concerns

A sexual difficulty may occur anywhere in the sexual response sequence. A man's penis may not become erect; a woman's vagina may not become moist. A man may lose his erection while attempting to penetrate; the woman's vagina may dry up with penetration. Some men and women become excited, enjoy the plateau stage, but then cannot achieve orgasm. Or, the sexual cycle may be too long or too short for one of the partners. Sometimes the cause of the problem is alcohol or drugs, disease, injury, or chronic pain. Often it's the result of fear, anxiety, or ignorance.

#### Sexual Anxiety

One of the most common feelings associated with sex—along with curiosity, desire, and love—is anxiety. No one is born knowing about sex. We learn by doing. And, as with most activities—from skiing to speaking French—our first attempts tend to be awkward. A caring, loving relationship can make all the difference.

#### Problems with Arousal

The most frequent problem sex therapists and marriage counselors see is lack of sexual desire. Perfectly healthy couples, with no physical impairment, simply become bored with sex, despite the fact that they love each other and find their partners attractive and enjoyable. The problem may develop after the honeymoon or after the couple's twenty-fifth anniversary. Men and women are equally likely to lose interest in sex, and often neither partner has had previous arousal or orgasm problems.

Often stress—such as a recent move, a new baby, or a high-pressure job—is the real culprit. Severe stress can short-circuit normal sexual response. Couples who try to unwind by drinking or using tranquilizers usually make the problem worse by further dampening their sexual responses.

**STRATEGY FOR CHANGE**

**How to Keep Stress from Zapping Your Sex Life**

- Make time for a transition from your work-a-day world. Try walking, talking, or listening to music.
- Review your priorities. If other things have to come first for the time being, fine. If sex does have high priority, push other activities to the back burner.
- Be romantic. Create a sexy atmosphere: music, soft lights, a roaring fire. Try making love in places other than in bed.
- Make dates for sex. At first the idea of setting aside a time for sex may seem too businesslike, but it doesn't have to be. One sex therapist compares it to "lighting the pilot light so the furnace has time to warm up."
- Turn the pressure off. Sometimes a break from sex works wonders. During this time, you can kiss, hug, touch, and massage each other; but view each of these activities as an end in itself.

- Have fun together. The more time you spend enjoying yourselves (eating out, going to movies, playing tennis, hiking), the more you'll enjoy each other sexually.

### Impotence

An estimated 10 million American men suffer from **impotence,** or erection difficulties. This means they cannot perform sexually more often than once in four attempts. Psychological factors, such as anxiety about performance, may cause about half the cases of impotence. Just as often, the problem has physical origins. Diabetes and reactions to drugs—prescription and recreational—are the most frequent organic causes. Even cigarettes can create erection problems for men sensitive to nicotine. New treatments include implants (some inflatable, some permanently rigid) that enable impotent men to have sexual intercourse, and drugs that can be injected directly into the penis.

### Failure to Respond

Women probably fail to become aroused at least as often as men, but it doesn't seem to be as upsetting to them as the inability to become erect is to men—if only because it isn't as noticeable. Also, our culture allows women to say they simply "don't feel like sex." The myth that a man should become aroused at every opportunity urges many men to have sex—or try to—regardless of how they feel.

### Male Orgasm Problems

For men, a common concern is **premature ejaculation,** in which a man ejaculates within 30 to 90 seconds of inserting his penis into his partner's vagina or after 10 to 15 thrusts. A premature ejaculator cannot control ejaculation long enough to satisfy a responsive partner at least 50 percent of the time. By this definition, a man may be premature with some women but not with others.

To delay orgasm, men may try to think of baseball or other sports, but this just makes sex boring. Others masturbate before intercourse, taking advantage of the refractory period, during which a man cannot ejaculate again. Others bite their lips, dig their nails into their palms, or concentrate on squeezing the muscles in their groins. Usually this just results in premature ejaculators with bloody lips and scarred palms. Some physicians prescribe drugs, including antidepressants and androgens (male sex hormones), to cure this problem. Topical anesthetics used to prevent climax dull pleasurable sensations for the woman as well as for the man.

Men can learn to control ejaculation by concentrating on their sexual response rather than by trying to distract themselves or ignore their reaction. By learning to sense the feelings that precede ejaculation, recognizing the emission stage and the point of ejaculatory inevitability, a man can develop better control.

### Problems of Intercourse and Orgasm in Women

Some women have a problem with **dyspareunia,** or pain during intercourse. An extreme form of painful intercourse is **vaginismus,** in which involuntary contractions of the muscles of the outer third of the vagina are so intense that they totally or partially close the vaginal opening. This problem often derives from a fear of penetration.

The female orgasm has long been a controversial sexual topic. About 90 percent of sexually active women have experienced orgasm, but only 50 percent of these women achieve orgasm through intercourse. Even fewer reach orgasm if intercourse isn't accompanied by direct stimulation of the clitoris. Does a woman who fails to achieve orgasm through intercourse have a sexual problem? The best answer is that she does if she wants to have orgasm during intercourse and can't.

Many counseling programs urge women who have never had orgasms to masturbate. They are then encouraged to share with their partners what they've learned, communicating with words or gestures what is most pleasing to them. Some women regularly want or need more than a single orgasm during intercourse. Partners can help by varying positions and experimenting with sexual techniques. However, in sexual response, more is not necessarily better; the couple should keep in mind that no one else is counting.

## Drugs and Sex

Many recreational drugs, such as alcohol and marijuana, are believed to enhance sexual performance. In fact, these drugs often interfere with normal sexual response. Cigarette smoking can also impair sexual performance. According to the Impotence In-

**impotence** A sexual difficulty in which a man is unable to achieve erection.
**premature ejaculation** A sexual difficulty in which a man ejaculates so rapidly that his partner's satisfaction is impaired.
**dyspareunia** A sexual difficulty in which a woman experiences pain during sexual intercourse.
**vaginismus** A sexual difficulty in which a woman experiences painful spasms of the vagina during sexual intercourse.

formation Center, smoking ten or more cigarettes a day increases the likelihood of impotence.[15]

Medications can also cause sexual difficulty. In men, drugs used to treat high blood pressure, anxiety, allergies, depression, muscle spasms, obesity, ulcers, irritable colon, and prostate cancer can cause impotence, breast enlargement, testicular swelling, priapism (persistent erection), loss of sexual desire, inability to ejaculate, and reduced sperm count. In women, they can diminish sexual desire, inhibit or delay orgasm, and cause breast swelling or secretions.

## Atypical Behavior

Although sexual desire and response are universal, some individuals develop sexual appetites or engage in unusual activities that are not typical sexual behaviors.

### Sexual Addiction

Some men and women can get relief from their feelings of restlessness and worthlessness only through sex (either through masturbation or with a partner). Once the sexual high ends, they're overwhelmed by the same negative feelings and driven, once more, to have sex.

Some therapists describe this problem as sexual addiction; others, as sexual compulsion. Professionals continue to debate exactly what this controversial condition is, how to diagnose it, and how to overcome it.[16]

According to some sex therapists, as many as one in every twelve adults may suffer from it. Others believe it is much less common. But most agree that for some people, sex is more than a normal pleasure: It is an overwhelming need that must be met, even at the cost of their careers and marriages.

Sexual addicts can be heterosexual or homosexual, male or female. Some of the characteristics exhibited by sexual addicts are:

- a sexual preoccupation that interferes with a normal sexual relationship with a spouse or a lover
- a compulsion to have sex again and again within a short period of time and to engage in sexual behavior that results in feelings of anxiety, depression, guilt, or shame
- a great deal of time away from family or work, to look for partners or to engage in sex
- the use of sex to hide from troubles

Several organizations with names like Sexaholics Anonymous and Sexual Addicts Anonymous are operating around the country. Modeled on the highly successful Alcoholics Anonymous approach, they offer support from people who share the same problem.

#### Sexual Deviations

Sexual deviations listed by the American Psychiatric Association include the following:

*Fetishism*—Obtaining sexual pleasure from an inanimate object or an asexual part of the body, such as the foot

*Pedophilia*—Sex between an adult and a child

*Transvestism*—Becoming sexually aroused by wearing the clothing of the other sex

*Exhibitionism*—Exposing one's genitals to an unwilling observer

*Voyeurism*—Obtaining sexual gratification by observing people undressing or involved in sexual activity

*Sadism*—Becoming sexually aroused by inflicting physical or psychological pain

*Masochism*—Obtaining sexual gratification by suffering physical or psychological pain.

Psychiatrists distinguish passive sexual deviancy, which does not involve actual contact with another, and aggressive deviancy. Most voyeurs and obscene phone callers do not seek physical contact with the objects of their sexual desire. These behaviors are predominantly, but not exclusively, male. Transvestites, who enjoy wearing the clothing of the other sex and often masturbate while cross-dressed, also tend to be male (and heterosexual).

# SEXUAL ASSAULT

A crime may be a violation of the law, or it may be what the dictionary terms "a grave offense, especially against morality." Sexual crimes may fit either or both of these definitions because they attack the integrity and innermost being of another person.

## Rape

The crime of **rape** consists of sexual penetration of a female or a male by means of intimidation, force, or fraud for aggressive and sexual reasons. Some see rape as an expression of hostility, a violent act only incidentally triggered by sexual considerations. Rap-

**rape** Sexual penetration of a female or a male by means of intimidation, force, or fraud.

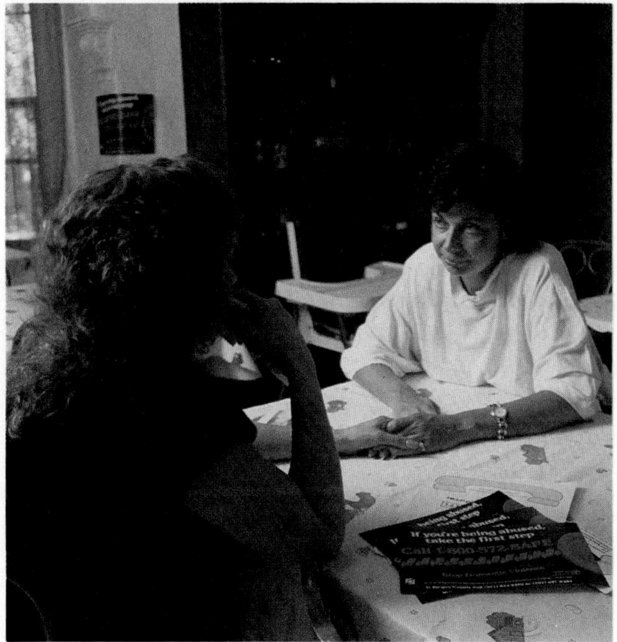


Counseling can help victims of sexual assault begin the slow process of healing.

ists have attacked children, old women, pregnant women, and nuns.

Within the broad category of rape are specific subcategories of the crime. **Statutory rape** refers to unlawful sexual intercourse between a male over the age of 16 and a female under the "age of consent," which ranges from age 12 to age 21 in different states. **Acquaintance rape** in which the rapist is known by the victim, is a growing danger.

The incidence of rape is increasing faster than any other crime of violence in America. Only one in every five to ten rapes is reported. More than 70 percent of all rapes are not spontaneous, but are deliberate, planned attacks.[17]

Physical and sexual abuse in marriage, including rape, is a problem that has come into the open only recently. There are now special programs and shelters for victimized wives in metropolitan areas. Any woman, married or not, can turn to local groups, as well as to police and health officials, for aid.

**If You Are Attacked** Only you can judge whether you can resist an attacker without risking serious harm. If your life is threatened by a gun, a knife, or sheer brawn, you may feel it's wisest to submit—but if you feel you can resist, fight as vigorously as possible. Police recommend yelling "Fire!" Kick the attacker in the groin, or grab his testicles and squeeze as hard as possible. His reaction to severe pain should be to release or loosen his grip on you. If you cannot get to his genitals, try for his eyes. You should bite, claw, and hit with any heavy object that's available. Do not rely on weapons, as they may be taken from you and used against you.

**statutory rape** Unlawful sexual intercourse between a male over 16 years of age and a female under the age of consent.
**acquaintance rape** Rape by a person known by the victim.

STRATEGY FOR CHANGE

## Reducing the Risk of Rape

The following list, prepared by the Queen's Bench Foundation of San Francisco, provides commonsense suggestions for preventing rape when you're out alone:

- Be aware of yourself and of areas of possible trouble, and plan ahead what you might do in case of attack.
- Vary your routes home, especially at night. Try to walk with other people or take public transportation, especially after dark. If you must walk alone, walk in the middle of the sidewalk, out of reach of people hiding in doorways or parked cars.
- Stay on well-lighted streets. If there is little traffic, you might want to walk in the middle of the street.
- If you suspect that you are being followed, look behind you. Cross the street, walk in a different direction, and vary the speed of your walk. If the person persists in following you, go into the nearest lighted house or open business, and call a friend, a cab, or the police. Don't be afraid to scream or make noise; you may scare a would-be attacker away.
- If you must walk in an unfamiliar area, get a map and plan your route in advance. Always walk briskly and confidently. Don't look lost, or as if your mind is a million miles away. Wear sensible clothes and shoes.
- If a car pulls up beside you, stay more than an arm's length away. Don't become involved in a long conversation.
- If you fear danger, yell "Fire" or "Call the police," rather than "Rape" or "Help." Run to the nearest lighted place and get inside quickly. Break a window instead of ringing a bell.

The following can stop an attack long enough so you can get away:

- *Lighted cigarette.* Use it on his face.
- *Plastic lemon filled with ammonia.* Aim for his eyes; it will induce temporary blindness.

- *Umbrella.* Put one hand in the center, the other at the end. Use a jabbing motion toward his neck or stomach.
- *Hat pin.* Carry one in your hand or clothing. Wrap your hand around it, and scrape his face or jab at his neck.
- *Keys.* Carry these with the ends sticking out through your fingers. Use a blow of the fist, or scrape the keys across his hand or face.
- *Hardbound book.* Hold it with both hands and smash the edge into the side of his nose or his throat.

**If You Are Raped** Following are some suggestions for dealing with a rape:

*During the Rape*—Stay calm. Talk sanely and quietly, to remind the attacker that you are a human being. Memorize the details of his face and clothing.

*If You Want to Report It to the Police*—Don't take a bath. Call a friend or a rape crisis center first, and then the police. Insist on going to the hospital. Give as clear and comprehensive a description of your attacker as possible.

*At the Hospital*—Ask for antibiotics for sexually transmitted diseases. Have your friend check all medication given you. Talk to the counselor about testing for HIV infection.

*If You Don't Want to Report It*—Call a friend or rape crisis center. Before you take a bath, go to a doctor; you may later decide to report the rape. Get treatment for sexually transmitted diseases. If you must go to a hospital, remember that you don't necessarily have to talk to the police.

### Date Rape

Any woman forced to have sexual intercourse against her will is a victim of rape, regardless of whether or not she knows her rapist. **Date rape** is a type of acquaintance rape that occurs when the victim is on a date with the attacker. Date rape, particularly on college campuses, may be more common than anyone has suspected. A survey of women on 32 college campuses reported that 15 percent of the women interviewed had experienced one rape, and 89 percent of these women had been raped by someone they knew.[18] Most of the women did not report the rape. One out of every 12 men admitted that he may have raped or attempted to rape a date or acquaintance.

The victims of date rape may feel confused about what happened. They are unlikely to notify the police because they fear that no one will believe their stories. Often, the emotional aftermath of the attack is devastating. The women suffer nightmares, anxiety, and flashbacks. They tend to blame themselves, questioning their judgment and wondering what they did to cause the rape.

Because they're often too ashamed to tell anyone what happened, they suffer alone, without skilled therapists or sympathetic friends to reassure them. Years after a rape, these women may still be struggling with rage against men and with problems establishing trusting relationships. Women who were raped in the past and remain haunted by the experience should seek professional help. A therapist can help them begin the slow process of healing. (See "Health Spotlight: Avoiding Date Rape.")

### Male Rape

Although many people think that men who rape other men are always homosexuals, most rapists of men consider themselves to be heterosexual and usually seek victims who at least appear straight. Young boys are not the only victims. The average age of male victims is 24 years—and probably as many men are raped outside of jail as inside.

## Sexual Abuse of Children

Sexual abuse of children can take many forms, including sexually suggestive conversations, prolonged kissing, petting, oral sex, or intercourse. These incidents often cause enormous psychological damage. Often the molesters are relatives, teachers, baby-sitters, or neighbors.

Sensing that they did something wrong, children often feel ashamed and blame themselves. They're afraid to confide in their parents for fear of being punished. To help child victims of sexual abuse, many schools and community organizations are sponsoring educational programs about "stranger danger" that teach children how to avoid being touched or fondled when or where they don't want to be.

## Sexual Harassment

Any unwanted sexual attention—leering, pinching, patting, repeated sexual comments, or pressure for dates or sexual intimacy—is **sexual harassment.** A 1989 survey by the Project on the Status and Education of Women of the Association of American Colleges found that 20 to 30 percent of undergraduate women and 30 to 40 percent of graduate students

**date rape** An acquaintance rape in which the rapist is someone with whom the victim has gone out on a date.

**sexual harassment** Unwanted sexual attention, including leering, pinching, patting, pressure for a sexual relationship, and lewd comments.

HEALTH SPOTLIGHT

## Avoiding Date Rape

Researchers have found that the best way for women to prevent date rape is to make clear early in the encounter that they are not interested in sex. Screaming, physical resistance, and claiming to have a sexually transmitted disease have also stopped would-be rapists. But the single most effective tactic of all is saying, "This is rape, and I'm calling the cops."

Here are other suggestions for reducing your risk:

**If You Are a Woman**

- Be wary if the man calls all the shots, ordering for you at restaurants, planning what you do on your date, and directing everything you do together. He may do the same thing when it comes to sex.
- Back away from a man who pressures you into other activities you don't want to do on a date, such as chugging beer or drag racing with his friends.
- Be very clear in communicating what you feel. Don't just say no. If a date is being sexually aggressive, insist that he leave—or you get up and leave.
- Avoid misleading messages. Don't tell him to stop touching you, talk for a few minutes, and then resume petting.
- Stay out of risky situations. Try to go on your first few dates with a group. Stay away from places so isolated you won't be able to get help. At any age, parking in a remote spot is not a good idea.
- If you know at the onset of a relationship that you do not want to have sex with this person, say so openly. Talk openly about your sexual expectations.
- Let your date know from the beginning how you feel about sexual involvement on first, second, third, or twentieth dates. State your feelings and fears clearly.
- Learn to resist. Many women expect someone they know and date to respond to, and respect, their no's. If your date doesn't get your message, shout, scream, scratch, kick—do whatever you have to do to show that you are serious about not wanting sex.
- If you are raped on a date, tell someone. You should also get a medical examination as soon as possible and talk to a counselor about the pros and cons of reporting the rape to the police.

**If You Are a Man**

- Remember that it's okay not to "score" on a date.
- Set limits. Think about what you're willing to do—how much sexual activity is enough. Remember, your partner will be making decisions about the same things.
- Talk to each other. Tell your partner your limits.
- Find out how she feels. Listen to your partner. If she says no—even if she says it quietly and shyly, she means no.
- Be aware of your partner's actions. If she pulls away, if she tries to get up, understand that she's sending you a message—one you should acknowledge and respect.
- Don't assume a sexy dress or casual flirting is an invitation to sex.

SOURCES: Goleman, Daniel. "When the Rapist Is Not A Stranger," *New York Times*, August 29, 1989. American College Health Association.

had experienced some form of sexual harassment on campus.[19] Because college administrations can be held legally responsible for allowing a "hostile" or "offensive" environment, many schools have set up committees to handle student reports and to take action against faculty members.

If harassment occurs at work and the harasser is a boss, client, supervisor, or coworker, victims should document their complaints by writing down specific incidents (including dates, times, places, and what happened). Many companies have established grievance procedures for handling sexual harassment complaints. It sometimes helps to confront the harasser, either in person or by writing a note, and state that you are not interested in his or her attention.

## THE BUSINESS OF SEX

Sex, without affection and individuality, becomes a product to be packaged, marketed, traded, bought, and sold. Two billion-dollar industries that treat sex as a product are prostitution and pornography.

### Prostitution

Prostitution, described as the world's oldest profession, is a nationwide industry grossing more than a billion dollars a year and employing 100,000 to 500,000 women. In every state except Nevada (and in all but a few counties there), prostitution is illegal. However, customers are rarely arrested. There is a relatively new danger for prostitutes and their clients: AIDS transmission. In some cities, as many as half of the prostitutes are infected with the AIDS virus, and some researchers see prostitution as a growing means of heterosexual transmission of the disease.

### Pornography

Most laws against pornography are based on the assumption that such materials can set off uncontrollable, dangerous sexual urges, ranging from promiscuity to sexual violence. Research does indicate that exposure to scenes of rape or other forms of sexual violence against women, or to scenes of degradation of women does lead to tolerance of these hostile and brutal acts.

## MAKING THIS CHAPTER WORK FOR YOU

### Responsible Sexuality

**Women and men have different sexual organs, hormones, and health problems. During a woman's menstrual cycle, her ovary releases an egg cell, or ovum, that travels through the fallopian tube to the**

## WHAT DO YOU THINK?

As you're walking through the campus, you see a couple making out on a bench. As you get closer, you realize both are men. How do you react? Why do you think you feel that way? Do you think others may be upset? How would you feel if it were a heterosexual couple?

One of your friends has just started going out with someone you've known since childhood. Your friend confided a while back that she has herpes. You're pretty sure that the guy she's dating doesn't know. You consider yourself friends with both. How would you feel about the friend who's not telling? Do you think it's any of your business? What would you do about it?

Many people think they're not at risk of HIV infection because they aren't gay, they don't use intravenous drugs, and they don't date anyone who is gay or uses IV drugs. "I could tell if someone is HIV-positive just by being with him or her," they tell themselves. What do you think of this attitude? Do you believe that people can "tell" whether they or other individuals have been exposed to HIV? If you became involved with someone, how would you find out if he or she is a "safe" partner? How would you feel if that person asked you about your sexual history?

uterus. If the egg is not fertilized, the uterine lining is shed during menstruation. Menstrual-cycle problems include premenstrual syndrome and tension; menstrual cramps (dysmenorrhea); and amenorrhea, a stopping of regular menstrual cycles. Between the ages of 45 and 55, menopause occurs, and a woman's menstrual cycle stops.

Circumcision, the surgical removal of the foreskin of the penis, has some health advantages as well as some potential complications for males. As they grow older, men are at risk for prostatitis, prostate enlargement, and prostate cancer. At mid-life, men experience the male menopause, a period of change and possible crisis.

Our sexual hormones—in the female, estrogen and progesterone; in the male, testosterone—play a key role in sexual development. At puberty, estrogen causes a girl to develop female secondary sex characteristics—including enlarged external genitals, and full breasts and hips—and prepares her body for conception and pregnancy. Testosterone stimulates the development of male secondary sex characteristics, which include a deeper voice, facial and body hair growth, and enlarged genitals.

A person's gender is determined, not only by his or her physiological sex, but also by psychological and sociological factors. Four absolute biological differences separate men and women: Only men can make sperm; only women can menstruate, become pregnant, and nurse a baby. As our recognition of sexual similarities has grown, more men and women are choosing roles and occupations that traditionally have been closed to them. Individuals who allow themselves to express both their masculine and feminine traits are androgynous.

Our interest in sex changes during our lives, depending on physical and emotional health, other activities, and needs. One's sexual orientation may be predominantly heterosexual, bisexual, or homosexual. Regardless of sexual preference, healthy sexuality involves an understanding of your own body, your partner's, and responsible sexual behavior.

Sexual options include celibacy, erotic fantasizing, kissing and touching, masturbation, intercourse, and oral sex. Whatever the type of sexual stimulation, the body's response always follows the same sequence: excitement, plateau, orgasm, and resolution.

Only safe sex practices can overcome the risk of acquired immune deficiency syndrome (AIDS) and other sexually transmitted diseases. The safest sex practices are abstinence and sexual relations with only one partner, who has never been exposed to the human immunodeficiency virus (HIV), which causes AIDS.

HIV is spread through contact with body fluids—semen, vaginal fluid, blood, and possibly saliva—from infected individuals. Repeated sexual contact, use of contaminated needles, and blood transfusions (received between 1978 and 1985) are the most common modes of transmission. The only way to know if you or your partner has been exposed to HIV is to take the HIV antibody test. Unsafe sex practices include sexual contact with a partner whose history is unknown and sexual contact without a condom.

Common sexual problems of both men and women include sexual anxiety, lack of sexual interest, sexual unresponsiveness, and sexual impairment due to the use of recreational drugs or medications. In men, common problems include impotence and premature ejaculation; in women, common problems are dyspareunia and vaginismus. A person who has never experienced excitement or orgasm is suffering from a primary sexual difficulty; a person is suffering from a secondary difficulty if he or she is not responding the way he or she used to or does in other circumstances. Sexual addiction and sexual deviations are considered atypical sexual behaviors.

Sex, a source of great pleasure, can also be a means of causing great pain. Rape, by acquaintances as well as strangers, is a growing danger. Sexual victims include the most vulnerable people in our society: children. Prostitution and pornography strip sex of its emotional, deeply human meaning and transform it into a business.

The days when sex seemed more of a recreational activity than an expression of deep needs and desires are past. As they look toward the twenty-first century, most sexually active people realize that sexual involvement is far too significant to be treated as a sport. Any time two people come close, they are expressing fundamental needs and desires. Whatever their sexual preference or experience, they are embarking on a very special form of sharing. They will touch each other, and their lives will be different, if only in the smallest ways. If they make love, they will be making much more: memories, emotional connections, and attachments.

By caring for your sexual health, you prepare yourself to become a responsible, responsive sexual partner. By avoiding the dangers of sexually transmitted diseases, you assume responsibility for your safety and health. By dealing with any sexual problems that arise, you take charge of a key aspect of your health and behavior.

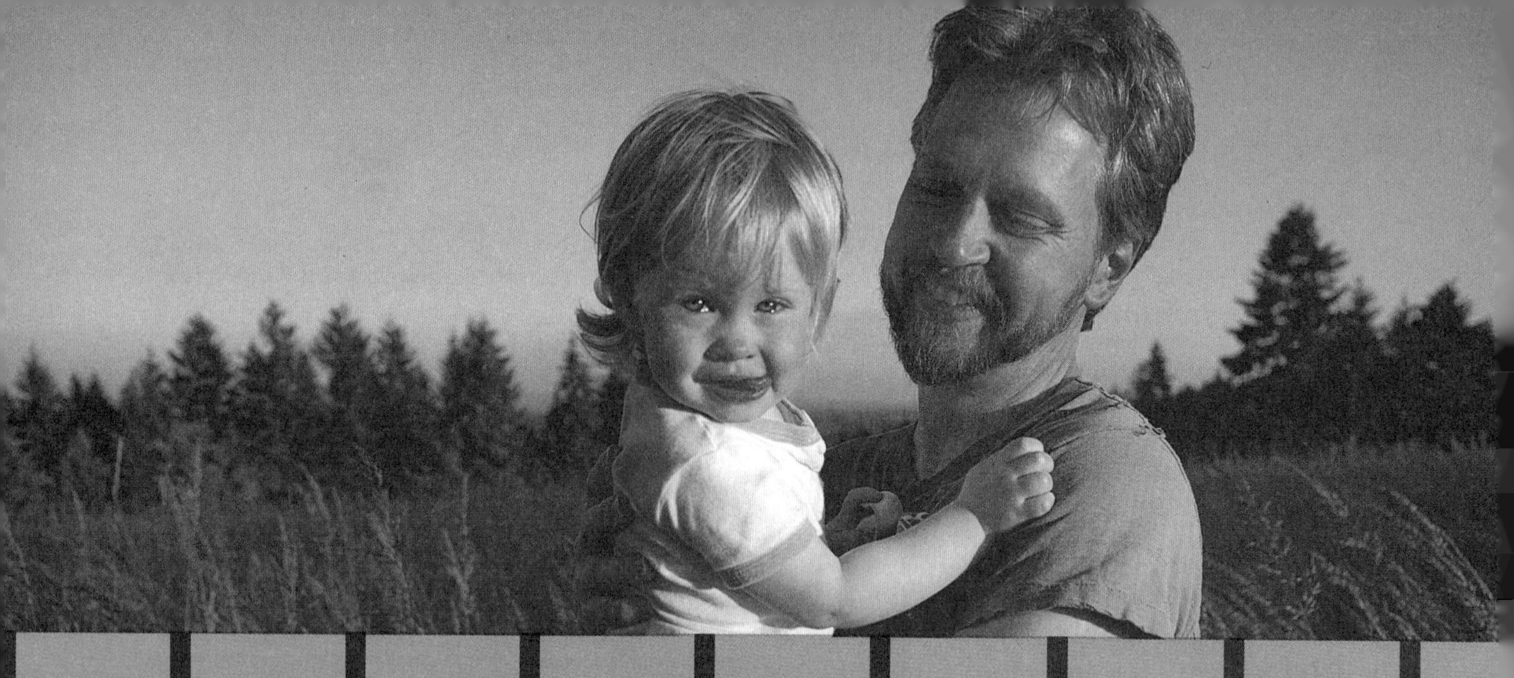

# 8 REPRODUCTIVE CHOICES

In this chapter

Conception

The basics of birth control

Abortion

Pregnancy

Childbirth

Infertility

Making this chapter work for you: Responsible reproductive choices now and in the future

*As human beings, we have a unique power: the ability to choose not to conceive.* No other species on earth can separate sexual activity and pleasure from reproduction. This option also means that anyone who engages in heterosexual intercourse must acknowledge responsibility for another life—the child who might be conceived. This chapter provides information on conception, contraception, and the processes by which a fetus develops and enters the world.

## CONCEPTION

Nature has stacked the deck in favor of reproduction. A single male ejaculation may contain 500 million sperm, all designed to fertilize a single egg (or ovum). The creation of sperm, or **spermatogenesis,** starts in the male at puberty (see Figure 8-1). Hormones regulate the production of sperm in the testes and of seminal fluid, or semen, in the prostate and seminal vesicles. Each of the sperm released into the vagina during intercourse moves on its own, propelling itself toward its target.

To succeed, the sperm must reach the uterus and then travel up one of the fallopian tubes. Just about every sperm produced by a man in his lifetime fails to accomplish its mission. **Fertilization** occurs only when the hardy sperm meets a ripe egg and merges with it.

The human egg is far more rare than the sperm. Each woman is born with her lifetime supply of ova, and usually 300 to 500 mature eggs eventually leave her ovaries. Each month, in one or the other of the woman's ovaries, an egg is released in the process called ovulation (see Figure 8-2 (a)). It is swept through

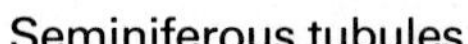


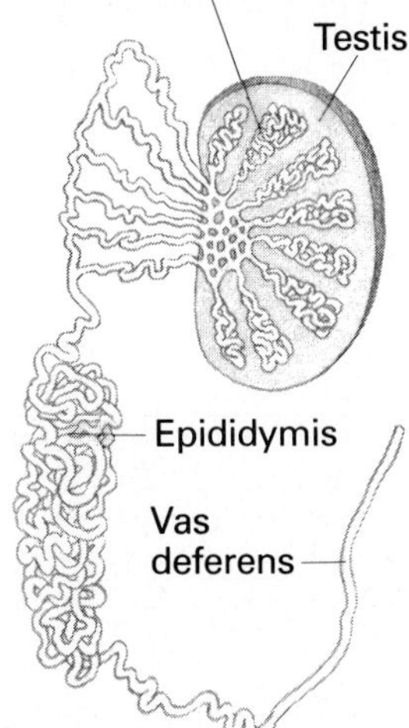


SOURCE: Hales, Dianne. *An Invitation to Health, Fourth Edition,* Benjamin/Cummings, 1989.

**FIGURE 8-1** Spermatogenesis. Sperm cells form in the seminiferous tubules and are passed into the coiled tubules of the epididymis, where they are stored until ejaculation.

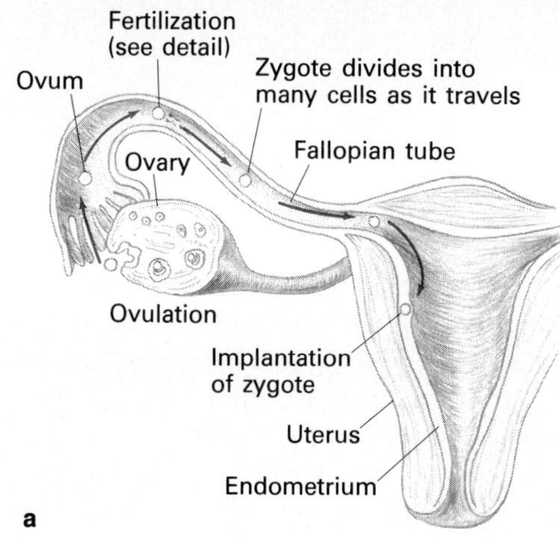


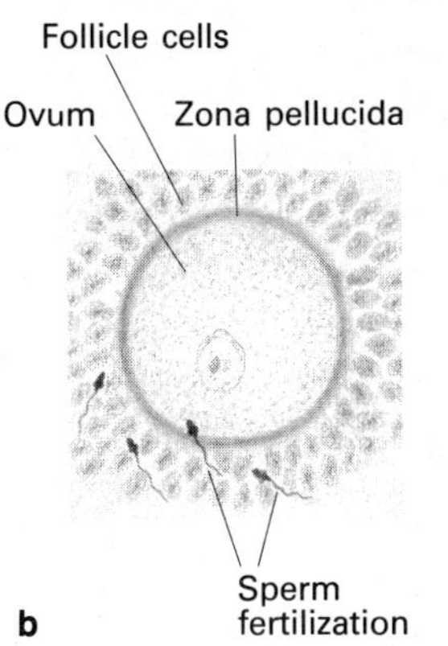


SOURCE: Hales, Dianne. *An Invitation to Health, Fourth Edition,* Benjamin/Cummings, 1989.

**FIGURE 8-2 (a)** The path of the ovum from ovulation to implantation. The ovum, released from the ovary into the fallopian tube, is fertilized by a sperm in the tube. The fertilized egg continues through the tube into the uterus, where it burrows into the endometrium, the lining of the uterus. **(b)** Successful fertilization requires the efforts of thousands of sperm. All the sperm that reach the egg deposit tiny amounts of an enzyme that helps break down first the protective outer layer of follicle cells and then the inner layer, the *zona pellucida,* surrounding the cell. A sperm can then enter the ovum through the break in the protective layers.

**spermatogenesis** The process by which sperm cells are produced.
**fertilization** The union of an ovum and a sperm.

the fallopian tubes to the uterus, a journey that takes 3 to 4 days. An unfertilized egg lives for about 24 to 36 hours, disintegrates and, during menstruation, is expelled along with the uterine lining.

If a sperm, which can survive in the female from 2 to 5 days, meets a ripe egg in a fallopian tube, it faces another barrier: a layer of cells and a jellylike substance that surrounds each egg (Figure 8-2 (b)). Each sperm that touches the egg deposits an enzyme that dissolves part of this barrier. When a sperm bumps into a bare spot, it penetrates the egg membrane and merges with the egg (fertilization).

As the fertilized egg travels down the fallopian tube, it divides to form a tiny clump of cells called a **zygote.** When it reaches the uterus, about a week after ovulation, it burrows into the endometrium, the lining of the uterus. This process is called **implantation.**

## THE BASICS OF BIRTH CONTROL

Ideally, sexual partners should together decide which form of birth control to use. However, you have to be realistic about your own situation. This may mean assuming full responsibility for your reproductive ability by and for yourself.

If you are a sexually active heterosexual, you are, or will be, a consumer of birth control services, advice, and devices—or else you are likely to become a consumer of obstetrical services. Not deciding to use birth control is in itself a decision for anyone who is sexually active. Why don't people use contraceptives? In many cases, ignorance is the reason. According to one survey, 70 percent of teenage girls engaging in intercourse without contraceptive protection felt that they could not become pregnant if they simply didn't want to; didn't have an orgasm; or had intercourse in certain positions, such as standing up.[1]

Every year 1.2 million to 3 million accidental pregnancies occur as a result of contraceptive failures, including problems with the drug or device itself or from failure to use it properly. However, no contraceptive works if you don't use it (see Table 8-1).

You also have to recognize the risks associated with various methods of contraception. If you are a woman, the risks are chiefly yours. Although most women never experience any serious complications, it is important to find out the potential for long-term risks, including infertility after years of IUD use. Risks that are acceptable to others may not be acceptable to you—or vice versa.

There is no "right" decision in these matters. However, good decisions are based on sound information. You should consult a physician or family-planning counselor if you have questions or want to know how certain methods might affect existing or familial medical conditions, such as high blood pressure or diabetes.

Always discuss contraception with your partner. Men should not shift this responsibility automatically to women simply because women become pregnant. It takes two people to conceive a baby, and two people should be involved in deciding *not* to conceive a baby (see Table 8-2).

**zygote** A fertilized egg.
**implantation** The embedding of the fertilized ovum in the uterine lining six to seven days after fertilization.

**TABLE 8-1** Birth Control in the 1990s: What Americans Choose

| METHOD | PERCENTAGE OF BIRTH CONTROL USERS WHO CHOOSE IT | PERCENTAGE OF FAILURE IN FIRST YEAR OF USE |
|---|---|---|
| Oral contraceptives | 32 | 3 |
| Female sterilization | 19 | 0.4 |
| Condoms | 17 | 12 |
| Male sterilization | 14 | 0.15 |
| Diaphragm | 4–6 | 2–23 |
| Rhythm | 4 | 20 |
| IUD | 3 | 6 |
| Contraceptive sponge | 3 | 18 |
| Vaginal foams, etc. | 2 | 21 |

**TABLE 8-2** Contraceptive Methods

| METHOD | ADVANTAGES | DISADVANTAGES | DON'T USE IF YOU |
|---|---|---|---|
| ORAL CONTRACEPTIVES Combination pill, multiphasic pill, mini-pill | May lower risk of ovarian and endometrial cancers and of tubal pregnancy, eases menstrual cramps, may protect against rheumatoid arthritis. Since the mini-pill contains no estrogen, it may cause fewer side effects. | May cause weight gain, tender and swollen breasts, light or absent periods, nausea, darkening of facial skin, headaches, and depression; may delay resumption of ovulation after stopping pill. May increase risk of breast cancer in women who use pill for several years in their teens and early twenties. Breakthrough or irregular bleeding more likely to occur with mini-pill, which also has a higher risk of tubal pregnancies. | Have a history of breast or endometrial cancer, high blood pressure, heart attacks, stroke, liver tumor or other serious liver disease, gall bladder disease, or phlebitis; have a tendency to form blood clots; are breast-feeding; are over age 35 and smoke; are over age 40; or suspect you are pregnant. Women who experience abnormal bleeding or who have had a tubal pregnancy should not use the mini-pill. |
| INTRAUTERINE DEVICE Progestasert/Paragard | Once inserted, requires no further action and doesn't interfere with lovemaking. | Increased risk of tubal pregnancy, infertility, and pelvic inflammatory disease (PID); may cause increased menstrual flow and cramps, possible perforation of uterine wall, or partial or complete expulsion; must be checked periodically for correct placement. Progestasert must be replaced yearly. | Have a history of PID or other pelvic infections, have never had a child, or have multiple sex partners. |
| DIAPHRAGM | Fully reversible, with no side effects, may protect against some sexually transmitted diseases. | Spermicide must be reapplied for each episode of intercourse, some women find it difficult to insert and unaesthetic, may become dislodged during sex, must be checked periodically for tears, requires periodic refitting by doctor. | Are allergic to rubber or spermicide. |
| CONDOM | Available without a prescription at low cost, no side effects, protects against AIDS and other sexually transmitted diseases. | Have to interrupt lovemaking, reduces sexual pleasure for some men. Condoms can break or leak. | Are allergic to rubber. |
| VAGINAL SPONGE | Widely available without a prescription, may be inserted up to 24 hours in advance of lovemaking, does not require additional spermicide, may protect against some sexually transmitted diseases. | May cause burning sensation from spermicide, some women have difficulty removing the device, possible risk of toxic shock. | Are menstruating (because of toxic-shock risk), have cervical or vaginal infections, have given birth within previous six weeks. |

**TABLE 8-2** Contraceptive Methods *(Continued)*

| METHOD | ADVANTAGES | DISADVANTAGES | DON'T USE IF YOU |
|---|---|---|---|
| SPERMICIDES Foams, jellies, creams, suppositories, and tablets | Inexpensive and widely available without a prescription, fully reversible, may protect against some sexually transmitted diseases. | Must be inserted 10 to 30 minutes before each act of intercourse, some women find them unaesthetic. | Are allergic to nonoxynol-9 or other chemicals in spermicides |
| VAGINAL CONTRACEPTIVE FILM (VCF) | Available without a prescription; thin film dissolves in vagina, releasing spermicide, and need not be removed. | Must be inserted at least 5 minutes before intercourse; effective for up to 2 hours, then new film must be inserted. | Are allergic to spermicide. |
| NATURAL FAMILY PLANNING Rhythm, calendar, basal body temperature, cervical mucus observation | Does not violate religious bars against artificial birth control, requires no medication or devices. | Restricts sexual activity to specific time of woman's menstrual cycle, less reliable for women with irregular cycles, vaginal infections can interfere with mucus observation. | Are not highly motivated or are reluctant to abstain from sex for up to two weeks of a woman's cycle. |
| STERILIZATION Tubal ligation or occlusion | Permanent; woman does not have to use any other method of birth control. | Reversal sometimes possible, but should be considered permanent; risk of infection, bleeding, accidental perforation of or injury to uterus or vagina during operation; can be abdominal discomfort and bleeding for 48 hours after operation. | May later want to conceive. |
| Vasectomy | Permanent, after follow-up tests show no sperm remaining in semen; requires no other form of birth control. | Reversal sometimes possible, but should be considered permanent; temporary discomfort after the procedure is performed. | May eventually want to father a child; associate virility with reproductive capacity. |

SOURCE: Schrotenbauer/Subak–Sharpe, "A Complete Guide to Modern Contraceptives," *Family Circle*, April, 1987.

## The Birth Control Pill

The **oral contraceptive,** usually referred to as "the pill," is the method of birth control preferred by unmarried women and by those under age 30. More than 50 million women around the world, including 8 to 10 million in the United States, take the pill. Women 15 to 24 years old are most likely to choose oral contraceptives. In use for 30 years, the pill is one of the most researched, tested, and followed-up medications in medical history—and one of the most controversial.

Three types of oral contraceptives are available in the United States: a combination pill, a multiphasic pill, and a mini-pill. The **combination pill** contains two hormones, synthetic estrogen and progestin, which play important roles in controlling ovulation and the menstrual cycle.

The **multiphasic pill** provides different levels of estrogen and progesterone at different times of the month, to mimic the normal hormonal fluctuations of the natural menstrual cycle. These pills reduce the total hormonal dose and side effects.

**oral contraceptive** A preparation of synthetic hormones that inhibit ovulation; also referred to as the birth control pill or "the pill."

**combination pill** A type of oral contraceptive containing synthetic estrogen and progestin.

**multiphasic pill** A type of oral contraceptive that mimics the normal hormonal fluctuations of the menstrual cycle.

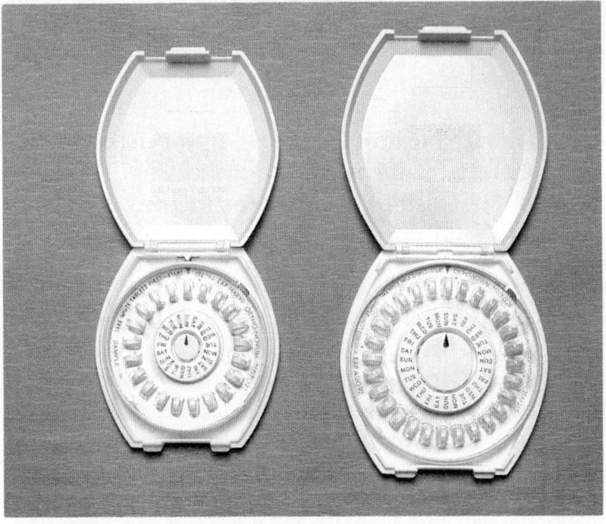

**FIGURE 8-3** Although most birth control pills come in packets of twenty-eight pills, some types come in twenty-one–day supplies. The woman taking the twenty-one–day type takes one tablet every day for twenty-one days, then begins a new packet seven days later. All twenty-one of the pills contain hormones. The twenty-eight–day packets contain twenty-one pills with hormones and seven placebos (inert pills). The woman takes a pill every day, beginning a new packet immediately after she finishes the old. With the twenty-eight–day packets, there is no need to remember to start taking the pills after a seven-day hiatus.

The combination and multiphasic pills block the release of hormones that would stimulate the process leading to ovulation. They also thicken and alter the cervical mucus, making it more hostile to sperm, and they make implantation of a fertilized egg in the uterine lining more difficult.

The **mini-pill** contains a small amount of progestin and no estrogen. Unlike the women who take combination pills, those using mini-pills probably do ovulate at least occasionally. The mini-pills make the mucus in the cervix so thick and tacky, though, that sperm cannot enter the uterus. Mini-pills may also interfere with implantation by altering the uterine lining.

Today, the pill usually comes in 28-day packets (see Figure 8-3): twenty-one of the pills contain the hormone(s) and seven are "blanks," included so that the woman takes a pill every day, even during her menstrual period. If a woman forgets to take one pill, she should take it as soon as she remembers it. If she forgets during the first week of her cycle or misses more than one pill, she should rely on another form of birth control until her next menstrual period.

### Is the Pill Safe?

In the past, pill use has been associated with a higher incidence of heart disease and strokes. The new generation of pills has cut the risk of heart disease and stroke among users by as much as 80 percent.[2] The danger may be lowest with the mini-pill. Yet there is still a very real risk of cardiovascular problems associated with use of the pill, primarily for women over 35; those who smoke; and those with other health problems, such as high blood pressure. Heart attacks strike an estimated one in 14,000 pill users between the ages of 30 and 39, and one in 1,500 between the ages of 40 and 44. Strokes occur five times more frequently among women taking oral contraceptives, and clots in the veins develop in one out of every 500 previously healthy women on the pill.

Women generally worry more about the newer pill's association with cancer than with cardiovascular disease. In 1989, studies linked pill use to an increased rate of breast cancer in women younger than 45.[3] According to the findings, women who take the pill when they are in their teens or early twenties could double their risk of breast cancer. Earlier studies had found no extra danger of breast cancer in pill users.[4] Some physicians advise women to consider other forms of birth control if they are young or have a family history of breast cancer and to avoid using the pill for more than a few years.

The pill has several advantages, reducing the likelihood of benign breast lumps, ovarian cysts, and cancer of the lining of the uterus. In addition, the pill is more effective than any form of contraception other than sterilization. In actual use, the failure rate is 1 to 5 percent for estrogen/progesterone pills and 3 to 10 percent for mini-pills.

### Choosing and Using the Pill

Before starting on the pill, you should undergo a thorough physical examination, including the following:

- routine blood pressure test
- pelvic exam, including Pap smear
- breast examination
- blood test
- urine sample

In describing your medical history, note any incidence of or family tendency toward hypertension or heart disease, diabetes, liver dysfunction, hepatitis, unusual menstrual history, severe depression, sickle-

**mini-pill** A type of oral contraceptive containing synthetic progestin.

cell anemia, cancer of the breast or uterus, high cholesterol levels, or migraine headaches.

You should also be aware of the following possible side effects of the pill:[5]

- *Breakthrough Bleeding*—This is an inconvenience, not a danger, caused while the body adjusts to the hormones in the pill. Your doctor may advise a different brand of pill to avoid the problem.
- *Nausea, Bloating, Fatigue, Breast Tenderness or Fullness*—These conditions may last up to three months. Also, you may gain or lose weight or experience mood swings.
- *Darkening of the Skin Across the Nose and Cheeks*—This condition also occurs in pregnancy, but it is rare and is not dangerous. When you go off the pill, the darkening usually fades.

Even if you experience no discomfort or side effects, see a physician at least once a year for an examination, which should include a blood pressure test and a pelvic and breast exam.

Notify your doctor at once if you develop severe abdominal pain, chest pain, coughing, shortness of breath, pain or tenderness in the calf or thigh, severe headaches, dizziness, faintness, muscle weakness or numbness, speech disturbance, blurred vision, a sensation of flashing lights, a breast lump, severe depression, or yellowing of your skin.[6]

Generally when a woman stops taking the pill, her normal menstrual cycle resumes within three months. However, 2 to 4 percent of pill users experience prolonged delays.[7] Women who become pregnant during the first or second cycle after discontinuing use of the pill may be at greater risk of miscarriage; they are also more likely to conceive twins. Most physicians advise women who want to conceive to change to another method of contraception for three months after they stop taking the pill.

## Barrier Contraceptives

As their name implies, these forms of birth control block the meeting of egg and sperm by means of a physical barrier: a diaphragm, cervical cap, or condom. They have become increasingly popular because they can do more than prevent conception; when the diaphragm or cervical cap are used with certain spermicides and are combined with the use of condoms, they can help protect users from sexually transmitted diseases, including HIV infection.[8] Another benefit is that they lower the risk of infertility in women. The reason may be that barrier contraceptives prevent infection, which can lead to infertility.

Barrier contraceptives may have one disadvantage. In 1989, researchers reported that women who'd relied on condoms and diaphragms for birth control prior to becoming pregnant are more than twice as likely to develop a serious pregnancy complication called preeclampsia, which is characterized by high blood pressure, fluid retention, and kidney problems.[9] The scientists speculated that frequent exposure to the prospective father's semen before conception may help prevent the mother's immune system from attacking her own fetus. With barrier contraceptives, this does not happen.

### The Diaphragm

A **diaphragm** is a bowllike rubber cup with a flexible rim, in sizes ranging from 2 to 4 inches (50 to 105 millimeters) in diameter. Used by itself, it is not an effective contraceptive. Its main function is to serve as a container for a sperm-killing foam or jelly. Used with a spermicide (available at pharmacies without a prescription) and properly fitted by a physician, a diaphragm acts as both a physical and a chemical barrier to the entry of sperm into the uterus (see Figure 8-4).

The effectiveness of the diaphragm in preventing pregnancy depends on strong motivation and a precise understanding of its use. If diaphragms with spermicide are used consistently and carefully, they can be 95 to 98 percent effective. Without spermicide, their effectiveness is far lower. When used with a spermicide containing nonoxynol-9 and a condom, diaphragms offer extra protection against sexually transmitted diseases, including HIV infection.

### The Cervical Cap

Like the diaphragm, the **cervical cap** acts as a physical barrier blocking the path of the sperm to the uterus. The rubber or plastic cap, which resembles a large thimble, fits snugly around the cervix (see Figure 8-5). Smaller and thicker than a diaphragm, it is about as effective. One advantage is that it can be left in place for several days (rather than hours). A primary disadvantage is that the caps are more difficult to insert and remove and may damage the cervix. Not all women can get a cap that fits properly.

---

**diaphragm** A round, flexible rubber disk that is inserted into the vagina to cover the cervix and prevent the passage of sperm into the uterus during sexual intercourse.
**cervical cap** A cup-shaped device that is inserted into the vagina to cover the cervix and prevent the passage of sperm into the uterus during sexual intercourse.

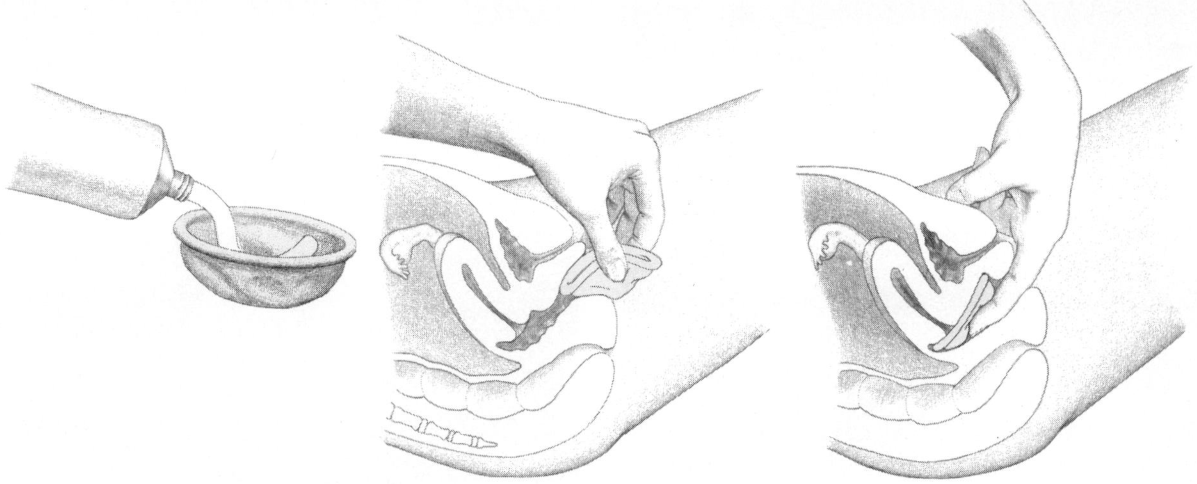

**FIGURE 8-4** How to use a diaphragm. First apply spermicide to the cup and around the rim. Holding the diaphragm by its outer rim and compressing its sides, slide it into the vagina until it lodges behind the pubic bone and covers the cervix. Check its position with your finger by feeling the cervix through the diaphragm.

The diaphragm can be inserted up to 4 hours before intercourse. If intercourse doesn't occur within 3 to 4 hours or if it occurs more than once, additional spermicide should be added, without removing the device. The diaphragm must be left in place for 6 to 8 hours after intercourse.

To remove the diaphragm, hook one or two fingers over the forward rim and pull down and out. Wash the diaphragm with warm water and mild soap, dry it thoroughly, and store it in a container for protection. Diaphragms last two to three years, but should be refitted if you gain or lose more than 10 pounds, give birth, or have a pelvic infection or pelvic surgery.

## The Condom

A **condom** covers the erect penis and catches the ejaculate, thus preventing sperm from entering the woman (Figure 8-6). A new type of condom uses a spermicidal lubricant that kills most sperm on contact and is thus more effective than other brands. Although the theoretical effectiveness rate for condoms is 97 percent, the actual rate is only 80 to 85 percent. The condom can be torn during the manufacturing process or during its use. Careless removal can also decrease effectiveness. However, the major reason that condoms have such a low effectiveness rate is that couples don't use them each and every time they have sex (see "Health Spotlight: Condoms: a Guide for Men and Women" later in this chapter).

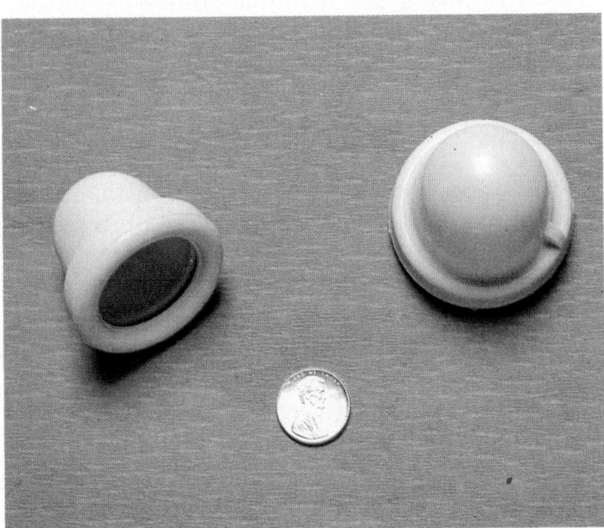

**FIGURE 8-5** Various sizes of cervical caps.

## The Contraceptive Sponge

The **contraceptive sponge** is a soft, disposable, polyurethane sponge, about 2 inches in diameter, that contains a spermicide (Figure 8-7). It is available, without a prescription, at pharmacies. The sponge, which has a concave surface that fits around the cervix, does not require individual fitting. Up to 24 hours before intercourse, a woman wets the sponge with water, compresses it, and inserts it by hand or with an applicator—a process that is not much more difficult than inserting a tampon. She leaves it in place for 6 hours after intercourse and removes it by pulling on an attached nylon loop. The sponge cannot be reused.

**condom** A sheath worn over the penis during sexual acts, to prevent conception and/or the transmission of disease.
**contraceptive sponge** A small polyurethane sponge that contains a spermicide and is designed to fit over the cervix to prevent conception.

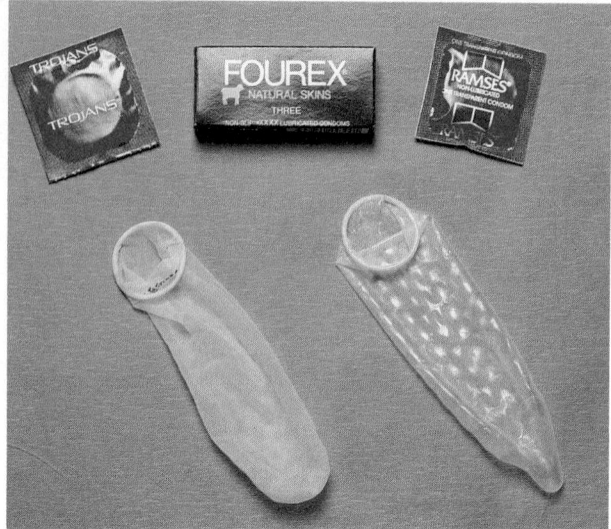


a

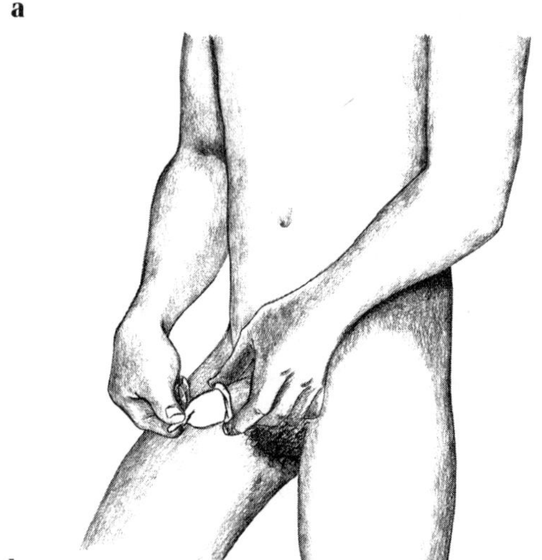

b

SOURCE: Hales, Dianne. *An Invitation to Health, Fourth Edition,* Benjamin/Cummings, 1989.

**FIGURE 8-6 (a)** Types of condoms. The one on the right is nipple-ended, which means that it has space to hold semen. The condom on the left is blunt-tipped (also referred to as a plain-end condom). The condoms shown here are unrolled. **(b)** Condoms should be put on the erect penis before it enters the vagina, to catch preejaculatory drops of semen. The end of a blunt-tipped condom needs to be twisted (see the illustration) as it is rolled onto the penis in order to leave space at the tip for semen. If inadequate space is left at the tip of the condom, semen can be forced out of the condom or down the sides, causing the condom to slip off. When withdrawing the penis from the vagina, hold the condom tight at the base of the penis (preferably while it is still erect) to prevent leakage.

The contraceptive sponge prevents conception by acting as a physical and chemical barrier to sperm and by absorbing and trapping semen. According to manufacturers, it is 85 percent effective (a 15 percent failure rate) if used properly. In preliminary studies its actual failure rate was 16.8 percent.

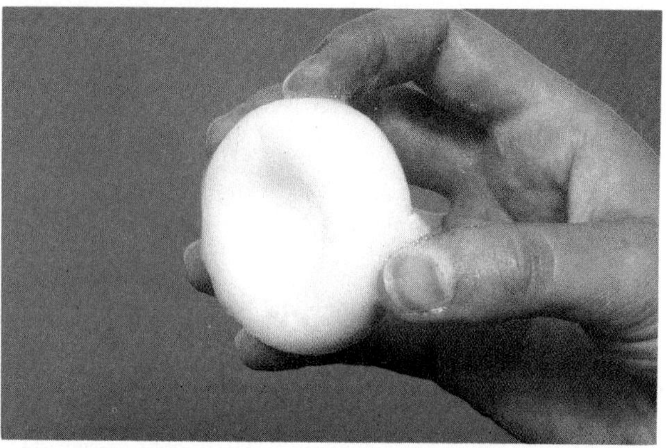

**FIGURE 8-7** The contraceptive sponge.

The most common side effects of the sponge are irritations, rashes, and allergic reactions to the spermicide. About 2 percent of users report an allergic reaction; another 2 to 3 percent have expelled the sponge, usually during a bowel movement. The sponge may also increase the risk of toxic shock syndrome (see Chapters 7 and 15), particularly if left in place for several days. The actual risk of toxic shock for those who use the sponge in accordance with the directions is unknown. (Manufacturers provide a toll-free number for women having difficulty with sponge removal.)

## The Intrauterine Device

Once a widely used form of birth control, the **intrauterine device (IUD)** is a small piece of molded plastic, with a string attached, that is inserted into the uterus through the cervix to interfere with implantation. The IUD became less common after most brands were removed from the market because of their serious complications. About 3 percent of American women using contraception currently rely on IUDs, according to manufacturers' estimates.

A physician or other trained health professional inserts an IUD during the woman's period, when the cervix is slightly softened and dilated, but it can be removed at any time during her cycle. A woman should check regularly, particularly after each menstrual period, for the string attached to the IUD, because she may not notice if the IUD is expelled.

**intrauterine device (IUD)** A device inserted into the uterus to prevent pregnancy.

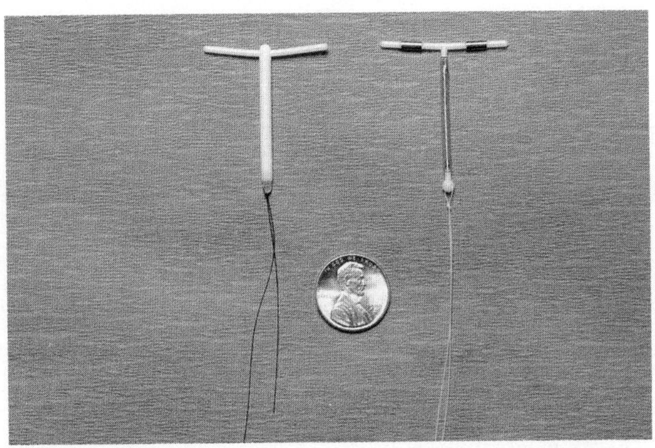

**FIGURE 8-8** The Progestasert intrauterine device and The Paragard IUD.

The two IUDs on the market are the Progestasert (Figure 8-8), a T-shaped device containing 38 mg of progesterone, which prevents implantation, and the Paragard (Figure 8-8), which contains copper and interferes with the growth of a fertilized egg by causing biochemical reactions with the uterine lining.

The IUD is highly effective, easy to reverse, and now causes fewer complications than the pill. However, because of the increased risk of pelvic inflammatory disease (PID), scarring, and infertility, many gynecologists recommend other forms of birth control for childless women who someday may want to start a family. Also, IUDs are not recommended for women with many sexual partners, because the IUD may increase the risk of sexually transmitted infection.

Almost 50 percent of all pregnancies beginning with an IUD in place end in miscarriage; if the IUD is removed early in the pregnancy, this risk drops to 30 percent. Because of the serious risks (including infection, premature delivery, and possibly a higher rate of birth defects) of continuing the pregnancy, doctors generally remove an IUD if pregnancy occurs and offer therapeutic abortion to the woman.

## Spermicides

### Vaginal Spermicides

Modern **vaginal spermicides** include chemical foams, creams, jellies, vaginal suppositories, and gels (Figure 8-9). Some creams and jellies are made for use with a diaphragm. Others can be used alone. Those containing nonoxynol-9 provide another benefit when used with condoms: they kill organisms that cause sexually transmitted diseases, such as chlamydia and HIV infection.

Several vaginal suppositories claim high effectiveness, but no American studies have confirmed these claims. In general, failure rates are as high as 10 to 25 percent. However, conscientious use of a spermicide in combination with another method of prevention, such as the condom, can provide very safe and very effective birth control.

The side effects of vaginal spermicides are minimal. For years scientists speculated about an increased risk of miscarriage and of birth defects in newborns of women who used spermicides near the time of conception. However, large-scale studies

**vaginal spermicide** A substance in the form of a cream, foam, jelly, or suppository that is inserted into the vagina to kill or neutralize sperm.

## HEALTH HEADLINE

### New Option for Birth Control

In December, 1990, the Food and Drug Administration approved the first new contraceptive method in decades. "Norplant" consists of six tiny silicone rubber tubes that release low doses of a synthetic form of the female hormone progesterone. Physicians using a needle and a local anesthetic, implant the tiny tubes directly beneath the skin of a woman's upper arm. The implants remain effective for up to five years. Fertility is restored soon after their removal.

Norplant has the highest effectiveness rate of any reversible form of contraception, including the birth control pill, and does not cause serious side-effects. Hormonal implants have been used by more than 500,000 women in 15 countries and have been tested by about 55,000 women in the U.S.

SOURCE: Hilt, Philips. "U.S. Approved 5-Year Implants to Curb Fertility," *New York Times*, December 11, 1990.

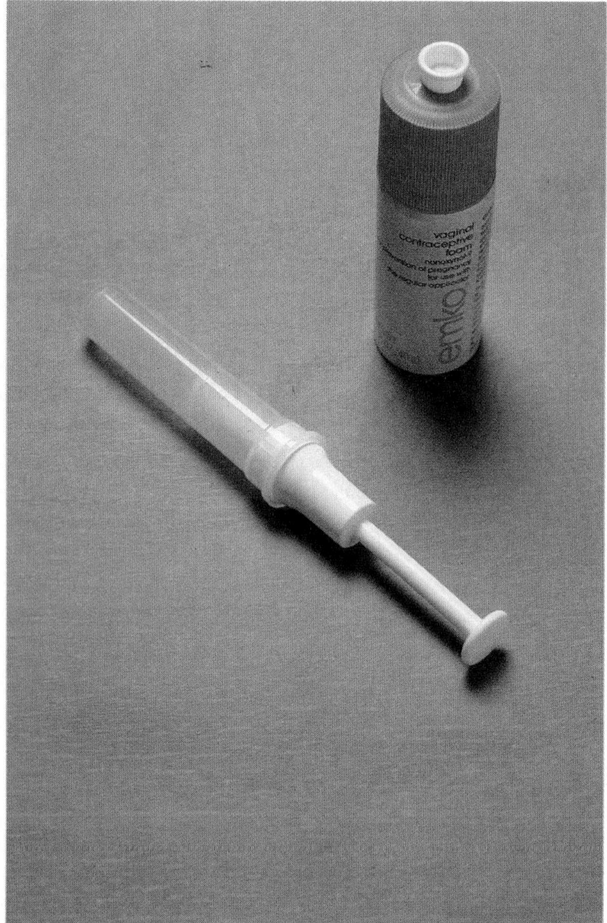


a

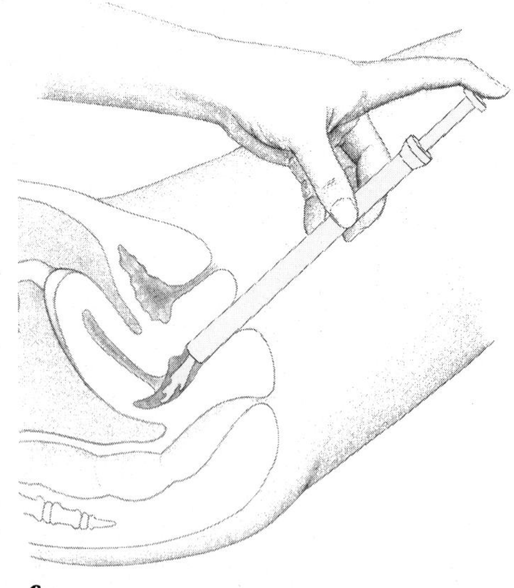

c

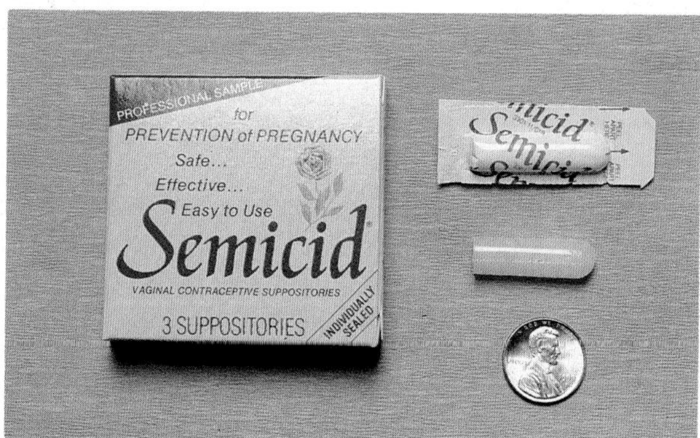


b

SOURCE (C): Hales, Dianne. *An Invitation to Health, Fourth Edition*, Benjamin/Cummings, 1989.

**FIGURE 8-9** Vaginal spermicides are available in pharmacies, without a prescription. **(a)** Foam and applicator. **(b)** How to use vaginal spermicides. The spermicide is inserted with an applicator no more than 1/2 hour before intercourse, and two applications are better than one. The spermicide is more likely to remain in place if the woman does not get up and walk around after inserting it. A fresh application is required if the woman has intercourse a second time. If she wants to douche, she should wait at least 8 hours to allow time for all the sperm to be killed. **(c)** The spermicidal suppository is inserted high into the vagina by hand.

showed that there is no relationship between spermicides and birth defects.[10,11] Some women and men are irritated by the chemicals used in spermicides, but often a change of brand solves this problem.

## Vaginal Contraceptive Film

Available from pharmacies, without a prescription, the 2-inch by 2-inch thin film known as the **vaginal contraceptive film (VCF)** is laced with spermicide (Figure 8-10). Once inserted into the vagina, it dissolves into a stay-in-place gel. A woman inserts the film by folding it and guiding it in with a finger so that it covers the cervix. The VCF can be inserted from a maximum of 90 minutes to a minimum of 5 minutes before intercourse.

A VCF is effective for up to 2 hours and need not be removed. A new film must be inserted if intercourse occurs again after 2 hours. Its theoretical effectiveness is similar to that of other forms of spermicide; paired with a condom, it is almost 100 percent. Advantages of the VCF include the fact that the film can be used by people allergic to foams and jellies and that it dissolves gradually and almost unnoticeably, unlike foams and jellies. Because the VCF contains nonoxynol-9, it also provides extra protection against sexually transmitted diseases.

**vaginal contraceptive film (VCF)** A small dissolvable sheet saturated with spermicide.

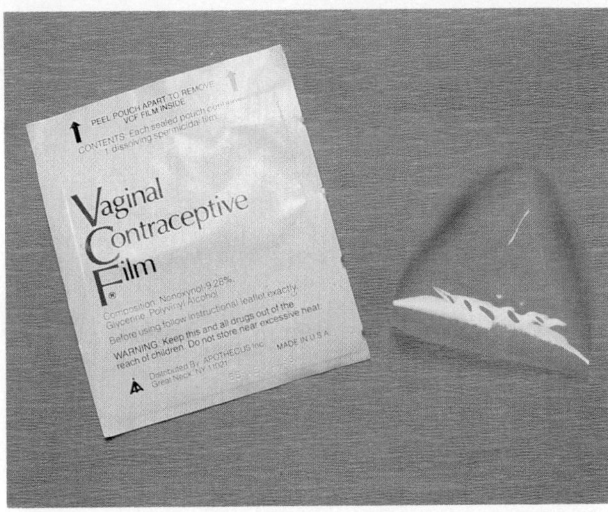


**FIGURE 8-10** Vaginal contraceptive film comes as a small sheet of dissolvable spermicide. Fold it before inserting it high into the vagina, where it will cover the cervix, thus preventing sperm from reaching the ovum.

STRATEGY FOR CHANGE

**Doubling Up for Safety**

There are certain times, including the following, when no one method of contraception may ensure protection from pregnancy:

- for the remainder of the cycle after forgetting more than one birth control pill or after forgetting just one pill in the first week of the cycle
- the first month after switching to a different brand of oral contraceptive
- when first learning to use a diaphragm

In such circumstances, the couple may choose not to have intercourse or to combine two methods of contraception.

## Sterilization

The most popular method of birth control among married couples in the United States is **sterilization** (surgery to end a person's reproductive capability). Each year an estimated 1 million men and women in the United States undergo sterilization surgery.

Sterilization has no effect on sex drive in either men or women. Many couples report that their sexual activity increases after sterilization, because they are free from the fear of pregnancy or the need to deal with contraceptives. And, the risks of sterilization are one-time risks.

Sterilization should be considered permanent and should be used only if both individuals are sure that they want no more children. Although sterilization does not usually create psychological or sexual problems, it can worsen existing problems, particularly marital ones. Couples should discuss sterilization, together and with a physician, to understand fully the possible physical and emotional consequences.

### Male Sterilization

A **vasectomy** is, literally, the cutting of the vas deferens, the tubes that carry sperm from the testicles into the urethra for ejaculation. A vasectomy, usually a 15- to 20-minute office procedure done under a local anesthetic, begins with two small incisions, one on each side of the scrotum. The doctor lifts up each tube, cuts it, and ties off the ends to block the flow of sperm (see Figure 8-11). Sperm continue to form but are broken down and absorbed by the body.

The man usually experiences some local pain, swelling, and discoloration for about a week. More serious complications, including the formation of a blood clot in the scrotum (which usually disappears without treatment), infection, and inflammatory reaction, occur in a small percentage of cases. The National Institute of Child Health and Human Development, in a 15-year follow-up of nearly 5,000 men, found that sterilization poses no increased danger of heart disease, even decades after the procedure.[12]

The pregnancy rate among the wives of vasectomized men is about 15 per 10,000 women per year; most result from failure to wait several weeks after

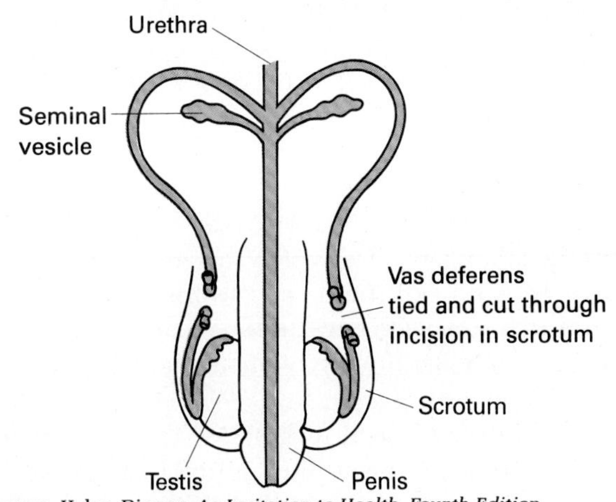


SOURCE: Hales, Dianne. *An Invitation to Health, Fourth Edition,* Benjamin/Cummings, 1989.

**FIGURE 8-11** Vasectomy

**sterilization** A surgical procedure that causes infertility.
**vasectomy** The cutting and tying shut of the vas deferens to stop the passage of sperm to the penis.

## HALES INDEX

Percentage of college students who know when a woman is most likely to conceive: Women: 40; men: 33

Percentage of American couples using contraception: 76

Percentage of women who use the pill: Unmarried: 48; married: 22

Percentage of married couples who've undergone sterilization for either spouse: 51

Percentage of Americans who think abortion should be legal under certain circumstances: 51

Percentage of abortion patients using birth control in the month they conceived: 50

Percentage of newborns whose mothers are 30 or older: 33

Percentage of women who drink at least once during pregnancy: 86

Percentage of women who smoke during pregnancy: 11

Percentage of teenage and unmarried women who do not receive adequate prenatal care: 33

Percentage of cesarean births: In 1960: 5; in 1990, 25

SOURCES: **1** "Conception Misconceptions," *Psychology Today,* April 1989. **2** Hilts, Philip. "Plan Offered to Stabilize Birth Rate in the 1990s," *New York Times,* February 24, 1990. **3, 4** Alan Guttmacher Institute, National Center for Health Statistics, 1990, interviews. **5** Salholz, Eloise. "The Future of Abortion," *Newsweek,* July 17, 1989. **6** Henshaw, Stanley and Jane Silverman. "The Characteristics and Prior Contraceptive Use of U.S. Abortion Patients," *Family Planning Perspectives,* July/August 1988. **7** Census Bureau, 1990. **8, 9** Rosenthal, Elisabeth. "When a Pregnant Woman Drinks," *New York Times,* February 4, 1990. **10** Lewin, Tamar. "Study Cites Deficiencies in Prenatal Care in U.S.," *New York Times,* November 2, 1989. **11** Brody, Jane. "Research Casts Doubts on Need for Many Cesarean Births as Their Rate Soars," *New York Times,* July 27, 1989.

the operation, until sperm stored in the vas deferens are ejaculated, before having unprotected coitus.

Sometimes men want to reverse their vasectomies, most commonly because they want to conceive children with a new spouse. Although anyone who chooses to have a vasectomy should consider it a permanent procedure, "vasovasotomy" (vasectomy reversal) is sometimes successful in restoring fertility. New microsurgical techniques have led to annual pregnancy rates for the wives of men undergoing vasovasotomies of about 40 to 60 percent, depending on many factors, including the doctor's expertise and the time elapsed since the vasectomy.

### Female Sterilization

Various sterilization procedures tie, cut, or otherwise seal the fallopian tubes, which each month normally carry an egg from the ovaries to the uterus. These operations may soon surpass the pill as the first contraceptive choice among women under, as well as over, age 30.

The two terms used to describe female sterilization are **tubal ligation** (the cutting or tying of the fallopian tubes) and **tubal occlusion** (the blocking of the tubes). The tubes may be cut or sealed with thread, a clamp, or a clip, or by coagulation (burning) to prevent passage of eggs from the ovaries. They can also be blocked with bands of silicone, which may be more effective than other devices.

The procedures used for sterilization are laparotomy, laparoscopy, and colpotomy. These techniques are discussed below.

**Laparotomy,** often done a few hours after childbirth, involves making an abdominal incision perhaps 2 inches long and cutting the tubes (see Figure 8-12). A laparotomy requires a 2- to 5-day hospital stay and up to several weeks of recovery. It leaves a scar and carries the same risks as all major surgical procedures: side effects of anesthesia, potential infection, and internal scars.

In a mini-laparotomy, an incision about an inch long is made just above the pubic hairline. Most often the tubes are tied and cut. They can also be sealed by electrical coagulation, which causes extensive damage to the tubes; there is also the risk of burns to nearby organs. The operation can be performed by a skilled physician in 10 to 30 minutes, usually under local anesthesia, and the woman can generally go home the same day. The failure (pregnancy) rate is only 1 per 1,000.

**tubal ligation** The suturing closed or tying shut of the fallopian tubes to prevent pregnancy.
**tubal occlusion** The blocking of the fallopian tubes to prevent pregnancy.
**laparotomy** A surgical sterilization procedure in which the fallopian tubes are ligated or occluded through an incision made in the abdomen.

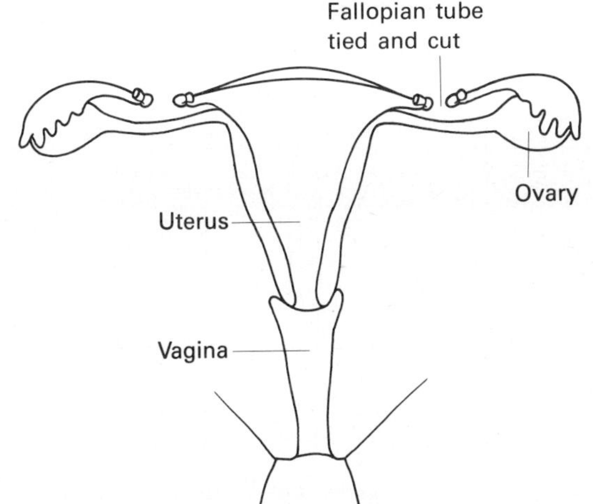


SOURCE: Hales, Dianne. *An Invitation to Health, Fourth Edition,* Benjamin/Cummings, 1989.

**FIGURE 8-12** Laparotomy

A **laparoscopy,** commonly called belly-button or band-aid surgery, can also be done on an outpatient basis and takes only 15 to 30 minutes. A lighted instrument inserted through a half-inch incision made in the lower rim of the navel (thus leaving no apparent scar) gives the doctor a view of the fallopian tubes.

First, the abdomen is inflated with carbon dioxide gas to allow an unobstructed view and to reduce the chances of injuring other organs. Using an operating laparoscope or a surgical tool, the doctor then cuts or coagulates the tubes. Most commonly the tubes are sealed by electrical coagulation. The possible complications are similar to those of mini-laparotomy, as is the failure rate.

A **colpotomy** provides access to the fallopian tubes through the vagina, behind the cervix. This leaves no external scar, but is somewhat more hazardous and less effective.

A **hysterectomy** (removal of the uterus) is a major surgical procedure that is too dangerous to be used as a method of sterilization, unless there are other medically urgent reasons for removing the uterus.

## Rhythm

The only form of contraception considered totally natural, and therefore permitted by the Roman Catholic Church, is the **rhythm method,** the abstinence from intercourse during the fertile phase of the menstrual cycle—that is, during the days just preceding and just following ovulation. Rhythm requires careful timing to avoid the possible meeting of a ripe egg and active sperm in the woman's fallopian tube.

The rhythm method involves no expense, no side effects, no need for prescriptions or fittings. On the days when the couple can have sex, there is nothing to insert, swallow, or check. However, some couples may find sexual abstinence for eight or nine days each month a problem. Conscientious planning and scheduling are essential.

The three methods commonly used to determine timing for the rhythm method are (1) calendar notation of date of ovulation, (2) daily check of body temperature, and (3) examination of cervical mucus.

### The Calendar Method

This approach involves the counting of days after menstruation begins to calculate the estimated day of ovulation. Sperm are capable of fertilizing an egg for approximately two days after ejaculation. This figure is only an average; sperm can live for as long as eight days. Because the egg is receptive to sperm on the day of ovulation and for one day afterward, coitus any time from two days before ovulation through the day following ovulation could result in conception.

In theory, a couple would have to abstain for only four days. However, because it is virtually impossible to calculate which four days are unsafe, a couple must abstain for a longer period to allow for miscalculations.

### The Basal Body Temperature Method

In this method the woman measures her **basal body temperature,** the body temperature upon waking in the morning, using a rectal thermometer, which is more precise than an oral one. She records her temperature on a chart like that shown in Figure 8-13.

The basal body temperature remains relatively constant from the beginning of the menstrual cycle to ovulation. After ovulation, basal temperature rises by more than 0.5 degree Fahrenheit. The woman knows that her safe period has begun when her temperature has been elevated for three consecutive days.

**laparoscopy** A surgical sterilization procedure in which the fallopian tubes are first observed with a laparoscope inserted through a small incision and then ligated or occluded.
**colpotomy** A surgical sterilization procedure in which the fallopian tubes are ligated or occluded through an incision made in the wall of the vagina.
**hysterectomy** The surgical removal of the uterus.
**rhythm method** A type of birth control in which sexual intercourse is avoided during those days of the menstrual cycle in which fertilization is most likely to occur.
**basal body temperature** The body temperature upon waking, before any activity.

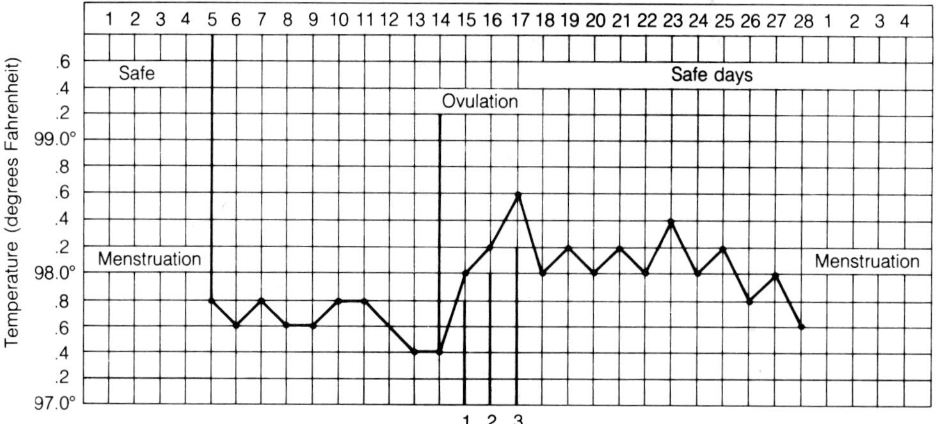


SOURCE: Hales, Dianne. *An Invitation to Health, Fourth Edition,* **Benjamin/Cummings**, 1989.

**FIGURE 8-13** Charting basal body temperature during a model menstrual cycle.

After eight to ten months, she should have a sense of her ovulatory pattern, in addition to knowing her daily readings.

### The Cervical Mucus Method

The mucus method, called **fertility awareness** by some and developed by Australian physicians Evelyn and John Billings, is based on observation of changes in the consistency of the mucus in the vagina. In the first days after menstruation, the vagina feels dry because of a decline in hormone production, indicating a safe period. Within a few days, estrogen levels rise, and the mucus begins to thin out and becomes less cloudy: the fertile period begins. At peak estrogen levels, the mucus is smooth, stretchable, and slippery (like a raw egg white), and very clear. Mucus with these characteristics is usually observed within 24 hours of ovulation and lasts one to two days, signaling maximum fertility. The mucus becomes sticky and cloudy again three days thereafter, and the second safe period begins. Most women using this method have to abstain from intercourse for about nine days out of each 28-day menstrual cycle.

A combination of the temperature and mucus methods may be 90 to 95 percent effective in preventing pregnancy. However, couples must be very conscientious to ensure that pregnancy does not occur. Because the length of the menstrual cycle varies among women, it may be hard to pinpoint by calendar alone the exact time of ovulation.

**fertility awareness** A way of determining a woman's fertile period by observing changes in the consistency of mucus in the vagina; also called the mucus method.

### Abstinence and "Outercourse"

Abstinence means abstaining from sexual activity or making love without having intercourse—and it is the only form of birth control that is completely safe. Some people refer to sexual activity not culminating in intercourse—kissing, hugging, massage, and oral-genital sex—as "outercourse."

Abstinence is 100 percent effective. "Outercourse" can prevent pregnancy, but couples must be careful to avoid direct vagina-to-penis contact, because sperm can swim up into the vagina and fallopian tubes to fertilize an egg. "Outercourse" also reduces the risk of contracting sexually transmitted diseases.

### Coitus Interruptus

Some couples use withdrawal of the penis before ejaculation (coitus interruptus) as a form of birth control. About half of the men who have tried coitus interruptus find it unsatisfactory. Some have difficulty realizing they're about to ejaculate or withdrawing quickly enough. Also, semen often leaks from the penis before ejaculation.

**STRATEGY FOR CHANGE**

**Choosing a Contraceptive**

You may choose different types of birth control at different stages of your life or switch contraceptives for various reasons (see Table 8-3). Here are some factors you and your partner should always consider and discuss:

- *Effectiveness.* Table 8-1 lists the failure rates for various contraceptives. Keep in mind that your own conscientiousness will play an important role. If you forget to take your daily pill or if you decide not to use a condom "just this once," you'll increase the odds of pregnancy by interfering with effective birth control.

- *Suitability.* If you don't have sex very often, a contraceptive with many risks, like an oral contraceptive, may be the wrong method for you. If you have many sexual partners and are at risk of contracting a sexual disease, a condom may provide protection against both pregnancy and infection, especially if used with a diaphragm or cervical cap.
- *Side effects.* Some complications related to contraceptives are serious threats to health. Be sure to ask questions and gather as much information as possible about what to expect.
- *Safety.* The risks of certain contraceptives, such as the pill, may be too great to allow their use if, for example, you have high blood pressure. Be honest in describing your medical history to your physician.
- *Future fertility.* Some women do not return to regular menstrual cycles for six months to a year after discontinuing oral contraceptives. These issues may or may not be important to you now, but you should try to look ahead.
- *Cost.* The only free contraceptive methods are abstinence and rhythm. If you're on a tight budget, you might consider the relative costs of a year's prescription of pills compared to a year's supply of spermicidal foam or jelly, or condoms.
- *Protection against sexually transmitted diseases.* The best contraceptive protection against HIV infection and other sexually transmitted diseases is a condom combined with a diaphragm or cervical cap, used with spermicides containing nonoxynol-9.

### After-Intercourse Methods

The so-called morning-after pill does not prevent conception; it interferes with the implantation of a fertilized egg. The pill currently used is ethinyl estradiol or conjugated equine estrogens. Morning-after pills are not recommended for use except in cases of rape, incest, or complicated high-risk pregnancy factors. If menstruation doesn't follow use of the morning-after pill, a **dilation and curettage (D and C)** procedure or an aspiration (suctioning) is performed to remove the contents of the uterus.

**Menstrual extraction**—considered a form of abortion by some—involves removing the contents of the uterus by suction with a device that does not require cervical dilation or anesthesia. Some women perform this procedure at home if their menstrual periods are a few days late. However, because the risk of infection is high, such home treatment is not recommended.

## ABORTION

Induced **abortion,** the purposeful termination of a pregnancy, should not be considered a form of contraception, but an alternative to the delivery of an unwanted child. It is too risky, too expensive, and too complex a procedure to be viewed as anything other than an emergency backup if contraception fails. More than 1.6 million abortions are performed in the United States every year. Three of every 100 American women between the ages of 15 and 44 choose to end a pregnancy.

**dilation and curettage (D and C)** A procedure in which the cervix is dilated and the contents of the uterus are removed with a scraping instrument (a curette).

**menstrual extraction** The removal of uterine contents, usually performed to hasten the menstrual process or to eliminate possible pregnancy.

**abortion** A procedure to remove uterine contents after pregnancy has occurred.

**TABLE 8-3** Why Women Switch Birth Control Methods

| | Method Abandoned | | |
|---|---|---|---|
| REASON | PILL/IUD | CONDOM/DIAPHRAGM SPERMICIDES | RHYTHM/ WITHDRAWAL |
| Side effects | 58% | 8% | 0% |
| Health concerns | 18 | 5 | 2 |
| Effectiveness | 10 | 48 | 86 |
| Inconvenience | 4 | 25 | 4 |
| Cost | 2 | 1 | 0 |
| Partner's objection | 2 | 6 | 7 |

SOURCE: Alan Guttmacher Institute.

SELF-SURVEY

## Which Contraceptive Method Is Best for You?

***Directions***

Check yes or no for each statement as it applies to you and, if appropriate, your partner:

| | Yes | No |
|---|---|---|
| 1. You have a set routine. | ____ | ____ |
| 2. You prefer a method with little or no bother. | ____ | ____ |
| 3. You have a good memory. | ____ | ____ |
| 4. You are forgetful. | ____ | ____ |
| 5. You have heavy, crampy periods. | ____ | ____ |
| 6. You are a risk taker. | ____ | ____ |
| 7. You have sexual intercourse frequently. | ____ | ____ |
| 8. You need a birth control method right away. | ____ | ____ |
| 9. You are comfortable with your own sexuality. | ____ | ____ |
| 10. You dislike doctors and pelvic exams. | ____ | ____ |
| 11. You are concerned about sexually transmitted diseases. | ____ | ____ |
| 12. You have a cooperative partner. | ____ | ____ |
| 13. You have premature ejaculations. | ____ | ____ |
| 14. You have patience and a sense of humor. | ____ | ____ |
| 15. You have sexual intercourse infrequently. | ____ | ____ |
| 16. You have a lot of privacy. | ____ | ____ |
| 17. You are a nursing mother. | ____ | ____ |

***Scoring***

Recommendations here are based on yes answers to the following numbered items:

- 1, 2, 3, 5, 7—The birth control pill might be a good choice for you.
- 4, 8, 10, 12, and 14—Contraceptive foams might be most appropriate for you.
- 6, 8, 9, 11, and 13—Condoms might be the best choice for you.
- 9, 15, 16, and 17—Consider using a diaphragm with cream or jelly.

If your responses indicated that there is more than one appropriate method of birth control for you, remember you can use various methods of birth control throughout your life. If your responses do not suggest any of these birth-control methods, you might want to consider abstinence or a natural family planning method. Though this score is not absolute, it should assist you and your physician in making the best choice for you.

SOURCE: Adapted from Cox, Doyle, Kammerman, and Valois, *Wellness R.S.V.P.*, Benjamin/Cummings, 1981.

## The Abortion Pill

More than 50,000 women, mostly in France, have taken a hormonal compound called RU 486, which ends a pregnancy if used in the first five weeks after conception. RU 486 blocks progesterone, the hormone that prepares the uterine lining for pregnancy. If a woman takes the pill, the lining breaks down and is expelled along with the fertilized egg. Women have compared the discomfort to severe menstrual cramps. According to a 1990 report in *The New England Journal of Medicine*, the drug effectively induced abortion in 96 percent of 2,115 French women who took RU 486 within 49 days of their last menstrual period.[13]

Considered safer than surgical abortion, RU 486 has been opposed by abortion foes but may become available in the U.S. within a few years. It is undergoing testing as a contraceptive that would be taken after ovulation, in the second half of a woman's menstrual cycle, to induce menstruation and as a treatment for endometriosis, cancer, and other disorders.

## Abortion Methods

Medically, first-trimester abortion is less risky than childbirth. However, the likelihood of complications increases when abortions are performed in the second trimester (that is, the second three-month period) of pregnancy rather than in the first trimester.

**Suction curettage,** developed in China, involves gradual dilation (opening) of the cervix, often by inserting into the cervix one or more sticks of laminaria (a sterilized seaweed that absorbs moisture and expands, thus gradually stretching the cervix). Some women feel pressure or cramping with the laminaria in place. Occasionally the laminaria itself starts to bring on a miscarriage.

At the time of abortion, the laminaria are removed; dilators are used to enlarge the cervical opening farther, if needed. The doctor inserts a suction tip into the cervix, and the uterine contents are drawn out into the vacuum system (see Figure 8-14). A curette (a surgical instrument shaped like a spoon) is used to check for complete removal. With these methods, the risk is low. Major complications, such as perforation of the uterus, occur in fewer than 1 in 100 cases. About 90 percent of the abortions performed in this country are by this technique.

Most medical centers perform suction curettage until week 12 of the pregnancy, when the risks to the woman increase. Between weeks 13 and 15, doctors generally use a technique called **dilation and evacuation (D and E),** in which they open the cervix and use medical instruments to remove the fetus from the uterus. D and E procedures are performed under local or general anesthesia, and account for about 6 percent of U.S. abortions.

To induce abortion from week 16 to week 20, prostaglandins, natural substances found in most body tissues, are administered as vaginal suppositories or injected into the amniotic sac by inserting a needle through the abdominal wall. They induce uterine contractions, and the fetus and placenta are expelled within 24 hours.

A variety of other methods are used for second-trimester abortions. Included among these are injections of saline or urea solutions into the amniotic sac. They kill the fetus and trigger contractions that expel the fetus and placenta. Sometimes vaginal suppositories or drugs that help the uterus contract are used. Complications from abortion techniques that induce labor include nausea, vomiting, diarrhea, tearing of the cervix, excessive bleeding, and possible shock and death.

A **hysterotomy** involves surgically opening the uterus and removing the fetus. It is generally done

**suction curettage** The removal of the contents of the uterus by means of suction and scraping.
**dilation and evacuation (D and E)** The removal of the contents of the uterus through use of medical instruments.
**hysterotomy** The surgical opening of the uterus.

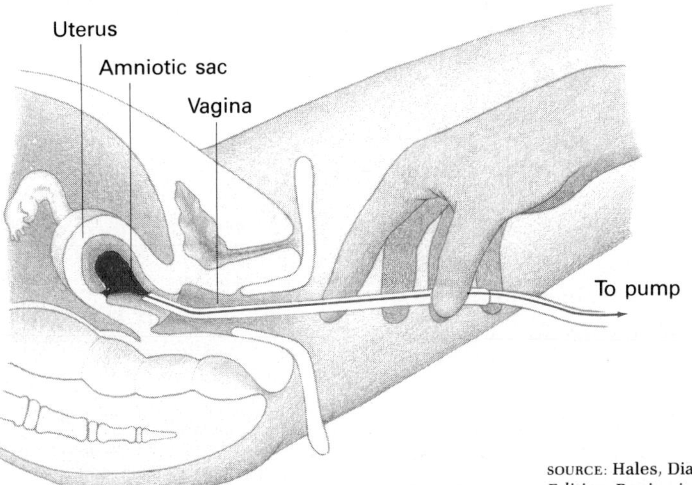


SOURCE: Hales, Dianne. *An Invitation to Health, Fourth Edition,* Benjamin/Cummings, 1989.

**FIGURE 8-14** Suction curettage. The contents of the uterus are extracted through the cervix with a vacuum apparatus.

HEALTH SPOTLIGHT

## Condoms: A Guide for Men and Women

Every sexually active adult should know about condoms, which may well become basic "survival gear" for the twenty-first century.

### What Condoms Can Do

- *Prevent HIV infection.* According to laboratory studies, the tiny human immunodeficiency virus (HIV), which causes AIDS, cannot penetrate a condom made of latex. Condoms are most effective in combination with spermicides containing nonoxynol-9.
- *Protect against other sexual diseases.* Among the sexually transmitted diseases for which condoms can lower risk are syphilis, gonorrhea, chlamydia, and herpes. Condoms appear to lessen a woman's risk of pelvic inflammatory disease; prevent transmission of the human papilloma virus, which has been implicated in genital warts and cervical cancer; and may protect against some parasites that cause urinary tract and genital infections.
- *Prevent pregnancy.* Their theoretical effectiveness is about 90 percent; combined with a spermicide, it's higher.

### What Condoms Can't Do

Condoms cannot provide 100 percent protection against pregnancy or sexually transmitted diseases, including HIV infection. For anyone not in a faithful, long-standing, monogamous relationship—heterosexual or homosexual—condoms can make sex safer, but not absolutely safe. Condoms fail, not only because couples don't use them correctly, but also because they aren't always manufactured properly.

If 100 couples use condoms correctly and consistently for a year, two of the women will still become pregnant within that time—in theory. In real life, ten women are likely to get pregnant. The failure rate for protection from HIV infection may well be higher than that for pregnancy.

### A User's Guide

- Buy only American-made latex condoms, not natural sheepskin, which may leak. Most physicians recommend prelubricated, spermicide-treated condoms.
- Keep condoms cool and dry.
- Before using a condom, make sure it is soft and pliable. If it is yellow or sticky, throw it out.
- Don't check for leaks by blowing up a condom before using it. You may weaken or tear it.
- The condom should be put on at the beginning of sexual activity, before genital contact occurs. There should be a little space at the top of the condom to catch the semen. Wait until just before intercourse to apply spermicide. Choose a brand containing nonoxynol-9. Any vaginal lubricant should be water-based. Petroleum-based creams or jellies, such as Vaseline, can deteriorate the latex.
- After ejaculation, the condom should be held firmly against the penis so it doesn't slip off or leak during withdrawal. Couples engaging in anal intercourse should use a lubricant as well as a condom, but should never assume that a condom will protect them from HIV infection or other sexually transmitted diseases.

SOURCES: Centers for Disease Control. "Condoms for Prevention of Sexually Transmitted Diseases," *Journal of the American Medical Association*, vol. 259, no. 13, April 1, 1988. Kaplan, Helen Singer. *The Real Truth About Women and AIDS*. New York: Simon and Schuster, 1987. Rinzler, Carol Ann. "The Return of the Condom," *American Health*, July 1987. "Rubber Sales Expanding," *Psychology Today*, October 1988.

from week 16 to week 24 of the pregnancy, primarily in emergency situations when the woman's life is in danger or when other methods of abortion are considered too risky.

Late-pregnancy abortions increase the risk of spontaneous abortion or premature labor in subsequent pregnancies and should be avoided. Table 8-4 summarizes medical techniques for abortion, when they can be used, where they're performed, and their possible side effects.

### The Politics of Abortion

Abortion is one of the most controversial political, religious, and ethical issues of our time. In the United States, abortions were illegal in some states until 1973, when the U.S. Supreme Court, following a 1970 ruling on the case of *Roe* versus *Wade* by the New York Supreme Court, said that an abortion in the first three months (the first trimester) of pregnancy is a decision between a woman and her physician and is protected by privacy laws. The court ruled that, during the second trimester, abortion could be performed on the basis of health risks; during the final trimester, it could be performed only for the sake of the mother's health.

In 1989 the Supreme Court narrowed the interpretation of *Roe* versus *Wade* by upholding a law that sharply restricted publicly funded abortions and required doctors to test if a fetus could survive at 20 weeks of pregnancy. The court also paved the way for states to enact laws limiting access to abortion.

The abortion issue continues to stir passionate emotion. Both advocates and opponents have marched, picketed, and protested to spread their views. In some cases, abortion foes have bombed, burned, or vandalized abortion facilities.

## PREGNANCY

The early 1990s are seeing a record number of births—about 4 million a year—as post–World War II "baby boomers" who'd delayed having babies finally start their families. The Census Bureau expects the birth rate to decline somewhat—to around 3.8 million births—by the late 1990s.[14] The average age of mothers has risen, but about 70 percent of babies are still born to women in their twenties. Today's mothers are averaging slightly fewer than two children each.

**TABLE 8-4** Abortion Methods

| GESTATIONAL AGE | ABORTION METHOD | POSSIBLE SIDE EFFECTS | FACILITY |
|---|---|---|---|
| Week 5–7 | Menstrual extraction | Allergic reactions, mild cramping, minimal vaginal bleeding, or incomplete removal of tissue | Physician's office or family-planning clinic recommended |
| Week 7–12 | Vacuum aspiration (suction curettage) | Mild cramping and minimal bleeding | Physician's office, family-planning clinic, or hospital |
| | Dilation and curettage (D and C) | Uterine or cervical trauma, incomplete evacuation, or infection | Physician's office, family-planning clinic, or hospital |
| Week 13–15 | Dilation and evacuation (D and E) | Uterine or cervical trauma, infection, reaction to general anesthetic | Hospital |
| | Prostaglandin vaginal suppository | Vomiting, diarrhea, or temperature elevation | Hospital |
| Week 16–24 | Prostaglandin injection | Headache, vomiting, or diarrhea; retained placenta with hemorrhage; allergic reaction to drug; bronchial constriction | Hospital |
| | Hysterotomy | Future pregnancies may require repeat cesarean delivery | Hospital |
| After week 24 | Abortion inadvisable | | |

But not every couple is opting for parenthood. A third of all married couples say they plan not to have children; a generation ago, only a fifth of all married couples were childless—often not by choice. Childless couples are at least as likely—if not more likely—to be content with their marriages as couples with children. In various studies, the happiest spouses are those who have either no children or no more children than they want. Those who conceive accidentally are the most likely to feel regrets.

Of course, you don't have to be part of a couple to want or to conceive a child. The number of never-married women who are becoming single parents has risen dramatically. They want children—with or without an ongoing relationship with a man.

## Your Genetic Legacy

Every human cell (with the exception of the gametes—the egg and the sperm) contains twenty-three pairs of **chromosomes** (the rodlike structures within the nucleus of a cell on which genes are located), forty-six chromosomes in all (Figure 8-15). Each parent contributes one set of twenty-three chromosomes (one member of each pair).

**Genes,** a cell's instructions for life, determine a person's sex, hair, eye color, and many other traits. They are made up of **deoxyribonucleic acid,** or **DNA.** Each cell possesses two genes, occupying the same position on each chromosome of the pair, for each inherited characteristic.

The two genes for a given characteristic may express themselves in the same way or differently. If the actions of the two genes are alike, the person is said to be **homozygous** for that trait. If the actions are different, the person is called **heterozygous.** Of a heterozygous pair of genes, one will be dominant over the other, and the trait it determines will appear in the individual. The other gene for the trait is called recessive (see Figure 8-16). A homozygous pair of genes may be made up of two dominant or two recessive genes. For example, brown eyes are a **dominant trait;** blue eyes are a **recessive trait.** If one parent contributes a gene for brown eyes and the other a gene for blue (a heterozygous pairing), the child's eyes will be brown. If both contribute a brown-eye gene (a homozygous dominant pairing), the eyes will again

**chromosomes** The structures in the cell nucleus that carry the heredity factors (genes); composed of DNA and protein.
**genes** The biologic units of heredity located on the chromosomes; transmitters of hereditary information.
**deoxyribonucleic acid (DNA)** A complex protein found in all living cells; carries the organism's genetic information.
**homozygous** Possessing identical genes for a given inherited trait.
**heterozygous** Possessing different genes for a given inherited trait.
**dominant trait** A specific trait, determined by a gene on a chromosome, that will prevail over another, recessive trait.
**recessive trait** A specific trait, determined by a gene on a chromosome, that will not occur in offspring unless matched at fertilization by an identical gene on the pairing chromosome.

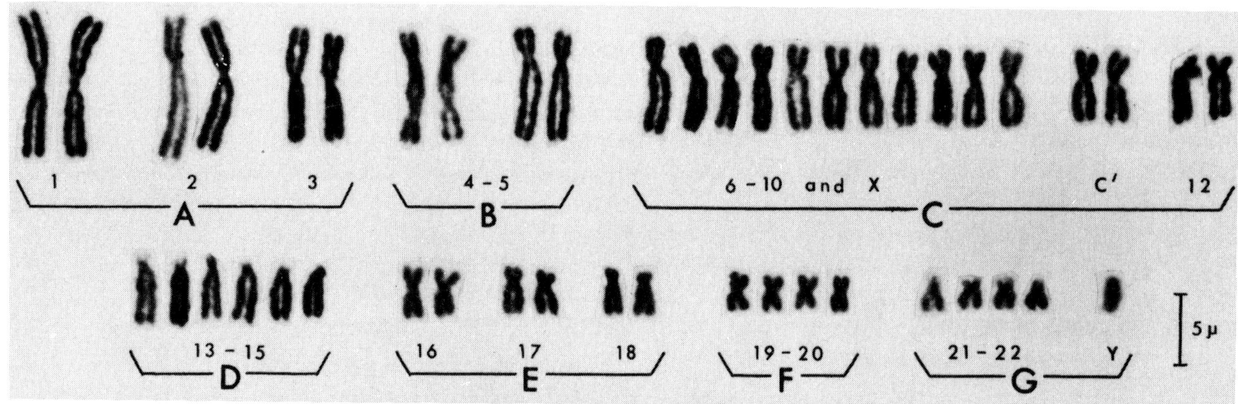


SOURCE: Hales, Dianne. *An Invitation to Health, Fourth Edition,* Benjamin/Cummings, 1989.

**FIGURE 8-15** The twenty-three pairs of human chromosomes. The chromosomes are photographed through a microscope during cell division. (Note that each chromosome has already divided.) The photograph is then cut up and the chromosomes arranged by size in an orderly pattern. Without more elaborate techniques than have been used here, a number of chromosomes of similar appearance cannot be distinguished; so they are arranged in groups. The X chromosome is a member of the C group. One of the smallest chromosomes is the Y chromosome in group G, which indicates that this individual is a male.

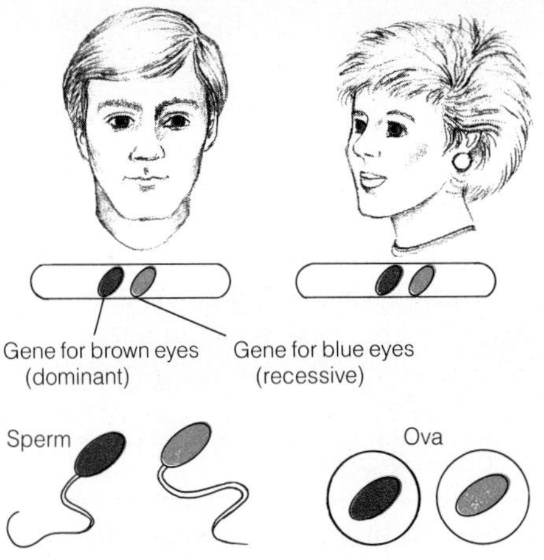


One sperm combines with one ovum to produce a new individual. The child receives one chromosome from each pair (23 in all) from each parent. So the children of this couple can carry the following combinations of eye color genes and have the following eye colors.

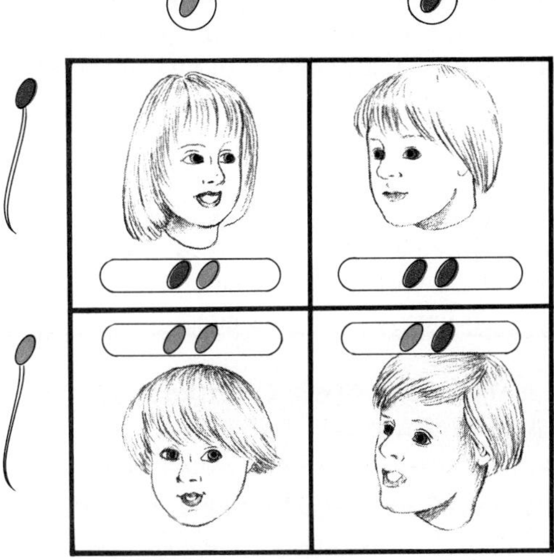

Thus we expect one-fourth of the children of this couple to have blue eyes. We expect one-half of their children to be brown-eyed carriers of a gene for blue eyes.

SOURCE: Hales, Dianne. *An Invitation to Health, Fourth Edition*, Benjamin/Cummings, 1989.

**FIGURE 8-16** Recessive and dominant genes: how two heterozygous brown-eyed parents can have both brown-eyed and blue-eyed children.

be brown. However, if both contribute a blue-eye gene (a homozygous recessive pairing), the eyes will be blue.

### How Sex Is Determined

Chromosomes 1 through 22 are similar in size, shape, and gene makeup to any of the other sets. The sex-determining chromosomes, pair 23, are both X chromosomes in the female. In the male, there is one X and one Y chromosome.

When the female produces an egg, it gets one of the two X chromosomes. A sperm gets either an X or a Y chromosome. When an X-bearing egg combines with an X-bearing sperm, the resulting XX zygote (fertilized egg cell) develops into a female. When an X-bearing egg combines with a Y-bearing sperm, the resulting XY zygote develops into a male. But the process of actually becoming male or female is a long and complex one.

In the beginning, all human embryos are alike, with all-purpose gonads—structures that contain future reproductive cells—that can become either testes or ovaries and with growth buds for male or female genitals. Without a Y chromosome, an embryo remains neuter for its first twelve weeks of life; the go-

## HEALTH HEADLINE

### The Psychological Impact of Abortion

**Legal abortion early in pregnancy is not hazardous to a woman's mental health, according to an American Psychological Association panel that reviewed studies of hundreds of women of different ages and social and economic groups. All the studies reached the same conclusion: that severe negative mental responses after abortion are rare.**

**After first-trimester abortions, women are most likely to report feelings of relief and happiness. Only 17 percent said they felt any guilt—the most common negative emotion. However, women who aborted pregnancies that they'd wanted, who lacked support from partners or parents, or who were less sure of their decision beforehand were more likely to have negative emotional responses.**

**According to the panel, most women do not find the decision to have an abortion difficult, unless they choose abortion later in pregnancy. In one study, only 12 percent of 100 first-trimester patients found it difficult to decide on abortion, compared to 51 percent of 200 second-trimester patients.**

SOURCE: Adler, Nancy et al. "Psychological Responses After Abortion," *Science*, April 6, 1990.

nads then develop into ovaries. For an embryo to become male, the Y chromosome must signal the gonads about six weeks after conception and instruct them to become testes.

From this point on, the sex hormones produced by the gonads, not the chromosomes, play the crucial role in the making of a male or female. Testosterone, the primary male hormone, virilizes an embryo and sculpts male genitals. Estrogen, the dominant female hormone, directs the development of a girl's reproductive system. Because of its mother's estrogen, an embryo—even with XY chromosomes—will develop into a girl if it produces no hormones of its own or if it fails to respond to testosterone.

## The Beginning of Life

At the midpoint of a menstrual cycle, a woman's ovary releases one of its stored eggs. When one sperm penetrates the cell membrane of the ovum (see Figure 8-17), the fertilized egg multiplies into a cluster of cells (see Figure 8-18) and floats down the fallopian tube to embed itself in the endometrium, the lining of the wall of the uterus.

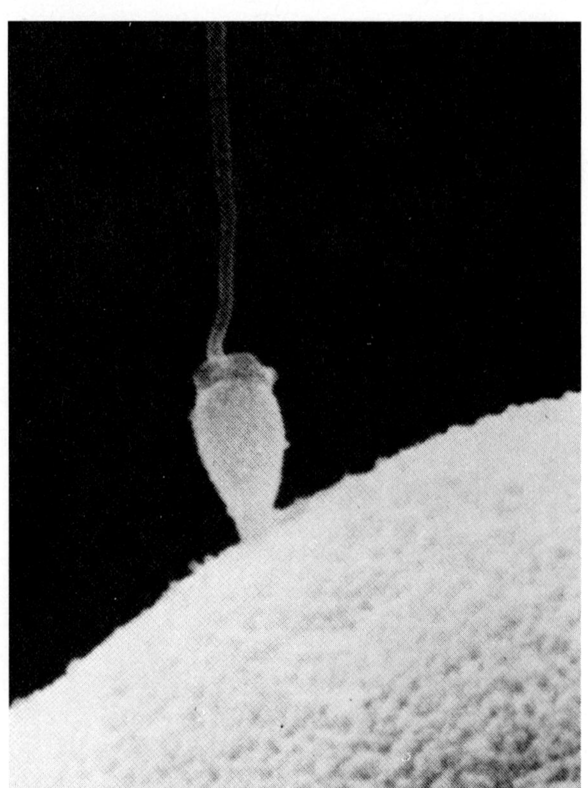

SOURCE: Bloom, W. and D. W. Fawcett. *A Textbook of Histology,* Tenth Edition. Philadelphia: Saunders, 1975.

**FIGURE 8-17** A sperm about to penetrate an ovum.

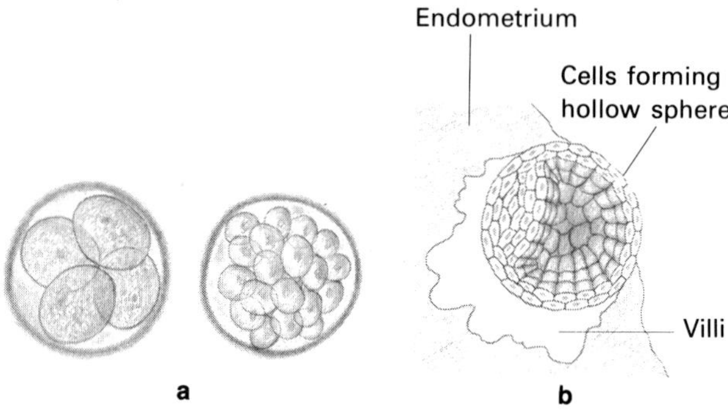


SOURCE: Hales, Dianne. *An Invitation to Health, Fourth Edition,* Benjamin/Cummings, 1989.

**FIGURE 8-18 (a)** Division of the zygote into many cells. **(b)** Implantation.

Small fingerlike projections, called **villi,** burrow into the uterine blood supply. These villi produce a chemical messenger that signals the ovaries to continue their output of progesterone. This messenger substance, called **human chorionic gonadotropin (HCG),** appears in a woman's body only during pregnancy. The uterus becomes slightly larger; the cervix, softer and blueish because of the increased blood flow to it. Progesterone and estrogen trigger changes in the milk glands and ducts in the breasts, which increase in size and feel somewhat tender. The pressure of the growing uterus against the bladder causes a more frequent need to urinate.

### How a Woman's Body Changes During Pregnancy

Pregnancy transforms how a woman looks and feels. The most common physiological changes are the following:

*First Trimester:*

- increased urination because of hormonal changes and the pressure of the enlarging uterus on the bladder
- enlarged breasts as milk glands develop
- darkening of the nipples and the area around them
- nausea or vomiting, particularly in the morning
- fatigue
- increased vaginal secretions
- pinching of the sciatic nerve, which runs from the buttocks down through the back of the legs, as the pelvic bones widen and begin to separate
- irregular bowel movements

**villi** Short vascular projections attaching the fetus to the uterine wall.
**human chorionic gonadotropin (HCG)** A hormone produced by the chorionic villi.

*Second Trimester:*

- thickening of the waist as the uterus grows
- weight gain
- increase in total blood volume
- slight increase in size and change in position of the heart
- darkening of the pigment around the nipple and from the navel to the pubic region
- darkening of face
- increased salivation and perspiration
- secretion of colostrum from the breasts (Mothers planning to breast-feed should massage their nipples regularly.)
- indigestion, constipation, and hemorrhoids
- varicose veins

*Third Trimester:*

- increased urination because of pressure from the uterus
- tightening of the uterine muscles (called Braxton-Hicks contractions)
- breathlessness because of increased pressure by the uterus on the lungs and diaphragm
- heartburn and indigestion
- trouble sleeping because of the baby's movements or the need to urinate
- "dropping" of the baby's head into the pelvis about 2 to 4 weeks before birth
- navel pushed out

### How a Baby Grows

Silently and invisibly, a fertilized egg develops into a human being. When the cluster of cells reaches the uterus, it is still smaller than the head of a pin. Once nestled into the spongy uterine lining, it becomes an **embryo.** The embryo takes on an elongated shape, rounded at one end. A sac (the **amnion**) envelops it. As water and other small molecules cross the amniotic membrane, the embryo floats freely in the absorbed fluid, cushioned from shocks and bumps.

A primitive placenta forms. The **placenta** is an organ that will supply the growing baby with food, water, and nutrients from the maternal bloodstream and carry waste back to the mother's body for disposal.

Figure 8-19 and the remaining text in this section describe the major steps that occur during the nine months a baby spends in the womb.

**First Month:** The embryo grows to about 1/4 inch in length and 1/7 ounce in weight. Foundations are formed for the nervous system, genital-urinary system, skin, bones, and lungs. Arm and leg buds begin to form. Rudiments of the eyes, ears, and nose appear. The head is disproportionately large because of brain development.

**Second Month:** The embryo's length is now 1.2 inches and the weight approximately 1/6 ounce. Fingers and toes are distinct. The circulatory system is complete. In medical terms, the embryo becomes a **fetus** around the eighth week.

**Third Month:** The fetus's length is 2 inches; fetal weight is 1/2 ounce. The fetus is clearly male or female. Its kidneys excrete urine. The heart beats. The nose and palate take shape.

**Fourth Month:** The fetus's length is 4 inches; fetal weight is 2 ounces. The mother can feel fetal movements. Heart sounds can be heard through a special stethoscope.

**Fifth Month:** The fetus's length is 8 inches; fetal weight 1.4 pounds. The skin appears wrinkled. Eyebrows and fingernails develop.

**Sixth Month:** The fetus's length is 11.5 inches; fetal weight is 2.1 pounds. The skin is red. If born, the infant will cry and breathe, but rarely survives.

**Seventh Month:** The fetus's length is 14 to 15 inches; fetal weight is 3 pounds. The fetus can survive outside the womb. Eyelids open. Fingerprints are set. The fetus moves vigorously.

**Eighth Month:** The fetus's length is 15 to 17 inches; fetal weight is 4 to 5 pounds. The face and body have a loose, wrinkled appearance.

**Ninth Month:** The fetus's length is 16 to 19 inches; fetal weight is 6 to 7 pounds. The skin is smooth. The bones of the skull have hardened. The baby is ready to survive on its own outside the womb.

### Emotional Aspects of Pregnancy

Expecting a child can change the way a man and a woman look at themselves, each other, and the world.

---

**embryo** An organism in its early stage of development; in humans, the embryonic period lasts from about the second to the eighth week of pregnancy.
**amnion** The innermost membrane of the sac enclosing the embryo or fetus.
**placenta** An organ that develops after implantation and to which the embryo attaches, via the umbilical cord, for nourishment and waste removal.
**fetus** The child in the uterus from the eighth week until birth.

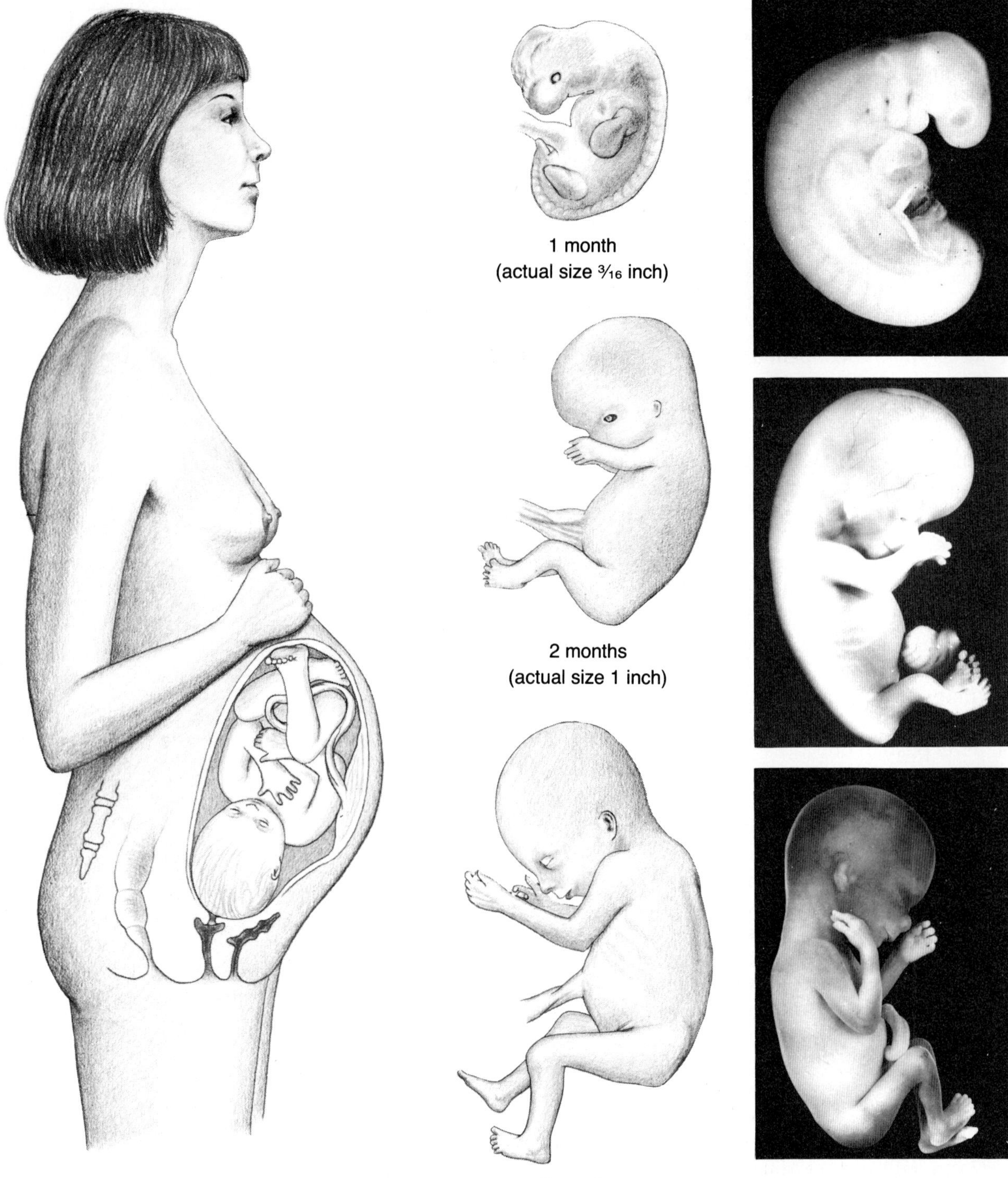


**Figure 12-7** Growth of a fetus.

SOURCE: Hales, Dianne. *An Invitation to Health, Fourth Edition,* Benjamin/Cummings, 1989.

**FIGURE 8-19** Growth of a fetus.

Almost all would-be parents worry about their ability to care for a helpless newborn. By talking openly about their feelings and fears, they can strengthen the bonds between them so they can work together as parents as well as partners.

**The Mother's Experience** The physiological changes of pregnancy can affect a woman's mood. In early pregnancy, she may feel weepy, irritable, or emotional. As the pregnancy continues, she may become calmer and more energetic. Despite the inevitable concerns for their unborn children and their changing bodies, many women feel that pregnancy is one of the most exciting and fulfilling times of their lives.

**The Father's Perspective** Like their partners, men feel a range of intense emotions about the prospect of having a child: pride, anxiety, hope, fears for their unseen child and for the woman they love. Although many men want to be as supportive as possible, they may think they have to be strong and calm and pull away from their wives. What's best for both partners is honest communication about what they're feeling—the bad as well as the good—and reassurance of each other's love. The more involved fathers become in preparing for birth, the closer they feel to their partners and babies afterward.

## Prenatal Care: Taking Care of Yourself—and Your Baby

A pregnant woman has to take good care of herself to provide good care for her unborn child. That means regular medical checkups. A woman should have her first prenatal visit as soon as she discovers she is pregnant. Most women see their obstetricians or nurse-midwives once a month until the twenty-eighth week of pregnancy. As they enter the last trimester, they see their doctors every other week until the thirty-sixth week, then every week until labor begins.

### Nutrition

Women who take a simple daily multivitamin before conception can cut in half the risk that their children will suffer neural tube defects, including spina bifida, which stem from faulty formation of the spinal column, according to the federal Centers for Disease Control.[15]

Throughout pregnancy, a well-balanced diet is critical for a mother and her baby before and at birth. The National Research Council recommends a weight gain of 24 to 27 pounds for a pregnant woman (see Figure 8-20). If the woman gains much less, the risk to the infant is high.

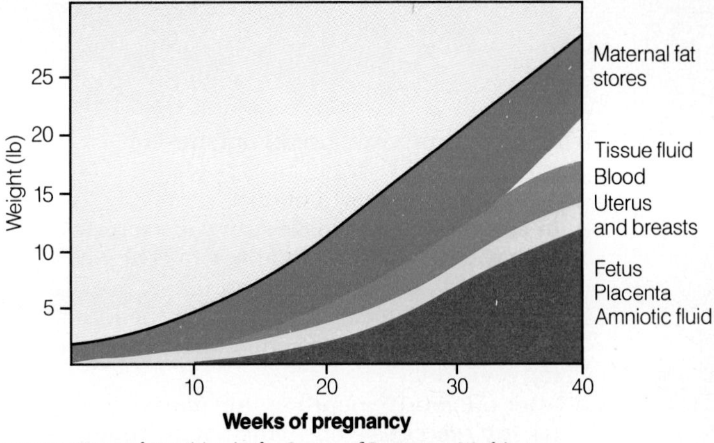


SOURCE: *Maternal Nutrition in the Course of Pregnancy.* Washington, D.C.: National Academy Press, 1970. Adapted with permission.

**FIGURE 8-20** Accounting for weight gain during pregnancy.

> **STRATEGY FOR CHANGE**
>
> **Eating for Two**
>
> Here are nutrition guidelines the American College of Obstetrics and Gynecology has developed for mothers-to-be:
>
> - Consume about 300 more calories a day than before pregnancy.
> - Do not restrict salt.
> - Drink six to eight glasses of liquids each day, including water, fruit and vegetable juices, and milk.
> - Concentrate on eating the right foods, not on watching your weight. Never diet during pregnancy.
> - Eat four or more servings each day from these food groups: fruits and vegetables, whole-grain or enriched bread and cereal, and milk and milk products. Also eat at least three servings of meat, poultry, eggs, fish, nuts, or beans.

### Exercise

Almost all pregnant women can benefit from exercise throughout pregnancy—as long as they don't push too hard or too far. Regular exercise (three times a week) is better, safer, and more effective than occasional workouts. One of the best activities for a mother-to-be is brisk walking.

> **STRATEGY FOR CHANGE**
>
> **Exercising During Pregnancy**
>
> These are some of the guidelines for safe exercise developed by the American College of Obstetricians and Gynecologists:
>
> - Don't exercise strenuously for more than 15 minutes.

- Avoid vigorous exercise in hot, humid weather.
- Avoid jerky, bouncy motions.
- In aerobics classes make sure you exercise on a wooden or carpeted floor to cushion shock and ensure a firm footing.
- Stretch and flex carefully because the joints and connective tissue soften and loosen during pregnancy.
- After the fourth month of pregnancy, don't do any exercises while lying flat on your back.
- Drink plenty of fluids before and after exercising.
- Don't let your body temperature rise above 100 degrees Fahrenheit or your heart rate climb above 140 beats per minute.
- Walk, swim, and jog in moderation; play tennis only if you played before pregnancy. Ski only if you're experienced, and stick to low altitudes and safe slopes. Do not water-ski or surf.

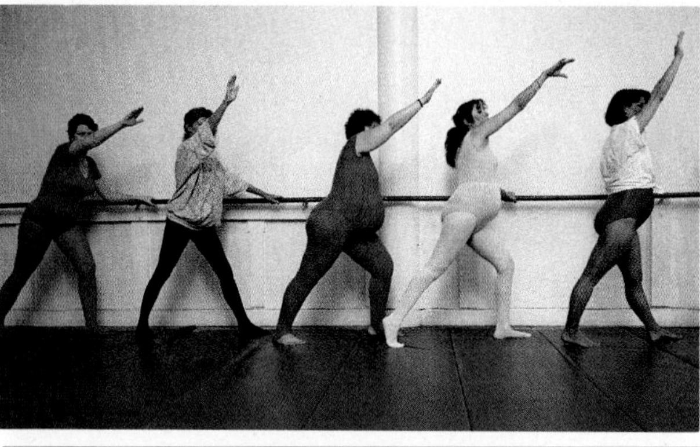

Almost all pregnant women can benefit from exercise—as long as they don't push themselves too far or too hard.

### Smoking

Smoking increases the risk of miscarriage, stillbirth, low birth weight, heart defects, and premature birth; smoking impairs growth, also. The sooner a mother-to-be stops smoking, the better the baby's chances of developing normally.

### Alcohol

In 1990 the federal Centers for Disease Control estimated that more than 8,000 alcohol-damaged babies are born every year.[16] One of every 750 newborns has a cluster of physical and mental defects called the fetal alcohol syndrome. Many more babies suffer fetal alcohol "effect": low birth weight, irritability as newborns, various complications of pregnancy, and lifelong mental impairment as a result of their mothers' alcohol consumption.

In a 1989 study of 2,278 highly educated women, 30 percent had more than one drink a week while pregnant.[17] The risk of fetal alcohol syndrome is greatest if a mother drinks 3 ounces or more of pure alcohol (the equivalent of six or seven cocktails) a day. However moderate drinking—one or two daily cocktails—may also have an effect. The National Institute on Alcohol Abuse and Alcoholism and the U.S. Surgeon General advise pregnant women—and those trying to become pregnant—not to drink at all.

### Caffeine

Moderate to heavy caffeine users are at greater risk of miscarriage than women who use little or no caffeine. Some evidence has linked caffeine with low birth weight and premature labor.[18] The Food and Drug Administration advice is for pregnant women to "avoid caffeine-containing products or use them sparingly."

### Illegal Drugs

At least one of every ten newborns is exposed to illegal drugs before birth. The consequences of drug use during pregnancy include severe damage to the baby's brain and nervous system and other birth defects.

Compared to mothers who did not smoke pot, marijuana smokers have smaller, sicker babies and a higher risk of stillbirths, according to preliminary research data. Drug use may also lead to neurochemical birth defects by disrupting normal development of the brain. Cocaine use increases the risk of premature birth, stillbirths, and malformations. Physicians urge prospective mothers to stay drug-free for at least three months before they conceive, as well as throughout their pregnancies.

### Radiation and Other Environmental Risks

High levels of radiation of the type used for cancer therapy have been associated with birth defects. Diagnostic X-rays should be avoided if possible but are not a significant threat, particularly after the first trimester. At least in theory, the rapidly developing fetus is especially vulnerable to pollutants, toxic wastes, heavy metals, pesticides, gases, and other hazardous compounds.

## Genetic Disorders

Major genetic disorders may be responsible for 33 to 50 percent of all miscarriages, and 2 to 4 percent of newborns have a genetic abnormality. The most common genetic problem among American whites is cystic fibrosis, a disabling abnormality of the respiratory system and the sweat and mucous glands. Among the other genetic disorders that occur are the following:

- *Down Syndrome*—**Down syndrome,** caused by an extra number 21 chromosome, occurs in one of every 600 to 1,000 births. Infants with Down syndrome are born with varying degrees of physical and mental retardation. The chance of a woman delivering a Down syndrome infant increases with her age. At age 25, the chances are 1 in 1,200; at age 35, they rise to 1 in 365; at age 40, they are 1 in 100.
- *Sickle-Cell Anemia*—About 8 to 10 percent of North America's 25 million blacks carry a gene for **sickle-cell anemia,** a blood disorder that occurs when **hemoglobin,** the oxygen-carrying proteins of red blood cells, is abnormal and causes red blood cells to assume a crescent, or sickle, shape. Unable to provide adequate oxygen to vital organs of the body, sickled cells cause tiredness, loss of interest and appetite, pain, and a host of other symptoms. Blood transfusions can prolong a victim's life, but there is no cure. About half the victims die before age 20.
- *Phenylketonuria*—**Phenylketonuria (PKU)** is a genetic disease in which the liver enzyme needed by the body for the metabolism of the amino acid phenylalanine is absent. If both parents are carriers, there is a one-in-four chance the child will develop the disease. In most states, the law requires testing of newborns for PKU. If PKU is detected, an immediate, long-term therapeutic diet can reduce the effects of the disorder. If untreated, the victim becomes severely mentally retarded.
- *Tay-Sachs Disease*—**Tay-Sachs disease** is caused by an enzyme deficiency that occurs almost exclusively among young children of Eastern European Jewish ancestry. Tay-Sachs victims appear normal at birth but gradually deteriorate physically and mentally. Death usually occurs before the fifth birthday. Carriers can be identified by a blood test.

## Prenatal Testing

All parents worry whether their unborn baby is normal and healthy. Sophisticated tests can answer some, but not all, of their questions and can identify more than 250 diseases and defects. The most common prenatal tests are:

- *Ultrasonography,* which uses high-frequency sound waves to draw a picture of a fetus. Ultrasonography can check fetal age and spot certain birth defects.
- *Alpha-fetoprotein (AFP) screening,* which measures in the mother's blood a substance produced by the baby's kidneys between the thirteenth and twentieth week of pregnancy. Levels that are too high could indicate a neural tube defect; levels that are too low may signal Down syndrome.
- *Amniocentesis,* performed from the fourteenth to sixteenth week of pregnancy, removes a small amount of the amniotic fluid surrounding the fetus. The fluid contains cells shed by the fetus, which

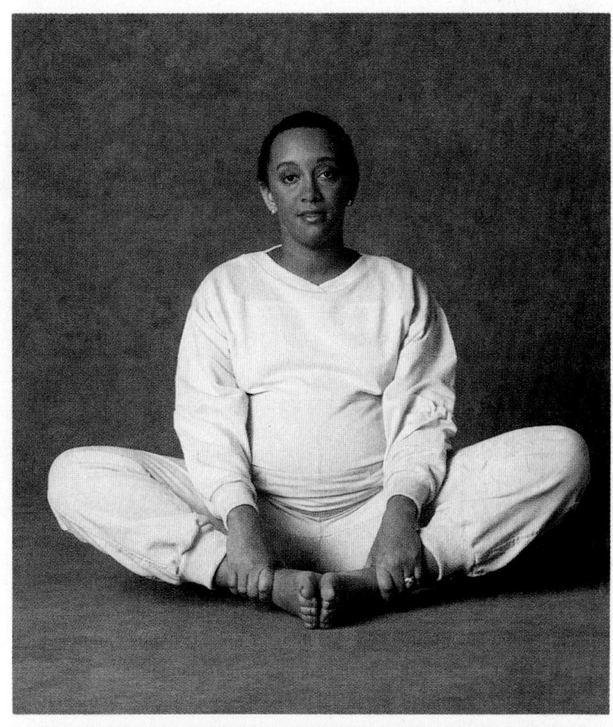

No responsibility is greater than that of bringing another human being into this world.

**Down syndrome** A genetic disorder leading to some degree of physical and mental retardation, caused by an extra number 21 chromosome.
**sickle-cell anemia** A debilitating genetic disorder of the blood characterized by sickle-shaped red blood cells, primarily affecting blacks.
**phenylketonuria (PKU)** A genetic disorder in which a crucial liver enzyme is absent, resulting in severe mental retardation if not treated.
**Tay-Sachs disease** A genetic disorder resulting in death by age 5 or 6; occurs almost exclusively among Jews of Eastern European ancestry.

**TABLE 8-5** Some Diseases That Can Be Detected by Amniocentesis and Chorionic Villi Sampling

| DISEASE | SYMPTOMS | INCIDENCE* |
|---|---|---|
| Cystic fibrosis | Liver, lung, pancreas disease | 1 in 2,000 Caucasians |
| Duchenne's muscular dystrophy | Wasting muscle disease | 1 in 5,000 males |
| Fragile X syndrome | Mental retardation | 1 in 1,000 males (primarily) |
| Hemophilia | Bleeding disorder | 1 in 5,000 males |
| Huntington's chorea | Fatal brain disease | 1 in 20,000 |
| Polycystic kidney disease | Kidney failure | 1 in 1,000 |
| Tay-Sachs disease | Fatal enzyme deficiency | 1 in 3,600 Eastern European Jews |
| Sickle-cell anemia | Hemoglobin affected | 1 in 400 U.S. blacks (primarily) |
| Beta thalassemia | Spleen and blood affected | Varies with race and origin |

*Estimated cases per number of live births.

are grown in tissue culture and then checked for any chromosomal or genetic defects.

- *Chorionic villi sampling,* performed at eight to ten weeks of pregnancy, involves suctioning of a small sample of the chorionic villi, the tissue surrounding the fetus, for laboratory analysis. Results are generally available within a week.

There are no known risks for sonography and AFP testing. For both chorionic villus sampling and amniocentesis, there is about a 1 percent risk of miscarriage. These tests are usually recommended only if the mother is over age 35, has already had a child with a genetic disorder, or is known to be a carrier of a detectable genetic disorder (see Table 8-5).

## Complications of Pregnancy

In about 10 to 15 percent of all pregnancies, there is increased risk of a problem, such as a baby's failure to grow normally. **Perinatology,** or maternal-fetal medicine, focuses on caring for the special needs of high-risk mothers and their unborn babies. Perinatal centers, with state-of-the-art equipment and 24-hour staffs of specialists in this field, have been set up around the country. Several of the most frequent complications of a pregnancy are discussed below.

### Ectopic Pregnancy

Any woman who is of childbearing age, has had intercourse, and feels abdominal pain with no reasonable cause may have an ectopic pregnancy, one that is not in the uterus. Ectopic, or tubal, pregnancies have tripled over the last 12 years, although no one understands why.[19] Risk factors include previous pelvic surgery, particularly involving the fallopian tubes; pelvic inflammatory disease; infertility; and use of an IUD.

The misplaced egg develops normally, producing the usual signs of pregnancy, until the cramped amniotic sac bursts. The woman bleeds internally and feels lower abdominal pains, or she may feel an aching in her shoulders as the blood flows upward toward the diaphragm. If the bleeding is substantial, the woman can go into shock, with a low blood pressure and high pulse rate. Symptoms are hot and cold flashes, nausea, dizziness, fainting, pelvic pain, and irregular bleeding.

The usual treatment for the burst tube is removal, but microsurgery can often save a damaged tube. However, ectopic pregnancies can lead to permanent infertility. About 50 percent of the women who have had an ectopic pregnancy conceive again; 10 percent have another misplaced pregnancy.

### Miscarriage

A **miscarriage,** or **spontaneous abortion,** is a pregnancy that ends before the twentieth week of gestation. About one of every ten pregnancies ends in miscarriage. An estimated 70 to 90 percent of women who miscarry eventually become pregnant again.[20]

Physicians typically recommend bedrest if a woman begins bleeding or cramping early in pregnancy. In some cases, the cramping stops, and the pregnan-

**perinatology** The medical specialty concerned with the diagnosis and treatment of pregnant women with high-risk conditions and their fetuses.
**miscarriage** A pregnancy that terminates before the twentieth week of gestation.
**spontaneous abortion** See *miscarriage.*

cy continues normally. In others, the bleeding becomes intense, the cervix widens, and the embryo passes out of the woman's body. If the miscarriage is complete, the bleeding stops; the uterus returns to its normal state and shape. If it is incomplete, a physician has to remove any bits of tissue remaining in the uterus by performing a dilation and curettage (D and C).

### Infections

The infectious disease most clearly linked to birth defects is **rubella** (German measles). All women should be vaccinated against this disease at least three months prior to conception to protect themselves and any children they may bear.

The most common prenatal infection today is cytomegalovirus, which causes very mild flulike symptoms in adults but can cause brain damage, retardation, liver disease, cerebral palsy, hearing problems, and other malformations in unborn babies.

Sexually transmitted diseases—such as syphilis, gonorrhea, and genital herpes—can be particularly dangerous during a pregnancy if not recognized and treated. If a woman has a herpes outbreak around the date her baby is due, her physician will deliver the baby by cesarean section to prevent infection of the baby. HIV infection endangers both a pregnant woman and her unborn baby. An infected woman's child has a 15 percent to 50 percent chance of contracting HIV before, or at, birth.[21] (See Chapter 15 for a full discussion of sexually transmitted diseases and their risks in pregnancy.)

### Premature Labor

Approximately 10 percent of all babies are born too soon (before the thirty-seventh week of pregnancy). Thrust into the world before they are ready to survive on their own, they are among the most vulnerable of newborns. Bedrest, close monitoring, and, if necessary, medications can buy more time in the womb for babies if their mothers recognize the warning signs of premature labor (a dull, low backache; a feeling of tightness or pressure on the lower abdomen; and intestinal cramps, sometimes with diarrhea) early enough to get treatment.

**rubella** An infectious disease often causing birth defects in pregnant women; also called German measles.

**STRATEGY FOR CHANGE**

**Warning Signs of Problems**

Notify a physician if any of the following symptoms develop during pregnancy:

- vaginal bleeding
- abdominal pain
- persistent nausea and vomiting
- unusual thirst
- chills or fever
- swelling of the face or fingers
- severe or continuous headaches
- dimness or blurring of vision
- fluid leaking from the vagina

## Teen Pregnancy: Children Having Children

The United States has the highest rates of adolescent pregnancy and abortion of any developed country, even though teen pregnancy and birth rates dropped in the 1980s.[22] Every year approximately 1.1 million girls become pregnant; 45 percent undergo abortions. Of those who carry to term, 90 percent keep their babies. In the past, most teenage mothers were married. Today most are not.

Pregnancy poses health risks for the teenager and her child. She is more likely to develop complications in pregnancy, and her child is more likely to have a low birth weight and to die in its first year of life. However, some risks can be overcome. According to a study by the National Institute of Child Health and Development, pregnant teenagers who receive adequate prenatal care gain more weight during pregnancy and deliver fewer premature or low-birth-weight babies.[23] Yet nearly one in ten adolescents doesn't start prenatal care until the third trimester or receives none at all.

# CHILDBIRTH

A generation ago delivering a baby was something a doctor did in a hospital. Today parents are active participants who can choose from an almost bewildering array of options.

The first decision parents-to-be face is choosing a "birth attendant," who can be a physician or a nurse-midwife. Certified nurse-midwives in the United States deliver more than 90,000 babies a year, mostly in hospitals and birth centers. Their approach is based on the belief that the typical pregnant woman can deliver her baby naturally, without technological inter-

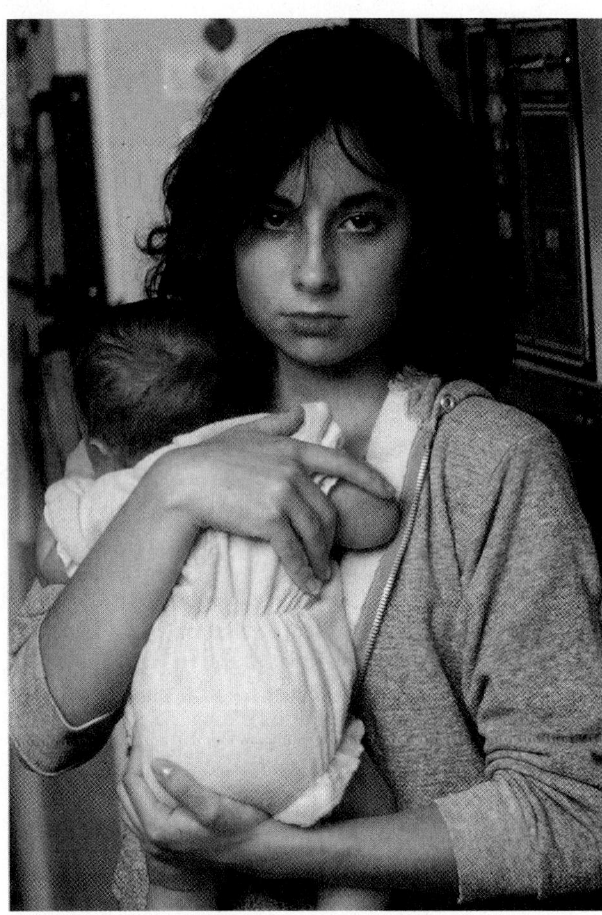

The United States has the highest rate of teenage pregnancy of any developed country.

vention. Lay midwives have a similar orientation but less formal training; only a handful of states permit lay midwives to deliver babies.

**STRATEGY FOR CHANGE**

**Who Should Deliver Your Baby?**

When you are interviewing physicians or midwives, look for the following:

- experience in handling various complications
- extensive prenatal care
- a commitment to be at the mother's side for the entire labor, to spot complications quickly and to provide assistance
- a philosophy toward childbirth and medical interventions that is compatible with your own

## Where to Have Your Baby

A hospital with trained specialists and a nursery for newborns is recommended for high-risk women. However, if their pregnancies are normal and uncomplicated, mothers-to-be can consider alternatives almost unheard of a generation ago, including in-hospital birthing rooms decorated to look like comfortable bedrooms; "birthing chairs," specially molded so a woman can stay in an upright position to push her baby into the world; and independent birth centers that offer a homelike setting to low-risk mothers.

Only about one percent of babies are born at home. The American College of Obstetricians and Gynecologists opposes home births because of "potential hazards" to mother and child, but a study of 4,054 home births in Missouri found that the mortality rate for babies born at home was virtually the same as in hospitals—provided a doctor or trained midwife was in attendance.

## Preparing for Childbirth

The most widespread method of childbirth preparation is **psychoprophylaxis,** or the **Lamaze method.** Fernand Lamaze, a French doctor, instructed women to respond to labor contractions with prelearned, controlled breathing techniques. As the intensity of each contraction increases, the laboring woman concentrates on increasing her breathing rate in a prescribed way. Her partner coaches her during each contraction and helps her cope with her discomfort. Studies have shown that women who've gone through childbirth preparation have fewer complications and require fewer drugs.

## Labor and Delivery

There are three stages of labor. The first starts with the **effacement** (thinning) and **dilation** (opening up) of the cervix, the neck of the uterus. Effacement is measured in percentages, dilation in centimeters or finger widths. This stage ends when the cervix is completely dilated to 10 centimeters (or five fingers) and the baby is ready to come down the birth canal (see Figure 8-21). The second stage ends with the birth of the baby. The third ends with the delivery of the placenta.

**psychoprophylaxis** A method of childbirth preparation taught to expectant parents to help the woman cope with the discomfort of labor; combines breathing and psychological techniques.
**Lamaze method** See *psychoprophylaxis*.
**effacement** The thinning of the cervix before delivery.
**dilation** The opening up of the cervix before delivery.

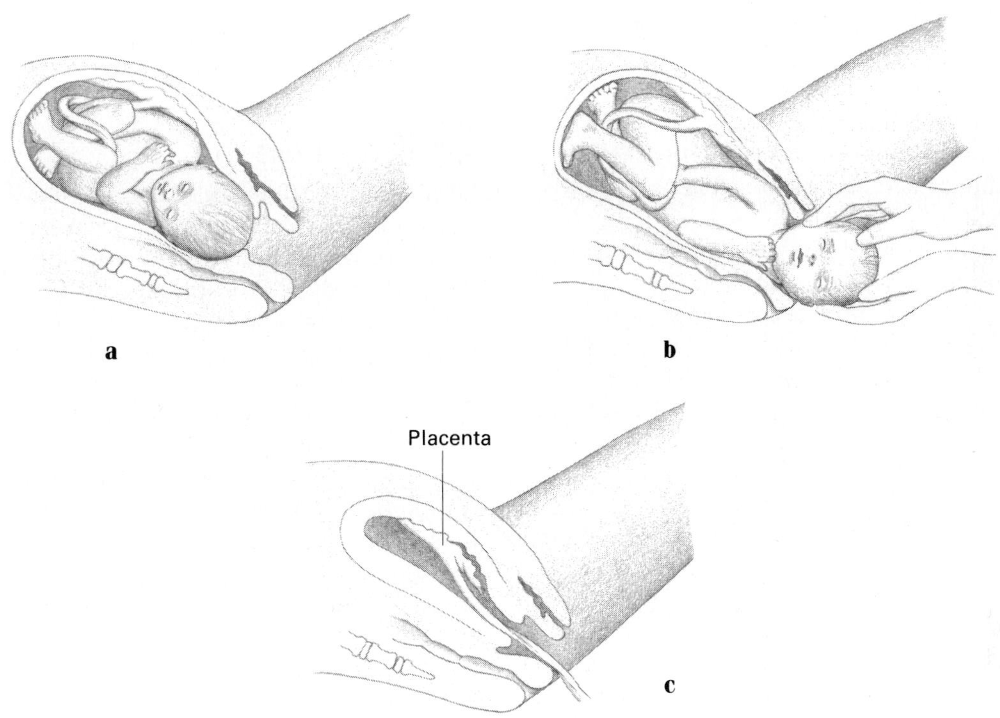


SOURCE: Hales, Dianne. *An Invitation to Health, Fourth Edition,* Benjamin/Cummings, 1989.

**FIGURE 8-21** The three stages of labor. **(a)** Opening of the birth canal by progressive dilation and effacement of the cervix. **(b)** The birth of the baby. **(c)** The delivery of the placenta (afterbirth).

### First Stage

The first contractions of the early, or latent, phase of labor are usually not uncomfortable and last 15 to 30 seconds, occurring every 15 to 30 minutes and gradually increasing in intensity and frequency. As the cervix dilates a total of 5 to 8 centimeters, many women rely on breathing exercises to overcome discomfort.

The most difficult contractions come after the cervix is about 8 centimeters dilated. During this transition phase, the last part of the cervical dilation, the contractions are more painful because the woman feels greater pressure from the fetus. For first babies, first-stage labor averages 12 to 13 hours. Women who are having a second or subsequent child have shorter first-stage labor.

### Second Stage

When the cervix is completely dilated, the second stage of labor begins. The baby moves into the vagina, or birth canal, and out of the mother's body. This stage can take up to an hour or more. Strong contractions may last for 60 to 90 seconds and occur every 2 to 3 minutes.

As the baby's head descends, the mother feels an urge to push. By bearing down, she helps the baby complete its passage to the outside. Women who have gone through prepared childbirth training often feel a sense of relief from the acute pain of the transition phase and at the prospect of delivery.

As the baby's head appears, or crowns, the doctor may perform an episiotomy, an incision made from the lower end of the vagina toward the anus to enlarge the vaginal opening. The purpose of the episiotomy is to prevent the head from causing an irregular tear. Sometimes women can avoid an episiotomy by good nutrition throughout pregnancy, exercise, trying different birth positions, or having an attendant massage the perineal tissue; but the skin's elasticity and the baby's size are also factors.

Under usual circumstances, the birth of the baby is gradual: head first, shoulders, then body. With each contraction, a new part is born. However, the baby can be in a more difficult position, facing up rather than down or with feet or buttocks first (a breech birth).

### Third Stage

In the third stage of labor, the uterus contracts firmly after delivery of the baby; usually within 5 minutes, the placenta separates from the uterine wall. The woman may bear down to help expel the placenta, or the doctor may exert gentle external pressure. If an episiotomy has been performed, the doctor sews up the incision. The uterus may be massaged, or the baby may be put to the mother's breast to stimulate contraction of the uterus, because breast-feeding causes the uterus to contract and hastens its return to normal size.

In some hospitals, mother and child are never separated. In others, there are modified lying-in arrangements in which the mother receives help in taking care of her baby. In still others, babies, particularly those with a low birth weight or those who have suffered serious birth traumas, are kept in nurseries.

### Cesarean Birth

In a **cesarean delivery,** a doctor lifts the baby out of the woman's body through an incision made in the uterus and lower abdomen. In the last ten years, the cesarean delivery rate has more than doubled—increasing for all age groups, all marital statuses, and all racial groups, and in all types and sizes of hospitals.[24]

About 25 percent of all babies are delivered by cesarean "section" every year. The United States has a cesarean rate 50 to 200 percent higher than that of other industrialized countries (except Canada and Australia). High-income women are 73 percent more likely to have cesareans than poor women, according to a 1989 report by University of California researchers in *The New England Journal of Medicine.*[25, 26]

About 36 percent of cesareans are performed because the woman has had a previous cesarean delivery. Yet the latest research indicates that more than two-thirds of women who undergo cesarean deliveries because of failure to progress in labor and approximately four-fifths of those who have cesarean sections for other reasons can have successful vaginal deliveries in subsequent pregnancies.

The most common reason for cesareans is "failure to progress," a vague term indicating that labor has gone on too long and may put the baby at risk. Other reasons include the baby's position (if feet or buttocks are first) and signs that the fetus is in danger.

In most cesarean deliveries, the mother, given a regional anesthetic, is awake and aware of what's happening; the father can remain at her side. Some women feel more physical discomforts after a cesarean, including nausea, pain, and abdominal gas; others bounce back quickly. All must refrain from strenuous activity, such as heavy lifting, for several weeks.

Women can lower the likelihood of a cesarean delivery by using breathing techniques to relax, walking as much as possible in early labor, and trying different labor positions. However, under some circumstances, a cesarean delivery will remain the safest way for a baby to enter the world.

## Following Birth

For the mother, the high of delivery may be followed by a low known as postpartum depression. This time of fatigue, anxiety, and fluctuating moods is so common that it is listed in obstetrics texts as a normal consequence of delivery. For most women, it is a temporary feeling. For others, the depression, combined with fatigue and the new demands of the newborn, can persist for weeks and even months.

In addition, it takes a while for the mother's body to return to normal. The woman usually loses about 11 pounds at delivery and an additional 4 to 5 pounds in the following weeks. Usually four to eight weeks are required for the woman's reproductive organs, especially the uterus, to return to normal. (Breast-feeding hastens this process, and exercises help restore the abdomen to its original size, shape, and tone.) For three to six weeks, there is a discharge called lochia, a mixture of blood from the site in the uterus where the placenta was attached and from the uterine lining. If the mother doesn't nurse, menstruation resumes in about four to ten weeks.

### Breast-feeding Versus Bottle-feeding

A generation ago, most middle- and upper-class women bottle-fed their babies. Today, an increasing number of mothers and medical professionals feel that breast milk is best. Breast-fed babies have fewer illnesses and a much lower hospitalization rate. Their mortality rate is also lower. Breast milk seems not only to prevent or lessen disease, but also to help bring infection under control. When breast-fed babies do get sick, they recover more quickly. Breast-fed babies are also less likely to become obese or to develop allergies. In addition, the process of nursing more closely bonds mother and child.

According to the American Council on Science and Health, at least 20 percent of women are unable to breast-feed after their first deliveries; 50 percent of new mothers encounter significant difficulties in nursing. Sometimes the woman's breasts become inflamed, or she must take medications that would be

---

**cesarean delivery** The surgical procedure in which an infant is delivered through an incision made in the abdominal wall and uterus.

dangerous to her infant; sometimes the infant is unable to suckle vigorously enough to get an adequate milk supply. Another problem is that, in certain areas of the country, the levels of pesticides and other chemical contaminants in mother's milk can be high.

### Crib Death: Sudden Infant Death Syndrome

Sudden Infant Death Syndrome (SIDS), or "crib death," is the most common cause of death in infants less than a year old. Each year, 10,000 to 18,000 babies die as a result of this syndrome. Premature and very small babies are the most vulnerable.

Typically, a seemingly healthy infant, usually one to seven months old, is put to bed according to the daily routine. The baby may have some signs of a cold or cough. When the parents return to the crib, they find that the child is dead. There is no sign of a struggle, nor does the baby suffocate in the blankets. Determining the cause of death often proves impossible.

Physicians know of no way to predict or prevent crib death. Highly sensitive electronic monitors can be set up to alert parents if their baby stops breathing during sleep. These are recommended if a baby has had a "near-miss" episode—that is, if the child stopped breathing before but was discovered in time.

## INFERTILITY

Of the couples who marry this year, 20 percent will not be able to conceive a child; 10 percent of couples already married will not be able to have additional children.[27] **Infertility** is a problem of the couple, not of the individual man or woman. Often neither partner is fully fertile. If either were married to a more fertile partner, their **subfertility** might never be noticed.

In women, the most common causes of subfertility or infertility are abnormal menstrual patterns, suppression of ovulation, and blocked fallopian tubes.

In men, infertility is usually linked to either the quantity or the quality of sperm. Normal fertility has been defined as the presence of more than 20 million sperm per milliliter of semen in an ejaculation of 3 to 5 ml. Sometimes the problem is ejaculatory incompetence (the inability to ejaculate or difficulty therewith) or retrograde ejaculation, in which some of the semen travels in the wrong direction, back into the body of the male.

Medical treatment can identify the cause of infertility in about 90 percent of affected couples. The odds of successful pregnancy range from 30 to 70 percent, depending on the specific cause of infertility.

### Alternatives for Childless Couples

Since the 1960s, artificial insemination has led to an estimated 250,000 births in the United States, primarily in couples in which the husband is infertile. However, some states do not recognize such children as legitimate; others do, but only if the woman's husband gave his consent for the insemination.

Some women practice artificial insemination on their own by inserting sperm from a man into their vaginas at the time they're ovulating. No data are available on how successful this approach is, but women have reported becoming pregnant in this fashion.

New approaches to infertility include microsurgery, sometimes with lasers, to open destroyed or blocked egg and sperm ducts; new hormone preparations to induce ovulation; and the use of sound waves to monitor ovulation. Home ovulation kits help by pinpointing ovulation with an accuracy never before possible.

Among the most promising techniques that can help couples overcome fertility problems are:

- *In vitro fertilization,* which involves removing the ova, often with a long needle, from a woman's ovary just before normal ovulation would occur. The woman's egg and her mate's sperm are placed in a special fertilization medium for a specific period of time and are then transferred to another medium to continue developing. If the fertilized egg cell shows signs of development, within several days it is returned to the woman's uterus by means of a hollow tube placed through the vagina and cervix. The egg cell implants itself in the lining of the uterus, and the pregnancy continues as normal. The success rate varies from center to center but is generally less than 20 percent.
- *Gamete intrafallopian transfer (GIFT),* which involves placing sperm and eggs into the fallopian tubes. Less time-consuming and less expensive than in vitro fertilization, GIFT mimics nature by allowing fertilized eggs to develop in the fallopian tubes

---

**infertility** The inability to conceive a child.
**subfertility** Difficulty conceiving a child.

according to a normal timetable. The success rate is about 20 percent.

- *Embryo transfer,* in which the sperm of the husband of an infertile woman is placed in another woman's uterus during ovulation. Five days later, the fertilized egg is transferred to the uterus of the infertile woman, who then carries and delivers the developing embryo. Embryos may be frozen for later implantation in a process (called cryopreservation) that is highly controversial because of the legal issues over the "ownership" of the unborn.
- *Host uterus,* in which the sperm from a man and the egg from a woman are combined in a laboratory. The fertilized egg is implanted in a second woman who agrees to bear the child, which is not genetically related to her.
- *Surrogacy,* in which a woman is artificially inseminated with the sperm of an infertile woman's husband. She carries the baby to term, usually for a fee ($5,000 to $10,000). After delivery, the surrogate mother turns the baby over to the couple. Ever since the widely publicized "Baby M" case, in which a surrogate mother went to court to keep her child, surrogacy has become less common.

## Adoption

Parents can be "made" as well as born. Adoption matches parents yearning for youngsters to love with children who need loving. Couples interested in adoption can work either with public agencies or with private counselors who contact obstetricians directly.

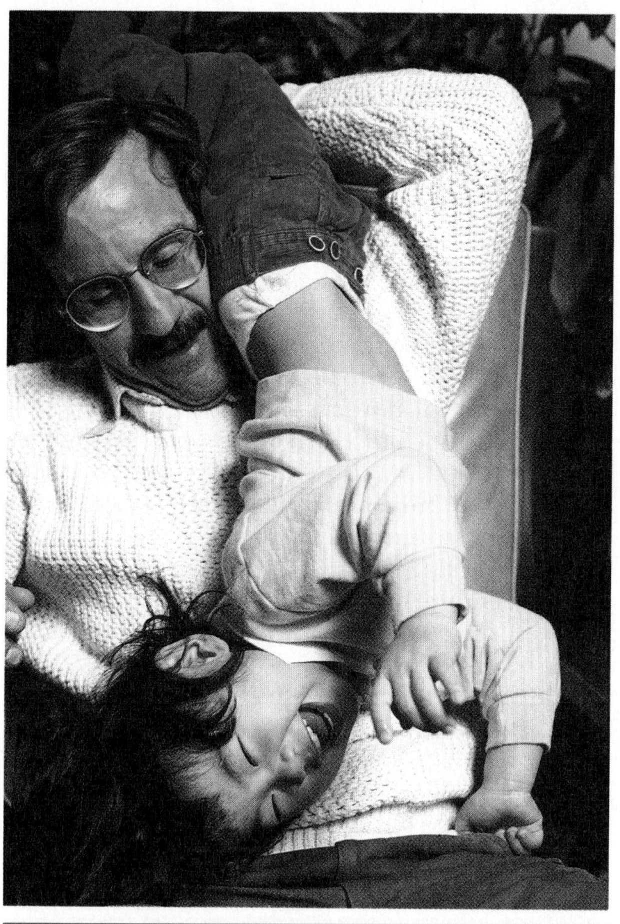

Adoption matches parents yearning for youngsters with children who need loving.

## WHAT DO YOU THINK?

Jennifer has obtained a diaphragm, spermicide, and condoms, but she hates carrying birth control devices in her purse. She thinks if a date ever saw them, he'd assume she wanted sex. And even though she worries about sexually transmitted diseases, she feels too embarrassed to ask a partner to wear a condom. Can you understand her feelings? If you're a woman, how would you handle a similar situation? If you're a man, how would you react?

Fearing a ban on legal abortions, some women are learning techniques for performing home abortions, often by a process of suctioning the contents of the uterus called menstrual extraction. They argue that women should not have to depend on medical professionals for abortion. Critics point out that home abortions can be dangerous and lead to serious complications. What do you think? What would you do if abortion became illegal and you or your girlfriend got pregnant and did not want to continue the pregnancy?

Pregnant women who use hard drugs or alcohol have been arrested and put on trial for abusing their unborn children. Prosecutors feel this is their last hope for defending innocent victims of substance abuse. Health officials argue that addicted or alcoholic pregnant women need help, not punishment. What do you think?

Adoption poses some problems that prospective adoptive parents should consider in advance. Because of improved birth control methods and the legalization of abortion, there are fewer healthy newborns available for adoption. Some agencies have one- to seven-year waiting lists.

An increasing number of people support "open" adoptions, which allow for visiting and communication with the natural parents even though the adoptive parents retain legal custody. Even after a "closed" adoption the "birth parents" may at some point search for their children, if only to explain why they put them up for adoption. Alternatively, as they get older, adopted children may want to find their natural parents.

## MAKING THIS CHAPTER WORK FOR YOU

### Responsible Reproductive Choices Now and in the Future

Human beings have the unique ability to choose whether or not to conceive. However, simply not wanting to conceive is never enough to halt conception. Before you become sexually active, you have to decide about birth control. The fact that women bear children does not mean that men are not equally responsible for birth control. A sexually active couple that does not use contraception has an 80 percent chance of conceiving a child within a year. If you decide to take that gamble, you use as stakes your future, your partner's future, and the life of the person you may conceive.

To prevent conception, you can eliminate sperm from the ejaculate, or you can prevent the sperm and ejaculate from entering the vagina. You can make the survival of sperm in the vagina more difficult, or you can block the sperm's path into the uterus and fallopian tubes. By preventing ovulation, you can make sure that the sperm does not find a ready, ripe egg. Or, you can prevent the fertilized egg from implanting itself in the uterine wall.

The various methods of birth control use one or more of these tactics to prevent conception. Though today's contraceptives are relatively effective, safe, and convenient, none is 100 percent safe, 100 percent effective, or 100 percent convenient.

One of the most effective birth control methods is the oral contraceptive pill, which inhibits ovulation, alters the cervical mucus so that sperm are prevented from entering the uterus, and interferes with implantation. The barrier contraceptives, which include the diaphragm, cervical cap, and condom, prevent sperm from reaching the egg. When they are used with a condom and spermicides containing nonoxynol-9, they can help protect users from sexually transmitted diseases. Because of their risks, intrauterine devices are no longer a popular contraceptive method.

Users of the rhythm method of birth control abstain from intercourse during the days just preceding and just following ovulation. Other options include the spermicide-saturated contraceptive sponge, vaginal spermicides, vaginal contraceptive film, abstinence, and sexual activities that do not involve intercourse. The most popular and effective, but permanent, birth control method among married couples is sterilization—either by vasectomy in a man or blocking, cutting, or tying the fallopian tubes in a woman.

After-intercourse methods of birth control include the morning-after pill, which prevents implantation of a fertilized egg; menstrual extraction, in which the uterine lining is suctioned out; and dilation and curettage (D and C), in which the uterine contents are scraped out.

One of the most controversial and divisive issues today is legalized induced abortion, the termination of pregnancy by the removal of the uterine contents. A hormonal compound, RU 486, often called "the abortion pill," is being used in Europe as a method of terminating pregnancy in its first weeks. Commonly used abortion methods in the United States are suction curettage, dilation and evacuation, prostaglandin injection, and hysterotomy.

The decision to conceive a child is only the first of many. Even before the child's birth, parents are responsible for its well-being. They need to make responsible decisions about where the child will be born, what they can do to prepare for childbirth, and who will deliver the baby.

Having a healthy baby depends on good nutrition; rest and exercise; and avoiding risks, such as smoking, alcohol, caffeine, harmful drugs, and exposure to radiation. Among the serious complications of pregnancy are ectopic pregnancies, which occur when the fertilized egg implants itself at sites other than in the uterus; miscarriages, which usually occur before the sixteenth week of pregnancy; infections, which may cause disease, brain damage, and malformations of the baby; and premature labor, which occurs after week 20 and before week 37 of the pregnancy.

Labor consists of three stages: the thinning and opening of the cervix to 10 centimeters; the passage of the baby through the cervix and vagina into the world; and the delivery of the placenta. A cesarean, or surgical, delivery may be necessary to overcome certain risks. After birth, the woman's body begins to return to its prepregnant state. Breast-feeding can protect the baby from various illnesses and promotes bonding between mother and baby.

One in every five couples has problems conceiving a child. Infertile couples may decide to attempt to have a child by such medical procedures as in vitro fertilization, gamete intrafallopian transfer, or artificial insemination. Another alternative is adoption. Because many adopted children seek out their biological parents and many biological parents try to find the child they gave up for adoption, the policy of open adoption is gaining support.

Choices about sex invariably lead to choices about reproduction. Sexual responsibility means recognizing that fact and acting with full awareness of the consequences of sexual activity. You must think, not just of yourself, but also of your partner, because your decisions and actions may affect both of you, now and in the future. You must also consider the baby you might conceive if you don't use contraception. If you should decide to have a child, your responsibility as a sexual partner and parent extends to the new life you help to create.

SECTION IV

# YOUR LIFE-STYLE

Drug abuse is one of the greatest problems facing our society. Even if you don't rely on drugs to pick you up or bring you down, you drink very little, and you don't smoke, drugs remain part of your world. All of us constantly hear messages to take drugs, drink, and use tobacco. All of us live with the dangers and enormous costs of others' drug abuse. That's why it's important to know about the most commonly used drugs, how they work, and why people use them. This section provides information you can use to avoid or overcome habits that could destroy your health, happiness, and life.

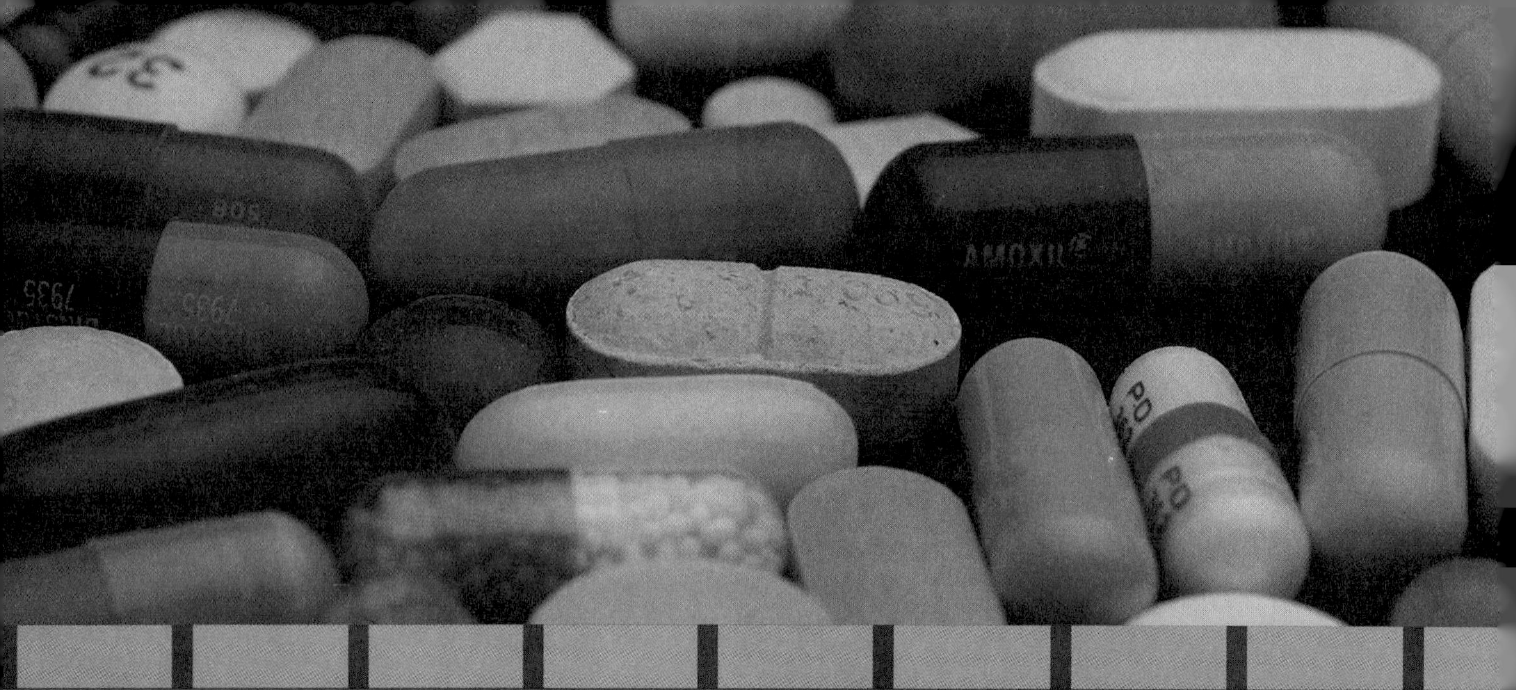

# 9 DRUG USE AND ABUSE: RECOGNIZING THE RISKS

In this chapter

Drug use, misuse, and abuse

Legal drugs

Illegal drugs

Psychoactive drugs

The toll of drug abuse

Overcoming drug dependency

Making this chapter work for you: Staying drug-free

*All drugs—legal or illegal, over-the-counter (OTC) or prescription—are chemicals that interact with your body's own chemistry and with other drugs.* The caffeine in your morning coffee is a drug, as is the nicotine in your cigarette and the alcohol in your beer or wine. And all three of these drugs are potentially addictive. Chapters 10 and 11 focus on two widely used and accepted "legal" drugs, alcohol and nicotine. This chapter provides information on the most common drugs of abuse and how they affect the body and mind.

## DRUG USE, MISUSE, AND ABUSE

A **drug** is any chemical other than food that is purposely taken to affect body processes. Drugs can extend and improve life by treating or preventing illness or by providing relief from physical or mental distress—but if they're misused or abused, they can shorten life.

Using a drug for a purpose other than that for which it was originally intended is **drug misuse**. Taking more of a drug than prescribed or using a friend's prescription of penicillin when your throat feels scratchy is an example of misuse.

Excessive drug use inconsistent with acceptable medical practice is **drug abuse**. Taking anabolic steroids to look more muscular is an example of abuse.

This chapter focuses on **psychoactive,** or mood-altering, drugs. Misuse of a psychoactive drug can grow into abuse and physical or psychological **addiction,** the compulsion for repetitive use of the drug. You are addicted if you rely on any drug to cope with life or if the drugs you take are interfering with normal living.

### Why People Abuse Drugs

People often start abusing drugs—illegal as well as legal—without realizing why. Some common reasons follow.

- *Curiosity*—Many young adults try drugs out of curiosity and may not try them again. Others who start because they're curious continue to use drugs for other reasons.
- *Boredom*—Some people see drugs as a recreational activity, but abuse is never recreational.

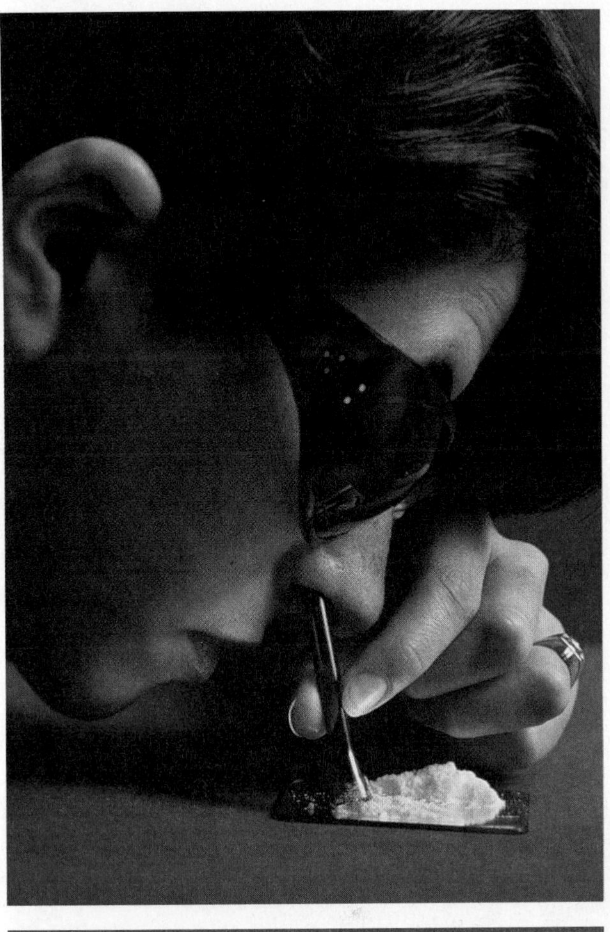

Many people who try psychoactive drugs out of curiosity may end up with a habit

- *Peer Influence*—If your friends use drugs, you may be likely to use them to remain part of the group.
- *Imitating Parents*—If your parents drink, smoke, or use drugs to alter their moods, you may model your behavior on theirs.
- *Availability of Drugs*—People who work in situations in which drugs are readily available, such as health care professionals, are more prone to abuse them.

**drug** Any substance other than food that, when taken, affects body functions and structures.
**drug misuse** The use of a drug for a purpose other than its original intent.
**drug abuse** The excessive use of a drug that has dangerous side effects.
**psychoactive** Affecting mood and/or behavior.
**addiction** A state of compulsive physiological need for a habit-forming substance.

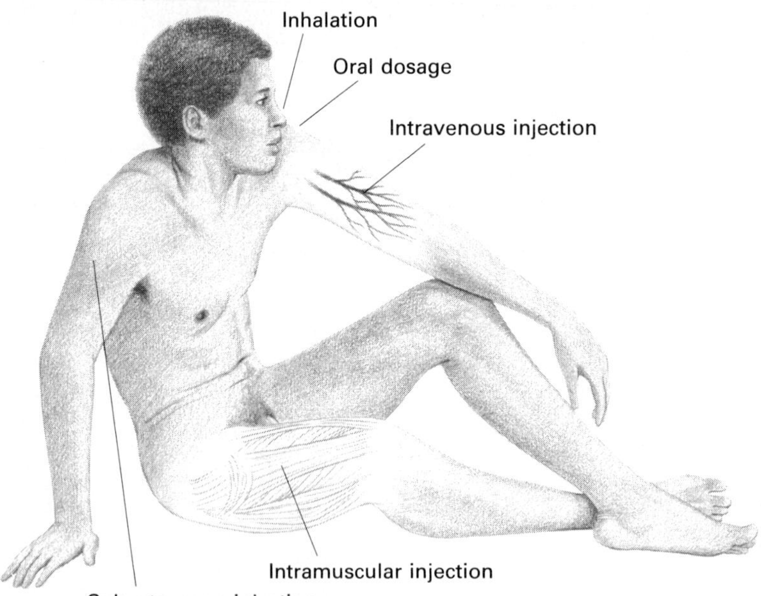


SOURCE: Hales, Dianne. *An Invitation to Health, Fourth Edition,* Benjamin/Cummings, 1989.

**FIGURE 9-1** Routes of administration of drugs.

- *Psychological Needs*—Some people turn to drugs because they want to feel better about themselves or because they feel powerless and hopeless.
- *Genetics or Childhood Environment*—The children of drug abusers may be at greater risk, possibly because of some genetic vulnerability or influences during childhood.
- *Socioeconomic Status*—The despair bred by poverty may drive some people to use drugs, but individuals from all economic levels abuse drugs.
- *Mental Illness*—Nearly a million Americans suffer the combined burdens of mental illness and chemical dependency.

**STRATEGY FOR CHANGE**

**Before You Can Say No**

You can take steps to protect yourself from the temptation to use drugs.

- Learn how to cope with stress. Try some of the coping techniques—such as exercise, visual imagery, or meditation—described in Chapter 3.
- Strengthen your self-esteem. Take pride in your achievements, particularly when setbacks may bruise your confidence.
- Develop a range of interests. Get into the habit of finding pleasure in swimming, dancing, or taking long walks.
- Practice assertiveness. Cultivate the art of speaking up and voicing your opinion—regardless of the subject.

## How Psychoactive Drugs Work

The effects of psychoactive drugs depend on several factors, including how the drug enters the body, drug action, and the presence of other drugs in the body.

### Routes of Administration

The most common way of taking a drug is by swallowing a tablet, capsule, or liquid. Drugs taken by mouth don't reach the bloodstream as quickly as drugs introduced by other means. A drug taken orally may not have any effects for 30 minutes or more. (See Figure 9-1.)

Drugs can enter the body through the lungs, either by sniffing a powder, like cocaine, or by inhaling gases, aerosol sprays, or fumes from solvents or other compounds that evaporate quickly. Young users often soak a rag with such fluids and press it over their noses, or place inhalants in a plastic bag, put the bag over their noses and mouths, and take deep breaths, a practice called huffing. Inhaling drugs can produce serious, even fatal consequences.[1]

With a syringe drugs can be injected **subcutaneously** (beneath the skin), **intramuscularly** (into muscle tissue, which is richly supplied with blood vessels), or **intravenously** (directly into a vein). Intravenous (IV) injection gets the drug into the bloodstream immediately (within seconds in most cases), intramuscular injection moderately fast (within a few

**subcutaneous** Under the skin.
**intramuscular** Into or within a muscle.
**intravenous** Into a vein.

minutes), and subcutaneous injection more slowly (within 10 minutes).

The use of needles for drug administration is extremely dangerous because many diseases, including hepatitis and HIV infection, can be transmitted if needles are shared. IV drug users have become the second-highest risk group (after homosexual men) for contracting HIV, and they are the chief source of transmission of the virus among heterosexuals (see Chapter 15).

### Types of Action

A drug can act locally, as novocaine does, to deaden pain in a tooth; it can act generally, throughout a body system, as alcohol does on the central nervous system; or it can act selectively, as a drug such as a laxative does when it has a greater effect on one specific organ or system than on others. A drug that accumulates when it is taken in faster than the body can metabolize and excrete it, thus heightening its effects, is **cumulative**. (Alcohol is such a drug.) Some drugs turn down, or dampen, the central nervous system. Others speed it up, or stimulate it.

### Interaction with Other Drugs

A drug can interact with other drugs in four different ways:

1. An **additive** interaction is one in which the resulting effect is equal to the sum of the effects of the drugs used.
2. A **synergistic** interaction is one in which the total effect of the two drugs is greater than the sum of the effects the two drugs would have had if taken by themselves on separate occasions. Mixing barbiturates and alcohol, for example, has up to 4 times the depressant effect that either drug has alone.
3. A drug can be **potentiating**—that is, one drug can increase the effect of another. Alcohol, for instance, can increase the drowsiness caused by antihistamines, drugs taken to relieve allergy symptoms.
4. Drugs can interact **antagonistically**—that is, one drug can neutralize, or block, another drug with opposite effects. Tranquilizers, for example, may counter some of the nervousness and anxiety produced by cocaine.

### Toxicity

The **toxicity** of a drug is the level at which it becomes poisonous to the body, causing either temporary or permanent minor or major damage.

### Tolerance

The body's ability to withstand the effects of a drug is called **tolerance**. Continued use of a drug can result in increased tolerance (decreased responsiveness) to that drug, so that larger and larger doses become necessary to achieve a constant effect. A heroin user, for instance, may start with a 3-mg dose but in a few months' time needs a 1,000-mg dose to get the same results. Larger doses cost more money and increase the possibility of toxic side effects.

### Addiction

Dependence refers to the attachment—psychological or physical, or both—that a person may develop to a drug. **Physical dependence** occurs when physiological changes in the body's cells cause an overpowering, constant need for the drug. If the drug isn't taken, the user develops withdrawal symptoms, such as intense anxiety, extreme nausea, and deep craving for the drug. The use of tranquilizers, painkillers, barbiturates, or narcotics can result in physical dependence.

With **psychological dependence,** also called habituation, there is a strong craving for a drug because it produces pleasurable feelings or relieves stress or anxiety. Marijuana and LSD may not create physical dependence, but continued use of either can result in psychological dependence.

### Individual Differences

Each person responds differently to different drugs at different times and in different settings. Often, drugs intensify the emotional state a person is in. If you are feeling depressed, a drug may make you feel more depressed. A generalized physical problem, like

---

**cumulative** Characterized by an increase in effects upon successive additions of the same or another substance.
**additive** Characterized by a combined effect that is equal to the sum of the individual effects.
**synergistic** Characterized by a combined effect that is greater than the sum of the individual effects.
**potentiating** Making more effective or powerful.
**antagonistic** Opposing or counteracting.
**toxicity** Poisonousness.
**tolerance** The capacity to endure the effects of a substance.
**physical dependence** The physiological attachment to, and need for, a drug.
**psychological dependence** The emotional or mental attachment to the use of a drug.

having the flu, may make your body more vulnerable to the effects of a drug. Genetic differences among individuals may also account for varying reactions to drugs.

### Set

Personality and psychological attitude can play a role in drug effects, so that one person may have a frightening bad trip on the same LSD dosage that produces a "beautiful, profound" experience for another. To a certain extent, this depends on each user's **set** (or mind-set), his or her expectations or preconceptions about using drugs. Someone who snorts cocaine to enhance sexual pleasure may feel more stimulated simply because that is what he or she expects.

### Setting

The setting during drug use also influences its effects. Drinking beer with a rowdy group of friends while watching a football game on television is entirely different from sharing a bottle of wine with a date in a quiet restaurant. The alcohol affects your body in the same way, but you respond differently because of the setting.

## LEGAL DRUGS

Over-the-counter drugs and drugs obtained through a prescription from a physician are legal, but that doesn't mean they're safe.

### Caffeine: America's Favorite Drug?

Caffeine may be the world's most-used drug. When we think of caffeine, we usually think of coffee, but we get caffeine from many sources (see Table 9-1).

Because it is a stimulant, caffeine relieves drowsiness, helps in the performance of repetitive tasks, and improves capacity for work. Caffeine also raises metabolic rate, so a caffeine user burns 3 to 4 percent more calories in an hour than a nonuser.[2] Some athletes feel that caffeine gives them an extra boost that allows them to go farther and longer in endurance events. But in addition, caffeine can trigger anxiety, insomnia, irregular heartbeat, faster breathing, upset stomach and bowels, dizziness, and headaches. Those who use caffeine heavily and then suddenly stop may suffer headaches, irritability, and fatigue.

Although there is no conclusive proof that caffeine causes birth defects, it does cross the placenta into the tissues of a growing fetus; the U.S. Surgeon General has recommended that pregnant women avoid or restrict their use of caffeine. Caffeine may also lower a woman's likelihood of conceiving, so women who hope to become pregnant might also want to cut out caffeine.

**TABLE 9-1** Learning to Look for Hidden Caffeine

| | CAFFEINE (MG) |
|---|---|
| Cup of instant freeze-dried coffee | 66 |
| Cup of regular coffee | 100–150 |
| Cup of decaffeinated coffee | 5 |
| Cup of cocoa | 50 |
| Cup of instant tea | 20–58 |
| Cup of black tea | 28–50 |
| Cup of green tea | 9–36 |
| Soft drink, 12 oz. | 32–65 |
| Chocolate bar | up to 25 |
| Excedrin, 32 mg | 65 |
| Nōdōz | 100 |

Switching to decaffeinated coffee may create rather than eliminate problems. Stanford University researchers have reported that when middle-aged men switched to decaf, their levels of harmful LDL cholesterol rose an average of 7 percent.[3] The reason may be the stronger type of beans used for decaffeinated brewing.

### Over-the-Counter Drugs

Americans spend more than $4 billion each year on drugs available without a prescription, referred to as **over-the-counter (OTC) drugs.** Individuals who take higher doses than recommended or who rely on these drugs for purposes other than those for which they were intended are misusing them. As a result, they could suffer side effects, particularly if they use OTCs in combination with other drugs, including alcohol. Alcohol can enhance the effects of many OTCs; it deepens the effects of **antihistamines** (antiallergy medications that cause drowsiness) and worsens the stomach irritation produced by aspirin.

The OTCs most often abused—intentionally or not—are painkillers, sedatives, and stimulants. Painkillers, called **analgesics,** can be used internally or externally. Internal analgesics, such as aspirin and acetaminophen, are taken by mouth. Aspirin relieves

**set** A person's expectations or preconceptions about a situation or experience.

**over-the-counter (OTC) drug** A medication that can be obtained legally without a prescription from a medical professional.

**antihistamine** A medication used to treat allergic reactions and cold symptoms; inactivates histamine, a substance found in body tissues that plays a role in allergic reactions.

**analgesic** A medication that relieves pain without inducing a loss of consciousness.

pain, lowers fever, and reduces inflammation and swelling in joints, but it can upset the stomach or aggravate ulcers. Acetaminophen relieves pain and reduces fever without causing intestinal side effects, but it isn't effective against inflammatory pain, such as arthritis. External painkillers are rubbed or sprayed on the skin and have effects like those of aspirin.

Drugs that relax the central nervous system to relieve anxiety or induce sleep are **sedatives.** Most OTC sedatives are really allergy medications containing antihistamines, which cause drowsiness. Some antihistamine preparations also contain aspirin or acetaminophen.

OTC stimulants contain about as much caffeine as one or two cups of coffee. They can produce the same side effects as coffee, including increased alertness, irritability, and nervousness.

## Prescription Drugs

Prescription drugs can be obtained only by order of a licensed physician or, in some cases, a dentist. The psychoactive medications most likely to be abused are sleeping pills, antianxiety medications, opiates, amphetamines, and steroids.[4]

In small doses, sedatives, such as Seconal and Nembutal, are calming; in larger doses, they induce sleep. Valium, Librium, and similar compounds relax the muscles and relieve anxiety. One tablet is roughly equivalent to one alcoholic drink. Users, who may begin taking antianxiety drugs to ease tension during a life crisis, can easily become dependent on them. Prescription **opiates** are analgesics, or painkillers, composed of morphine or codeine.

### Amphetamines

Amphetamines, once widely prescribed for weight control because they suppress the appetite, stimulate the central nervous system. In hyperactive children, the amphetamine Ritalin helps increase attention span. In narcoleptics, who suffer from irresistible attacks of sleepiness, amphetamines can prevent sudden episodes of sleep in dangerous situations, such as driving a car.

The side effects of amphetamines include extra strain on the heart. People who use amphetamines for long periods of time without medical supervision may develop a form of paranoia called amphetamine psychosis[5] (see the section on amphetamines and methamphetamine ("ice") later in this chapter).

**sedative** A drug that depresses the central nervous system, resulting in sleep or a trancelike state.
**opiate** A drug derived from opium.

Valium is one of the prescription drugs most likely to be abused.

### Anabolic Steroids

Anabolic steroids, synthetic derivatives of the male hormone testosterone, are powerful compounds prescribed for treatment of burns or injuries. Increasingly, weight lifters, football players and other athletes, as well as people who simply want to look athletic, have been buying and using these drugs illegally (see Chapter 5).

The potential side effects of anabolic steroid use include an increased risk of heart disease or stroke; liver tumors and jaundice; acne; transmission, through shared needles, of the virus that causes AIDS; breast enlargement in men; atrophy of the testicles; impotence; and deepened voice, breast reduction, and beard growth in women.

Users can become increasingly aggressive and paranoid, and they may explode in violent outbursts. Recent studies have found that steroids can be addictive and create the same problems with dependence and withdrawal as cocaine.[6–9]

**STRATEGY FOR CHANGE**

**Avoiding Prescription Drug Misuse**

Always be sure you know the answers to the following questions before leaving your physician's office with a prescription:

- What is the name of the drug, and what is it supposed to do?
- When should it be taken and for how long?
- What foods, drinks, other medicines, or activities should I avoid while taking this drug?
- Are there any possible side effects?
- Is there any written information on the drug?
- Is there any other treatment that might be equally effective?

## ILLEGAL DRUGS

By the time they reach their middle twenties, as many as 80 percent of young adults have tried an illegal drug.[10,11] Young people between the ages of 14 and 24 are the most likely to experiment with them. Some are lucky enough to satisfy their curiosity without getting hurt or caught. Others pay a terrible price. They lose their self-esteem, friends, well-being, and sometimes their lives.

**HEALTH HEADLINE**

**More Drugs Hit World Market**

**According to the U.S. State Department, worldwide production of opium, cocaine, hashish, and marijuana is soaring. From 1985 to 1990, opium production increased 187 percent; cocaine, 43 percent; and marijuana, 502 percent. Despite record drug seizures and international cooperation in the war on drugs, the glut of drugs is expected to lead to much greater drug availability and more widespread addiction throughout the world in the 1990s.**

SOURCE: Sciolino, Elaine. "World Drug Crop Up Sharply in 1989 Despite U.S. Effort," *New York Times*, March 2, 1990.

**STRATEGY FOR CHANGE**

**Alternatives to Drugs**

If you're looking for something extra in your life, consider these alternatives instead of drugs:

- If you need physical relaxation, try athletics, exercise, or outdoor hobbies.
- If you want to stimulate your senses, train yourself to be more sensitive to nature and beauty. Take time to appreciate the sensations you experience when you're walking in the woods or embracing a person you love.
- If you're anxious, depressed, or uptight and want relief from emotional pain, turn to people: in some cases, friends; in others, professional counselors or support groups.
- If you want to be accepted, volunteer in programs in which you can assist others and not focus on yourself.
- If you want to escape mental boredom, challenge your mind through reading, classes, creative games, discussion groups, memory training, or travel.
- If you want to enhance your creativity or your appreciation of the arts, pursue training in music, art, singing, or writing. Attend more concerts, museum shows, or dance performances.
- If you want to promote political or social change, volunteer in political campaigns or join lobbying and political action groups.
- If you want to find meaning in life or expand your personal awareness, explore various philosophical theories through classes, seminars, and discussion groups. Study yoga or meditation.
- If you're looking for kicks or adventure, sign up for a wilderness survival outing; take up boardsailing or rock-climbing.

### The Making of a Drug Habit

Mental health professionals have described several stages of drug dependency:

- *Stage 0: The Call to Do Drugs*—The villain, if there is one, is our society, in which "doing drugs" is common in many communities, on college campuses, and even in certain businesses. Young adults may try drugs because of peer pressure, curiosity, the lure of excitement, the need to belong, or the desire to rebel. Without parental support, strong coping skills, and an informed attitude, many teens find it difficult, almost impossible, to say no—if not the first time they're offered a drug, the second or the seventeenth.

- *Stage 1*—New users experience a chemically induced "high," which may be surprising and pleasant. The drugs most teens try first are alcohol and marijuana, and many use them whenever they're offered. Soon they become regular weekend users (see Table 9-2).
- *Stage 2*—Users no longer are content to wait for an offer to share a "high." Casual users begin to beg or buy; and the drug—whether it's alcohol or pot—makes it easier to cope with the agony of not making the team, not having a date, or not passing a course. Behavior begins changing at this point: Users may drop out of activities; stop seeing old friends; and may try other drugs, such as inhal-

**TABLE 9-2** Clinical Stages of Progressive Drug Abuse

| STAGE | MOOD ALTERATION | FEELINGS | DRUGS | SOURCES | BEHAVIOR | FREQUENCY |
|---|---|---|---|---|---|---|
| **Stage 1** Learning the mood swing | Euphoria, normal, pain | Feeling good, with few consequences | Tobacco, marijuana, and alcohol | Friends | Little detectable change; moderate "after-the-fact" lying | Progression to weekend use |
| **Stage 2** Seeking the mood swing | Euphoria, normal, pain | Excitement and early guilt | All of the above, plus inhalants, hash oil, "uppers," "downers," and prescription drugs | Buying | Extracurricular activities and hobbies dropped; mixed friends (straight and drug users); attire change; erratic school performance and attendance; unpredictable mood and attitude swings; "conning" behavior | Weekend use, progressing to 4 or 5 times per week; some solo use |
| **Stage 3** Preoccupation with the mood swing | Euphoria, normal, pain | Euphoric highs; doubts, including severe shame and guilt, depression, and suicidal thoughts | All of the above, plus mushrooms, PCP, LSD, and cocaine | Selling | "Cool" appearance; straight friends dropped; family fights (verbal and physical); stealing/police incidents; pathologic lying; school failure, skipping, and expulsion; jobs lost | Daily; frequent solo use |
| **Stage 4** Using drugs to feel normal | Euphoria, normal, pain | Chronic guilt, shame, remorse, and depression | Any available | Any possible | Physical deterioration (weight loss and chronic cough); severe mental deterioration (memory loss and flashbacks); paranoia, volcanic anger, and aggression; quitting school; frequent overdosing | All day, every day |

SOURCE: National Institute on Drug Abuse, 1982.

ants, hashish, or prescription pills. Boys may use drugs to seduce girls; girls may do drugs to be accepted by boys.

Despite the excitement of the forbidden, young users begin to feel shame and guilt as they start to lead double lives. They may feel hung over or suffer other side effects of drug use. To handle psychological and physical discomfort, they turn again to drugs, using drugs on their own and during the week, as well as with others on weekends. This is the stage at which a user is "hooked." By the end of it, there is little, if any, hope of turning back without outside help.

- *Stage 3*—Users are preoccupied with getting high. They start having fights with parents, old friends, and teachers. Because drugs are costing them more, they may steal or deal, and often end up in trouble with the police. Depressed, guilty, even suicidal, they seek chemical comfort and try other drugs, including LSD, PCP, and cocaine.
- *Stage 4*—Users will try any drug they can get, and they'll do almost anything to get drugs. They use more drugs more often, and drug consumption is the focus of their lives. They either drop out or are forced out of school. Physically, they suffer fatigue, weight loss, chronic coughs, and continuous aches. They start having blackouts, flashbacks, and episodes of violent or bizarre behavior, often triggered by their increasing paranoia. The risk of overdosing and possible death rises steadily—and they cannot change until they are drug-free. They are addicts, and their drug dependency has taken control of their lives.

**STRATEGY FOR CHANGE**

**How Can You Tell If Someone Is Abusing Drugs?**

The National Institute on Drug Abuse lists the following behaviors as indications of a drug problem:[12]

- an abrupt change in attitude, including a lack of interest in activities once enjoyed
- frequent vague, withdrawn moods
- a sudden decline in work or school performance or the regular skipping of classes
- a sudden resistance to discipline or criticism
- secret telephone calls and meetings and a demand for greater privacy in terms of personal possessions
- increased frustration levels
- changes in sleeping and eating habits
- a sudden weight loss
- evidence of drug use (smell of marijuana, drug paraphernalia)
- frequent borrowing of money
- stealing
- disregard for personal appearance
- impaired relationships with family and friends
- disregard for deadlines, curfews, or other regulations
- unusual flare-ups of temper
- new friends, especially known drug users, and strong allegiance to these friends

### Polyabuse

Most users prefer a certain type of drug but use several others; this is called **polyabuse**. The average user who enters treatment is on five different drugs. The more drugs anyone uses, the greater the chance of side effects, complications, and possibly life-threatening interactions.

## PSYCHOACTIVE DRUGS

Legal or illegal, all psychoactive drugs affect the central nervous system. This chapter divides psychoactive drugs into the following partially overlapping categories: stimulants, depressants, antianxiety drugs, cannabis products, psychedelics and hallucinogens, narcotics, inhalants, and designer drugs (see Table 9-3).

### Stimulants

**Stimulants** act on the central nervous system and increase the heart rate, blood pressure, strength of heart contractions, blood sugar level, and muscle tension. These internal changes put extra stress on the body.

### Cocaine

Cocaine ("coke," "snow," "lady") is a drug extracted from the leaves of the South American coca plant and sometimes used as a surgical anesthetic. It is usually sold as a crystallike powder. Approximately 5 million Americans use cocaine regularly; almost 3 million may be addicted. As many as 30 percent of college students report trying cocaine before their fourth year of college. Though the number of people using

**polyabuse** The use of more than one drug.
**stimulant** Any substance that excites the central nervous system.

**Table 9-3** Common Drugs of Abuse

| DRUGS | WHAT THEY DO | HEALTH EFFECTS | LONG-TERM RISKS |
|---|---|---|---|
| **Cocaine and crack** | Speed up physical and mental processes; create sense of heightened energy and confidence | Headaches, exhaustion, shaking, blurred vision, nausea, seizures, loss of appetite, loss of sexual desire, impotence, impaired judgment, hyperactivity, babbling, extreme suspiciousness, violence. | Damage to nose (if snorted), blood vessels and heart; chest pain; heart attack; disruptions in heart rhythm; stroke; damage to liver and lungs (if smoked); hepatitis and HIV (if injected). If used in pregnancy, increased danger of miscarriage and physical and mental impairment for the fetus. |
| **Amphetamines** | Speed up physical and mental processes; lessen fatigue; boost energy; create sense of excitement | Loss of appetite, blurred vision, headache, dizziness, sweating, sleeplessness, trembling, anxiety, suspiciousness, delusions, hallucinations. | Malnutrition, skin disorders, ulcers, lack of sleep, depression, vitamin deficiencies, brain damage, high blood pressure, stroke, high fever, heart failure, violent behavior, fatal overdose. |
| **Barbiturates** | Produce mild intoxication, drowsiness and lethargy, decrease alertness | Drowsiness, poor coordination, slurred speech, cold skin, slowed breathing, weak and rapid heartbeat, impaired judgment, hangover, sleepiness, confusion, irritability. | Disrupted sleep; dangerously impaired vision. As users need higher doses, increased risk of fatal overdose. Withdrawal can produce extreme anxiety, insomnia, delirium, and convulsions. If used in pregnancy, can cause birth defects and behavioral problems. |
| **Antianxiety drugs (benzodiazepines, such as Valium and Librium)** | Slow down the central nervous system | Slurred speech, drowsiness, stupor. | Physical and psychological dependence, fatal overdose. Withdrawal can lead to coma, psychosis, death. |
| **Marijuana and hashish** | Relax the mind and body; alter mood; heighten perceptions | Faster heartbeat and pulse, dry mouth and throat, impaired perception and reactions, lethargy, nausea, possible hallucinations, panic attacks, decreased motivation. | Psychological dependence; impaired thinking, perception, memory and coordination; increased heart rate and blood pressure; dampened immunity. If used in pregnancy, babies are more likely to have small heads, poor growth, lower birth weight, and other abnormalities. |

*(Continued)*

**Table 9-3** Common Drugs of Abuse *(Continued)*

| DRUGS | WHAT THEY DO | HEALTH EFFECTS | LONG-TERM RISKS |
|---|---|---|---|
| **Psychedelics (LSD, mescaline, PCP, designer drugs)** | Alter perceptions and produce hallucinations, which may be frightening or pleasurable | Increased heart rate, blood pressure and body temperature, headache, nausea, sweating, trembling, "bad trips" on LSD. PCP can produce delusions of great strength and invulnerability and trigger violent attacks. | With LSD, disturbing flashbacks, psychological dependence. Effects on fetus not known. With PCP, stupor, increased heart rate and blood pressure, coma, convulsions, heart and lung failure, ruptured blood vessels in the brain, death. MDMA can lead to brain damage. |
| **Opiates (opium, morphine, heroin, or synthetic narcotics)** | Relax the central nervous system, relieve pain, produce temporary sense of well-being | Restlessness, nausea, vomiting, slowed breathing, weight loss, lethargy, mood swings, slurred speech, sweating. | Physical dependence, malnutrition, lower immunity, infections of the heart lining and valves, skin abscesses, congested lungs, hepatitis, tetanus, liver disease, AIDS (from infected needles), fatal overdose. |
| **Inhalants** | Produce temporary feelings of well-being, giddiness, hallucinations | Nausea, sneezing, coughing, nosebleeds, lack of coordination, loss of appetite, decreased heart and breathing rates, impaired judgment, loss of consciousness. | Hepatitis, liver failure, kidney failure, respiratory impairment, blood abnormalities, irregular heartbeat, possible suffocation. |

cocaine occasionally has dropped, the number who use cocaine more than once a week has grown.[13,14]

Once cocaine was an exotic drug of the very rich, the "champagne" of recreational drugs. Today newer, less expensive (and more dangerous) forms of cocaine have made it the drug of choice among the urban poor and among suburban teenagers, as well as among performers, athletes, and executives. Crack (a smokeable form of cocaine) once was mainly an inner-city problem; now this drug—like many others—has spread to the suburbs and to the middle and upper class.

The typical cocaine user is a young man with a higher-than-average income. The highest rates of cocaine use are among young white men (18 to 25 years of age) in the West and Northeast, most of whom also use alcohol and marijuana. However, cocaine use among women, particularly young ones, is on the rise.

The immediate effects of cocaine last for only 5 to 15 minutes because it is rapidly metabolized by the liver. With repeated use the brain becomes tolerant of cocaine's stimulant effects, so users must take more of the drug to get high. Its physical effects include headaches, exhaustion, shaking, blurred vision, nausea, seizures, loss of appetite so severe that it can lead to dramatic weight loss and malnutrition, loss of sexual desire, and impotence (Figure 9-2).

**Crack** This smokeable mixture of cocaine and baking soda or a similar substance is known as **crack,** for the popping sound it makes when burned, or **rock,** for its appearance. Smoked in a glass water pipe, a small piece, or "quarter rock," of crack produces a 20- to 30-minute high and sells for as little as $10 to $15. It is often purchased at "crack houses," where eager buyers slip their money through a slot in the door and receive crack in return. Because it sets off rapid

**crack** A smokeable form of cocaine that is highly addictive.
**rock** See *crack*.

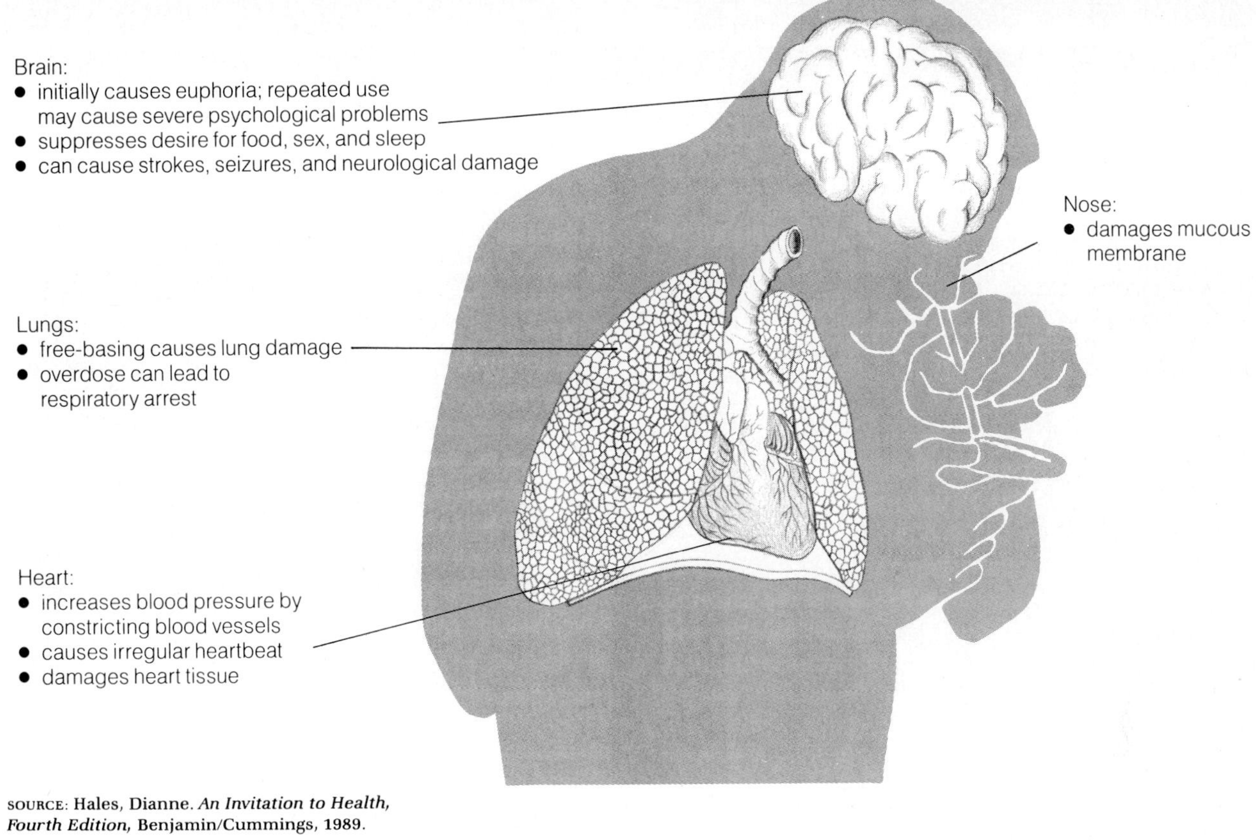


SOURCE: Hales, Dianne. *An Invitation to Health, Fourth Edition,* Benjamin/Cummings, 1989.

**FIGURE 9-2** Effects of cocaine on the body.

ups and downs, crack causes a powerful chemical and psychological dependence. As soon as users come down from one high, they want more crack. A heroin addict may shoot up several times a day, but crack addicts need another hit within minutes. Thus a crack habit can quickly become more expensive than heroin addiction. Some addicts have $1,000-a-day habits.

Crack makes its users active, paranoid, and dangerous. Police in big cities have traced many brutal crimes, including murders, to young crack addicts. Smoking crack doused with liquid PCP, a practice called "space-basing," has especially frightening effects on behavior.

**Methods of Cocaine Use** The three common methods of cocaine ingestion are snorting, smoking (called free-basing), and injection. All can produce serious ill effects, but smoking and injection are the most dangerous.

When sniffed or snorted, cocaine anesthetizes the nerve endings in the nose. It then relaxes the lung's bronchial muscles. Smoking cocaine speeds its absorption. The blood vessels constrict and the heart muscles are overstimulated; the result can be a heart attack or respiratory failure.[15]

Many cocaine users inject the drug, at least occasionally. However, because the cocaine high lasts only 20 minutes, addicts must shoot up so frequently that

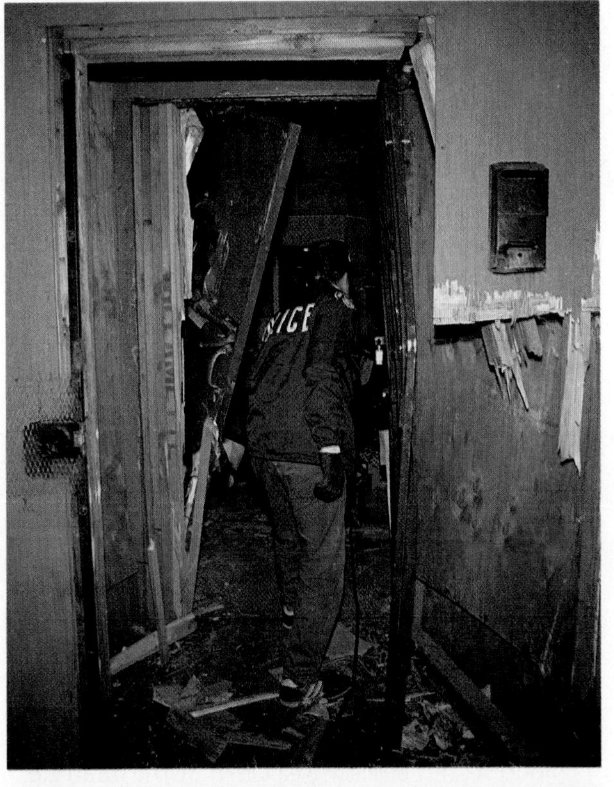

"Crack houses" have turned many neighborhoods into dangerous places for children and families.

## HALES INDEX

Number of times medications are not taken as prescribed: 1 in 4

Number of male high school seniors who've used anabolic steroids: 1 in 20

Amount users spend on illicit drugs a year: $79 billion

Number of college students who've used an illegal drug at least once: 1 in 2

Number of Americans who use cocaine regularly: 5 million

Number of Americans who've tried cocaine at least once: 30 million

Number of people who try crack who become addicted: 1 in 6

Number of Americans who've tried marijuana: 1 in 3

Number of college students who've used MDMA (ecstasy) at least once: 1 in every 3 to 5

Number of Americans who would report their best friend if he or she was selling cocaine: 1 in 3

Annual costs of drug abuse, including treatment, reduced productivity, lost employment, welfare payments, and imprisonment: $60 billion

SOURCES: **1** Cramer, Joyce et al. "How Often Is Medication Taken as Prescribed?" *Journal of the American Medical Association,* June 9, 1989. **2** Kashkin, K. B. and H. D. Kleber. "Hooked on Hormones?," *Journal of the American Medical Association,* January 11, 1990. **3** "Survey Says Drug Use Down Among Young," *San Francisco Chronicle,* February 14, 1990. **4** "At Last, Some Good News," *Time,* February 26, 1990. **5, 6** Altman, Lawrence. "Cocaine's Many Dangers: The Evidence Mounts," *New York Times,* January 26, 1988. **7** Kolata, Gina. "Experts Finding New Hope on Treating Crack Addicts," *New York Times,* August 24, 1989. **8** Carper, Jean. *Health Care U.S.A.* New York: Prentice-Hall, 1989. **9** Phillips, Pat. "Ecstasy Makes Clouded Comeback," *Medical World News,* March 13, 1989. **10** "Public Polled on Attitudes about Cocaine Users, Sellers," *American Medical News,* February 16, 1990. **11** National Institute of Drug Abuse.

they severely damage their veins. A particularly dangerous, and often deadly, practice is injection of a "speedball," a combination of cocaine and heroin. If cocaine users share needles, they put themselves at risk for another lethal problem: infection that causes AIDS virus (see Chapter 15 for a complete discussion of AIDS). Other complications of injecting cocaine include skin infections, hepatitis, inflammation of the arteries, and infection of the lining of the heart.

**Cocaine's Effects on the Brain and Body** As recent research has shown, cocaine, which may be deadlier than heroin, can trigger heart attacks (even in young, healthy people), strokes, destruction of the liver, and other serious complications, including the following:[16]

- *Heart and Blood Vessels*—Cocaine causes blood vessels to tighten, the heart rate to speed up, and blood pressure to rise suddenly. It can also trigger potentially fatal disruptions of the heart's rhythm. These effects can lead to a shortage of oxygen for the heart, which can cause chest pain (angina) or a heart attack. Cocaine can also cause spasms that reduce or shut the flow of blood that nourishes the heart. A sudden rise in blood pressure can damage and even rupture or break the walls of blood vessels already weakened by the build-up of fatty deposits (this condition is called atherosclerosis). Researchers have found that cocaine directly and permanently damages heart muscle by creating red streaks called contraction bands that impair the normal beating of the heart. (See Chapter 13 for more information on the heart.)
- *Brain*—A powerful stimulant to the central nervous system, cocaine produces feelings of soaring well-being (euphoria) and boundless energy. Users feel overly confident of their physical and mental ability. Repeated or high doses can lead to impaired judgment, hyperactivity, nonstop babbling, and paranoia (extreme feelings of suspicion) so severe it could trigger violence. The brain never learns to tolerate cocaine's negative effects, so users become increasingly anxious and suffer hallucinations and suicidal ideas.[17]

  Cocaine can also cause blood vessels in the brain to clamp shut and can trigger a stroke, bleeding in the brain, and potentially fatal brain seizures. Cocaine users can also develop psychiatric or neurological complications.
- *Reproductive System*—Although some users initially try cocaine as a sexual stimulant, it does not enhance sexual performance. At low doses, it may delay ejaculation and orgasm and cause heightened sensory awareness. However, men who use cocaine regularly have problems maintaining erections and ejaculating. Both male and female

cocaine users tend to lose interest in sex and have difficulty in reaching orgasm.

- *Nasal Passages*—Frequent snorting can irritate and damage the mucous membrane in the nose and destroy a user's sense of smell.
- *Other Organ Systems*—Cocaine can damage the liver and cause lung damage in free-basers. Some smokers have died of respiratory complications, such as pulmonary edema (the buildup of fluid in the lungs).
- *Pregnancy*—Cocaine, which is dangerous for pregnant women and their babies, causes miscarriages, developmental disorders, and life-threatening complications during birth. Women who use cocaine while pregnant are more likely to miscarry in the first 3 months of pregnancy than women who don't use drugs and than heroin and narcotic users.[18]

  Infants born to cocaine users suffer major complications, including withdrawal and permanent disabilities. Because cocaine affects blood pressure, it can deprive a fetal brain of oxygen or cause brain vessels to burst, so the fetus suffers the prenatal equivalent of a stroke, which can cause permanent physical and mental damage. Cocaine babies have higher-than-normal rates of respiratory and kidney troubles and may be at greater risk of sudden infant death syndrome. Visual problems, lack of coordination, and developmental retardation are common.[19]

**Dependence** Five to 20 percent of coke users—a group as large as the estimated number of heroin addicts—are dependent on cocaine and experience nervousness, nausea, sleep loss, weight loss, increased blood pressure and heart rate, paranoia, hallucinations, and even general convulsions. An hour after these behavioral and physical effects subside, a heavy coke user may experience anxiety, shakiness, irritability, fatigue, depression, and a craving for more cocaine. These withdrawal symptoms are referred to as "crashing."

Cocaine is a hard habit to break. Some psychiatrists are trying a medical approach by using antidepressant drugs that block cocaine's impact on the brain. Crack users have enormous difficulty overcoming their addiction. One new approach for crack addicts is acupuncture—the use of carefully placed needles, which may stimulate brain chemicals called endorphins that block the pain of withdrawal.[20,21]

## Amphetamines

Amphetamine pills are sold under a variety of names: amphetamine (trade name Benzedrine, or "bennies"), dextroamphetamine (Dexedrine, or "dex"), methamphetamine (Methedrine, or "meth" or "speed"), and Desoxyn ("copilots"). Related uppers include methylphenidate (Ritalin), pemoline (Cylert), and phenmetrazine (Preludin).

Amphetamines lessen fatigue, and improve concentration and physical performance. In addition, abuse of these drugs can produce **euphoria,** a feeling of well-being or elation. In pure form, amphetamines are tablets or capsules. Abusers may grind and sniff the capsules or make a solution and inject the drug. A new, smokeable form of methamphetamine is known as "ice."

**Effects** Amphetamines increase heart and breathing rates and blood pressure, dilate pupils, and decrease appetite. Users may experience a dry mouth, sweating, headache, blurred vision, dizziness, sleeplessness, and anxiety. Extremely high doses can cause a rapid or irregular heartbeat, tremors, loss of coordination, and even collapse.

Psychologically, amphetamines make users feel restless, anxious, irritable, and moody. Higher doses make the user feel "wired"—talkative, confident, and powerful. Prolonged use of large amounts of amphetamines can induce psychosis: seeing, hearing, and feeling things that don't exist; having delusions (irrational thoughts or beliefs); and feeling paranoid (as if everyone is out to get you). People in this suspicious state may become violent.

The long-term effects of amphetamine abuse include malnutrition; skin disorders; ulcers; lack of sleep; depression; vitamin deficiencies; and, in some cases, brain damage resulting in speech and thought disturbances. Amphetamines taken intravenously, rather than in tablet form, and in high doses over a long period of time can create a sudden increase in blood pressure that can cause death from stroke, very high fever, or heart failure.[22]

Users may develop tolerance and dependence and continue to take the amphetamine in larger doses to prevent the "down" mood when its effects wear off. When a person has been using amphetamines in high doses (100 mg or more a day for several weeks) and then stops, deep sleep occurs. It can last for days and is followed by withdrawal; symptoms include lethargy, intense hunger, emotional depression, disturbed sleep, and increased dreaming. These symptoms usually peak within four days of quitting, but depression and irritability may persist for months.

---

**euphoria** A feeling of well-being or elation.

### Ice

A smokeable form of methamphetamine ("ice", "crystal," "crystal meth"), a synthetic stimulant popularly known as "speed," may become a major drug of abuse in the 1990s. Smoking ice increases heart rate and blood pressure; high doses can cause permanent damage to blood vessels in the brain. Other physical effects include blurred vision, dry mouth, and increased breathing rate. Prolonged use can cause fatal lung and kidney disorders and psychological problems, including amphetamine psychosis, a state of paranoia in which users lose touch with reality and believe they're being watched or chased. Some users experience terrifying sensations, such as the feeling that spiders are crawling under their skin. Babies born to ice-using mothers show severe behavioral disturbances, including tremors and prolonged crying.[23]

Produced in the Philippines, Taiwan, Korea, and Japan, ice first became popular in Hawaii, where police describe Honolulu as being trapped in an "Ice Age."[24] The drug is cheaper to produce than crack, is more addictive than heroin, and produces an intense physical and psychological high that can last from 4 to 14 hours. Ice is odorless and cannot be easily detected in public.

### Crank

*Crank* is the street term for propylhexedrine, a central nervous system stimulant that is less potent than amphetamine. Abusers often extract the drug from decongestant inhalants and inject it intravenously. The injections produce effects similar to those of amphetamine. Users may feel high or may hallucinate and lose contact with reality. Injecting propylhexedrine can lead to convulsions, strokes, and respiratory and kidney failure. Also, abusers can develop infected veins; if they share needles, they can be infected with the virus that causes AIDS.

### Look-alikes and Act-alikes

Drugs manufactured to look like real amphetamines and to mimic their effects are called **look-alikes**. They usually contain legal stimulants, such as caffeine, ephedrine, and phenylpropanolamine (used in diet pills). **Act-alikes**—manufactured to get around new state laws prohibiting look-alikes—contain the same ingredients as look-alikes but don't physically resemble any legal drugs. They're sold on the street as "speed" or "uppers," even though they're not as strong as amphetamines. Young people who buy them are often told they're legal, safe, and harmless. However, in large quantities, they can produce all the negative effects of amphetamines.

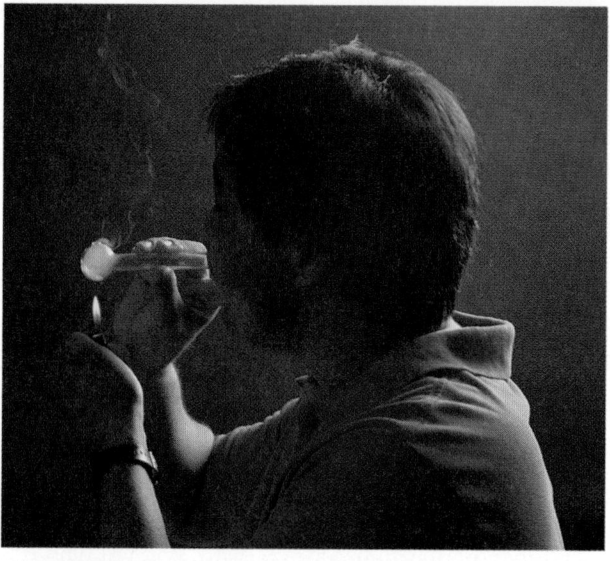

"Ice," a smokeable form of methamphetamine, is cheaper than crack and more addictive than heroine.

## Depressants

Drugs that relax the central nervous system are called **depressants,** sedatives or **hypnotics;** the most widely used is alcohol (see Chapter 10). Others are the barbiturates, both long- and short-acting; nonbarbiturate sedatives; and antianxiety medications. The lowest dose may relieve you of anxiety, but increasing doses can cause disinhibition, sedation, sleep, anesthesia, coma, and death.

Depressants have a synergistic effect when they are mixed together. If your driving ability is already impaired by alcohol, taking barbiturates will make your driving even worse. As you develop tolerance for one sedative or become dependent on it, you will also develop tolerance for other sedatives. This is an example of **cross-tolerance** or **cross-addiction.**

### Barbiturates and Related Drugs

Barbiturates, which are used medically for inducing relaxation and sleep, relieving tension, and treating epileptic seizures, are usually taken by mouth in tablet, capsule, or liquid form. When used as a general anesthetic, they are administered intravenously.

**look-alike** A drug manufactured to look like real amphetamine and to mimic its effects.
**act-alike** A drug manufactured to get around state laws prohibiting look-alikes.
**depressant** A drug that relaxes the central nervous system.
**hypnotic** A drug that induces sleep or a trancelike state.
**cross-tolerance** The capacity to endure the effects of psychoactive substances similar to one for which a tolerance has developed.
**cross-addiction** A state of physical dependence in which physiological need for one psychoactive substance leads to dependence on similar substances.

Barbiturates such as pentobarbital (trade name Nembutal, or "yellow jackets"), secobarbital (Seconal, or "reds"), and thiopental (Pentothal) are rapidly absorbed into the brain. The longer-acting barbiturates, such as amobarbital (trade name Amytal, or "blues" or "downers") and phenobarbital (Luminal, or "phennies"), take longer to penetrate the brain and keep a person drowsy for several hours.

Used in low dosages, barbiturates produce mild intoxication and euphoria and decrease alertness and muscle coordination. With a higher dosage, a person may show slurred speech, slow respiration, cold skin, and a weak and rapid heartbeat, and may become unconscious. A user's mind-set definitely affects the amount of relief barbiturates bring from anxiety or depression.

Side effects include drowsiness, impaired judgment and performance, and a hangover that may last for hours or even days. Eventually barbiturates lead to a physical dependence. People addicted to barbiturates tend to be sleepy, confused, or irritable.

Barbiturates are a factor in nearly a third of all reported drug-related deaths. As the user builds up tolerance, the likelihood of a potentially fatal overdose increases. Withdrawal is time-consuming and difficult to manage medically. Symptoms include anxiety, insomnia, delirium, and convulsions. Occasionally, an abrupt ending of barbiturate use leads to the user's death.

Barbiturates can easily cross through the placenta and cause birth defects and behavioral problems. Babies born to women who abused sedatives during pregnancy may be physically dependent on the drugs and may develop breathing problems, feeding difficulties, disturbed sleep, sweating, irritability, and fever.

### Methaqualone

Methaqualone, often called "the love drug," because it once was considered an aphrodisiac, is marketed under a variety of trade names, such as Quaalude ("ludes" or "Q") and Sopor ("sopors"). Its dangers include physical and psychological dependence, injury or death from car accidents caused by faulty judgment and drowsiness, convulsions, coma, and death from overdose. The combination of methaqualone and alcohol is particularly dangerous.

## Antianxiety Drugs

The primary antianxiety drugs, used for tension or muscular strain, are benzodiazepines. They are sold in a variety of compounds such as chlordiazepoxide (Librium), diazepam (Valium), oxazepam (Serax), and flurazepam (Dalmane). Another group of tranquilizing drugs are the dicarbamates—including meprobamate, which is sold under such trade names as Equanil and Miltown. These drugs produce sedation for up to 10 hours or longer.

The benzodiazepines, absorbed slowly into the bloodstream, take a while to reach the brain, but they have an effect for several days. Like the barbiturates, high doses of these drugs produce slurred speech, drowsiness, and stupor. You can become both psychologically and physically dependent on these drugs within 2 to 4 weeks. Withdrawal symptoms may include coma, psychosis, and even death.

**HEALTH HEADLINE**

**More Students Saying No to Drugs**

**The percentage of high school seniors and college students who use drugs has fallen to about half of what it was a decade ago, according to a University of Michigan poll. The percentage using drugs in 1989 was 19.7, down from 21.3 percent in 1988 and about 40 percent in 1979. In 1979, nearly 11 percent of high school seniors smoked marijuana daily; in 1989, only 2.9 percent did. In 1979, 33.5 percent of seniors thought trying cocaine once or twice was risky; a decade later 54.9 percent were wary of trying cocaine even once.**

SOURCE: Jones, Laurie. "U.S. Teen Drug Use Dropped in 1989, Survey Finds," *American Medical News*, February 23, 1990.

## Cannabis Products

Marijuana ("pot," "grass") is a mixture of the crushed leaves and flowers of *Cannabis sativa*, or hemp, one of the oldest cultivated nonfood plants. Hashish is an extract of cannabis that is 2 to 10 times as concentrated as marijuana. In both, the primary psychoactive ingredient is **tetrahydrocannabinol (THC).**

Marijuana use has been falling ever since the late 1970s. In 1990, 42 percent of college students reported using it, compared to 51 percent in 1980. Nearly one of every three Americans over age 12 has tried marijuana at least once.[25]

**tetrahydrocannabinol (THC)** The primary psychoactive ingredient in marijuana and hashish.

Cannabis is being used experimentally as a legal medical therapy for severe nausea in cancer patients undergoing chemotherapy. Researchers are also continuing studies of marijuana's possible usefulness in reducing pressure within the eye in glaucoma and in treating muscle spasticity.

Usually, marijuana is smoked in a cigarette ("joint") or pipe; it may also be eaten along with other foods (as in brownies), though with a less predictable effect. The high depends on how long a person can hold the marijuana smoke in the lungs, which means that experienced smokers usually feel stronger effects. Also, different types of marijuana have different percentages of THC. Due to careful cultivation, the strength of today's marijuana is about 10 times greater than that of the pot used in the 1970s; the physical and mental effects are also greater.

Marijuana smoke contains more than 400 chemicals besides THC, including some similar to the tobacco tars implicated in lung cancer. Smoking about five marijuana cigarettes a day narrows the air passages and inflames their lining. Heavy, long-term use can lead to bronchitis, just as tobacco smoking does. Being in a room with pot smokers can make nonusers experience similar psychoactive effects—and cause their urine to test positive for drug use.

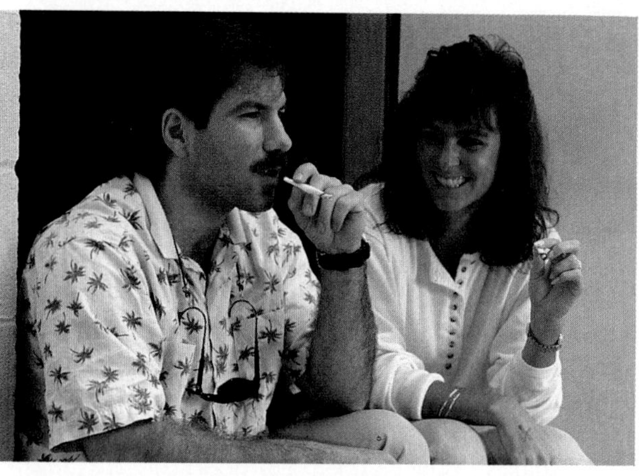

A single joint may be as damaging to the lungs as smoking five tobacco cigarettes.

**Effects of Marijuana** At low to moderate doses, marijuana acts somewhat like alcohol and some tranquilizers and it takes effect within minutes. Unlike alcohol, marijuana at low doses does not dull sensation, but it may cause slight alterations in perception. It is not safe to drive a car for as long as 4 to 6 hours after a single joint.

The immediate physical effects of marijuana include faster heartbeat and pulse rate, bloodshot eyes, and dry mouth and throat. High doses diminish the ability to perceive and to react and may intensify all the reactions experienced with low doses: sensory distortion and, in the case of hashish, vivid hallucinations and LSD-like psychedelic reactions. Some people suffer acute panic attacks.

Long-term regular users of marijuana may become psychologically dependent. Some experience "burnout," a dulling of their senses and responses. Teenagers who smoke pot regularly often lose interest in school and don't remember what they learned when they were high. Marijuana seems to impair thinking, reading comprehension, and verbal and mathematical skills.

Smoking a single joint may be as damaging to the lungs as smoking five tobacco cigarettes. Marijuana smokers absorb nearly 5 times as much carbon monoxide into their blood streams and inhale 3 times as much tar as tobacco smokers.

Among marijuana's other physiological and psychological effects are the following:

- *Central Nervous System*—Marijuana impairs coordination and short-term memory, slows learning, and distorts sensory perception.
- *Respiratory System*—Marijuana users show signs of impaired lung functioning when compared to nonusers.
- *Cardiovascular System*—Marijuana increases the heart rate and sometimes the blood pressure, posing greatest risk to those with hypertension and heart disease.
- *Reproductive System*—Marijuana may suppress ovulation and alter hormone levels in female users and may impair fertility of male users. The frequent use of marijuana during pregnancy can lower birth weight and cause abnormalities similar to those of the fetal alcohol syndrome. Women who smoke pot while pregnant are more likely to have babies with problems such as small head size, irritability, and poor growth.
- *Immune System*—Animal studies have suggested that marijuana can dampen the body's resistance to disease.
- *Gateway to Other Drugs*—Fewer than 1 percent of people who've never used marijuana ever use cocaine. Many people who try marijuana just a few times never experiment with other drugs. However, 73 percent of those who've smoked pot at least 1,000 times have also used cocaine.[26]

SELF-SURVEY

## Do You Have a Drug Problem?

To assess whether you have a drug problem, answer the following questions, based on the American Psychiatric Association's *Diagnostic and Statistical Manual of Mental Disorders*, 3d edition, revised.

- Have you tried repeatedly to cut down or control drug abuse?
- Are you unable to fulfill social or work obligations because of your drug use? For example, do you skip classes because you're high or crashing?
- Do you need to take more of the drug to get its desired effects? If you use a constant amount of the drug, do you feel diminished effects?
- Do you feel specific symptoms if you cut back or stop using the drug?
- Are you preoccupied with getting or taking the drug?
- Do you forego important social, occupational, or recreational activities in order to get or take the drug?
- Do you frequently take another psychoactive substance to relieve withdrawal symptoms (a drink to relieve shakiness, for instance)?
- Do you frequently use the drug in larger doses or over a longer period than is recommended?
- Do you continue to use the drug despite a physical or mental disorder, or a significant problem that you realize is exacerbated by drug use (such as low grades or family conflict)?
- Have you developed a mental or physical disorder or condition because of prolonged drug use (for example, nasal problems because of cocaine sniffing)?

If you answered yes to three or more of these questions, you are dependent on a drug and should seek professional help.

Marijuana is illegal in most places. Under federal law, a person can be sentenced to up to one year in jail or ordered to pay a $5,000 fine, or both, for possession of marijuana.

## Psychedelics and Hallucinogens

Some **psychedelics** and **hallucinogens**, including peyote and psilocybin, have long been used in the religious rituals of some North American and Central American Indians. Others, such as LSD and PCP, have become widespread within only the last two decades.

### Peyote, Mescaline, and Derivatives

Peyote is a spineless cactus with a small crown, or button, that is dried and then swallowed. The active ingredient in peyote is **mescaline.** When eaten, mescaline affects the brain within 30 to 90 minutes, and effects may persist for 12 hours. The average dose may produce vivid hallucinations, including brightly colored lights, animals, and geometric designs.

**psychedelic** A drug that produces a heightened sense of reality; visual hallucinations; and, in some instances, psychoticlike behaviors.
**hallucinogen** A drug that causes hallucinations.
**mescaline** A drug obtained from the mescal cactus; causes hallucinations, euphoria, and a heightened sense of awareness.

### LSD

LSD (lysergic acid diethylamide, or "acid"), initially used as a tool to explore mental illness, became popular among the hippies and flower children of the 1960s. LSD is taken orally, usually with another substance such as a sugar cube, because the dosage needed is so small—100 to 200 micrograms. (A shirt button is about the size of a gram; a microgram is one-millionth the size of the button.) LSD is 1,000 times more potent than most other drugs.

LSD produces hallucinations, including bright colors and altered perceptions of reality. These effects begin within 30 to 60 minutes and last 10 to 12 hours. During this time, there are slight increases in body temperature, heart rate, and blood pressure; sweating, chills, and goose pimples appear. Some users develop a headache and nausea. The most common disturbing reaction to the drug is a "bad trip," an acute anxiety reaction that may trigger panic, depression, confusion, fear of insanity, and distorted thoughts and perceptions. LSD users have injured or killed themselves by jumping out of windows, swimming out to sea, or throwing themselves in front of cars. In some unstable persons, LSD may trigger psychotic episodes. Although there is no evidence that LSD creates physical dependence, it may well create psychological dependence. The most common delayed reaction is the flashback, in which individuals reexperience the perceptual and emotional changes originally produced by the drug. LSD's potential impact on a fetus is unknown.[27]

### Psilocybin

Obtained from the so-called magic mushroom *Psilocybe stunzii*, psilocybin is not as potent as LSD, but it can produce hallucinations and distortions of time and space at doses of 5 to 15 mg. Psilocybin is popular among Indians in Central America for religious use, but the psilocybin sold on the streets in the United States is likely to be LSD or supermarket mushrooms sprayed with LSD or PCP.

### PCP

PCP (phencyclidine—trade name Sernyl, "angel dust," "peace pill," "lovely," or "green") is manufactured as a tablet, capsule, liquid, flake, spray, or crystallike white powder that can be swallowed, smoked, sniffed, or injected. Sometimes it is sprinkled on crack, marijuana, tobacco, or parsley, and smoked. A fine powdered form of PCP can be snorted or injected.

Once PCP was thought to have medicinal value as an anesthetic. But its side effects, including delirium and hallucinations, made it unacceptable for medical use. PCP and similar anesthetics resemble, but are not true psychedelics.

PCP use peaked in the 1970s, but it is still a popular drug of abuse in both inner-city ghettos and suburban high schools. According to the National Institute of Drug Abuse, while use of other drugs has generally declined, PCP use has increased among teenagers.[28]

PCP's greatest danger is its **behavioral toxicity**—what it causes users to do to themselves and to others. It can trigger psychotic attacks that turn normal people temporarily insane and sometimes violent. Because of its delusional effects, users feel they have superhuman strength and abilities; because of its anesthetic effects, they feel no pain.

The effects of PCP are utterly unpredictable. It may trigger violent behavior or irreversible psychosis the first time it is used, or the twentieth, or never. In low doses (5 to 10 mg), PCP produces changes—from hallucinations to feelings of emptiness or drowsiness—similar to those produced by other psychoactive drugs. As with alcohol, the user may experience double vision, nausea, and muscular incoordination. Higher doses may produce a stupor that lasts several days, increased heart rate and blood pressure, flushing, sweating, dizziness, and numbness. Taking large amounts can lead to convulsions, coma, heart and lung failure, ruptured blood vessels in the brain, and death.

## Narcotics

Although the word *narcotics* is often used to refer to all illicit drugs, **narcotics** are really only one type of psychoactive drugs. Narcotics include the opiates—opium and its derivatives, morphine, codeine, and heroin—and some other nonopiate synthetic drugs, all of which have sleep-inducing and pain-relieving properties. Narcotics are used medically to relieve pain, but they have a high potential for abuse. Some narcotics, including opium, morphine, heroin, and codeine, come from a resin taken from the seedpod of the Asian poppy. Others, such as meperidine (Demerol), are manufactured.

All of the opiates relax the user. When injected, they may produce an immediate rush. They can also produce restlessness, nausea, vomiting and "nodding" (shifting from alertness to drowsiness). With large doses, the pupils become smaller. The skin becomes cold, moist, and bluish. Breathing slows down; the user cannot be awakened and may die. Over time, opiate users may develop infections of the heart lining and valves, skin abscesses, and congested lungs. Infections from unsterile solutions, syringes, and needles can lead to hepatitis, tetanus, liver disease, and infection with the virus that causes AIDS.

Dependence is very likely, especially among those who use a lot of the drug or use it over a long time. If a narcotics addict stops taking the drug, withdrawal begins within 4 to 6 hours, producing uneasiness, abdominal cramps, diarrhea, chills, sweating, and nausea. The intensity of the symptoms depends on the extent of the addiction; they may get stronger for 24 to 72 hours and subside within 7 to 10 days.

### Opium

Opium, a natural derivative of the opium poppy, may be smoked, long the custom in Asian cultures, or it may be sniffed as a powder. In both cases, it affects

**behavioral toxicity** Having harmful effects on an individual's actions and attitudes.

**narcotic** An addictive drug that relieves pain and induces sleep; derived from opium, or is chemically similar to such derivatives.

the central nervous system very rapidly. Two organic substances that can be extracted from it, morphine and codeine, are used extensively in medicine.

**Morphine** Morphine—which acts primarily on the central nervous system, eyes, and digestive tract—masks pain by producing mental clouding, drowsiness, and often euphoria. It does not decrease the physical sensation of pain as much as it alters a person's awareness of the pain; in effect, a patient no longer cares about pain.

Use of morphine may result in nausea and vomiting and in a decrease in the rate of respiration; in high doses it can depress respiration to the point of death. Its effects vary greatly, depending on the individual. Some people experience very unpleasant feelings, such as anxiety and fear.

**Codeine** Codeine appears naturally in opium, but most of it is produced from morphine. A weaker painkiller and sedative than morphine, it is distributed in liquid products for relieving coughs and in tablet and injectable form for relieving pain.

### Heroin

Two percent of Americans are addicted to heroin. The primary attractions of heroin ("horse," "junk," "smack," or "downtown") are the euphoria and pain relief it produces. Some addicts also report a kick or rush when heroin is injected directly into their veins. The effects of heroin do not last long—usually only 2 to 4 hours—so addicts have to shoot up four or five times a day.[29]

Although heroin is principally still a ghetto drug, its use has become more widespread among those in the middle class or at least among those who try whatever recreational drug is new and trendy. These users tend to prefer "skin-popping" (subcutaneous injection) to "mainlining" (intravenous injection). Or, they snort heroin as a powder, or dissolve it and inhale the vapors. To try to avoid addiction, some users begin by "chipping," taking small or intermittent doses. Regardless of the method of administration, tolerance can develop rapidly.

The primary danger associated with its use is that the addict, who is consuming ever larger doses, may overdose and stop breathing completely. Another danger is the transmission of HIV among heroin users who share needles.

Heroin addiction is marked by lethargy, weight loss, loss of sexual appetite, and the continual attempt to avoid withdrawal symptoms. These symptoms include sweating, fever, chills, cramps, diarrhea, vomiting, and severe aches and pains. In addition, there is extreme anxiety; insomnia; restlessness; and, of course, a craving for the drug. Addicts continue to use heroin as much to avoid pain as to experience pleasure.

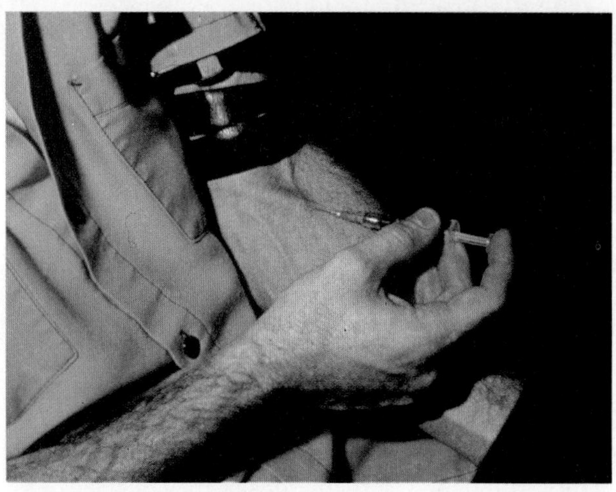

Heroin addicts must shoot up several times a day to prevent severe withdrawal symptoms.

### Other Synthetic Narcotics

Methadone (Dolophine, or "meth" or "dollies") is a synthetic narcotic that helps heroin addicts kick their habit by switching to methadone. In some urban areas, addicts are kept on methadone indefinitely. More than 100,000 ex-heroin addicts have taken methadone. Some have resumed normal, socially productive lives. However, methadone itself has become a drug of abuse; some believe it is even more damaging to the body than is heroin. Many addicts in methadone treatment centers continue to use heroin.[30]

Two semisynthetic derivatives of morphine are hydromorphone (trade name Dilaudid, or "little D"), with 2 to 8 times the painkilling effect of morphine, and oxycodone (Percodan, or "perkies"), similar to codeine but more potent. The synthetic narcotic meperidine (Demerol, or "demies"), which is addictive, is now probably second only to morphine in popularity for use in relieving pain. It is also used by addicts as a substitute for morphine and heroin.

The synthetic narcotic propoxyphene (Darvon) is a somewhat less potent painkiller than codeine, no more effective than aspirin in usual doses. Nevertheless, it has been one of the most widely prescribed drugs for headaches, dental pain, and menstrual cramps. At higher doses, Darvon produces a euphoric high, which may make its misuse tempting. The National Institute of Drug Abuse has estimated that Darvon kills more people each year than does heroin.

### Inhalants

**Inhalants** are chemicals that produce vapors with psychoactive effects. Most commonly abused inhalants—such as solvents, aerosols, model-airplane glue, cleaning fluids, and petroleum products like kerosene and butane—were never meant to be used as drugs. But some anesthetics and nitrous oxide (laughing gas) are also abused. Most inhalants produce the same effects as anesthetics in slowing down the body's functions. At low doses, users may feel slightly stimulated; at higher doses, they may feel less inhibited.

Use of inhalants is growing among high school students, who may not have money for, or access to, other drugs. Although some young people think inhalants safe, they're anything but. Because users cannot think clearly, they may act aggressively or put themselves in dangerous situations.

Regular use of inhalants leads to tolerance, so that the sniffer needs more and more to attain the desired effects. Side effects of their use include nausea, sneezing, coughing, nosebleeds, bad breath, lack of coordination, loss of appetite, decreased heart and breathing rates, and impaired judgment.

Inhalants can also cause serious medical complications, such as hepatitis with liver failure, kidney failure, respiratory impairment, destruction of bone marrow and skeletal muscles, blood abnormalities, and irregular heartbeats (arrhythmias). (Several youngsters have died of fatal arrhythmias while running away from police who discovered them using inhalants.) Inhalation of butane from cigarette lighters displaces oxygen in the lungs, causing suffocation. The heart stops because of a lack of oxygen to circulate the blood.

Two inhalants abused by adults are amyl nitrate and butyl nitrate. Amyl nitrate is used by heart patients to dilate (widen) the blood vessels and increase heart rate. When sold illegally, this clear, yellowish liquid is packaged in a cloth-covered, sealed bulb, which, when broken, makes a snapping sound—hence the street names "snappers" and "poppers." Butyl nitrate ("locker room" or "rush") produces a high that lasts from a few seconds to several minutes. The immediate effects of these inhalants include decreased blood pressure, followed by increased heart rate, flushed face and neck, dizziness, and headache.

### Designer Drugs

Produced in chemical laboratories, **designer drugs** are sold illegally. Easy to manufacture from available raw materials, the drugs themselves were once technically legal because the law had to specify the exact chemical structure of an illicit drug. However, a law now bans all chemical cousins of illegal drugs.

Synthetic narcotics are particularly dangerous because they're far more potent than those derived from natural substances. Derivatives of fentanyl, an anesthetic widely used for surgery in the United States, are 20 to 2,000 times as powerful as heroin; therefore, the risk of a fatal overdose or brain damage is much greater.[31]

### MDMA

MDMA (methylene dioxymethylamphetamine, commonly called "ecstasy") is somewhat related to mescaline and amphetamine. Psychiatrists have experimented with MDMA in patients, because it alters a user's social and personal perceptions. The Drug Enforcement Agency has classified it, along with heroin and LSD, as a drug with "high potential for abuse and no medical usefulness."[32]

Use of MDMA, particularly by college-age Americans, has increased. An estimated 500,000 to 4 million people use the drug, which creates feelings of warmth and openness. However, the day after MDMA use, people report insomnia, muscle aches, fatigue, and problems concentrating. MDMA destroys brain cells in animals and may cause brain damage in humans.

## THE TOLL OF DRUG ABUSE

Drug users pay a heavy price—physically, psychologically, mentally, financially, and socially. They become fatigued, cough constantly, lose weight, and ache from head to toe. They may suffer blackouts; flashbacks; and episodes of increasingly bizarre behavior, often triggered by escalating paranoia. Their risk of overdose rises steadily. They may also lose or jeopardize everything they hold dear: their families, their jobs, their friends, their financial security. Deep down they may yearn to change, but they can't—until they become drug-free.

Drug abuse also takes a toll on people who don't use or abuse drugs. Addicts may turn to crime and violence to get the money they need to support their habits. They put the lives of others at risk when they drive, operate machinery or do shoddy work while on drugs. As a society, we have to pay the financial

**inhalant** A substance that produces vapors that has psychoactive effects when sniffed.
**designer drug** An illegally manufactured psychoactive drug that has dangerous physical and psychological effects.

HEALTH SPOTLIGHT

## Coaddiction: Are You Helping a Drug User?

John uses cocaine regularly and often can't get up and moving in the morning. Rather than confront him, his wife Joan wakes him up, pulls him out of bed and into the shower, and drops him off at work. If he's late, she makes excuses to his boss. John is the one with the drug problem; but, without realizing it, Joan is helping him stay on drugs. In fact, he might not be able to keep up his habit without her unintentional cooperation.

Drug experts have discovered that often the spouses, parents, and friends of users suffer from coaddiction and, without meaning to, allow or enable their loved one to remain chemically dependent. In one research study psychologist Dr. Charles Nelson identified six styles of enabling:

- *Avoiding and shielding.* Coaddicts may cover up for abusers or prevent them from experiencing the full impact of the harmful consequences of drug use. For example, a coaddict may say the user is working on a project and can't be disturbed so friends don't visit when the user is strung out on drugs.
- *Attempting to control.* A coaddict may try to take control of the significant other's use of drugs personally—for instance, by withholding sex or using sex as a reward for cutting drug use.
- *Taking over responsibilities.* A coaddict may take over the user's household chores, such as grocery shopping or running errands, or may get money to pay the user's drug-related debts.
- *Rationalizing and accepting.* Coaddicts try to understand, explain, and accept their partner's drug use. They may tell themselves that the drugs are giving the user more energy or helping him or her be more open.
- *Cooperating and collaborating.* The coaddict may become involved in buying, selling, testing, preparing, or using the drug.
- *Rescuing.* The coaddict may be overprotective, allowing a user to use drugs at home to avoid the risk of an accident elsewhere.

SOURCES: Blau, Melinda. "Codependency: No Life to Live," *American Health,* May 1990. H. Julia. *Letting Go with Love: Help for Those Who Love an Alcoholic/Addict Whether Practicing or Recovering.* Los Angeles: Tarcher, 1987. Sorenson, James and Guillermo Bernal. *A Family Like Yours: Breaking the Patterns of Drug Abuse.* San Francisco: Harper & Row, 1987.

costs for their lost jobs, damaged health, medical treatment, and rehabilitation.

STRATEGY FOR CHANGE

### Saying No to Drugs

If people offer you a drug, here are some ways to say no:

- Anticipate situations when you might be offered drugs and prepare possible responses.
- Let them know you aren't interested.
- Have something else to do: "No, I'm going for a walk now."
- Be prepared for different types of pressure. If your friends tease you, tease back.
- If the pressure seems threatening, simply walk away.
- Keep it simple. "No, thanks," "No," or "No way" gets the point across.
- Give them the cold shoulder and ignore them.
- Change the subject.
- Hang out with people who won't ask you questions you have to say no to.

## Drugs and Driving

One often unrecognized impact of drugs is their effect on driving ability. Here are the facts from the National Institute on Drug Abuse.[33]

- *Alcohol*—Affects perception, coordination, and judgment. Increases the sedative effects of tranquilizers and barbiturates.

- *Marijuana*—Affects a wide range of driving skills, including the ability to "track" (stay in the lane) through curves, brake quickly, and maintain speed and a safe distance between cars. Slows thinking and reflexes; normal driving skills remain impaired for 4 to 6 hours after smoking a single joint.
- *Tranquilizers*—Slow reaction time and interfere with hand-eye coordination and judgment. The greatest impairment occurs in the first hour after taking the drug.
- *Sedatives*—A variety of effects, depending on the particular sedative. Dalmane, a popular medication for inducing sleep, builds up in the body and can impair driving skills the morning after its use. Barbiturates and Quaaludes make drivers very sleepy and, therefore, incapable of driving safely.
- *Stimulants*—With repeated use, stimulants impair coordination. Amphetamines can make a driver more edgy and less coordinated, and thus more likely to be involved in an accident.
- *Hallucinogens*—Distort judgment and reality, cause confusion and panic, and make driving extremely dangerous.

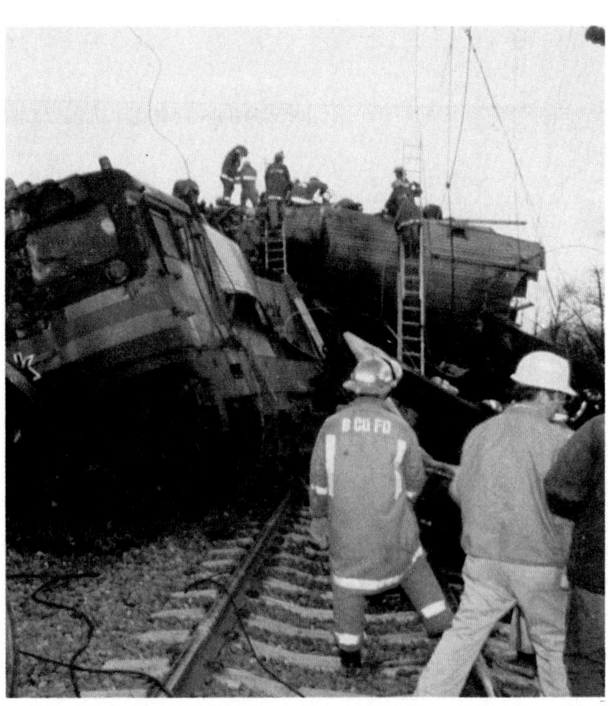

Using drugs on the job can lead to serious consequences.

### Drugs on the Job

Workers of every variety—from truck drivers to stockbrokers—use drugs. Current estimates are that 5 to 13 percent of the U.S. work force abuse drugs other than alcohol, and cocaine has replaced marijuana as the primary drug of abuse on or off the job.[34] As a result of this widespread drug use, the military and a growing number of companies are requiring drug tests of job applicants and employees.

## OVERCOMING DRUG DEPENDENCY

Drug abuse doesn't have to be a life—or, as it sometimes turns out, a death—sentence. More users than ever before—"potheads" and "coke-aholics" and pill-poppers—are realizing that drugs aren't solutions, but problems in themselves. These users are seeking help in record numbers. However, many detoxification programs do not have adequate funding, and addicts (including pregnant women hoping to break their habits for their babies' sakes as well as their own) often have to wait months for treatment.

Users often seek help because of an overdose, a medical emergency, or some other crisis—but that's only the beginning of the long path to recovery. Even after their physical dependence has been overcome, users need to rebuild their daily lives.

The basic approaches to drug-abuse treatment are:

- *Detoxification*—The supervised withdrawal from drug dependence, either with or without medication, in a hospital or as an outpatient.
- *Therapeutic Communities*—Highly structured, drug-free environments in which abusers live under strict rules while participating in group and individual therapy.
- *Outpatient Drug-Free Programs*—Many, including Narcotics Anonymous and Pills Anonymous, follow the philosophy of Alcoholics Anonymous, in which users admit their helplessness and put their faith in a "higher power."

Different forms of intervention help different kinds of people. Although valid statistics are difficult to obtain, most professionals do feel that drug treatment works. (See the health directory in the appendix for more information.)

**STRATEGY FOR CHANGE**

**If Someone You Love Has a Drug Problem**

- Get as much information as you can so you understand what you—and your loved one—are up against.

- Get some intervention training. Specially trained counselors work at most chemical dependency units; some offer advice by phone.
- Confront the user. Along with other loved ones and, if possible, a professional counselor, detail incident after incident in which the drug abuse affected or hurt you, other members of your family, or the user.
- Don't expect a drug abuser to quit without help. Chemical dependency is a medical and psychological disorder that requires professional treatment.
- Offer your support, but make it clear that you expect your loved one to undergo therapy.
- If your loved one agrees to treatment, make sure that the program is based on a complete evaluation that checks for medical or emotional problems as well as chemical dependency.
- Don't believe abusers who say they've learned to "control" their drug use. Absolute abstinence is a cornerstone of any good rehabilitation program.
- Encourage a user to attend support groups, such as Cocaine Anonymous or Narcotics Anonymous, for at least a year after rehabilitation.
- Get help for yourself. Most hospitals and chemical-dependency programs offer educational programs for coaddicts.

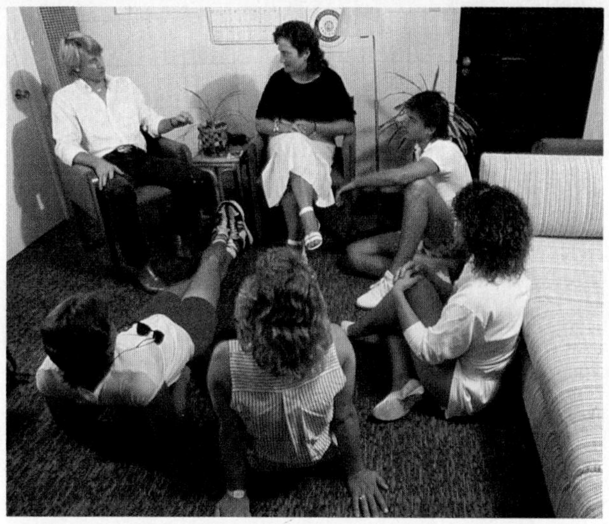

Overcoming a drug habit isn't easy; many former addicts find support from others with the same problem.

## MAKING THIS CHAPTER WORK FOR YOU

### Staying Drug-free

Drugs—chemicals taken to alter physiological or psychological processes—can be misused (used for a purpose other than that for which it was originally

## WHAT DO YOU THINK?

When cramming for an exam, you take a double dose of OTC stimulants. The next night, you can't get to sleep, so you have a few drinks and take some of the Valium a doctor prescribed when you pulled a muscle several months ago. Do you consider your behavior drug misuse? Why? Is it dangerous?

A medical journal reported the case of "B," a quiet 23-year-old construction worker and youth minister, who became interested in bodybuilding and began taking anabolic steroids. One day he ripped a telephone booth from its base and threw it to the ground. Then he and his companions picked up a hitchhiker and drove him to a wooded area, where B beat the man to death with a board. After his arrest and subsequent end of drug use, B once again became shy and peace-loving. Does steroid rage excuse B's behavior? Should he be imprisoned for his crime? Why or why not?

A growing number of employers require drug testing for employees and job applicants. Do you think potential employers have the right to require drug screening? How would you feel about undergoing a drug test? Would you want airline pilots or train engineers to be tested regularly? Do you think that anyone who objects must be using drugs? Why else would someone refuse a drug test?

intended) or abused (used excessively or inappropriately). The misuse or abuse of psychoactive drugs can lead to physical and psychological addiction.

Physical dependence occurs when physiological changes caused by a drug result in an intense need for the drug. Psychological dependence occurs when users crave a drug for the emotional or mental changes it produces.

Drugs that are available legally, such as caffeine, over-the-counter (OTC) drugs, and prescription drugs, can be misused or abused. The OTCs most often abused include pain relievers, sedatives, and stimulants. Prescription medications such as amphetamines and anabolic steroids are often misused and lead to serious physical risks.

People turn to psychoactive drugs for many reasons, including curiosity, boredom relief, peer influence, availability of drugs, psychological or emotional problems, and genetic or childhood influences. Initially, users discover the pleasure of feeling high. They then begin using drugs to help them cope with problems and become more preoccupied with drugs. Eventually, drug use takes over their lives.

Stimulants include amphetamines and cocaine, which produce feelings of high energy. Cocaine may be snorted as a powder, smoked (or free-based) in a form called crack or rock, or injected. The effects of cocaine use include impaired judgment, psychological disorders (including psychosis), headaches, nausea, damaged nasal membranes in snorters, weight loss, liver damage, heart attack, strokes, brain seizures or hemorrhage, complications during pregnancies, and mental and physical damage to infants born to cocaine users.

Amphetamine abusers may suffer from tremors, irregular heartbeat, loss of coordination, psychosis and paranoia, malnutrition, skin disorders, ulcers, depression, brain damage, and heart failure. A new form of smokeable methamphetamine, known as ice, increases heart rate and blood pressure; high doses can cause permanent damage to blood vessels in the brain. Like ice, crank produces effects similar to those of amphetamines.

Alcohol, barbiturates, antianxiety drugs, and marijuana and hashish are depressants or sedatives that depress the central nervous system. Barbiturate use can result in physical dependence. And because the addict needs increasingly larger doses, the risk of fatal overdose is high. Antianxiety medications such as Valium and Librium can produce dependence, drowsiness, and slurred speech. Withdrawal from them can produce coma, psychosis, and even death.

THC, the primary psychoactive ingredient in marijuana and hashish, can produce an increased heart rate, dry mouth and throat, and altered perception; high doses may result in distorted perception, hallucinations, and acute panic attacks. Long-term marijuana use may result in psychological dependence; lung damage; impairment of the central nervous system, reproductive system, and immune system; use of other drugs; mental and emotional dulling; loss of drive; and legal consequences.

Psychedelics and hallucinogens—including peyote and its active ingredient mescaline, lysergic acid diethylamide (or LSD), psilocybin, and phencyclidine (or PCP)—can produce hallucinations and, in some users, panic, paranoia, and psychotic episodes. PCP is a dangerous psychoactive drug because of its effects on behavior.

The narcotics—including opium, morphine, heroin, and codeine—may lead to infections of the heart; skin abscesses; congested lungs; tetanus; liver disease; hepatitis; and, from using unsterile syringes and needles, HIV infection. A narcotics addict who stops taking the drug experiences withdrawal sickness—nausea, abdominal cramps, fever, sweating and chills, diarrhea, and severe aches and pains. The most abused synthetic narcotics are Demerol, Darvon, and methadone, which is used to help heroin addicts break their dependency, but is also addictive and physically harmful.

Inhalants, including amyl nitrate and butyl nitrate, can lead to serious complications. Designer drugs are illegally manufactured drugs that are far more potent than natural substances.

Drugs can affect users' abilities to drive and work and cause accidents involving themselves and others. A person desiring treatment for drug dependency has three alternatives: detoxification in a hospital or as an outpatient, admission to a therapeutic community, or admission to an outpatient drug-counseling program.

Drugs are a fact of life in our society, and sooner or later you have to decide whether they will be part of your life. If drugs ever seem appealing as a quick fix to whatever is troubling you, consider positive addictions that can help you solve your problems without creating new and bigger ones. A positive addiction—whether it is to mountain-climbing or music—can produce a very real high. But there's a crucial difference between this sort of stimulation and drug dependency: With one, you're in control; with the other, drugs are.

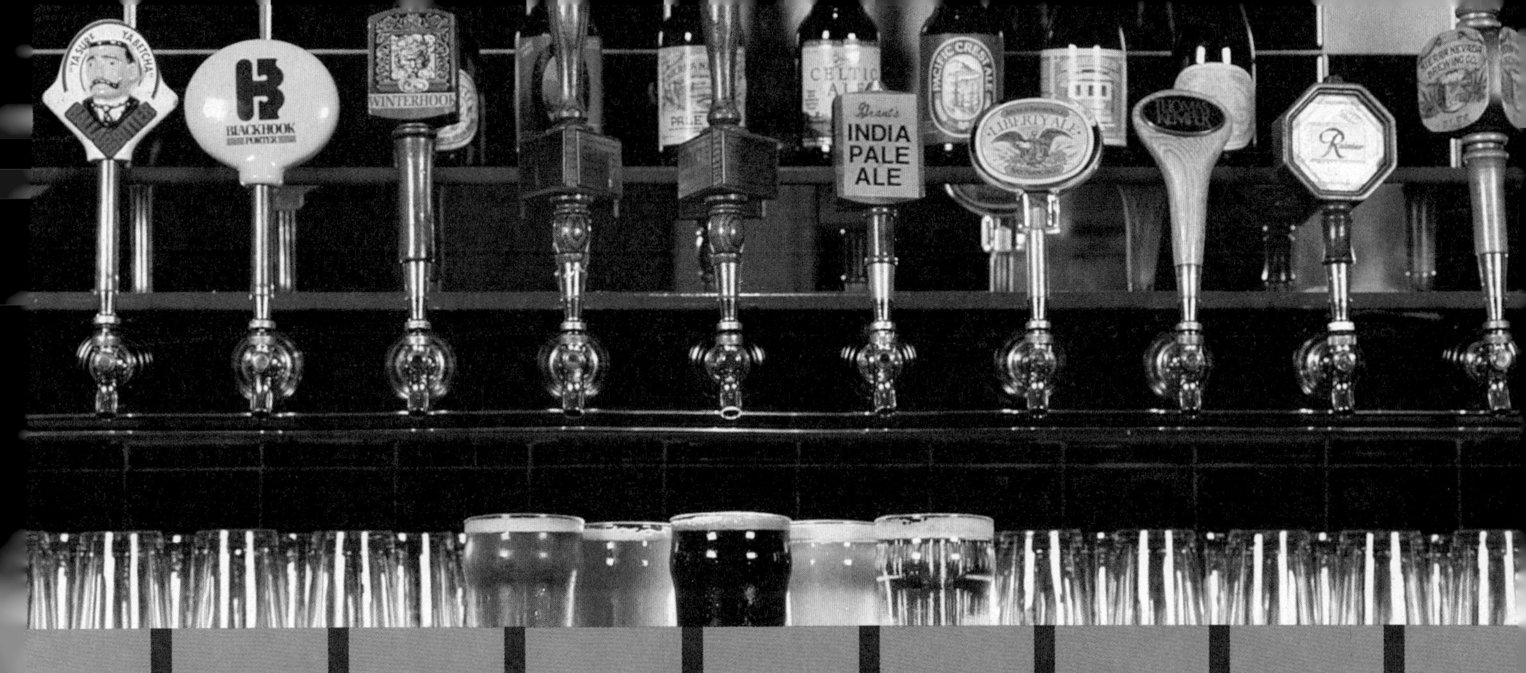


# 10 ALCOHOL: RESPONSIBLE DRINKING

**In this chapter**

**Drinking today**

**Moderate drinking**

**Effects of alcohol on the body and brain**

**The disease of alcoholism**

**Making this chapter work for you: Responsible drinking**

*Alcohol is a powerful and potentially dangerous drug, and you may decide not to drink at all or only rarely.* If you don't want to live without alcohol, you must learn to live with it—to use, not abuse it. The key to responsible drinking is knowing when to say "No more." This chapter provides information about moderate drinking; alcohol's effects on body, brain, and behavior; and the diagnosis, impact, and treatment of alcoholism.

## DRINKING TODAY

America is sobering up. In 1989 alcohol consumption reached its lowest level in 30 years.[1] Slightly more than half (56 percent) of Americans drink alcoholic beverages, a significant decline from the early 1980s. Executives are wary of dulling their competitive edge by mixing business and booze. Amateur athletes figure the extra bottle of beer may put them out of the running in marathons. Dieters tallying up the calories in a glass of wine fear for their weights and their waists (see Table 10-1). Most men and women who use alcohol are light drinkers who down fewer than three alcoholic drinks a week.[2]

Although more people are drinking less, alcohol remains the most widely used drug in America, topping even cigarette tobacco in popularity. According to the Department of Health and Human Services (HHS), 10.5 million adults exhibit some symptoms of alcoholism or alcohol dependence. Another 7.2 million abuse alcohol but do not yet show symptoms of dependence. Projections for 1995 indicate that 11.2 million adults will exhibit symptoms of alcohol dependence.[3]

According to HHS, a minimum of 3 percent of deaths can be attributed to alcohol-related causes. Alcohol use contributes to a variety of illnesses, including liver disease, cancer, and heart problems. Exposure to alcohol before birth is one of the leading known causes of mental retardation. Nearly half of violent deaths are alcohol-related. More than 20,000 motor vehicle fatalities each year are due to alcohol abuse.

### Who Drinks?

Among people of all ages, about three-fourths of the men and about three-fifths of the women are drinkers. Although women are less apt to drink and generally drink less, the proportion of women who drink, particularly among those under age 35, has increased. Men and women are most likely to drink between the ages of 21 and 34. At all ages, 2 to 5 times more men than women are heavy drinkers. Among those age 65 and over, more people abstain than drink; only 7 percent of older men and 2 percent of older women are heavy drinkers.[4]

The more money and education people have, the more likely they are to drink either moderately or heavily. The greatest percentage of abstainers have less than an eighth-grade education. The proportion of drinkers goes up with increasing level of education, although there are slightly fewer "heavy" drinkers among people with postgraduate, as opposed to college, educations. Farm owners have the lowest proportion of drinkers, whereas professionals and businessmen have the highest.

There are proportionately more drinkers in New England, in the middle Atlantic area, and on the West Coast than elsewhere. Cities and suburbs have nearly double the proportion of moderate drinkers that small towns and rural areas have.

### College Drinkers

Most young people drink, including 76 percent of college students. Despite the change in legal drinking age from 18 to 21, alcohol remains the most pop-

**TABLE 10-1** Average Number of Calories in Alcoholic Drinks*

| BEVERAGE | SERVING SIZE, OZ | CALORIES PER SERVING |
|---|---|---|
| Wine | 5 | 110 |
| Light wine | 5 | 65 |
| Wine cooler | 12 | 220 |
| Sherry | 3 | 125 |
| Beer | 12 | 150 |
| Light beer | 12 | 100 |
| Gin, vodka, rum, rye, or whiskey (80 proof) | 1.5 | 100 |
| Cordials or liqueurs (25–100 proof) | 1 | 50–100 |
| Martini | 2.5 | 156 |
| Bloody Mary | 5 | 116 |
| Tom Collins | 7.5 | 121 |
| Daiquiri | 2 | 111 |

*All figures are for drinks without ice.

SOURCE: Christian, Janet and Janet Greger. *Nutrition for Living*, Benjamin/Cummings, 1987. Adapted from "To drink or not to drink? That's one of the questions," *Tufts University Diet and Nutrition Letter*, 1986.

**TABLE 10-2** Drinking in College

Percentage of college students saying that they had had at least one drink within the past 30 days and the percentage saying that they had had five or more drinks in a row in the past two weeks.

| YEAR | 1 IN 30 DAYS | 5 OR MORE IN 2 WEEKS |
|---|---|---|
| 1980 | 81.8 | 43.9 |
| 1981 | 81.9 | 43.6 |
| 1982 | 82.8 | 44.0 |
| 1983 | 80.3 | 43.1 |
| 1984 | 79.1 | 45.4 |
| 1985 | 80.3 | 44.6 |
| 1986 | 79.7 | 45.0 |
| 1987 | 78.4 | 42.8 |
| 1988 | 77.0 | 43.2 |
| 1989 | 76.2 | 41.7 |

SOURCE: Based on confidential surveys of 1,200 college students by the Institute for Social Research, 1989. Copyright 1990 by the New York Times Company. Reprinted by permission.

ular drug on campus. According to a survey by the University of Michigan's Institute of Social Research in 1990 (see Table 10-2), three of every four students drink alcohol at least once a month. Two of every five have five drinks or more in one sitting at least once every two weeks. About 4 percent—down from a high of 7 percent in 1984—drink daily. Nearly one in every five college women shows signs of alcohol dependency.[5–7]

### Younger Drinkers

According to the National Institute on Alcohol Abuse and Alcoholism (NIAAA), the average age at which children take their first drink is now just under 13; 40 percent have tasted alcohol by the age of 10.[8] Alcoholism has become the number one drug problem among the nation's youth.

In a national survey, one of every three high school seniors reported drinking five or more drinks in a row at least once in the preceding two weeks. About 30 percent of teenagers experience negative consequences of alcohol abuse, including alcohol-related accidents, arrests, or impaired health or school performance.[9]

### Why People Drink

The most common reason people drink is to relax. Because alcohol turns down the central nervous system, a drink can make people feel less tense. However, there are many other reasons people reach for a drink, including the following:

- *Celebration*—Unless alcohol use violates family, ethnic, or religious values, people raise their glasses together on life's important occasions—births, graduations, weddings, promotions.
- *Friendship*—When friends visit, you may offer them a drink, or you may meet them somewhere "for a drink." Drinking is one of the most common rituals of friendships.
- *Romance*—Because alcohol lowers inhibitions, some people see it as a prelude to seduction. Yet alcohol can interfere with sexual response.
- *Social Ease*—When we use alcohol, we may seem bolder, wittier, sexier. At the same time, the people drinking with us become more relaxed and seem to enjoy our company more.
- *Role Models*—Athletes, some of the most admired celebrities in our country, have a long history of appearing in commercials for alcohol. Young boys grow up thinking that they should do as their heroes do, on the field and off, and learn to hold their liquor "like a man."
- *Advertising*—Brewers and beer distributors spend $15 million to $20 million a year promoting their products to college students. Their message: If you want to have a good time, you need a drink.

## Understanding Alcohol

Pure alcohol is a colorless liquid obtained by fermentation of a liquid containing sugar. **Ethyl alcohol,** or **ethanol,** is the type of alcohol in alcoholic beverages. The type you may keep in your medicine cabinet—methyl alcohol, or wood alcohol—is a poison that should never be drunk.

Any liquid containing from 0.5 to 80 percent ethyl

**ethyl alcohol** The intoxicating agent in alcoholic beverages.
**ethanol** See *ethyl alcohol.*

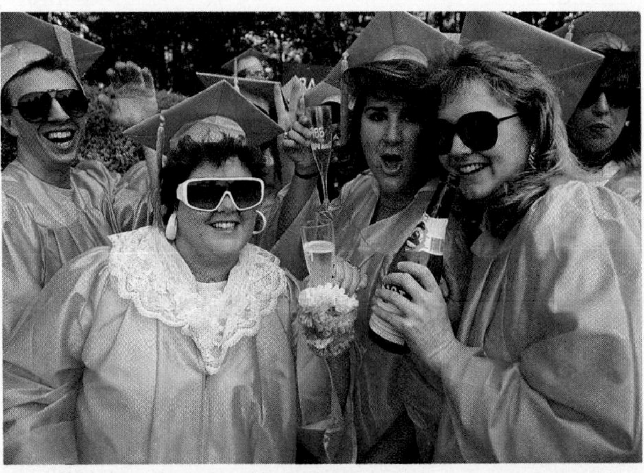

Toasts are a time-honored way of celebrating life's important occasions.

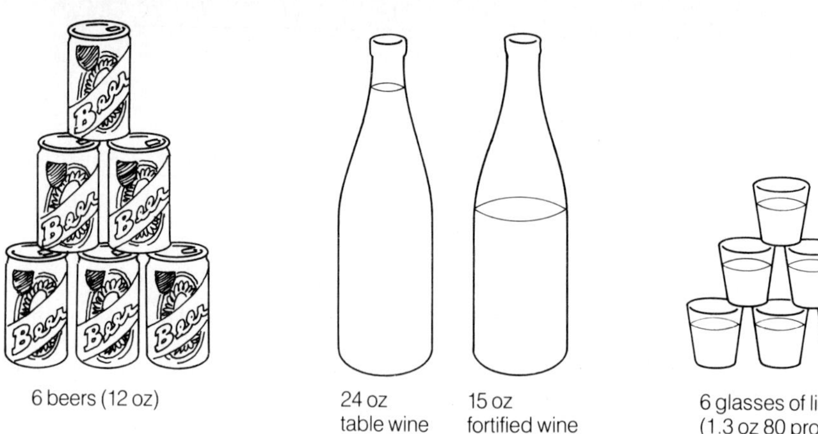


**FIGURE 10-1** These amounts of these alcoholic beverages, when consumed within a 2-hour period, would result in a blood alcohol concentration of 0.1 percent in a 160-pound person. That person would be legally drunk in most states.

alcohol by volume is an alcoholic beverage. As Figure 10-1 shows, different drinks contain different amounts of alcohol.

- *Beer*—Regular brews contain 5 percent alcohol; malt liquor beers may contain 8 or 9 percent alcohol.
- *Wine*—Most table wines contain 10 to 13 percent alcohol.
- *Fortified Wine*—Extra alcohol is added to wines like sherry and port; their alcohol content is about 20 percent.
- *Distilled Liquor*—"Hard" drinks, such as whiskey, gin, vodka, brandy, and most liqueurs, contain 40 to 50 percent alcohol.

## What's in Your Drink?

One drink can be any of the following:

- one bottle or can (12 oz) of beer with 5 percent alcohol
- one glass (4 oz) of table wine, such as burgundy, with 12 percent alcohol
- one small glass (2-1/2 oz) of fortified wine with 20 percent alcohol.
- one shot (1 oz) of distilled spirits, such as whiskey or vodka or rum, with 50 percent alcohol (100 proof) (With distilled spirits such as bourbon, scotch, vodka, gin, and rum, alcohol content is expressed in terms of **proof,** a number that is twice the percentage of alcohol. Thus 100-proof bourbon is 50 percent alcohol, and 80-proof gin is 40 percent alcohol.)

All these drinks contain close to the same amount of alcohol—that is, if the number of ounces in each drink is multiplied by the percentage of alcohol, each drink contains the equivalent of approximately 1/2 oz of straight 100 percent ethyl alcohol. Terms such as *bottle* and *glass* can be deceiving. Drinking a 16-oz can of malt liquor with 9 percent alcohol is not the

**proof** The alcoholic strength, measured as twice the percentage of alcohol present.

**TABLE 10-3** Alcohol Content in Drinks

| | SERVING SIZE | ALCOHOL BY VOLUME, %* | ALCOHOL CONTENT PER SERVING, OZ |
|---|---|---|---|
| Light beer | 12-oz can | 2.4 | 0.29 |
| | 12-oz can | 4.8 | 0.58 |
| Regular beer | 12-oz can | 3.2 | 0.38 |
| | 12-oz can | 5.0 | 0.60 |
| Wine | 4-oz glass | 12.0 | 0.48 |
| Martini | 3-oz glass (1.5 oz each of 80 proof gin and vermouth) | 40.0 | 1.20 |
| Eggnog | 8-oz glass (3 oz of 80 proof rum) | 15.0 | 1.20 |

*Varies by brand.

SOURCE: *Washington Post,* December 15, 1987.

same as drinking a 12-oz can of 5 percent beer (see Table 10-3).

## Types of Drinkers

Some people drink once a month and have one drink or less at a time. Others drink three or four times a month, and have two to four drinks at a time. So-called moderate drinkers usually drink a small amount (one drink or less) at least once a week, or have two to four drinks three or four times a month.

People with a drinking problem usually exhibit one of three main patterns of chronic alcohol abuse:

- daily intake of large amounts of alcohol
- regular heavy drinking on weekends
- long periods of sobriety, followed by binges of daily heavy drinking for weeks or months

The traditional definition of an **alcoholic** is a person whose drinking interferes with a major aspect of his or her life on a continuing basis. As you'll see later in this chapter, alcoholics are victims of a biological disease that impairs or destroys their ability to control their drinking.

# MODERATE DRINKING

Although 67 percent of American adults drink, fewer than 10 percent ever develop drinking problems. Studies conducted during the past several decades have indicated that moderate drinkers live longer, healthier lives than both alcoholics and those who abstain from alcohol altogether. In his landmark research on alcoholism, psychiatrist George Vaillant of Dartmouth University found that moderate drinkers (who, by his definition, averaged less than four drinks a day) often turned out to be better adjusted socially than total abstainers.[10]

### STRATEGY FOR CHANGE

#### How to Drink Moderately

- Set a limit and stick to it. Two drinks per day or drinking occasion is a reasonable amount.
- Learn to say no. A simple "Thank you, but I've had enough" will do.
- When you drink, enjoy everything about it, from the taste to the good company to the pleasant setting. Savor each sip.
- Don't cluster your drinks, having seven beers on Saturday instead of one each evening of the week.
- Always eat before going to a party.
- Have a nonalcoholic beverage to quench your thirst.
- If you're going out with friends, always designate a driver who will not drink at all during the evening.
- Don't drink on your own. Although it may be tempting to pour yourself a drink after a hard day, try to develop alternative means of unwinding: exercise, meditation, listening to music.

## How Much Can You Drink?

The best indicator for safe drinking is the amount of alcohol in your blood at any time; this amount is called your **blood alcohol concentration (BAC)**. This is the measure that highway patrol officers use (from breath or urine samples) to determine if a driver is drunk. BAC is expressed in terms of the percentage

**alcoholic** A person whose drinking interferes on a continuing basis with a major aspect of his or her life.
**blood alcohol concentration (BAC)** The amount of alcohol in a person's blood.

### HEALTH HEADLINE

#### Alcohol's Fatal Attraction

The twenties and the sixties are the high-risk ages for dying as a result of alcohol abuse. In a study of 105,095 Americans who died from diseases or accidents linked to drinking, epidemiologist James Shultz of the University of Miami found that alcohol tends to kill at two different stages of life—through injuries in young adulthood and through chronic illnesses later in life.

Deaths from injuries, mostly car accidents, rise steadily throughout the teen years but peak at 6,000 a year between the ages of 20 and 24. Deaths from cirrhosis of the liver, hepatitis, and other alcohol-linked illnesses rise slowly from age 20 to age 60.

SOURCE: U.S. Centers for Disease Control, March 1990.

**TABLE 10-4** Effects of Blood Alcohol Concentrations

| BLOOD ALCOHOL CONCENTRATION, % | PSYCHOLOGICAL AND PHYSICAL EFFECTS |
|---|---|
| 0.02–0.03 | No overt effects, slight feeling of muscle relaxation, slight mood elevation |
| 0.05–0.06 | No intoxication, but feeling of relaxation and warmth; slight increase in reaction time; and slight decrease in fine muscle coordination |
| 0.08–0.09 | Balance, speech, vision, and hearing slightly impaired; feelings of euphoria; and increased loss of motor coordination |
| 0.11–0.12 | Coordination and balance becoming difficult, and distinct impairment of mental facilities and judgment |
| 0.14–0.15 | Major impairment of mental and physical control: slurred speech, blurred vision, and lack of motor skill |
| 0.20 | Loss of motor control (must have assistance in moving about) and substantial mental confusion |
| 0.30 | Severe intoxication, and minimum conscious control of mind and body |
| 0.40 | Unconscious and at threshold of coma |
| 0.50 | Deep coma |
| 0.60 | Death from respiratory failure |

SOURCE: Girdano and Dusek, *Drug Education: Content and Methods, Third Edition*, 1980.

of alcohol in a person's blood: A BAC of 0.05 indicates approximately 5 parts alcohol to 10,000 parts of other blood components. Most people reach this level after one or two drinks and experience all the positive sensations of drinking—relaxation, euphoria, and well-being—without feeling intoxicated (see Table 10-4).

Table 10-5 shows approximate BAC reached according to how much you weigh and how many drinks you have had during 1 or 2 hours. To use this table, find your weight in it, and run your finger down the column to see what your BAC would be for varying numbers of drinks taken within 1 or 2 hours. For example, if you weigh 160 pounds and you have six drinks (six bottles of beer, for instance) within two hours, your BAC is 0.10 percent.

Many factors affect your BAC and your response to alcohol.

- *How Much and How Quickly You Drink*—The more alcohol you put into your body, the higher your BAC. If you chug drink after drink, your liver, which processes about 1/2 oz of alcohol an hour, won't be able to keep up; your BAC will soar.
- *What You're Drinking*—The stronger the drink, the faster and harder the alcohol hits. Straight shots of liquor and cocktails such as martinis will get into your bloodstream faster than beer or table

**TABLE 10-5** Approximate BAC According to Body Weight and Number of Drinks Consumed

| | BODY WEIGHT, POUNDS | | | | | | | |
|---|---|---|---|---|---|---|---|---|
| NUMBER OF DRINKS | 100 | 120 | 140 | 160 | 180 | 200 | 220 | 240 |
| **For 1 Hour of Drinking** | | | | | | | | |
| 1 | 0.03 | 0.03 | 0.02 | 0.02 | 0.02 | 0.01 | 0.01 | — |
| 2 | 0.06 | 0.05 | 0.04 | 0.04 | 0.03 | 0.03 | 0.03 | 0.02 |
| 3 | 0.10 | 0.08 | 0.07 | 0.06 | 0.05 | 0.05 | 0.04 | 0.04 |
| 4 | 0.13 | 0.10 | 0.09 | 0.08 | 0.07 | 0.06 | 0.06 | 0.05 |
| 5 | 0.16 | 0.13 | 0.11 | 0.10 | 0.09 | 0.08 | 0.07 | 0.07 |
| 6 | 0.19 | 0.16 | 0.13 | 0.12 | 0.11 | 0.10 | 0.09 | 0.08 |
| 7 | 0.23 | 0.19 | 0.16 | 0.14 | 0.13 | 0.11 | 0.10 | 0.09 |
| 8 | 0.26 | 0.22 | 0.18 | 0.16 | 0.14 | 0.13 | 0.12 | 0.11 |
| **For 2 Hours of Drinking** | | | | | | | | |
| 1 | 0.01 | 0.01 | — | — | — | — | — | — |
| 2 | 0.04 | 0.03 | 0.02 | 0.01 | 0.01 | 0.01 | — | — |
| 3 | 0.08 | 0.06 | 0.04 | 0.03 | 0.03 | 0.02 | 0.02 | 0.01 |
| 4 | 0.11 | 0.09 | 0.07 | 0.06 | 0.05 | 0.04 | 0.03 | 0.03 |
| 5 | 0.15 | 0.12 | 0.10 | 0.08 | 0.07 | 0.06 | 0.05 | 0.04 |
| 6 | 0.18 | 0.14 | 0.12 | 0.10 | 0.09 | 0.08 | 0.07 | 0.06 |
| 7 | 0.22 | 0.18 | 0.15 | 0.12 | 0.11 | 0.09 | 0.08 | 0.07 |
| 8 | 0.25 | 0.20 | 0.17 | 0.15 | 0.13 | 0.11 | 0.10 | 0.09 |

wine—drinks that not only contain less alcohol, but also contain nonalcoholic substances that slow the rate of **absorption** (passage of the alcohol into your body tissues).

If the drink contains water, juice, or milk, the rate of absorption will be slowed. However, carbon dioxide—whether it's in champagne, ginger ale, or a cola—whisks alcohol into your bloodstream. Alcohol in warm drinks, such as a hot rum toddy or sake, moves into your bloodstream more quickly than that in chilled wine or scotch on the rocks.

- *Your Size*—If you're a large person (whether due to fat or to muscle), you will get drunk more slowly than someone smaller who is drinking the same amount of alcohol at the same rate. Heavier individuals have a larger water volume that dilutes the alcohol they drink.
- *Your Sex*—Pound for pound, women are more sensitive to alcohol than men. Hormone levels also affect the impact of alcohol. Women are more sensitive to alcohol just before menstruation. Birth control pills and other forms of estrogen can intensify alcohol's impact. (See the section "Special Concerns for Women" later in this chapter for more on alcohol and women.)
- *Your Age*—The same amount of alcohol produces higher BACs in older drinkers, who have lower volumes of body water to dilute the alcohol, than in younger drinkers.[11]
- *Your Race*—Many members of certain ethnic groups, including Asians and American Indians, are unable to break down alcohol as quickly as Caucasians. This results in higher BACs as well as uncomfortable reactions, such as flushing and nausea, when they drink.
- *Family History of Alcoholism*—Some children of alcoholics don't register alcohol's impact in the usual ways and don't get the normal warning signals, such as light-headedness, that they're drinking too much.[12]
- *Eating*—Food slows absorption by diluting alcohol, covering some of the membranes through which alcohol would be absorbed, and prolonging the time the stomach takes to empty.
- *Expectations*—In various experiments, volunteers who believed they were drinking alcoholic beverages but who were actually drinking nonalcoholic drinks acted as if they were guzzling the real thing. They became more talkative, relaxed, and sexually stimulated.
- *Physical Tolerance*—If you drink regularly, your brain becomes accustomed to a certain level of alcohol. You may be able to look and behave in a seemingly normal fashion, even though you drink as much as it would take to intoxicate someone your size. However, your driving ability and judgment will be impaired.

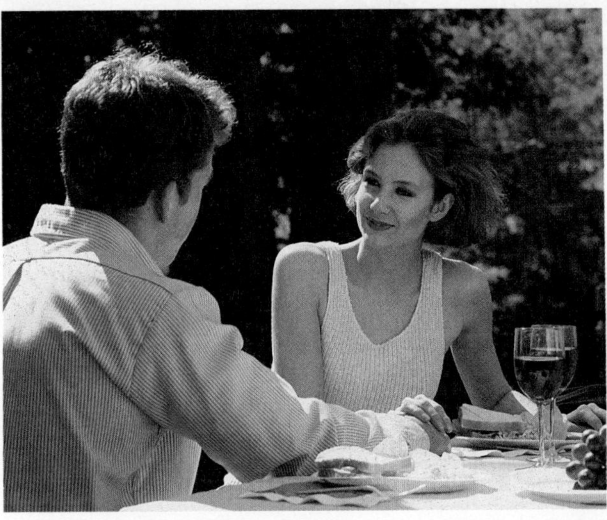

Because food in the stomach slows absorption of alcohol, eat before, and while, drinking.

Once you develop tolerance, you may drink more to get the desired effects from alcohol. In some people, this dependence can lead to abuse and alcoholism. After years of drinking, some people become exquisitely sensitive to alcohol. Such "reverse tolerance" means that they can become intoxicated after drinking only a small amount of it.

**STRATEGY FOR CHANGE**

**How to Drink Without Getting Drunk**

- When you're mixing a drink, measure the alcohol.
- Drink slowly. Never have more than one drink an hour.
- Eat before, and while, drinking.
- Choose foods high in protein (cheese, meat, eggs, or milk).
- Stay away from fizzy mixers, like club soda and ginger ale, which speed alcohol to the brain.

## The Danger Zone

With alcohol, more is definitely not better. Heavy drinking destroys the liver, weakens the heart, elevates blood pressure, damages the brain, and multiplies the risk of cancer. Individuals who have three to five drinks a day have a 50 percent higher mortality rate than those who have two or fewer drinks a day.

**absorption** The passage of substances into or across membranes or tissues.

The American Heart Association recommends that alcohol account for no more than 15 percent of the total calories consumed by an individual every day, up to an absolute maximum of 1.75 oz of alcohol a day.[13] That is the equivalent of three beers, two mixed drinks, or three-and-a-half glasses of wine. Your own limit may well be less, depending on your sex, size, and weight.

**STRATEGY FOR CHANGE**

**How to Help Others Drink Moderately**

When you're entertaining and serving alcohol, follow these guidelines:

- Avoid an open bar. Serve drinks yourself, or enlist a friend's help as bartender.
- Measure the amount of alcohol you put into mixed drinks, and figure out how many ounces your wine and beer glasses hold.
- Always serve food when serving drinks—but not the salty nuts, chips and pretzels bars serve to increase thirst.
- Make sure nonalcoholic alternatives are available.
- Avoid pushing drinks on guests and refilling glasses quickly.
- Stop serving alcohol one hour before the evening is to end.
- Never serve alcohol to a guest who seems intoxicated, and never let an intoxicated person drive home. You could be legally, as well as morally, responsible in the case of an accident.

## Hangovers

The more you drink and the faster you drink, the greater the chance of a hangover. Because your liver doesn't have time to break it down, alcohol accumulates in your bloodstream. The higher your peak blood alcohol level, the more likely you are to end up hung over.

Hangovers hit in many ways: headache, caused by dilation of the blood vessels of the head; nausea, caused by alcohol-induced secretion of hydrochloric acid, which irritates the stomach lining; thirst, caused by alcohol-induced dehydration through frequent urination; muscle aches, caused by overdoing while under alcohol's influence; or dizziness, caused by an alcohol-induced drop in blood sugar.

Usually it takes about 12 hours for your body to recover from alcohol poisoning. Solid food, bed rest, and aspirin will make the discomfort somewhat more bearable; but time, alone, will do the job. Neither black coffee nor cold showers speed up the process of sobering up.

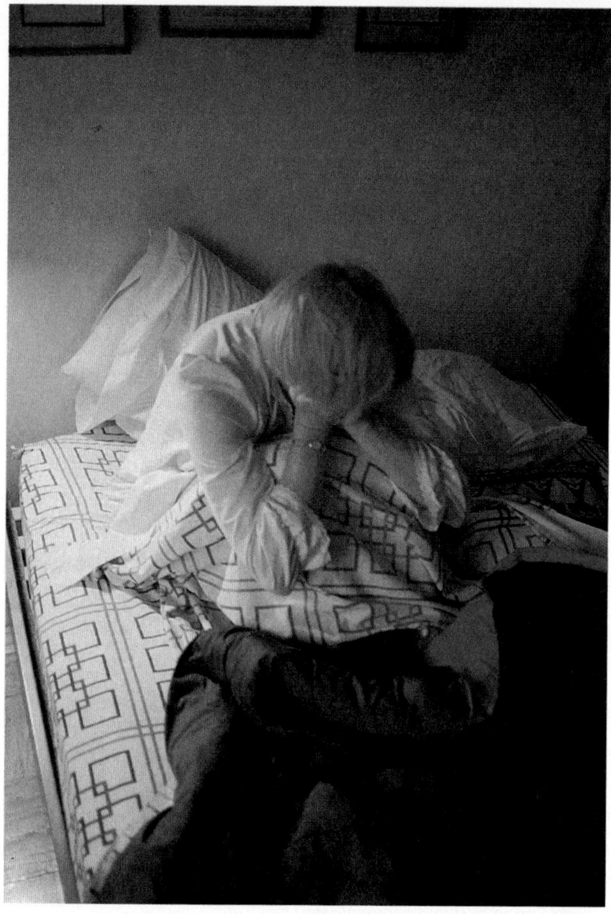

It may feel fun and relaxing at the time, but excessive drinking can lead to headache and illness the next day.

**STRATEGY FOR CHANGE**

**How to Handle a Hangover**

A Food and Drug Administration panel on over-the-counter hangover remedies recommends preparations with a combination of ingredients, such as pain relievers for headaches, antacids for stomach distress, and caffeine for fatigue or dullness. Following are alternatives for specific symptoms:

- *For headache.* Caffeine, aspirin or acetaminophen, a hot towel on your head, a hot shower
- *For nausea.* Bland foods, such as a soft-boiled egg or dry toast
- *For thirst.* Slightly salty liquids, such as chicken soup, to replace fluids lost through urination
- *For dizziness or weakness.* Orange juice

## EFFECTS OF ALCOHOL ON THE BODY AND BRAIN

Unlike drugs in tablet form or food, alcohol is directly and quickly absorbed into the bloodstream through the stomach walls and upper intestine. A typical drink reaches the bloodstream in 15 minutes and rises to peak level in about an hour. The bloodstream carries the alcohol to the liver, the heart, and the brain.

### Effects on the Body

Alcohol is a diuretic, a drug that speeds up the elimination of fluid from the body. However, most of the alcohol you drink can leave your body only after metabolism by the liver, which converts about 95 percent of the alcohol to carbon dioxide and water. The other 5 percent is excreted unchanged, mainly through urination, respiration, and perspiration.

#### Liver

The liver, because it must break down alcohol, is especially vulnerable to its effects. (See Figure 10-2.) Alcohol stimulates liver cells to attract white blood cells, which normally travel throughout the bloodstream engulfing harmful substances and wastes. If they begin to attack and invade body tissue, like the liver, they can cause irreversible damage. This may explain why continued drinking leads to **cirrhosis,** or severe scarring of the liver, for about 10 percent to 15 percent of chronic drinkers. (See the section "Liver Damage" for more on cirrhosis.)

**cirrhosis** A chronic disease, especially of the liver, characterized by a degeneration of cells and excessive scarring.

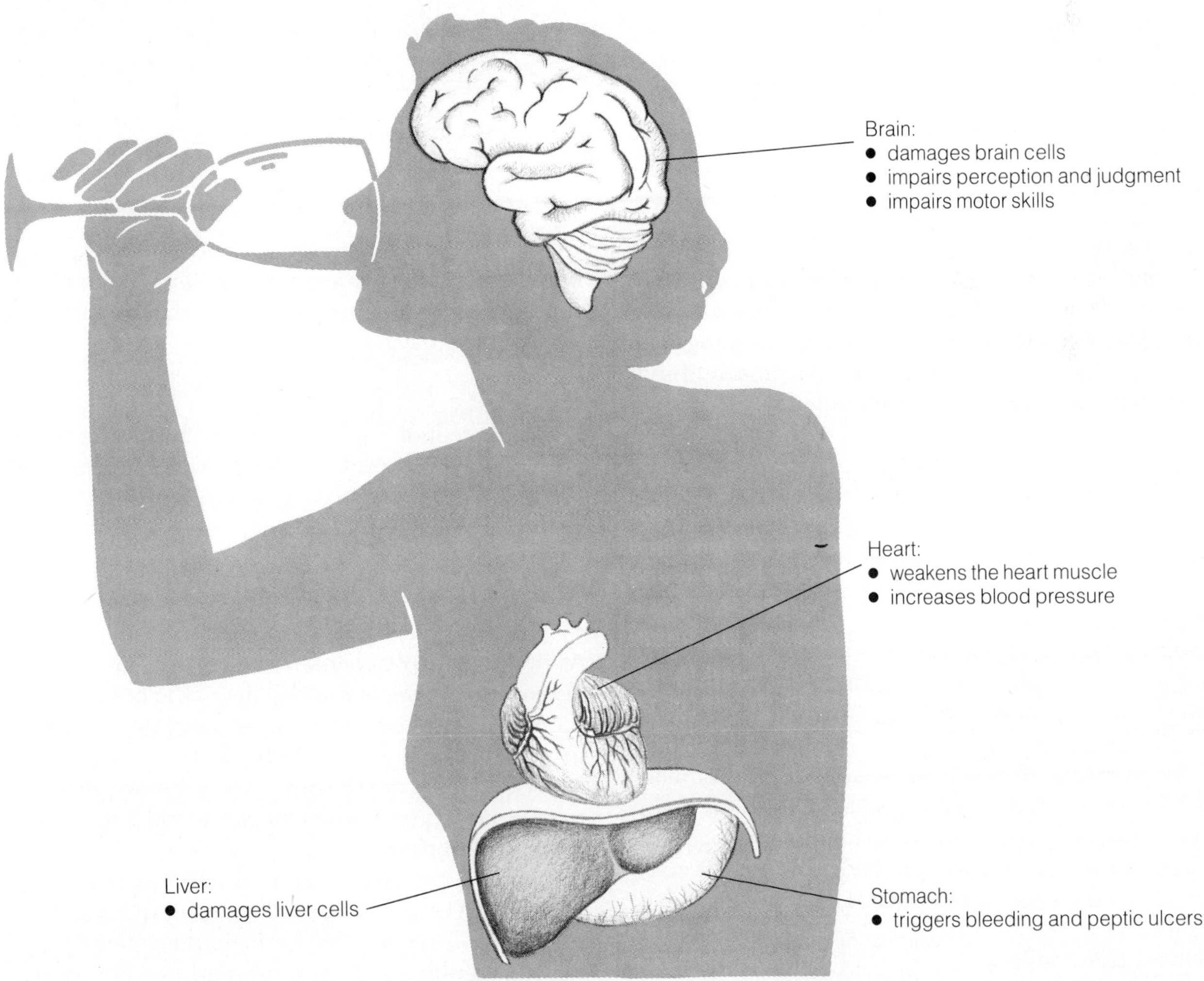


**FIGURE 10-2** Some of the effects of alcohol abuse.

**HALES INDEX**

Percentage of college students who drink alcohol at least once a month: 76

Percentage who have five drinks or more at a time at least once every two weeks: 42

Percentage who drink every day: 4

Percentage of college women who have a drinking problem: 20

Percentage of Americans who don't drink at all: 44

Percentage of people who drink who plan to cut down or quit: 25

Percentage of people who use alcohol who develop alcoholism: 10

Percentage of Americans who will be involved in an alcohol-related accident: 40

Percentage of drivers on the road at any time who are drunk: 10

Number of drunk drivers who are ever arrested: 1 of every 2,000

Costs of alcoholism in lost employment, reduced productivity, and health care every year: $128.3 billion

SOURCES: **1, 2, 3** University of Michigan Institute of Social Research. **4** "Twenty Percent of College Women Have a Drinking Problem," *San Francisco Chronicle*, April 18, 1990. **5, 6** Colasanto, Diane and Zeglarski, John. The Gallup Organization, 1989. **7** National Institute on Alcohol Abuse and Alcoholism. **8, 9, 10** Brody, Jane. "Personal Health," *New York Times*, December 29, 1988. **11** *Seventh Special Report to the U.S. Congress on Alcohol and Health*, Department of Health and Human Services, 1990.

### Stomach

Alcohol triggers the secretion of acids in the stomach, which irritate its lining. Excessive drinking at one sitting may result in nausea; chronic drinking may result in peptic ulcers (breaks in the stomach lining) and bleeding from the stomach lining.

### Cardiovascular System

Moderate drinkers have healthier hearts, suffer fewer heart attacks, have less buildup of cholesterol in their arteries, and are less likely to die of heart disease than heavy drinkers or teetotalers. In studies of participants in northern California's Kaiser-Permanente health program, individuals who averaged two drinks a day had a 40 percent lower chance of hospitalization for heart problems than those who had less than one drink a month.

Some researchers remain unconvinced that alcohol, in any amount, provides real benefits to the heart, and all agree that excessive drinking endangers it. Alcohol use can weaken the heart muscle directly, causing a disorder called cardiomyopathy.

### Blood Pressure

Alcohol may raise blood pressure. Whereas women in one study who averaged fewer than two drinks a day had lower blood pressures than nondrinkers, women and white men who had more than two drinks had higher blood pressures. In black men, blood pressures were highest in those who had three to five drinks a day.[14]

### Blood

Chronic alcohol use can inhibit the production of both white blood cells, which fight off infections, and red blood cells, which carry oxygen to all the organs and tissues of the body.

## Effects on the Brain and Behavior

At first, when you drink, you feel "up." In low dosages, alcohol affects the regions of the brain that inhibit or control behavior. So, you feel looser and act in ways you might not otherwise. However, you also experience loss of concentration, memory, discrimination, and fine motor control; mood swings; and emotional outbursts.

Alcohol is actually a central nervous system depressant, which means it depresses the activity of the neurons (nerve cells) in the brain, gradually dulling the responses of the brain and nervous system. One or two drinks act as a tranquilizer or relaxant. Additional drinks result in a progressive reduction in behavioral activity. This can lead to sleep, general anesthesia, coma, and even death. Alcohol is particularly dangerous when combined with other drugs, such as depressants and antianxiety medications (see Chapter 9).

### The Senses

Moderate amounts of alcohol have disturbing effects on perception and judgment, including the following:

- *Impaired Visual Acuity*—Glare bothers you more because you are less able to readjust your eyes to bright lights.
- *Muddled Hearing*—Although you can still hear sounds, you can't distinguish between sounds or judge their direction well.
- *Dulled Smell and Taste*—Because alcohol interferes with taste and smell, which are strong stimulators of appetite, drinkers often tend to skip meals.

## HEALTH HEADLINE

### Are Alcoholics Born or Made?

Scientists at the University of California, Los Angeles, and the University of Texas Health Sciences Center in San Antonio have identified a gene that puts people at risk for alcoholism. This finding, which provides the most solid evidence yet that alcoholism can be a hereditary disease, may pave the way for development of a blood test to identify high-risk individuals. However, as health experts note, "Genetics accounts for only part of the vulnerability to alcoholism." Not everyone with this gene becomes alcoholic, and some alcoholics do not carry this specific gene. Earlier studies have found that children of alcoholics have four times the risk of developing alcoholism that children of nonalcoholics have.

SOURCES: Blum, K. et al. "Allelic Association of Human Dopamine $D_2$ Receptor Gene in Alcoholism," *Journal of the American Medical Association*, vol. 263, no. 15, April 18, 1990. Gordis, E. et al. "Finding the Gene(s) for Alcoholism," *Journal of the American Medical Association*, vol. 263, no. 15, April 18, 1990.

Alcohol itself may cause vitamin deficiencies. For heavy drinkers with poor eating habits the result can be nutrition problems (see the section "Vitamin Deficiencies" later in this chapter).

- *Diminished Pain Perception*—You may walk outside without a coat on a freezing winter night and not feel the cold.
- *Altered Sense of Time and Space*—You may not realize, for instance, that you have been in one place for several hours.
- *Impaired Motor Skills*—Alcohol impairs your abilities to write, type, drive, and perform any other activities involving your muscles. This is why highway patrol officers sometimes ask a suspected drunk driver to touch his or her nose with a finger or to walk a straight line. Drinking large amounts of alcohol impairs reaction time, speed, accuracy, and consistency, as well as judgment.

### Sexual Performance

Drinking may increase interest in sex, but it may impair a man's ability to achieve or maintain an erection.

## Interaction with Other Drugs

Alcohol can interact with other drugs you use—OTC and prescription, legal and illegal. Of the 100 most frequently prescribed drugs, more than half contain at least one ingredient that interacts adversely with alcohol. Because alcohol and other psychoactive (mood-altering) drugs may work on the same areas of the brain, combining them can produce an effect much greater than that expected of either drug. The consequences can be fatal (see Table 10-6).

**STRATEGY FOR CHANGE**

**Think Before You Drink**

If you want to drink while taking medication, be sure you do the following:

- Read the warnings on nonprescription-drug labels or prescripton-drug containers.
- Ask your doctor about possible alcohol-drug interactions.
- Check with your pharmacist if you have any questions about your medications, especially OTC products.

## Special Concerns for Women

Eight out of every ten working women between the ages of 21 and 34 drink. In addition to the general problems alcohol can cause, these women may face special dangers.

**TABLE 10-6** Interactions of Alcohol and Some Common Drugs

| DRUG | POSSIBLE EFFECTS OF INTERACTION |
|---|---|
| Analgesics | |
| Narcotic (for example, codeine, Demerol, and Percodan) | Increase in central nervous system depression, possibly leading to respiratory arrest and death |
| Nonnarcotic (for example, aspirin and Tylenol) | Irritation of stomach, resulting in bleeding, and increased susceptibility to liver damage |
| Antabuse | Nausea, vomiting, headache, high blood pressure, and erratic heartbeat |
| Antianxiety drugs (for example, Valium and Librium) | Increase in central nervous system depression, resulting in decreased alertness and impaired judgment |
| Antidepressants | Increase in central nervous system depression; certain antidepressants in combination with red wine possibly causing a sudden increase in blood pressure |
| Antihistamines (for example, Actifed, Dimetapp, and other cold medications) | Increase in drowsiness, which makes driving more dangerous |
| Antibiotics | Nausea, vomiting, headache, and some medications rendered less effective |
| Central nervous system stimulants (for example, caffeine, Dexedrine, and Ritalin) | Stimulant effects of these drugs possibly reversing depressant effect of alcohol, but not decreasing intoxicating effects of alcohol |
| Diuretics (for example, Diuril and Lasix) | Reduction in blood pressure, resulting in dizziness when a person rises |
| Sedatives (for example, Dalmane, Nembutal, and Quaalude) | Increases central nervous system depression, possibly leading to coma, respiratory arrest, and death |

According to research by scientists in Italy and the U.S., reported in the *New England Journal of Medicine* in 1990, women have far less of a protective chemical that breaks down alcohol in the stomach. As a result, women absorb about 30 percent more alcohol into their bloodstream than men do. The alcohol travels through the blood to their brains, so that women become intoxicated much more quickly, and to their livers. In alcoholic women, the stomach seems to stop digesting alcohol at all, which may explain why women alcoholics are more likely to suffer liver damage than men. For a woman of average size, one drink has the same effect as two for the average-sized man.[15,16]

### Breast Cancer

In a report by researchers at Harvard Medical School, women who in one week consumed as few as three drinks (of beer and hard liquor, not wine) had a 30 percent greater chance of developing breast cancer than those who seldom or never drank. Another study, by National Cancer Institute investigators, found a 50 percent higher risk of breast cancer among women drinking any alcohol at all and a 100 percent increase in breast cancer among those having three or more drinks a week. Many physicians feel that those at high risk for breast cancer should stop or at least reduce their consumption of alcohol.[17–19] (See Chapter 14 for more on breast-cancer risks.)

### Osteoporosis

Alcohol can block the absorption of many nutrients, including calcium. As women become older, their risk of osteoporosis, a condition characterized by calcium loss and bone thinning, increases. Heavy drinking may worsen this condition.

### Pregnancy

When a woman drinks during pregnancy, her unborn child "drinks" too. Approximately 50 percent of women who are heavy drinkers (those who have three drinks a day 3 or more times a week) may deliver a baby with at least some of the disorders associated with **fetal alcohol syndrome:** small head, abnormal facial features (see Figure 10-3), jitters, poor muscle tone, sleep disorders, sluggish motor development, failure to thrive, short stature, delayed speech, mental retardation, or hyperactivity. (See Chapter 8 for more information about alcohol use during pregnancy.)

**fetal alcohol syndrome** A condition distinguished by specific physical and mental abnormalities in infants born to mothers who drank heavily during pregnancy.

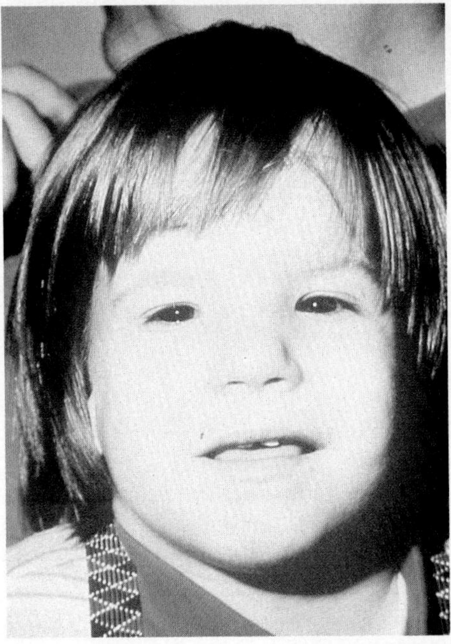

**FIGURE 10-3** A child with fetal alcohol syndrome has distinctive facial characteristics that vary with the severity of the disease. These characteristics include droopy eyelids, a thin upper lip, and a wide space between the nose and the upper lip.

## THE DISEASE OF ALCOHOLISM

Addiction specialists have developed a new definition of alcoholism as "a primary, chronic disease with genetic, psychological, and environmental factors influencing its development and manifestations. The disease is often progressive and fatal. It is characterized by continuous or periodic: impaired control over drinking, preoccupation with the drug alcohol, use of alcohol despite adverse consequences, and distortions in thinking, most notably denial."[20]

About 7 to 10 percent of Americans are alcohol-dependent, and about 17 million of those are alcoholics.[21] In general, alcoholism first appears between the ages of 20 and 40, although children can become alcoholics. Over time, dependence develops. When alcoholics stop drinking, they suffer serious withdrawal symptoms, including physical trembling, sweating, high blood pressure, delusions, and hallucinations.

The American Medical Association recognized alcoholism as a disease more than 20 years ago. Though it may be hard to think of alcoholism as a disease, because people don't catch it from a germ, alcoholics are just as ill as people with heart disease or diabetes.

### Are You at Risk?

No one knows alcoholism's exact cause. It may be that there are metabolic, biochemical, or even dietary factors involved in alcoholism. Heredity plays a definite but undefined role. According to researchers, alcoholism is 4 to 5 times more common among the children of alcoholics. Alcoholics, especially men, are more likely than nonalcoholics to have alcoholic parents and siblings.

The child of an alcoholic, adopted at birth by nonalcoholic parents, is at greater risk of developing alcoholism than is the child of a nonalcoholic placed in a similar home. Also, drinking habits may be handed down from one generation to the next; children who see their parents drinking heavily may do the same when they grow up.

Stress and traumatic experiences can trigger heavy drinking, even in those with no family predisposition to alcoholism. (Indeed, 30 percent of alcoholics may have no family history of the disease.) Some people start drinking heavily as a way of treating psychological problems, such as depression. Whatever the reason they start, some keep drinking out of habit. Once they develop physical tolerance and dependence—the two hallmarks of addiction—they may not be able to stop drinking on their own.

**STRATEGY FOR CHANGE**

**Recognizing the Warning Signs of Alcoholism**

- Experiencing the following symptoms after drinking: frequent headaches, nausea, stomach pain, heartburn, gas, fatigue, weakness, muscle cramps, or irregular or rapid heartbeats
- Needing a drink in the morning to start the day
- Denying any problem with alcohol
- Doing things while drinking that are regretted afterward
- Dramatic mood swings, from anger to laughter to anxiety
- Sleep problems
- Depression and paranoia
- Forgetting what happened during a drinking episode
- Changing brands or going on the wagon to control drinking
- Having five or more drinks a day

Family attitudes toward alcohol also influence children's drinking patterns. When drinking is part of rituals or ceremonies, such as family meals and religious occasions, and there is great disapproval of public drunkenness, there is a lower incidence of heavy drinking. Italians, the southern French, Span-

SELF-SURVEY

## Do You Have a Drinking Problem?

These twenty-six questions were developed by the National Council on Alcoholism, based on information from medical authorities around the world.

| | Yes | No |
|---|---|---|
| 1. Do you occasionally drink heavily after a disappointment or a quarrel, or when your parents give you a hard time? | ____ | ____ |
| 2. When you have trouble or feel pressured at school, do you always drink more heavily than usual? | ____ | ____ |
| 3. Have you noticed that you are able to handle more liquor than you did when you were first drinking? | ____ | ____ |
| 4. Did you ever wake up on the "morning after" and discover that you could not remember part of the evening before, even though your friends tell you that you did not pass out? | ____ | ____ |
| 5. When drinking with other people, do you try to have a few extra drinks that others don't notice? | ____ | ____ |
| 6. Are there certain occasions when you feel uncomfortable if alcohol is not available? | ____ | ____ |
| 7. Have you recently noticed that when you begin drinking you are in more of a hurry to get the first drink than you used to be? | ____ | ____ |
| 8. Do you sometimes feel a little guilty about your drinking? | ____ | ____ |
| 9. Are you secretly irritated when your family or friends discuss your drinking? | ____ | ____ |
| 10. Have you recently noticed an increase in the frequency of your memory blackouts? | ____ | ____ |
| 11. Do you often find that you wish to continue drinking after your friends say that they have had enough? | ____ | ____ |
| 12. Do you usually have a reason for the occasions when you drink heavily? | ____ | ____ |
| 13. When you are sober, do you often regret things you did or said while drinking? | ____ | ____ |
| 14. Have you tried switching brands or following different plans for controlling your drinking? | ____ | ____ |
| 15. Have you often failed to keep the promises you've made to yourself about controlling or cutting down on your drinking? | ____ | ____ |
| 16. Have you ever tried to control your drinking by changing jobs or moving to a new location? | ____ | ____ |
| 17. Do you try to avoid family or close friends while you are drinking? | ____ | ____ |
| 18. Are you having an increasing number of financial and academic problems? | ____ | ____ |
| 19. Do more people seem to be treating you unfairly without good reason? | ____ | ____ |
| 20. Do you eat very little or irregularly when you are drinking? | ____ | ____ |
| 21. Do you sometimes have the shakes in the morning and find that it helps to have a little drink? | ____ | ____ |
| 22. Have you recently noticed that you cannot drink as much as you once did? | ____ | ____ |
| 23. Do you sometimes stay drunk for several days at a time? | ____ | ____ |
| 24. Do you sometimes feel very depressed and wonder whether life is worth living? | ____ | ____ |
| 25. Sometimes after periods of drinking, do you see or hear things that aren't there? | ____ | ____ |
| 26. Do you get terribly frightened after you have been drinking heavily? | ____ | ____ |

Those who answer yes to two or three of these questions may wish to evaluate their drinking in these areas. "Yes" answers to several of these questions indicate the following stages of alcoholism:

- *Questions 1–8: Early Stage.* Drinking is a regular part of your life.
- *Questions 9–21: Middle Stage.* You are having trouble controlling when, where, and how much you drink.
- *Questions 22–26: Beginning of the Final Stage.* You no longer can control your desire to drink.

iards, Portuguese, Greeks, and some Chinese groups have a low incidence of alcoholism; the northern French, Swiss, Swedes, Poles, northern Russians, and Americans have higher alcoholism rates. In societies where traditional rituals have broken down, such as in Japan, alcoholism is on the rise. The societies with the lowest rates of alcoholism are those that restrict the amount of alcohol sold, making it relatively hard to obtain, or impose cultural restrictions on its use.[22]

## What Is an Alcoholic?

Although some people distinguish between problem drinkers and alcoholics, both are individuals whose lives are in some way impaired by their drinking. The only difference is one of degree.

Alcohol becomes a problem and you become an alcoholic when you're no longer in control of when you begin and when you stop drinking. The drinker spends more and more time anticipating the next drink, planning when and where to get it, buying and hiding alcohol, and covering up for secret drinking.

Probably fewer than 5 percent of alcoholics and problem drinkers are skid-row drunks. The other 95 percent are all around us every day. No one—not students, college professors, physicians, politicians, lawyers, or priests—is immune to alcoholism.

Medical professionals base the diagnosis of alcoholism on the presence of at least three of the following symptoms, persisting for a month or more, or occurring repeatedly over a longer period of time:

- alcohol taken in large amounts over a longer period than the person intended
- the persistent desire to quit drinking, or one or more unsuccessful attempts to cut down or quit
- a great deal of time spent getting, using, or recovering from alcohol
- giving up important social, occupational, or recreational activities because of drinking
- continued drinking despite social, psychological, or physical problems, such as ulcers, caused or worsened by alcohol
- because of tolerance, needing at least 50 percent more alcohol than in the past to achieve intoxication
- withdrawal symptoms
- drinking to relieve or avoid withdrawal symptoms

Alcoholism can be categorized by severity as follows:

- *Mild*—few, if any, symptoms beyond those required to make the diagnosis and no more than mild impairment in work, social activities, and relationships with others
- *Moderate*—symptoms or impairment between "mild" and "severe"
- *Severe*—many more symptoms than the three required to make the diagnosis and marked interference with work, social activities, or relationships with others

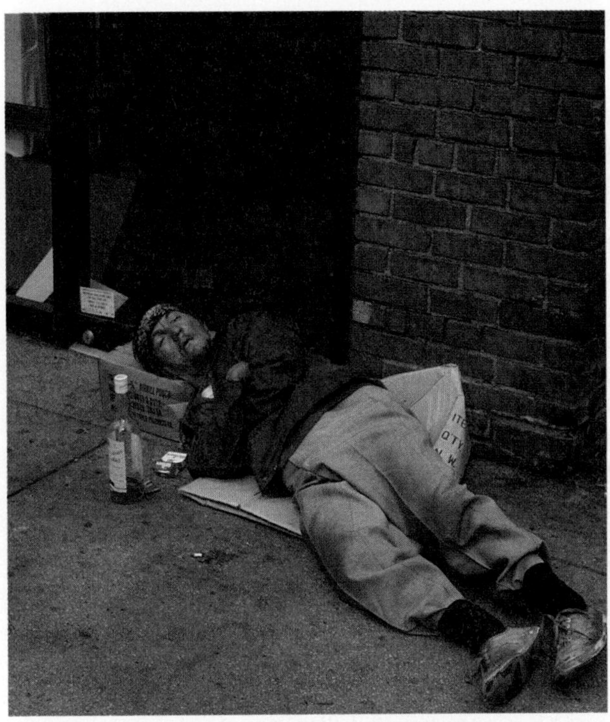

Although some "street" people are alcoholics, they make up only a small fraction of problem drinkers.

## Medical Complications

Over time, alcohol alters brain cell function, causes nerve damage, shrinks parts of the brain, and throws off normal hormonal balance. The liver is one of its primary targets; the heart and other vital organs also suffer. Among the medical problems associated with alcoholism are:

- cancer of the liver, larynx, esophagus, stomach, colon, and breast, as well as malignant melanoma, a deadly form of skin cancer (see Chapter 14 for more on cancer risks)
- high blood pressure, stroke, and heart disease
- damage to the brain, pancreas, and kidneys
- diabetes
- kidney failure
- ulcers
- colitis (inflammation of the colon)
- birth defects and fetal alcohol syndrome
- impotence and infertility

- diminished immunity to disease
- sleep disturbances

### Liver Damage

Chronic heavy drinking can lead to alcoholic hepatitis (inflammation and destruction of liver cells) and, in the 15 percent of people who continue drinking beyond this stage, cirrhosis (irreversible scarring and destruction of liver cells). In its early stages, cirrhosis causes very few symptoms. However, as more scarring occurs and liver cells are destroyed, the liver loses its ability to remove yellow pigment, called bilirubin, from the body; this results in a condition called **jaundice,** in which the skin appears yellow. Eventually a person's fingers and toes begin to swell because of fluid accumulation (**edema**). Uncontrolled bleeding may occur. The liver eventually fails completely, resulting in coma and death.

### Vitamin Deficiencies

Alcoholism is often associated with vitamin deficiencies, especially of thiamine ($B_1$), a deficiency which may be responsible for diseases of the neurological, digestive, muscular, and cardiovascular systems. Lack of thiamine may also result in Wernicke's syndrome, which is characterized by a clouding of consciousness and paralysis of eye nerves, and Korsakoff's psychosis, which is characterized by disorientation, memory failure, and hallucinations.

### Brain Damage

Chronic brain damage resulting from alcohol consumption is second only to Alzheimer's disease as a cause of mental deterioration in adults. Long-term heavy drinkers may suffer memory losses, may be unable to think abstractly or recall names of common objects, and may not be capable of following simple instructions. The deterioration caused by alcohol can be stopped or even reversed if drinking stops.

### Cancer

Alcohol may be a cocarcinogen, enhancing tobacco's cancer-causing effects. The risk of cancer generally increases with the amount of alcohol consumed and number of cigarettes smoked.

---

**jaundice** A condition in which accumulation of pigments in the blood produces a yellowing of the skin.
**edema** An abnormal accumulation of fluid in body parts or tissues; swelling.

### Accidents

Alcohol may contribute to almost half of the lives lost each year in car accidents, burns, falls, drownings, and choking accidents.

## The Cost to Society

Here are some of the ways in which alcohol takes its toll:[23]

- Drunk drivers are responsible for about 50 percent of driving-related deaths each year. (See Chapter 14 for more on car accidents.)
- Alcohol plays a role in up to 70 percent of the 4,000 drowning deaths each year. (See Chapter 14.)
- Alcoholics have a suicide rate 6 to 15 times greater than average. Alcohol plays some role in about 30 percent of all suicides.
- The mortality rate for alcoholics is 2.5 times higher than that for nonalcoholics of the same age.
- Drinking contributes to 45 to 68 percent of the cases of spouse abuse and to 38 percent of the cases of child abuse.
- Alcohol is involved in 83 percent of all arrests. About 30 percent of the nation's state prison inmates drank heavily before committing rapes, assaults, or burglaries.
- Of all males admitted to state mental hospitals, 40 percent suffer from alcoholism.

### The Children's Burden

Alcoholism shatters families, and often the children suffer the most, physically and psychologically. According to psychotherapists, children tend to adopt one of several roles in response to a parent's drinking:

- the adjuster, or "lost" child, who does whatever the parent says without thinking or feeling
- the responsible child, or family hero, who takes over many household tasks and never acknowledges his or her own feelings, fears, and needs
- the placater, who worries constantly about the family's hurt and pain
- the acting-out child, who shows anger early in life by causing trouble at home or in school
- the mascot, who disrupts tense situations by focusing attention on himself or herself, often by clowning, and hides his or her true feelings

Alcoholics' children are also prone to learning disabilities, eating disorders, compulsive achievement, and other compulsive behavior. The nightmare of their parents' drinking may haunt them long after they've grown up. Adult children of alcoholics are more likely to have difficulty solving problems, identifying and

HEALTH SPOTLIGHT

## The Crusade Against Drunk Driving

Every 21 minutes, someone in the United States is killed by a drunk driver—a total of 70 men, women, and children every day. Over the last few years, families of victims of drunk drivers have organized to change the way America treats its drunk drivers. Because of the efforts of MADD (Mothers Against Drunk Driving), SADD (Students Against Drunk Driving), and other lobbying groups, cities, counties, and states are cracking down on drivers who drink.

Because courts have held bars liable for the consequences of allowing drunk customers to drive, many bars and restaurants have joined the campaign against drunk driving. (There is even a group called Bartenders Against Drunk Driving, known as BADD.) Many communities now provide free rides home on holidays and weekends for people who've had too much to drink.

These people are working to save *your* life. If you are under age 35, the principal cause of death for people in your age group is motor vehicle accidents—and more than half of those accidents are caused by drinking drivers.

To keep drunk drivers off the road, many cities set up checkpoints to stop automobiles and check for drunk drivers. The U.S. Supreme Court has ruled that a driver's refusal to submit to a blood alcohol test at such checkpoints or at any other time can be used to prosecute him or her for drunk driving.

An increasing number of states have toughened their enforcement of drunk-driving penalties. These tougher policies seem to be working, and drunk driving has declined substantially, at least on weekend nights.

**What You Can Do To Prevent Drunk Driving**

- When going out in a group, always designate, to serve as driver, one person who will not drink at all.
- Never get behind the wheel if you've had more than two drinks within two hours, especially if you haven't eaten.
- Never let intoxicated guests drive home. Call a taxi, drive them yourself, or have them spend the night.

expressing feelings, trusting others, and being intimate. In addition to their increased likelihood of becoming alcoholics, the children of alcoholics are also more likely to marry alcoholics and keep on playing out the roles of childhood.

STRATEGY FOR CHANGE

### If Someone Close to You Drinks Too Much

- Try to remain calm, unemotional, and factually honest in speaking about the drinker's behavior.
- Discuss the situation with someone you trust: a clergyman, a social worker, friends, or an individual who has experienced alcoholism directly.
- Try to include the drinker in family life.
- Encourage new interests and participate in leisure time activities that the drinker enjoys.
- Be patient, and live one day at a time.
- Try to accept setbacks and relapses calmly.
- Refuse to ride with the drinker when he or she is intoxicated.
- Never cover up or make excuses for the drinker or shield him or her from the consequences of drinking.
- Don't assume the drinker's responsibilities; that takes away dignity and a sense of importance.

## Treatment for Alcoholism

The most difficult step for an alcoholic is to admit that he or she is one. Family, friends, and coworkers often shield the alcoholic from the truth for their own reasons—embarrassment, loyalty, or hope. Unconsciously they conspire to keep an alcoholic alcoholic. If alcoholics are not made aware of their disease through some unexpected trauma, such as being fired or jailed for drunk driving, those who care—family, friends, boss, physician—may have to confront them and insist that they do something about their alcoholism. Often this intervention can be the turning point for alcoholics and their families.

### Getting Help

There are more than 7,000 treatment programs for alcoholics. The most successful combine different approaches and provide ongoing support for people learning to live without alcohol.[24,25]

**Detoxification** Many alcoholics require help in overcoming their physiological addiction to alcohol. Withdrawal symptoms usually develop 6 to 24 hours after a person stops drinking. Symptoms include the following:

- irritability
- agitation
- difficulty concentrating
- tremor of the hands, tongue, and eyelids
- nausea and vomiting
- weakness or achiness
- sweating and elevated blood pressure
- anxiety
- depression
- headache
- dry mouth
- puffy and blotchy skin
- fitful sleep disturbed by bad dreams
- brief hallucinations
- fever
- seizures, particularly in individuals with epilepsy

Withdrawal symptoms almost always disappear within 5 to 7 days.

Many heavy drinkers have their first withdrawal symptoms in their thirties or forties. After ten or more years of heavy drinking, withdrawal may lead to delusions, hallucinations, and agitated behavior. This condition, referred to as **delirium tremens (DTs)**, is most likely to occur in drinkers suffering from malnutrition, fatigue, depression, or another physical illness.

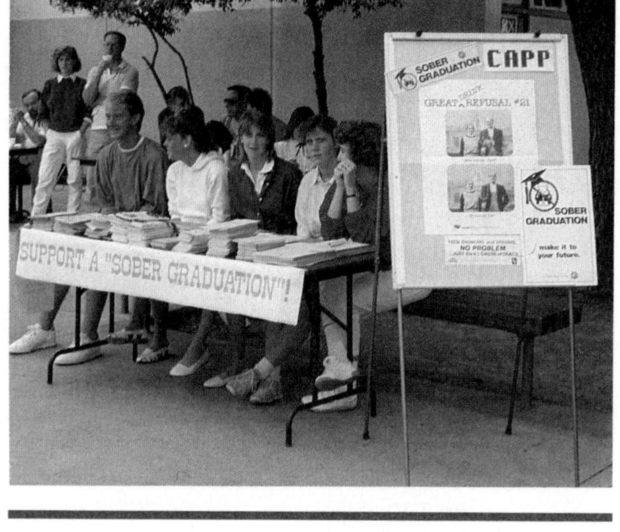


In recent years, more schools and businesses have sponsored alcohol awareness campaigns.

To allow careful monitoring of the individual and to prevent potentially fatal withdrawal reactions, **detoxification** is generally carried out in a medical or psychiatric hospital. Usually, patients begin treatment for their psychological addiction immediately after detoxification.

**Intermediate Care Units** Located in a hospital or at a separate facility, intermediate care units provide 2 to 6 weeks of intensive treatment, which usually includes individual and group psychotherapy, family therapy, fitness, relaxation exercises, biofeedback, spiritual counseling, and Alcoholics Anonymous meetings, as well as formal instruction in the nature of alcoholism. In a controlled environment with little stress, patients can prepare to reenter the alcohol-using world.

**Small-group Therapy** Participating in a small group with other alcoholics may be especially valuable because the members can confront each other. A professional therapist can keep members of the group from ganging up on one person. Some small groups use role playing or psychodrama, in which individuals play other people's roles (such as that of the

**delirium tremens (DTs)** The delusions, hallucinations, and agitated behavior following withdrawal from long-term chronic alcohol abuse.

**detoxification** The removal of a poisonous or harmful substance (such as a drug) from the body; a therapy for alcoholics in which they are denied alcohol in a controlled environment.

long-suffering spouse) and often reveal hidden emotions.

**Alcoholics Anonymous** Founded in 1935, Alcoholics Anonymous (AA) is a fellowship of recovering alcoholics in which members help each other maintain sobriety. Its basic precept is that alcoholics are powerless when it comes to drinking.

AA does not recruit members; it recognizes that the desire to stop drinking must come from the alcoholic. An individual who wants to solve his or her drinking problem can call Alcoholics Anonymous, which is listed in the telephone book, and find out when the next nearby meeting will be held. The AA representative may offer to send someone to the caller's house to talk about the problem and to escort him or her to the next meeting.

Meetings are held daily in almost every city in the country. There are no dues or fees for AA membership; the only requirement is a desire to stop drinking. Many AA members have additional drug problems, such as use of marijuana, cocaine, or barbiturates.

The average age of entry into AA is 30; about 60 percent of the members are men. Members generally come from a wide range of ages, occupations, nationalities, and socioeconomic classes. All learn the Twelve Steps of AA (see Figure 10-4). According to some studies, AA is the most effective means of overcoming alcoholism.

**FIGURE 10-4** The Twelve Steps of Alcoholics Anonymous

1. We admitted we were powerless over alcohol—that our lives had become unmanageable.
2. We came to believe that a Power greater than ourselves could restore us to sanity.
3. We made a decision to turn our will and our lives over to the care of God, as we understood Him.
4. We made a searching and fearless moral inventory of ourselves.
5. We admitted to God, to ourselves, and to another human being the exact nature of our wrongs.
6. We were entirely ready to have God remove all these defects of character.
7. We humbly asked Him to remove our shortcomings.
8. We made a list of all persons we had harmed and became willing to make amends to them all.
9. We made direct amends to such people wherever possible, except when to do so would injure them or others.
10. We continued to take personal inventory and when we were wrong promptly admitted it.
11. We sought through prayer and meditation to improve our conscious contact with God, as we understood Him, praying only for knowledge of His will for us and the power to carry that out.
12. Having had a spiritual awakening as the result of these steps, we tried to carry this message to alcoholics and to practice these principles in all our affairs.

SOURCE: "The Twelve Steps," in *Twelve Steps and Twelve Traditions.* Reprinted with permission of Alcoholics Anonymous World Services, Inc. Please see additional source information on page A-50.

**Women for Sobriety** Founded in 1975, this national self-help program is based on the premise that women alcoholics have different and often more severe problems than do male alcoholics. Most Women for Sobriety groups are no larger than ten members. A group meets once a week in a member's home.

**Family Therapy** A person's alcoholism may be a symptom of a poor family relationship or marriage. An apparently long-suffering wife, for instance, may secretly delight in her feelings of contempt for her alcoholic husband. Family therapy deals with both the drinking problem and such underlying problems.

One national self-help group, called Al-Anon, helps an alcoholic's adult family members cope with the problem of alcoholism in the family, teaching them how to leave behind guilt feelings about the alcoholic; how to become less judgmental and moralistic; how to understand their powerlessness over the drinking problem; and how to do what needs to be done for themselves, as well as for the alcoholic. A similar self-help group, Alateen, provides support for the teenage children of alcoholics.

**STRATEGY FOR CHANGE**

### What to Do If a Loved One Is Alcoholic

Here are some do's and don'ts from Al-Anon for dealing with a loved one who's an alcoholic. Do:

- forgive
- be honest with yourself
- be humble
- take it easy (Tension is harmful.)
- play (Find recreation and hobbies.)
- keep on trying whenever you fail
- learn the facts about alcoholism
- attend support-group meetings, like meetings of Al-Anon
- pray

Don't

- be self-righteous
- try to dominate, nag, scold, complain, or lose your temper
- try to push anyone but yourself
- keep bringing up the past
- keep checking up on your alcoholic
- wallow in self-pity
- make threats you don't intend to carry out
- be overprotective
- be a doormat

**Aversion Therapy** Small electric shocks have been used as a means of treating alcohol abuse since 1925, but this approach has not proven effective. Another aversive technique is the use, for a period of about ten days, of drugs that induce vomiting in combination with several drinks. Follow-up studies have shown successful one-year abstinence rates ranging from 35 to 60 percent.[26]

The drug disulfiram (Antabuse) causes nausea when alcohol is consumed. If the persons taking the drug never drink, they suffer no negative effects. However, if they drink at all while taking the drug, they will become extremely nauseated. If they drink a large amount of alcohol, they may become dangerously ill.

**Other Medications** Antianxiety and antidepressive drugs are sometimes useful, at least in beginning treatment for alcoholism. Scientists are testing drugs that block some of the effects of alcohol. Vitamin supplements can help overcome some of the nutrition deficiencies linked with alcoholism.

### Can Alcoholics Ever Drink Again?

Controversial studies have shown different success rates for controlled drinking. In a long-term study of more than 1,200 alcoholics treated in medical and psychiatric facilities, only 1.6 percent—mostly women with less severe alcoholism—were able to keep their drinking at a moderate level.[27] Some counselors feel that people who drink heavily but have not yet become totally dependent on alcohol may be able to learn how to drink moderately. However, most feel that once alcoholics have reached the point of requiring treatment, they can never return to symptom-free drinking.

### Recovering

Most treatment programs report that 80 percent of their patients remain on the wagon for at least a year; 60 percent, for two years. Estimates on long-term success range from a gloomy 12 percent to about 50 percent. Those most likely to remain sober after treatment are those with the most to lose by continuing to drink: employed, married, upper-middle-class men and women. Even years after their last drink, many ex-alcoholics, painfully aware of alcohol's power, describe themselves as "recovering."

## WHAT DO YOU THINK?

During the week, Mario doesn't drink at all. But on the weekend, which he says is his time to "relax and party," Mario drinks at least a six-pack of beer a day as he visits, goes to bars, or plays football with his friends. Does Mario have a drinking problem?

Driving home from a high school graduation party, an 18-year-old who has had too much to drink crosses the dividing line on a two-lane road. The driver of an oncoming car—a young mother with her two toddlers in the back seat—swerves to avoid a collision and hits a concrete wall. She dies instantly; both children suffer severe injuries that will leave them crippled for life. The young man has no record of drunk driving. Is he guilty of a criminal offense, perhaps murder? Should he be jailed? How would you feel if you were the victims' husband and father? If you were the drunk driver's friend?

Whenever he saw his father fly into a drunken rage, Jeff would swear he'd never drink when he grew up. Now, in college, Jeff's gone out with friends a few times and gotten terribly drunk. He feels funny turning down offers of a beer, but he's terrified of turning into an alcoholic like his dad. Yet he also wants to live as normally as possible. If he confided in you, what would you say? Do you think a support group for adult children of alcoholics might help? Why?

## MAKING THIS CHAPTER WORK FOR YOU

### Responsible Drinking

In recent years society's attitude toward drinking has become more sober. Alcoholism used to be called an "iceberg problem," because there was more to it below the surface than appeared above. Now that it's been exposed—in part by celebrity alcohol abusers like former First Lady Betty Ford, Elizabeth Taylor, and Liza Minnelli—we're coming to grips with the real dimensions of the problem.

Because people are concerned about the effects of alcohol use, there has been a decrease in beer and hard-liquor consumption. Most college students still drink, but less than in the past and with greater awareness of the dangers of drinking binges and driving while drunk.

When comparing amounts and types of alcohol, consider one drink to contain the equivalent of 1/2 oz of 100 percent ethyl alcohol. The percentage of alcohol in a person's blood, or blood alcohol concentration, is the measurement used by law enforcement officials to determine whether someone is legally drunk.

The rate of alcohol absorption depends on how strong a drink is; the drinker's size, sex, age, and race; family history of alcoholism; whether there is food in the stomach; and the drinker's expectations and tolerance to alcohol. Hangovers result from drinking more alcohol than can be metabolized by the liver; the excess alcohol accumulates in the bloodstream.

Moderate amounts of alcohol may have a positive effect on the cardiovascular system. In excess, however, alcohol can weaken the heart muscle, increase blood pressure, increase the risk of stroke, and inhibit the production of white and red blood cells. Alcohol, a central nervous system depressant, also impairs thinking, vision, motor skills, hearing, smell and taste, pain perception, sense of time and space, speech, and sexual performance. When combined with other drugs, alcohol can have more serious adverse effects.

Women, who don't neutralize alcohol as rapidly as men, feel its impact much more quickly and severely. Women who drink face increased danger of breast cancer and osteoporosis. Even moderate drinking can put the babies of pregnant woman at risk for impaired growth in the womb, premature birth, and physical abnormalities. Children of heavy drinkers may suffer from fetal alcohol syndrome or from some of the disorders associated with the condition, including mental retardation, birth defects, and hyperactivity.

Although the exact cause of alcoholism is not known, certain factors—including a biochemical imbalance in the brain, heredity, cultural acceptability, and stress—may play a role in the disease.

Chronic heavy drinking can cause severe liver damage, hepatitis, or cirrhosis. Vitamin deficiencies, which commonly occur with alcoholism, can result in severe neurological, muscular, digestive, and cardiovascular diseases. Excessive alcohol consumption can damage the brain, causing mental deterioration, and is also associated with heart damage and several types of cancer.

The economic, social, and personal costs of alcohol-related crimes, accidents, illnesses, and deaths are profound. Children of alcoholics are more likely to suffer abuse, to have psychological or emotional problems, to become alcoholics, and to marry alcoholics.

Withdrawal symptoms after prolonged drinking range in severity from weakness and irritability to DTs. Because withdrawal reactions may be fatal, detoxification is usually carried out in a medical facility. Alcohol treatment may involve small-group or family therapy, attendance at meetings held by Alcoholics Anonymous or Women for Sobriety, behavior therapy, hospital detoxification programs, or drug therapy. Most experts believe that complete abstinence from alcohol is the only treatment for alcoholism.

Responsible drinking is always an individual, as well as a societal, matter. As you decide about the role alcohol should play in your life, you might want to follow these guidelines, proposed by BACCHUS, a volunteer college-student organization that promotes responsible alcohol-related behavior:

- Set a limit ahead of time on how many drinks you're going to have—and stick to it.
- Develop alternatives to drinking so you don't turn to alcohol whenever you're depressed or upset. Exercise is a wonderful release for tension; meditation and relaxation techniques can also help you cope.
- During or after drinking, avoid performing tasks that require skilled reactions.
- Keep in mind that drinking should not be the primary focus of any activity. Responsible drinking is a matter of you controlling your drinking, rather than the drinking controlling you.

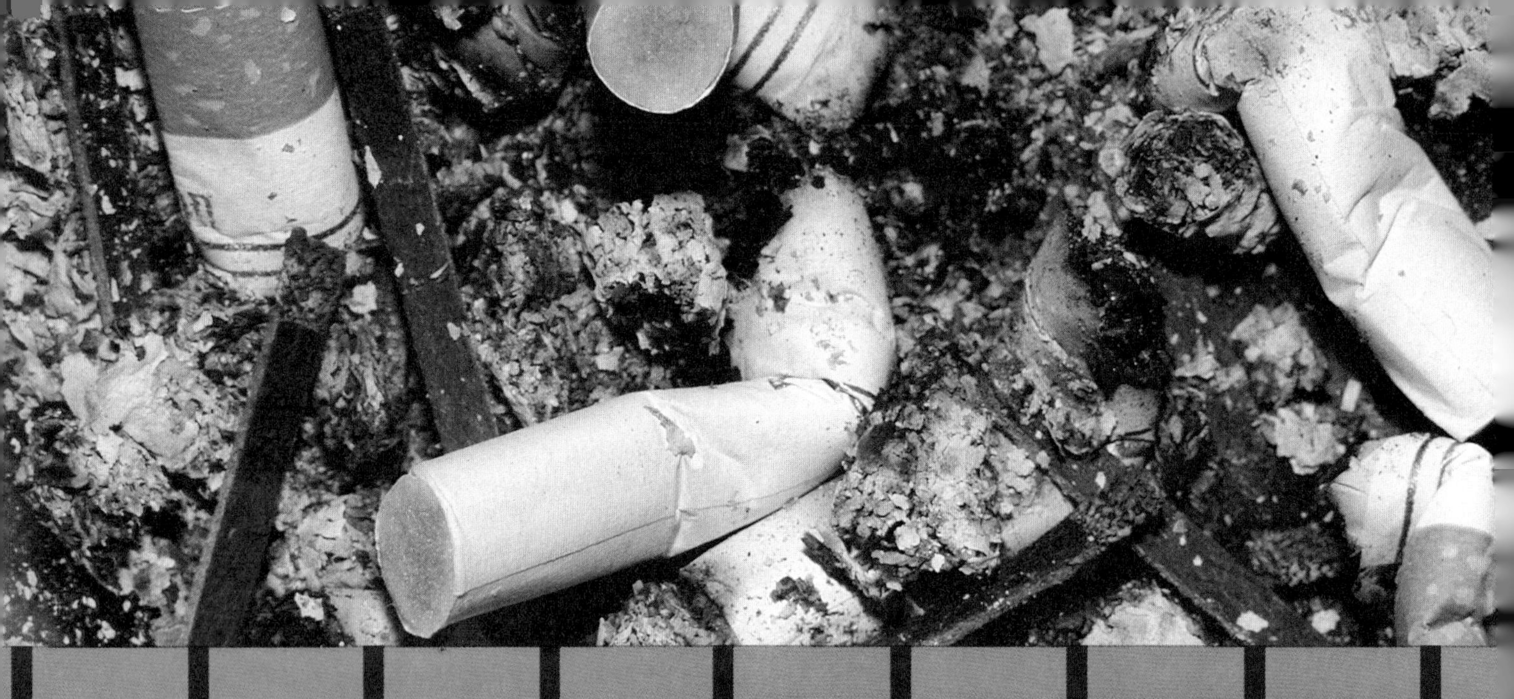

# 11 TOBACCO: BREAKING A DEADLY ADDICTION

In this chapter

Smoking today

Tobacco: What it is and what it does

The health effects of smoking

Other forms of tobacco

Passive smoking

Quitting

Making this chapter work for you: Breathing easier

*Tobacco use is the most serious and widespread addiction in the world and the major cause of preventable deaths in the U.S.* Each year, smoking claims more lives than alcohol and drug abuse combined. More Americans die because of smoking-related health problems every year than the total of all the American soldiers and sailors killed in World War I, World War II, and the Vietnam war.[1] Although tobacco dependency is an addiction—one some claim is more powerful than heroin addiction—it can be overcome. If you're a smoker or a user of smokeless tobacco, this chapter may provide the information you need to stop. Even if you don't smoke or chew tobacco, you have reason to be concerned: Passive smoke is a danger to all who breathe, and the costs of tobacco use are something we all bear and share.

## SMOKING TODAY

In the last ten years, the ranks of smokers have begun to dwindle. The Department of Health and Human Services (HHS) Office on Smoking and Health reports that the percentage of Americans who smoked dropped throughout the 1980s.[2] According to *Smoking and Health,* published by HHS in 1990, 26.5 percent of Americans age 17 or older smoke—the lowest percentage ever recorded (see Figure 11-1). Since the actual number of smokers has grown with the population, there are more smokers today than two decades ago. However, almost half of all Americans—48.9 percent—have never had a cigarette.

As a social behavior, smoking has become increasingly unpopular, even unacceptable. Corporations, cities, states, and communities are restricting smoking. Restaurants and airlines have banned smoking. National polls have found that the majority of Americans—including smokers—think smoking in the workplace should be restricted to designated areas.

### Who Smokes?

Men are still more likely to smoke than women. According to HHS, 29.5 percent of adult men are smokers; 40 percent have never smoked; and 30.4 percent are former smokers. Among adult women, 23.8 percent are smokers; 56.9 percent have never smoked; and 19.3 percent have quit. Blacks are more likely to smoke than whites: 28.4 percent of black Americans are current smokers, compared to 26.4 percent of whites. More men (36.2 percent) than women (23.4 percent) are heavy smokers. A third of white smokers are heavy smokers, but only 11.4 percent of blacks smoke 25 or more cigarettes a day.[3]

Today's smokers lit up their first cigarettes at a younger age than did smokers of the past. Half acquired the habit before they were 18 years old. This is important because the earlier you start smoking, the longer you're exposed to tobacco and the greater your risk. Young smokers also tend to become heavy smokers.

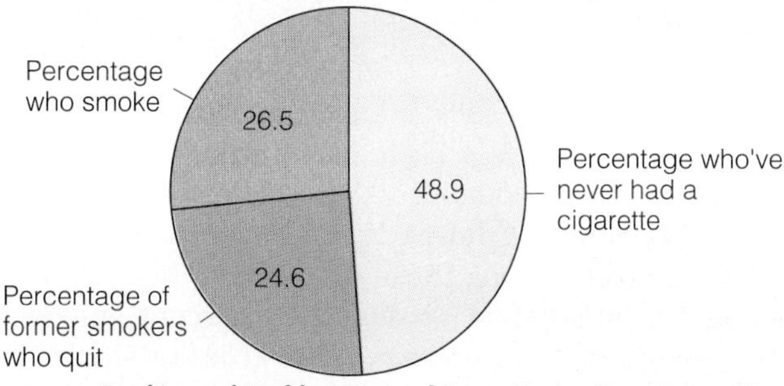


SOURCE: *Smoking and Health: A National Status Report,* Department of Health and Human Resources, 1990

**Figure 11-1** Who Smokes?

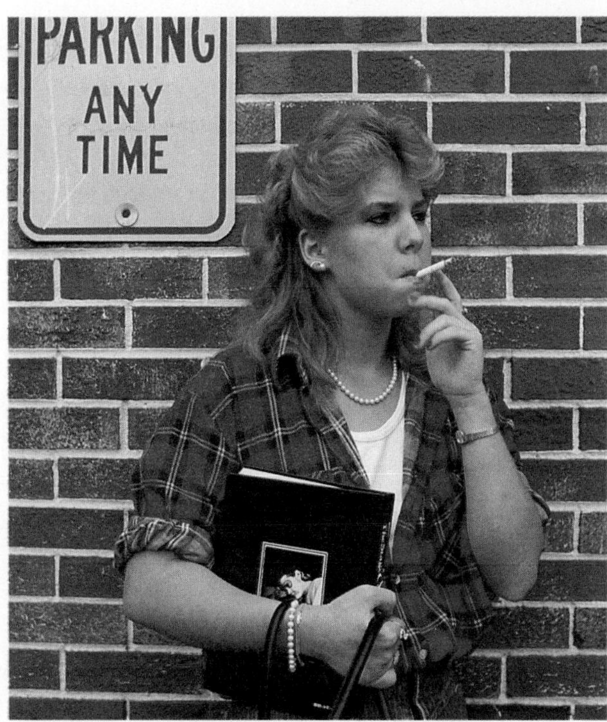


More than twenty percent of women smoke. Many lit up their first cigarette when they were in their teens.

The higher a person's educational and socioeconomic status, the less likely he or she is to smoke. Among college graduates, 16.3 percent smoke; however, 31.4 percent of those who never completed high school smoke. Among those whose total household income is more than $40,000, 21.8 percent smoke; 28.9 percent of those who earn $10,000 or less smoke.[4]

More than a third of current smokers (35.5 percent) have never tried to quit. Another 37.3 percent have made one or two attempts but resumed smoking. Almost 20 percent (18.9 percent) have quit three to five times, and 8.3 percent have tried to break their smoking habit six times or more but failed each time. The majority of ex-smokers (70.2 percent) made one or two attempts before quitting, 21.2 percent tried three to five times, and 8.6 percent tried six or more times before finally succeeding.[5]

## Why People Start Smoking

If you smoke, you may have started because of simple curiosity. But there are many reasons why people light up.

### Social Ease

Many people start smoking to imitate their parents or friends. They may want to be accepted by a group of people who smoke, or smoking may seem like a sign of maturity.

### Ignorance

Although most Americans are aware that there is a health risk associated with smoking, many don't know exactly what that risk is or how it might affect them: Nearly a third of the public still doesn't know that cigarette smoking can cause heart disease. Two out of five people don't know that smoking causes 80 percent of all lung cancer. Half of all women don't know that smoking during pregnancy increases the risk of stillbirth or miscarriage.

### Weight Control

According to recent research, smokers burn up 100 calories a day more than nonsmokers. (That number is about equivalent to the number of calories burned in walking a mile.) The increase probably happens because nicotine increases metabolic rate. When smokers quit, they are likely to gain 5 to 10 pounds, even if they eat the same amount of food as when they smoked. In a Memphis State University study of 209 student smokers, 39 percent of men and 25 percent of women said they smoked to control weight. However, smoking is more dangerous to health than

## HALES INDEX

Number of Americans who regularly use some form of tobacco: 1 in 3

Number of Americans who die of tobacco-related causes every day: 1,000

Minutes of life expectancy lost for each cigarette you smoke: 5-1/2

Number of smokers who started smoking by age 15: 1 in 2

Amount spent on cigarette advertising each year: $2.5 billion

Infants who die before their first birthday each year because their mothers smoked during pregnancy: 2,500

Cancers caused around the world by smoking each year: 900,000

Number of daily cigarettes linked to impotence in some men: 10

Each American's annual smoking-related costs: $221

Smoking's annual costs to the nation, including health care and insurance: $52 billion

Costs of smoking in lost productivity and health care per pack of cigarettes sold: $2.17

SOURCES: **1** "Tobacco Use by Adults," *Journal of American Medical Association*, November 3, 1989. **2** Work, Clemens. "Where There's Smoke," *U.S. News & World Report*, March 5, 1990. **3** American Cancer Society. **4, 5** Gallager, John. "Under Fire from All Sides," *Time*, March 5, 1990. **6, 7** American Cancer Society and National Cancer Institute. **8** "Coffee and Cigarettes: Facts on Helping and Hindering Sexual Potency," Impotence Information Center, January 23, 1990. **9, 10, 11** *Smoking and Health: A National Status Report*, Department of Health and Human Services, 1990.

5 or 10 extra pounds—and less attractive. And the American Cancer Society reports that smokers who combine a fitness program with their efforts to quit stay at the same weight or even lose several pounds.[6]

### Advertising

Cigarette companies spend more than $2.5 billion on advertisements and promotional campaigns. Recently, manufacturers have targeted ads at certain key groups, including minorities and women. The strategy seems to have worked; a higher proportion of women students in high school and college are becoming smokers.

Manufacturers have also aimed advertising efforts at black men (whose smoking rates are 8 to 10 percentage points higher than those for white men), Hispanics, blue-collar workers, and the military. Most troubling is a trend of advertising cigarettes in magazines and media aimed at teenagers and even young children.[7,8]

## Why People Keep Smoking

Whatever the reasons for lighting up the first cigarette, very different factors keep cigarettes burning—pack after pack, year after year. In fact, four out of five smokers want to quit but can't. The reason isn't a lack of willpower. In recent years, medical scientists have recognized tobacco dependence as an addictive disorder affecting more than 90 percent of all smokers.

### Pleasure

Most regular smokers enjoy smoking; nicotine is the reason. Researchers have shown that nicotine reinforces and strengthens the desire to smoke by acting on brain chemicals involved in feelings of well-being. Nicotine can also improve memory, help in performing certain tasks, reduce anxiety, dampen hunger, and increase pain tolerance.

### Dependence and Avoiding Withdrawal

If smokers do not get daily nicotine fixes, they suffer withdrawal symptoms, such as irritability and anxiety. Smokers find smoking relaxing because it reverses the very tensions triggered by the withdrawal from nicotine. In fact, after a few years of smoking, the most powerful incentive for continuing to smoke is to prevent withdrawal. Generally, ten cigarettes a day prevent withdrawal. For many who smoke heavily, however, signs of withdrawal, including changes in mood and performance, occur within 2 hours of their last cigarette. In this way nicotine has a more powerful hold on smokers than alcohol does on drinkers: About 10 percent of alcohol users lose control of their intake and become alcoholics. As many as 80 percent of all heavy smokers have tried to reduce or quit smoking but cannot overcome their dependency.[9]

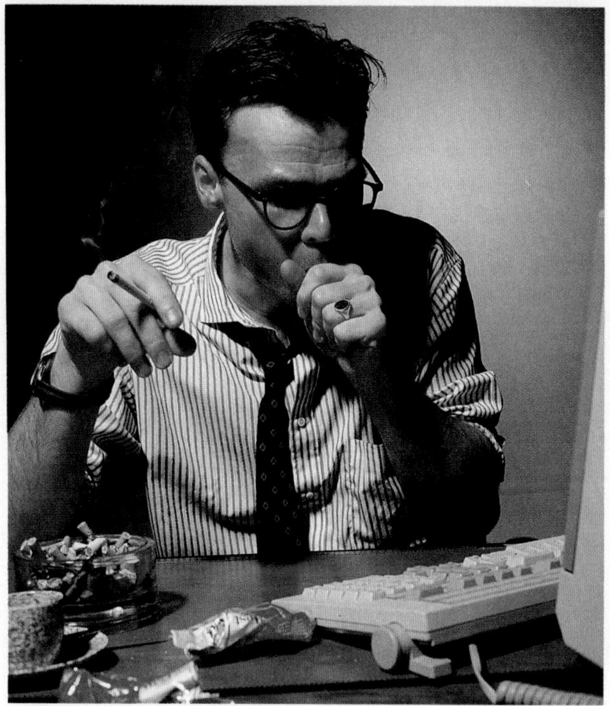

Eight of ten heavy smokers have tried to quit or cut down but cannot overcome their tobacco addiction.

### Addiction

Nicotine causes addiction because:

- It provides a strong sensation of pleasure.
- It leads to fairly severe discomfort during withdrawal.
- It stimulates cravings long after obvious withdrawal symptoms have passed.

Nicotine seems most addictive when absorbed by the lungs; it seems less addictive when absorbed through the linings of the nose and mouth. As with other drugs of abuse, continued nicotine intake results in tolerance (the need for more of a drug to maintain a constant effect), which is why only 2 percent of all smokers smoke just a few cigarettes a day or smoke only occasionally. The world's major medical groups have recognized tobacco dependence as an addictive disorder.[10]

**STRATEGY FOR CHANGE**

**Are You Hooked?**

- Have you tried unsuccessfully to stop smoking or to significantly reduce the amount of tobacco you use?

- When you stop using tobacco, do you develop withdrawal symptoms, such as a craving for tobacco, irritability, anxiety, difficulty concentrating, restlessness, a headache, drowsiness, and digestive disturbances?
- Do you continue to use tobacco despite a serious physical disorder (such as a respiratory disease) worsened by tobacco use?
- Do you resume tobacco use after quitting?

If you answer yes to any of these questions, you're a tobacco addict—whether or not you care to admit it. You may need help—from friends or family or from a stop-smoking group—to break your habit.

## TOBACCO: WHAT IT IS AND WHAT IT DOES

Tobacco is an herb that can be smoked or chewed and that affects the brain. Its primary active ingredient is nicotine, but there are almost 4,000 other compounds in tobacco smoke, including nicotine, tar, and carbon monoxide. The following section describes what goes into your lungs and how your body is affected (see Figure 11-2).

### Nicotine

A colorless, oily compound, **nicotine** is the addictive element in cigarettes. If you inhale, 90 percent of the nicotine in the smoke is absorbed into your body. But even if you draw smoke into your mouth only and not into your lungs, you absorb 25 to 30 percent of the nicotine. If you are a regular smoker, nicotine generally stimulates you when you begin smoking, but then tranquilizes you.

Nicotine increases your blood pressure, speeds up your heart rate 15 to 20 beats a minute, dampens hunger, irritates the membranes in the mouth and throat, and dulls the taste buds so that food does not taste as good as it would otherwise. Nicotine is also a major contributor to heart and respiratory diseases.

### Tar

**Tar,** a thick, sticky dark fluid produced when tobacco is burned, is made up of several hundred different

**nicotine** A poisonous alkaloid found in tobacco; one of the most toxic of all poisons; used in concentrated amounts as a powerful agricultural insecticide.
**tar** A substance present in the smoke of burning tobacco; composed of combustion by-products.

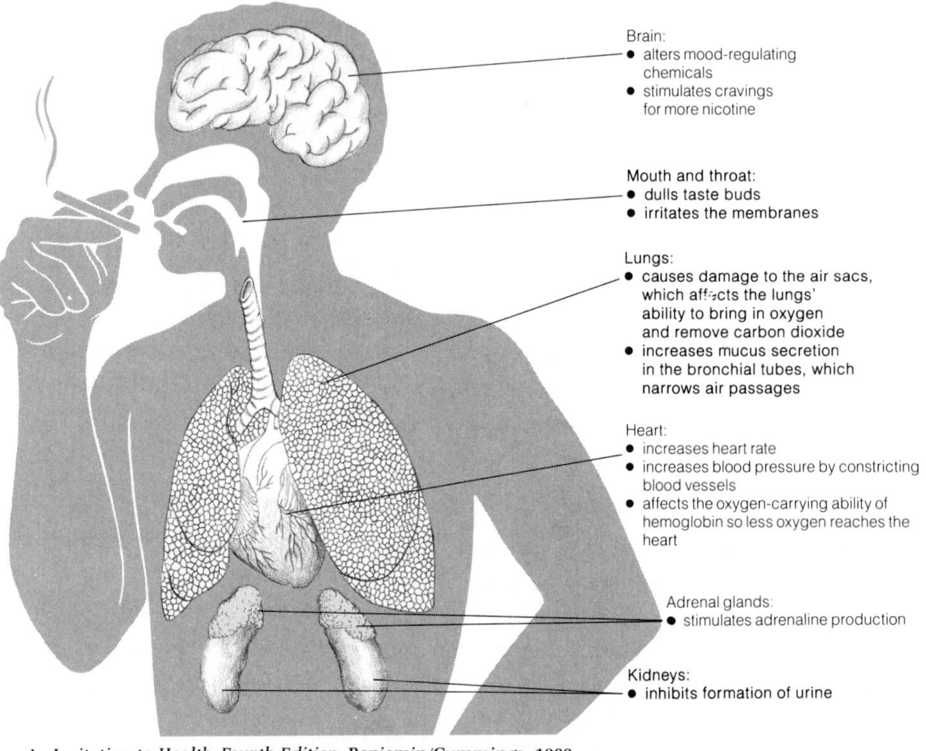


SOURCE: Hales, Dianne. *An Invitation to Health, Fourth Edition,* Benjamin/Cummings, 1989.

**Figure 11-2** Some of the effects of nicotine on the body.

chemicals—many of them poisonous, some of them **carcinogenic** (leading to the growth of cancerous cells).

As you inhale, tar settles in the forks of the branch-like bronchial tubes in your lungs; precancerous changes are apt to occur at these locations. In addition, tar and smoke damage the mucus and the cilia in the bronchial tubes, which are supposed to remove irritating foreign materials from the lungs.

### Carbon Monoxide

Smoke from cigarettes, cigars, and pipes contains **carbon monoxide,** the deadly gas that comes out of the exhaust pipes of cars, in levels 400 times those considered safe in industry. Carbon monoxide interferes with the ability of the blood to carry oxygen, impairs normal functioning of the nervous system, and is at least partly responsible for the increased risk of heart attack and strokes in smokers.

## THE HEALTH EFFECTS OF SMOKING

There's no longer any doubt that smoking stacks the deck against staying well and living longer (Figure 11-3). Every pack of cigarettes carries a warning about lung cancer and emphysema as well as injury to a fetus if the smoker is pregnant.

According to the federal Office on Smoking and Health, cigarette smoking, by contributing to heart and lung diseases, cancers, fires, and other causes of mortality, is responsible for almost 16 percent of all deaths in the United States each year. Among its victims are 2,500 infants who die before their first birthday, because their mothers smoked during pregnancy. Each year Americans who die of smoking-related

**carcinogen** A substance that produces cancerous cells or enhances their development and growth.
**carbon monoxide** A colorless, odorless gas that is a by-product of engine exhaust and burning tobacco; displaces oxygen on the hemoglobin molecules of red blood cells.

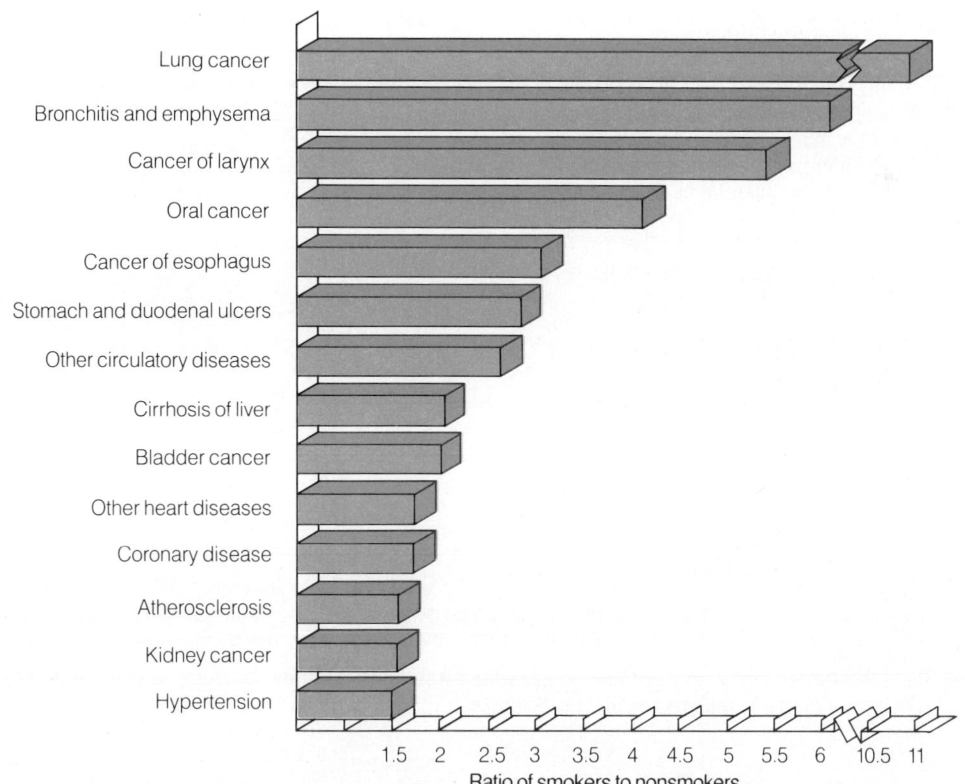


SOURCE: Chiras, Daniel D. *Environmental Science, Second Edition,* Benjamin/Cummings, 1987.

**Figure 11-3** Increased ratios of smoker deaths from fourteen disorders. A smoker is 10.8 times as likely to die of lung cancer as a nonsmoker: 108 smokers will die of lung cancer for every 10 nonsmokers in the general population.

SELF-SURVEY

## Why Do You Smoke?

This activity will help you identify smoking behaviors that, if recognized and controlled, could help you kick the habit. It will also advance your understanding of smoking behavior. If you do not smoke, have a friend who does smoke respond to these questions and discuss the results.

***Directions***

Respond to each question by circling one of the choices: 5 = Always, 4 = Frequently, 3 = Occasionally, 2 = Seldom, 1 = Never. Important: *Answer every question.*

| | Always | Frequently | Occasionally | Seldom | Never |
|---|---|---|---|---|---|
| A. I smoke cigarettes to keep myself from slowing down. | 5 | 4 | 3 | 2 | 1 |
| B. Handling a cigarette is part of the enjoyment of smoking it. | 5 | 4 | 3 | 2 | 1 |
| C. Smoking cigarettes is pleasant and relaxing. | 5 | 4 | 3 | 2 | 1 |
| D. I light a cigarette when I feel angry about something. | 5 | 4 | 3 | 2 | 1 |
| E. When I run out of cigarettes, I find it almost unbearable until I can get more. | 5 | 4 | 3 | 2 | 1 |
| F. I smoke automatically, without even being aware of it. | 5 | 4 | 3 | 2 | 1 |
| G. I smoke to stimulate myself, to perk myself up. | 5 | 4 | 3 | 2 | 1 |
| H. Part of the enjoyment of smoking a cigarette comes from the steps I take to light it. | 5 | 4 | 3 | 2 | 1 |
| I. I find cigarettes pleasurable. | 5 | 4 | 3 | 2 | 1 |
| J. When I feel uncomfortable or upset about something, I light a cigarette. | 5 | 4 | 3 | 2 | 1 |
| K. When I am not smoking a cigarette, I am very much aware of that fact. | 5 | 4 | 3 | 2 | 1 |
| L. I light a cigarette without realizing I still have one burning in the ashtray. | 5 | 4 | 3 | 2 | 1 |
| M. I smoke cigarettes to give me a lift. | 5 | 4 | 3 | 2 | 1 |
| N. When I smoke a cigarette, part of the enjoyment is watching the smoke as I exhale it. | 5 | 4 | 3 | 2 | 1 |
| O. I want a cigarette most when I am relaxed and comfortable. | 5 | 4 | 3 | 2 | 1 |
| P. When I feel blue or want to take my mind off cares and worries, I smoke. | 5 | 4 | 3 | 2 | 1 |
| Q. I get a real gnawing hunger for a cigarette when I haven't smoked for a while. | 5 | 4 | 3 | 2 | 1 |
| R. I've found a cigarette in my mouth and didn't remember putting it there. | 5 | 4 | 3 | 2 | 1 |

***Scoring***

1. In the spaces that follow, enter the number you have circled for each question, putting the number you have circled for question A over line A, for question B over line B, and so on.
2. Add the three scores on each line to get your totals. For example, the sum of your scores over lines A, G, and M gives you your score on Stimulation; lines B, H and N give the score on Handling; and so on.

| ______ + | ______ + | ______ = | ______ |
|---|---|---|---|
| A | G | M | Stimulation |
| ______ + | ______ + | ______ = | ______ |
| B | H | N | Handling |
| ______ + | ______ + | ______ = | ______ |
| C | I | O | Pleasurable relaxation |

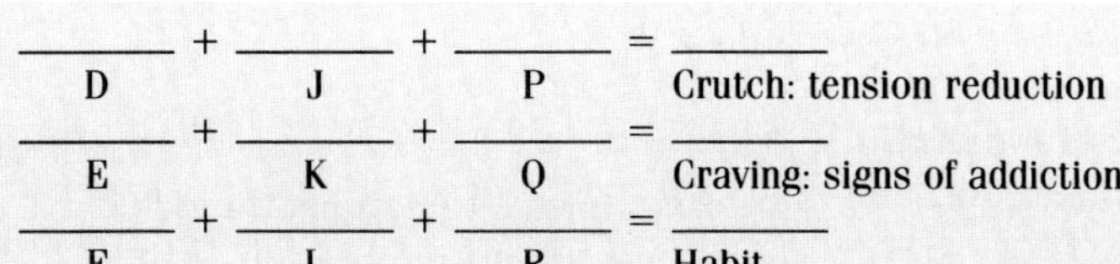

_____ + _____ + _____ = _____
D J P Crutch: tension reduction

_____ + _____ + _____ = _____
E K Q Craving: signs of addiction

_____ + _____ + _____ = _____
F L R Habit

Your total score in each category gives a rough indication of how important each factor is to you:

11–15 Highly important 7–10 Somewhat important 3–6 Not important

If you scored below 7 in every one of the six categories, it should be easy for you to quit smoking. If you scored higher in two or more, and particularly if you scored high in the "craving" and "habit" categories, you may have to use multiple strategies to counteract the reward that smoking currently gives you.

A score of 11 or above on any item indicates that this factor is an important source of satisfaction for you. The higher your score (15 is the highest), the more important a particular factor is in your smoking and the more useful the discussion of that factor can be in your efforts to quit.

***Explanation of Factors***

1. *Stimulation.* If you scored high on this factor, it means that you are one of those who is stimulated by the cigarette—that is, you feel that it helps you wake up, organize your energies, and keep you going. If you try to give up smoking, you may want a safe substitute—a brisk walk or moderate exercise, for example—whenever you feel the urge to smoke.
2. *Handling.* Handling things can be satisfying, but there are many ways to keep your hands busy without lighting up or playing with a cigarette. Why not toy with a pen or pencil? Try doodling, or play with a coin, a piece of jewelry, or some other harmless object.
3. *Accentuation of pleasure—pleasurable relaxation.* It is not always easy to find out whether you use the cigarette to feel good—that is, to get real pleasure out of smoking (factor 3)—or to keep from feeling so bad (factor 4). Those who do get real pleasure out of smoking often find that an honest consideration of the harmful effects is enough to help them quit. They substitute eating, drinking, social activities, and physical activities—within reasonable bounds—and find they do not seriously miss their cigarettes.
4. *Reduction of negative feelings or crutch.* Many smokers use the cigarette as a kind of crutch in moments of stress or discomfort, and on occasion it may work; the cigarette is sometimes used as a tranquilizer. However, those who smoke heavily, people who try to handle severe personal problems by smoking many times a day, are apt to discover that cigarettes do not help them deal effectively with problems.

   When it comes to quitting, this kind of smoker may find it easy to stop when everything is going well but may be tempted to start again in times of crisis. Again, physical exertion, eating, drinking, or social activity—in moderation—may serve as useful substitutes for cigarettes, even in times of tension.
5. *Craving or psychological addiction.* Quitting smoking is difficult for people who score high on the factor of psychological addiction. For them, craving for the next cigarette begins to build up the moment they put one out; so tapering off is not likely to work. They must go cold turkey. It may be helpful for these smokers to smoke more than usual for a day or two, so that the taste for cigarettes is spoiled, and then isolate themselves completely from cigarettes until the craving is gone. Giving up cigarettes may be so difficult and cause so much discomfort that once they do quit, they will find it easy to resist the temptation to go back to smoking.
6. *Habit.* This kind of smoker is no longer getting much satisfaction from cigarettes. Those who smoke from habit frequently light cigarettes without even realizing they are doing so. They may find it easy to quit and stay off them if they can break the habit patterns they have built up. Cutting down gradually may be quite effective if there is a change in the way cigarettes are smoked and in the conditions under which they are smoked. The key to success is becoming aware of each cigarette you smoke.

SOURCE: Adapted from Test III of the *Smoker's Self-Testing Kit*, which was developed by Dr. Daniel H. Horn and originally printed by the National Clearinghouse for Smoking and Health, Department of Health, Education, and Welfare, 1980.

causes before age 65 lose a total of 949,924 years of potential life. Also, smoking-related diseases annually account for $22 billion in health care costs and $43 billion in lost productivity.[11]

A cigarette smoker is more than 10 times more apt to develop lung cancer than is a nonsmoker and 20 times more likely to have a heart attack. Those who smoke two or more packs a day are 15 to 25 times more likely to die of lung cancer than are nonsmokers. The danger skyrockets when smokers are also exposed to known carcinogens, such as asbestos. This double threat increases the risk of lung cancer by as much as 92 times that for nonsmokers not exposed to asbestos. The Environmental Protection Agency lists tobacco smoke as the country's most dangerous airborne carcinogen.[12]

## Heart Disease

Although a great deal of publicity has been given to the link between cigarettes and lung cancer, smokers are most likely to die of heart disease (see Chapter 13), according to the U.S. Surgeon General. Smoking doubles the risk of heart disease, and smokers who suffer heart attacks have only a 50 percent chance of recovering. Smokers have a 70 percent higher death rate from heart disease than do nonsmokers; heavy smokers have a 200 percent higher death rate than smokers.

Smoking contributes to **aortic aneurysms** (a bulge in the large artery called the aorta, caused by a weakening of the walls) and **pulmonary heart disease** (a heart disorder caused by changes in blood vessels in the lungs).

The Surgeon General blames cigarettes for 1 out of every 10 deaths attributable to heart disease. Smoking is more dangerous than are the two best-known risk factors for heart disease: high blood pressure and a high cholesterol level. If smoking is combined with one of these, the chances of heart attack are 4 times greater. Women who smoke and use oral contraceptives have a 10 times higher risk of suffering heart attacks than do women who use neither.[13]

The number of years a person has smoked does not seem to have much bearing on the risk of heart attack. But if a person quits smoking, the risk falls to a level about the same as that for nonsmokers. In fact, even people who have smoked for decades can reduce their risk of heart attack if they quit smoking.

In addition to contributing to heart attacks, smoking causes a condition called cardiomyopathy, which weakens the heart muscle's ability to pump blood and results in the death of about 10,000 people a year. Although researchers don't know precisely how smoking poisons the heart muscle, they speculate that either nicotine or carbon monoxide has a direct toxic effect.

## Strokes

Smokers have 2 to 3 times the risk of stroke (interference with blood circulation in part of the brain)—after taking into account such factors as age, blood pressure, heart disease, and other risks. Subjects who quit smoking have only a slightly increased risk over nonsmokers.[14]

## Lung Cancer

Lung cancer, the leading cause of cancer deaths in the United States, kills more than 130,000 Americans a year—92,000 men and 44,000 women. As many as 83 percent the lung cancer cases could be avoided if individuals didn't smoke.[15]

The American Cancer Society estimates that tobacco smoking is the cause of 28 percent of all deaths from cancer and of more than 85 to 90 percent of all cases of lung cancer. Lung cancer—long the leading killer of American men—now claims more women's lives than breast cancer.[16]

More than fifty major scientific studies have confirmed the strong, direct correlation between smoking and lung cancer. The more people smoke, the longer they smoke, and the earlier they start smoking, the more apt they are to develop lung cancer. Smokers of two or more packs a day have lung cancer mortality rates 15 to 25 times greater than that for nonsmokers. If smokers stop smoking before cancer has started, their lung tissue tends to repair itself, even if there were already precancerous changes. Former smokers who have not smoked for 15 or more years have lung cancer mortality rates only somewhat above those for nonsmokers. Despite some advances in treating lung cancer, the prognosis for its victims is not good. Even with vigorous therapy, fewer than 10 percent survive for five years after diagnosis. This is one of the lowest survival rates for any type of cancer. If the cancer has spread from the lungs to other parts of the body, those surviving for five years after diagnosis drops to only 1 percent.

## Respiratory Diseases

Smoking quickly impairs the respiratory system. Even some high school smokers show signs of respiratory

---

**aortic aneurysm** A blood-filled sac in the aorta; caused by dilation or weakening of the blood vessel wall.

**pulmonary heart disease** A cardiovascular condition resulting from alterations in the blood vessels in the lungs.

difficulty—breathlessness, chronic cough, excess phlegm production—when compared with nonsmokers of the same age. Cigarette smokers are up to 18 times more likely than are nonsmokers to die of lung disease.[17]

Cigarette smoking is the major cause of **chronic obstructive lung disease (COLD),** which includes emphysema and chronic bronchitis, in men and women. COLD is characterized by progressive limitation of the flow of air into and out of the lungs. More than 10 million Americans suffer from bronchitis and emphysema; more than 60,000 die each year as a result of COLD.

In **emphysema,** the limitation of airflow is the result of disease changes in the lung tissue—changes affecting the smallest air passages and the walls of the alveoli, the tiny air sacs of the lung (see Figure 11-4). Eventually many of the air sacs are destroyed, and the lungs become much less able to bring in oxygen and remove carbon dioxide. As a result, the heart has to work harder to deliver oxygen.

In **chronic bronchitis,** the bronchial tubes in the lungs become inflamed. The inflammation thickens the walls of the bronchi, and the production of mucus increases. The result is the narrowing of the air passages. To some degree, the changes brought about by bronchitis are reversible.

Smoking is more dangerous than is any kind of air pollution, at least for most Americans—but exposure to both air pollution and cigarettes is particularly harmful. Although each may cause bronchitis, together they have a synergistic effect—that is, their combined effect exceeds the sum of their separate effects.

## Women and Smoking: Special Risks

Women have come a long way—in smoking, at any rate. More women smoke now than in the past, and they smoke more cigarettes. Although the percentage of women smoking has recently dropped somewhat,

**chronic obstructive lung disease (COLD)** Any one of several lung diseases, characterized by obstruction of breathing; includes emphysema and bronchitis.
**emphysema** A condition caused by overdistention of the pulmonary alveoli or by the abnormal presence of air or gas in the body's tissues.
**chronic bronchitis** A persistent inflammation of the bronchi due to irritation by air pollutants and tobacco smoke.

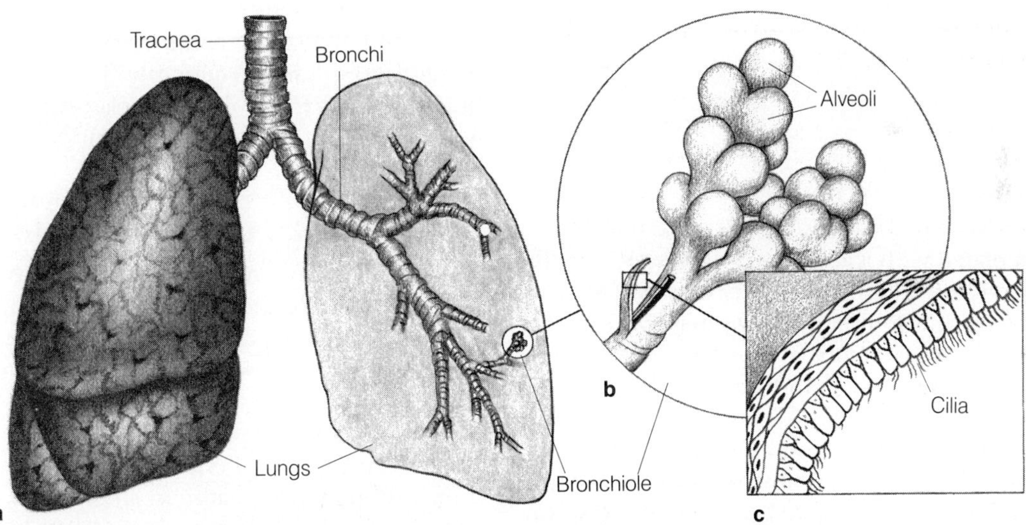


SOURCE: Hales, Dianne. *An Invitation to Health, Fourth Edition,* Benjamin/Cummings, 1989.

**Figure 11-4** The respiratory system and smoking. **(a)** Air travels down the trachea to the *bronchi,* large passageways that lead into the lungs. The bronchi branch off into smaller and smaller passageways; the smallest are called *bronchioles.* Smoking increases mucus secretion in the bronchial tubes, which narrows the air passages. This results in coughing and inflammation of the bronchi. **(b)** At the end of the bronchioles are clusters of *alveoli* (air sacs). When air reaches the alveoli, tiny capillaries pick up the oxygen, beginning its journey via the blood vessels to other parts of the body. Smoking damages the alveoli, which means less oxygen can be held in the lungs. As a result, less oxygen is available to the rest of the organs in the body. **(c)** Thousands of tiny cells, called *cilia,* line the bronchial passageways and sweep out foreign matter. Smoking destroys the cilia, allowing particles and bacteria to enter the alveoli and infect them.

this decrease is far smaller than the decline in percentage of male smokers. In the last 25 years, the number of male smokers has fallen by 21.4 percent; the number of female smokers has declined by only 5.8 percent.

Over a 20-year period the percentage of women smoking more than twenty-five cigarettes a day climbed from 13 percent to 23.4 percent. And women are starting to smoke at younger and younger ages. Of women smokers now between the ages of 28 and 37, 84 percent started smoking before the age of 20.[18]

The price women are paying for their smoking habit is high. Smoking directly affects women's reproductive organs and processes. Women who smoke are less fertile, and they experience menopause one or two years earlier than nonsmokers. Also, smoking boosts a woman's likelihood of developing cervical cancer and greatly increases the possible risks associated with taking oral contraceptives.[19] (See Chapter 8 for a complete discussion of the pill.)

A pregnant woman who smokes has a high risk of losing her baby before, during, or after birth (see Chapter 8). Her baby may be premature or underweight and may have heart and breathing problems and poor muscle tone. Possible long-term effects on children include impaired growth, abnormal intellectual and emotional development, and behavior problems.

## HEALTH HEADLINE

### Quitting: Once May Not Be Enough

**As many as 95 percent of people who manage to break their cigarette habit permanently do so on their own. The long-term abstinence rate for participants in formal stop-smoking programs is about 20 percent. However, most people who eventually quit on their own have tried other methods. According to therapists, quitting usually is not a one-time event but a "dynamic process" that may take several years.**

SOURCE: Cohen, Sheldon et al. "Debunking Myths about Self-quitting: Evidence from 10 Prospective Studies of Persons Who Attempt to Quit Smoking by Themselves," *American Psychologist*, November 1989.

## Other Smoking-related Problems

In addition to heart and lung disease, cigarette smoking is associated with a great many illnesses, including stomach and duodenal ulcers, various cancers, and cirrhosis of the liver. Smoking may worsen the symptoms or complications of allergies, diabetes, hypertension, peptic ulcers, and existing disorders of the lungs or blood vessels.

Smoking reduces a person's sex drive, produces bleeding gums and foul breath from trench mouth or gingivitis, and leads to early loss of teeth. Cigarette smokers tend to miss work one-third more often than do nonsmokers, primarily because of respiratory illnesses. In addition, each year an estimated 2,000 Americans lose their lives and more than 3,000 others are injured in cigarette-ignited fires.[20]

## Smoking and Medication

Smokers are more likely than nonsmokers to use medications: more aspirin, painkillers, sleeping pills, tranquilizers, cough medicines, stomach medicines, laxatives, diuretics, and antibiotics. But tobacco does not mix well with other drugs. According to the American Pharmaceutical Association, cigarette smoking interferes with the metabolism of drugs. Nicotine and other tobacco ingredients speed up the process by which the body uses and eliminates these drugs. So, the drug may not be able to do what it is supposed to do. As a result, smokers may have to take a medication more frequently than do nonsmokers. It is important to let your physician know if you smoke so that he or she can vary any prescriptions, if necessary.[21]

## The Financial Costs of Smoking

Cigarette smoking may cost $52 billion a year in health care and lost productivity. Business and industry pay more than $13 billion a year for smoking-related absenteeism, insurance premiums, disability payments, and training costs to replace employees who die prematurely from smoking.[22] Other social costs—the aggravation of allergies and other problems for nonsmokers who breathe in smoke, and the administration of smoking and nonsmoking sections in restaurants and theaters, for example—add to the direct costs.

In the course of a lifetime, the average smoker can expect to spend $10,000 to $20,000 on cigarettes—but that's only the beginning. The potential costs for medical services for a man between the ages of 35 and 39 who smokes heavily may be as high as $60,000. The greatest toll, of course, the pain and suffering of cancer victims and their loved ones, can't be measured in dollars and cents.

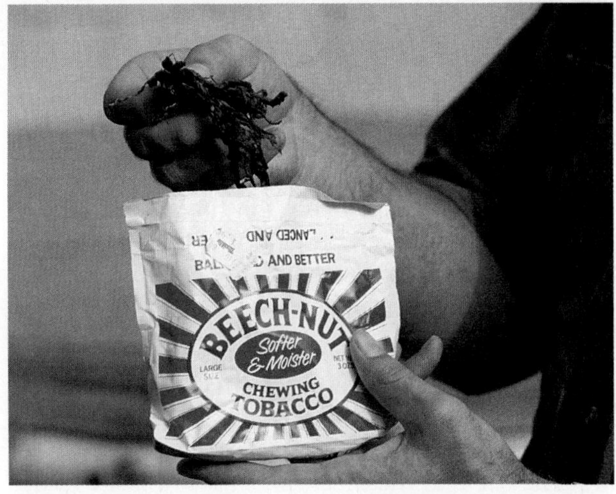


Although not as deadly as cigarettes, smokeless tobacco products like snuff and chewing tobacco are dangerous and can cause cancer.

## OTHER FORMS OF TOBACCO

Other forms of tobacco may be less deadly than cigarettes, but all are dangerous. Clove cigarettes, cigars, pipes, and smokeless tobacco put the user at increased risk of cancer of the lip, tongue, mouth, and throat.

### Clove Cigarettes

Sweeteners have long been mixed into tobacco; clove, a spice, is the latest ingredient to be added to the recipe for cigarettes. Clove cigarettes are becoming increasingly popular, with more than 150 million imported from Indonesia each year. Consumers of these cigarettes are primarily teenagers and young adults.

Clove cigarettes typically contain two-thirds tobacco and one-third cloves. Many users believe these cigarettes are safer because they contain less tobacco, but this isn't necessarily the case. The Centers for Disease Control report that people who smoke clove-containing cigarettes may be at risk for serious lung injury. Smoking clove cigarettes during a mild upper-respiratory illness can lead to severe breathing difficulty, and clove-cigarette smokers can become addicted to tobacco.[23]

Clove cigarettes may actually be more harmful than conventional cigarettes. Puff for puff, they deliver twice as much nicotine, tar, and carbon monoxide as moderate-tar American brands. Eugenol, the active ingredient in cloves (which dentists have used as an anesthetic for years), deadens sensation in the throat, allowing smokers to inhale more deeply and hold smoke in their lungs for a longer time. In addition, studies have shown that close chemical relatives of eugenol can produce the kind of cell damage that may eventually lead to cancer.[24]

### Pipes and Cigars

Many cigarette smokers switch to pipes or cigars to reduce their risk of health problems. But former cigarette smokers may continue to inhale, even though pipe and cigar smoke is more irritating than cigarette smoke.

People who have smoked pipes and cigars only and do *not* inhale are much less likely to develop lung and heart disease than are cigarette smokers. However, they are as likely as cigarette smokers to develop—and die of—cancer of the mouth, larynx, throat, and esophagus.

### Smokeless Tobacco

Other tobacco products may be taking the place of cigarettes in the mouths of Americans (see Figure 11-5). These include snuff and chewing tobacco.

*Snuff* is a finely ground tobacco that can be sniffed or placed inside the cheek and sucked. Nicotine is absorbed through the mucous membranes of the nose or mouth.

*Chewing tobacco* consists of leaves mixed with flavoring agents such as molasses. As the tobacco is chewed, nicotine is absorbed through the mucous membranes of the mouth.

An estimated 7 million to 22 million people, many of them young, use snuff and chewing tobacco.[25] In some parts of the country, as many as a third of high school students, especially teenage and young adult males, are users. One reason is that some professional baseball players often keep a wad of tobacco jammed in their cheeks—a practice many high school and college athletes imitate.

Although not as deadly as cigarette smoking, smokeless tobacco is dangerous. An advisory committee to the Surgeon General reported that "the oral use of smokeless tobacco represents a significant health risk. It is not a safe substitute for smoking cigarettes. It can cause cancer and a number of non-cancerous oral conditions, and can lead to nicotine addiction and dependence."

The report's overall conclusions included the following:[26]

- The use of snuff increases the likelihood of oral cancer by more than 4 times and the risk of cancer of the cheek and gum by 50 times. Experiments reveal powerful carcinogens in smokeless tobacco: nitrosamines, polycyclic aromatic hydrocarbons, and radiation-emitting polonium.

- Smokeless tobacco use can lead to the development of white patches on the mucous membranes of the mouth, particularly the site where tobacco is placed. These can develop into cancer.
- Nicotine, even when administered orally, can produce physiologic dependence.

Another danger for teenagers who use smokeless tobacco is that as they get older, and chewing tobacco and dipping snuff become less socially acceptable, they may switch to the deadliest form of tobacco of all: cigarettes. In the meantime, they're likely to develop bad breath, discolored teeth, missing teeth, cavities, gum disease, and nicotine addiction.

### STRATEGY FOR CHANGE

#### How to Stop Using Smokeless Tobacco

- Keep a record of when, where, and why you're most likely to use smokeless tobacco.
- Identify high-risk situations, such as while playing softball with your friends.
- Gradually reduce the amount of time you keep a wad of chewing tobacco or snuff in your cheek.
- As soon as you remove it, rinse your mouth with mouthwash or, if possible, brush your teeth. Use breath mints if you can't rinse or brush.
- Substitute sugarless chewing gum for chewing tobacco or snuff.
- If you're a young man (as most users of smokeless tobacco are), ask some of the women you know what they think of guys who chew tobacco or suck on snuff.
- When you're ready to quit, have your teeth cleaned. Talk to your dentist about staining, gum disease, and other hazards of smokeless tobacco.
- Drink a lot of fluids and exercise regularly to cleanse your system of nicotine.

## PASSIVE SMOKING

Maybe you don't smoke—never have and never will. That doesn't mean you don't have to worry about the dangers of smoking. If you live or work with people who do smoke, you are engaging in **passive smoking.**

On the average, a smoker inhales what is known as **mainstream smoke** 8 or 9 times with each cigarette, for a total of about 24 seconds. However, the cigarette burns for about 12 minutes, and everyone else in the room breathes in what is known as **sidestream smoke.** Sidestream smoke is even more hazardous than mainstream smoke: According to the American Lung Association, it has twice as much tar and nicotine, 5 times as much carbon monoxide, and 50 times as much ammonia. Researchers have found that if you are a nonsmoker sitting next to someone smoking seven cigarettes an hour, even in a ventilated room you will take in almost twice the maximum amount of carbon monoxide set for air pollution in industry—and it will take hours for the carbon monoxide to leave your body.[27]

The most vulnerable nonsmokers are those who live with smokers. Nonsmokers married to smokers have a much greater risk of lung cancer. The longer one spouse smokes, the greater the risk to the nonsmoking mate. A Pittsburgh study found that nonsmoking wives of smoking men died an average of four years earlier than did those whose husbands did not smoke.

Studies of children have shown that those whose parents smoke have a higher incidence of asthma, ear infections, respiratory infections, and lung impairment than do nonsmokers' children. A report in the American Heart Association journal, *Circulation,* in 1990 found that children regularly exposed to smoke may suffer the same adverse health effects as smokers, including increased risk of heart disease and stroke.[28]

The National Academy of Sciences and the American College of Physicians have called upon parents of small children to keep their houses smoke-free. Infants of parents who smoke are more often hospitalized for bronchitis and pneumonia than are youngsters in nonsmoking households.[29]

The Surgeon General has concluded that "the evidence is very solid" that passive smokers can suffer lung disease. According to the EPA, 500 to 5,000 people may die each year from cancer caused by inhaling other people's smoke, including 2,800 from lung cancer. The Surgeon General has warned that the risk of involuntary smoking may not be eliminated by simply separating smokers and nonsmokers within the same space.[30]

---

**passive smoking** Living or working with people who smoke.
**mainstream smoke** The smoke directly inhaled by a smoker.
**sidestream smoke** The smoke indirectly inhaled by a nonsmoker, usually as a result of being in the same room as a smoker.

STRATEGY FOR CHANGE

**How Nonsmokers Can Clear the Air**

Here are some ways to speak up for your rights to clean air:

- Let people know your feelings in advance by putting up "no smoking" plaques in your office, home, or car.
- When giving a party, designate a smoking room.
- Suggest that friends do the same for parties at their houses.
- If you're in a car and someone pulls out a cigarette, ask politely if the smoker can hold off until you reach your destination or stop for a break.
- If you're about to participate in a long meeting or class, suggest regular smoking breaks to avoid a smoke-filled room.
- At restaurants, always ask for a table in the nonsmoking section or, if there is none, one in a well-ventilated part of the restaurant.
- Whatever the circumstance, if someone's smoke is bothering you, speak up. Be polite, not pushy. Say something like "Excuse me, but smoke bothers me."

## QUITTING

If you inhale deeply and if you started smoking before age 15, you are trading a minute of life for every minute of smoking. Smoking not only kills, it also ages you. In a California survey 25-year-old men who smoked cigarettes had chronic illnesses serious enough to force them to limit their activity or take days of disability—illnesses that were the same as chronic illnesses in nonsmoking men twenty years their senior. Smokers even tend to have more wrinkles than nonsmokers.

Most smokers *want* to stop smoking but don't know how to go about it. Yet, the great majority of smokers eventually manage to quit on their own.[31] In the next few pages, we'll suggest some ways to stop smoking. If you're a smoker who desires to stop, try as many as necessary; some are bound to help.

### Cutting Down

Here are tips for smoking less—and less dangerously:

- Have your first cigarette of the day 15 minutes later than usual, then 15 minutes later than that the next day, then even later.
- When you feel a craving for a cigarette, distract yourself—talk to someone, drink a glass of water, or get up and move around.
- Establish nonsmoking hours and gradually extend them.
- If you usually smoke after eating, get up immediately, brush your teeth, wash your hands, or take a walk.
- Never smoke two packs of the same brand in a row.
- Buy cigarettes only by the pack, not by the carton.
- Make it harder to get to your cigarettes—lock them in a drawer, wrap them in paper, or leave them in your coat.
- Smoke with the hand you don't usually use.
- Smoke only half of each cigarette.
- Keep daily records so you can see how much progress you're making.
- Spend more time with nonsmokers.
- Don't empty ashtrays. Nothing smells worse than stale butts.

### Going Cold Turkey

If you are a heavily addicted smoker, psychologists recommend a sudden, decisive, and complete break, according to the American Cancer Society. You might try to stop for just one day at a time. Promise yourself 24 hours of freedom from cigarettes; and when the day is over, make a commitment for one more day. At the end of any 24-hour period, you can go back to smoking and not feel guilty.

STRATEGY FOR CHANGE

**How to Help a Smoker Quit**

Threats, tears, and complaints don't work. Here are some better techniques based on advice from Dr. Tom Ferguson, author of *The Smoker's Book of Health*:[32]

- Don't nag or tell smoking friends what to do. Encourage them to focus on what *they* think is best for taking more control of their smoking.
- Separate the smoking from the smoker. Let your friends know you'll continue to care, no matter what they do—or don't do.
- If you'd prefer that your smoking friends not smoke in your car, house, or presence, ask them—politely—to refrain. Be courteous and nonjudgmental.

Once a smoker decides to quit, here's how to help:

- Let your friend know how delighted you are and that you're confident things will work out.

- Offer to provide help with routine chores, such as preparing meals, doing household chores, or caring for children during the first tense, smoke-free days.
- Help keep your friend away from smokers and cigarettes.
- To join in the effort, consider giving something up yourself—such as coffee—for the first few days or weeks.
- Be prepared for a rough week, including the possibility of some verbal abuse. Try to forgive in advance.

## When You Need Help

The nicotine habit is one of the hardest addictions to overcome. And, as with other drug dependencies, people may be more successful in their efforts to quit if they have help. If you need help in learning how to change your behavior or in handling withdrawal symptoms or if you just need support from others who have the same problem, there are several options available to you.

### Stop-smoking Groups

Attending a stop-smoking group is one way of quitting. In this method, a large or small group meets regularly, and a leader conducts sessions designed to change your smoking pattern. Perhaps the strongest element is the support you get from others with the same problem. Regardless of the type of program, more smokers who sought help (37 percent) were able to maintain abstinence for a year than were those who tried to quit unaided (18 percent).[33]

The American Cancer Society runs about 1,500 stop-smoking clinics, each with about eight to eighteen members meeting for eight 2-hour sessions over four weeks. When there is a cost, it is nominal. Also, classes are available through health science departments and student health services on many college campuses, as well as through community public health departments.

Many businesses sponsor quit-smoking programs for employees. Most follow the approaches of professional groups. Motivation may be higher in these programs than in other stop-smoking groups, because companies may offer attractive incentives, such as lower rates on health insurance.

### Aversion Therapy

The theory behind **aversion therapy** is that if you have unpleasant thoughts or are punished every time you have a cigarette, you will finally stop smoking. This approach can involve taking drugs that make tobacco smoke taste unpleasant, undergoing electric shocks, having smoke blown at you, or experiencing rapid smoking (the inhaling of smoke every 6 seconds until you are dizzy or nauseated, a technique that can be dangerous because it causes rapid heartbeat).

### Nicotine Gum

A gum containing a nicotine resin that is gradually released as the gum is chewed helps some smokers break their habit. Each Nicorette pellet, a peppery-tasting gum, delivers about as much nicotine as a cigarette. Absorbed through the mucous membrane of the mouth, the nicotine doesn't produce the same rush as does a deeply inhaled drag. However, it maintains enough nicotine in the blood to diminish withdrawal symptoms. Available with a doctor's prescription, a month's supply costs roughly $120.

Although the gum is lightly spiced to mask nicotine's bitterness, many users say it takes several days to become accustomed to its unusual taste. Its side effects include mild indigestion, sore jaws, nausea, heartburn, and stomachache. Because Nicorette gum is heavier than regular chewing gum, it may loosen fillings or cause problems with dentures.

Nicotine in any form is harmful, and nicotine gum should *not* be used during pregnancy or by people who give up smoking because of heart disease. Chewing nicotine is less addictive than smoking, and most people who use it as a temporary crutch are able to stop chewing relatively painlessly. However, some transfer their dependence from cigarettes to the gum. When they stop using it, they go through withdrawal—although the symptoms may be milder than withdrawal from cigarettes.[34]

### Great American Smoke-out

Since 1976, a November day has been set aside for the annual Great American Smoke-out, an idea promoted by the American Cancer Society to encourage smokers to give up cigarettes for 24 hours. As many as 36 percent of American smokers have given up cigarettes on Smoke-out Day. According to a Gallup poll, more than 8 percent succeeded for the entire 24 hours; follow-up a year after previous smoke-outs indicated that 6 to 7 percent of those who quit for a day managed to break the habit permanently.

**aversion therapy** A treatment that attempts to help a person overcome a dependence or a bad habit by making the person feel disgusted or repulsed by the habit.

HEALTH SPOTLIGHT

## Breaking the Habit

Here's a six-point program to help you or someone you love toward a smokeless future. (Caution: Don't undertake the quit-smoking program until you have a 2- to 4-week period of relatively unstressful work and study schedules or social commitments.)

1. *Identify your smoking habits.* Keep a daily diary (a piece of paper wrapped around your cigarette pack with a rubber band will do) and record the time you smoke, the activity associated with smoking (after breakfast, or in the car), and your urge for a cigarette (desperate, pleasant, or automatic). For the first week or two, don't bother trying to cut down; just use the diary to learn the conditions under which you smoke.
2. *Get support.* It can be tough to go it alone. Phone your local chapter of the American Cancer Society, or otherwise get the names of some ex-smokers who can give you support.
3. *Begin by tapering off.* For a period of 1 to 4 weeks, aim at cutting down to, say, 12 to 15 cigarettes a day; or change to a lower-nicotine brand, and concentrate on not increasing the number of cigarettes you smoke automatically. In addition, restrict the times you allow yourself to smoke. Throughout this period, stay in touch, once a day or every few days, with your ex-smoker friend(s) and talk over your problems.
4. *Set a quit date.* At some point during the tapering period, announce to everyone—friends, family, and ex-smokers—when you're going to quit. Do it with flair. Announce it to coincide with a significant date, such as your birthday or anniversary.
5. *Stop.* A week before Q-day, smoke only five cigarettes a day. Begin late in the day, say after 4:00 P.M. Smoke the first two cigarettes in close succession. Then, in the evening, smoke the last three, also in close succession, about 15 minutes apart. Focus on the negative aspects of cigarettes, such as the rawness in your throat and lungs. After seven days, quit—and give yourself a big reward on that day, such as a movie or a fantastic meal or new clothes.
6. *Follow up.* Stay in touch with your ex-smoker friends during the following two weeks, particularly if anything stressful or tense occurs that might trigger a return to smoking. Think of the person you're becoming—the very person cigarette ads would have you believe smoking makes you. Now that you are quitting smoking, you are becoming sexier, more sophisticated, more mature, better looking, and healthier—and you deserve it.

SOURCES: American Cancer Society. National Cancer Institute.

### Other Methods

Hypnosis may help some people quit smoking. Hypnotists use their technique to create an atmosphere of strict attention and give smokers in a mild trance positive suggestions for breaking their cigarette habit.

Acupuncture, in which a circular needle or a staple is inserted in the flap in front of the opening to the ear, has also had some success. When smokers feel withdrawal symptoms, they gently move the needle or staple, which is supposed to increase the production of calming chemicals in the brain.

## WHAT DO YOU THINK?

Federal health officials have urged professional athletes to reject tobacco-industry support, such as funding for professional sports events, as blood money. Should athletes let their status and names be used to promote, even indirectly, a product that causes death? Should colleges refuse to host events sponsored by tobacco companies? Why or why not?

Cigarette companies have targeted advertising at groups whose smoking has increased in recent years: teenagers, young women, and minorities. They feel these individuals are less likely than others to be aware of tobacco's deadly effects. Should government restrict such advertising? Should all cigarette advertising be banned?

With smoking banned on airplanes, in many offices, and in more public places, smokers are beginning to feel discriminated against. Fighting back against smoking bans, they argue that they have a right to indulge in their habit. Those against smoking contend that no one has the right to cause others harm. What do you think? If you're a nonsmoker, would your opinion change if you were a smoker? If you're a smoker, would you think differently if you quit?

## MAKING THIS CHAPTER WORK FOR YOU

### Breathing Easier

Many people have stopped smoking because of the health risks associated with tobacco use and because, as a social behavior, it has become unpopular. Young people who begin smoking often do so because they believe they will be more accepted by, or appear more adult or attractive to, their peers. Smokers continue to smoke because they find smoking pleasurable, but they are also addicted to nicotine. If they don't receive regular daily doses, smokers suffer withdrawal symptoms, such as irritability, anxiety, headache, and changes in performance.

The incidence of heart attacks and cardiomyopathy is high among smokers, possibly because of the actions of nicotine (which increases blood pressure and constricts blood vessels) and carbon monoxide (which diminishes oxygen received by the heart).

Nicotine, the addictive element in cigarette smoke, affects mood, hunger, blood pressure, heart rate, and performance of certain mental tasks. Along with tar, nicotine contributes to heart and respiratory diseases.

In the United States more people die of lung cancer, usually caused by smoking, than of any other cancer. Also, smoking contributes to the development of other cancers, including cancer of the mouth and larynx, esophagus, bladder and kidney, and pancreas. Besides lung cancer, smoking can cause two types of chronic obstructive lung disease: emphysema and chronic bronchitis.

Women who smoke face the additional risk of developing reproductive disorders such as cervical cancer. Women who smoke during pregnancy are more likely than nonsmokers to miscarry and experience complications, including premature delivery, and to have babies with physical and intellectual impairments.

In addition to heart and lung diseases, cigarette smoking is associated with ulcers, liver disease, stroke, pulmonary heart disease, aortic aneurysm, gum disease and teeth problems, and reduced sex drive.

Clove cigarettes may be more dangerous than conventional cigarettes because they contain more nicotine, tar, and carbon monoxide. People who chew tobacco or use snuff are at risk for nicotine addiction, teeth and gum conditions, and cancer of the mouth and throat. Nonsmokers constantly exposed to cigarette smoke are at risk for developing lung diseases, including lung cancer.

One approach to quitting smoking is gradually cutting down the number of cigarettes smoked per day. Another is stopping all at once. For people who need help to stop smoking, methods of quitting include stop-smoking groups, aversion therapy, nicotine gum, hypnosis, and acupuncture.

Learning to live without tobacco requires great commitment. Instead of thinking about quitting something pleasant, see yourself as beginning something even more pleasant. With every healthy breath you take, you are renewing yourself, becoming better, making a new you.

SECTION V

# YOUR HEALTH RISKS

To some extent, you can influence how long you'll live. To an even greater extent, you can make choices that affect both the quantity and the quality of your life. The right choices aren't always easy. The chapters in this section can help by providing information you can use in making and following through on heathful decisions. By understanding the risks to your health, you can prepare to overcome them—and not simply live life, but celebrate it every day.

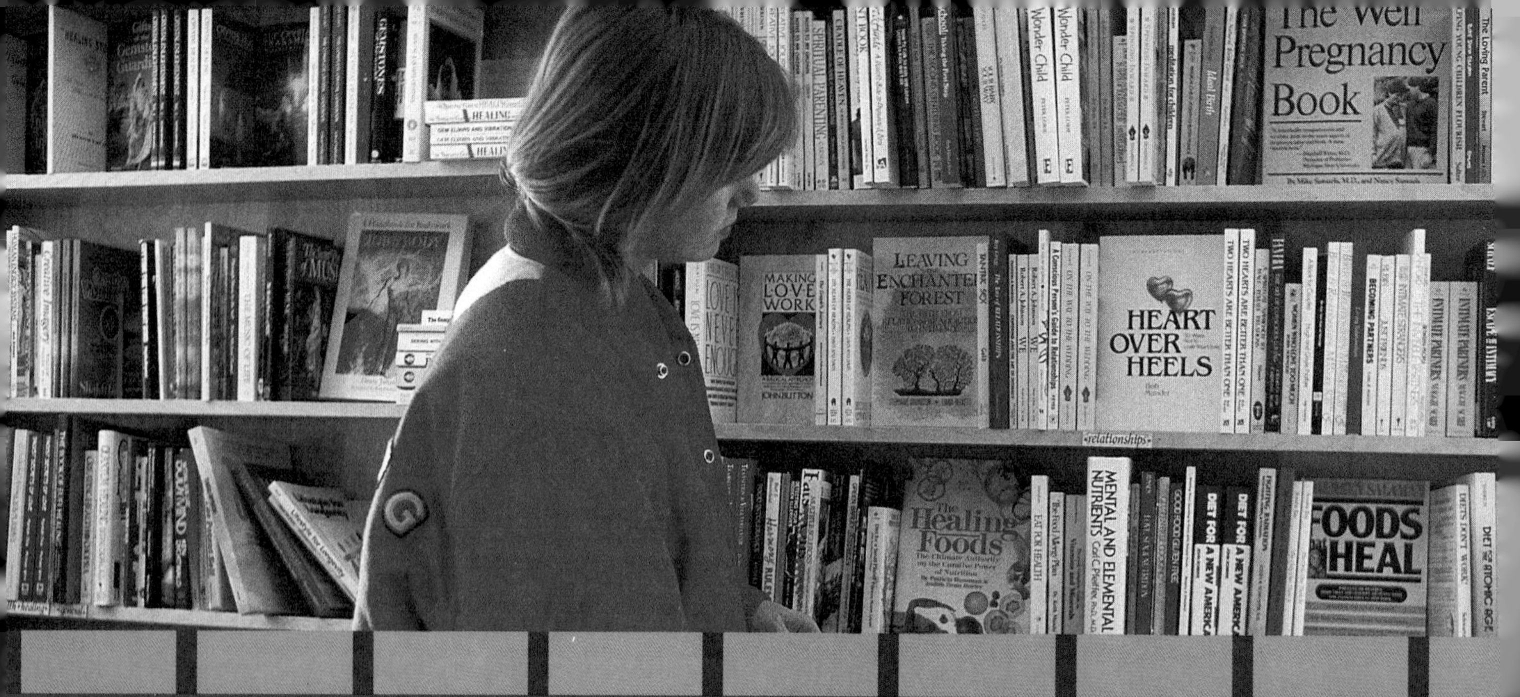


# 12 YOUR OPTIONS FOR HEALTH CARE: MAKING WISE CHOICES

**In this chapter**

**Patient, heal thyself**

**How to find care**

**When to seek care**

**Getting the most out of medical care**

**Paying for medical care**

**Alternative approaches to traditional medicine**

**Quackery**

**Making this chapter work for you: Making smart health-care decisions**

*Your body belongs to you.* The most sophisticated health-care delivery system, the newest breakthrough in medical science, cannot do as much good as you can for yourself. Modern medicine's finest hours generally come when the body is in crisis; only you can prevent such crises. Taking care of yourself involves common sense; conscientious care of minor problems; and proper use of health services, including screening for hidden diseases and regular physical examinations. This chapter will help you learn how to take better care of yourself—both on your own and with the help of health-care professionals.

## PATIENT, HEAL THYSELF

You, the patient, can do more for your well-being than any physician can. Every day you decide whether to smoke or exercise, what to eat, how much to drink, whether to wear your seat belt. If you play Humpty Dumpty and take too many chances with your health, doctors, nurses, and other therapists may be forced into the role of all the king's horses and all the king's men, desperately trying to put your shattered body together again. But even the best trained, most dedicated professionals might not succeed in restoring your health. That's why prevention is always the wisest course.

### Living Dangerously

Following are behaviors that increase your risk of health problems. (Also listed are the chapters in this text that discuss these behaviors and the ways to change them.)

- *Cigarette Smoking*—Possible consequences: emphysema, chronic bronchitis, lung cancer, and coronary artery disease (see Chapter 11)
- *Heavy Drinking*—Possible consequence: motor vehicle accidents (see Chapter 10)
- *Alcoholism*—Possible consequences: cirrhosis of the liver, malnutrition, and other complications (see Chapter 10)
- *Abuse of Drugs*—Possible consequences: drug dependence and adverse drug reactions, social withdrawal, loss of job, anxiety, malnutrition, suicide, homicide, overdoses, and accidents (see Chapter 9)
- *Careless Driving and Failure to Wear Seat Belts*—Possible consequences: accidents, injuries, and deaths (see Chapter 14)
- *Carelessness in Sexual Relationships*—Possible consequences: unwanted pregnancies and sexually transmitted diseases, including AIDS (see Chapters 7 and 8)
- *Poor Eating Habits*—Possible consequences: obesity, malnutrition, and heart disease (see Chapter 4)
- *Lack of Exercise*—Possible consequences: heart disease, osteoporosis, and obesity (see Chapter 5)

### Self-care

*Self-care* means learning about the body and its needs, how to respond quickly to emergencies, and when and how to use medical resources. Most people do treat themselves. You probably prescribe aspirin for a headache, chicken soup or orange juice for a cold, or a weekend trip to unwind from stress. Parents of young children clean and dress wounds; campers and climbers treat snakebites. Many people think of such tasks as first aid or coping until the physician comes; however, self-care emphasizes caring for such minor problems not *until* the doctor comes, but *instead* of the doctor coming. The essence of the self-care movement is individual decision making.

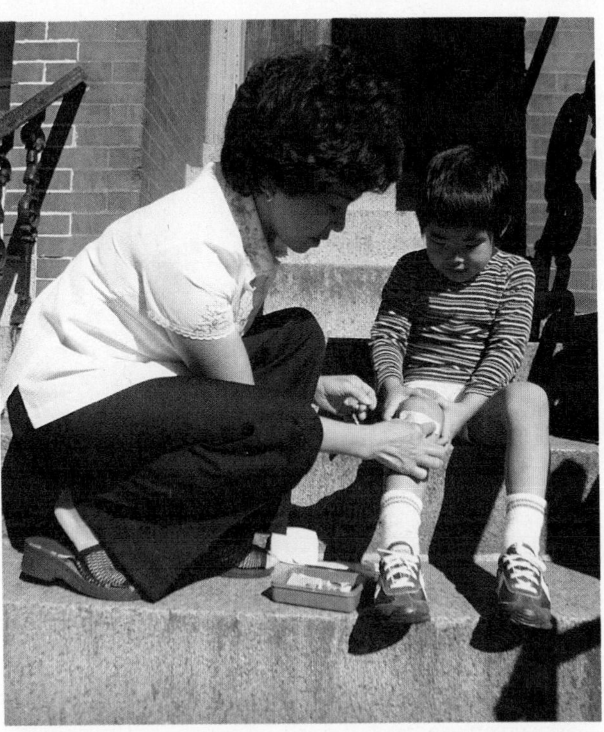

Parents of young children often become experts at treating minor injuries.

**TABLE 12-1** Home Medical Shelf: Essentials

| MEDICATION | AILMENT OR NEED |
|---|---|
| Aspirin and/or acetaminophen | For fever, headache, minor pain |
| Antacid | For stomach upset |
| Adhesive tape and bandages | For minor wounds |
| Hydrogen peroxide | For cleansing wounds |
| Sodium bicarbonate | For soaking and soothing |
| Liquid acetaminophen* | For pain and fever in small children |
| Syrup of ipecac* | To induce vomiting |

*For families with children under 12 years of age.

## Knowing What's Normal

At the very least, you should know what your **vital signs** are and what a normal reading should be:

- *Temperature* —98.6° Fahrenheit
- *Blood Pressure* —120/70 to 140/90, depending on age and sex
- *Pulse Rate* —72 beats per minute
- *Respiration Rate* —15 to 20 breaths per minute

You can measure your temperature (with a thermometer), pulse rate, and respiration rate yourself. If you want to invest in the equipment, you can monitor your blood pressure as well.

## Your Home Pharmacy

Your home pharmacy should contain only frequently needed medications. Know the uses, dosages, and possible side effects of any medication you purchase. You'll also need bandages, a thermometer, and tweezers. Table 12-1 lists the essential products for a home medical shelf; Table 12-2 gives a more complete list of agents that may sometimes be needed. Listed in alphabetical order in this section are some common medical problems and the drugs you'll need to treat them. Others are listed in "Minor Health Problems" in the appendix.

**Coughs** Medications include cough suppressants, which inhibit a cough, and expectorants (usually glyceryl guaiacolate), which liquify secretions and allow the cough to rid the body of bad material. Expectorants are a better choice, although suppressants are useful in the late stages of a dry, hacking cough. Avoid

**vital signs** Measurements of physiological functioning; specifically, temperature, blood pressure, pulse rate, and respiration rate.

**TABLE 12-2** Home Medical Shelf: Optional Items

| MEDICATION | AILMENT OR NEED |
|---|---|
| Antihistamines | Allergy |
| Nose drops and sprays | |
| Hydrogen peroxide, iodine | Antiseptic |
| Cold tablets, cough syrups | Colds and coughs |
| Bulk laxatives, milk of magnesia | Constipation |
| Sodium fluoride | Dental problems (preventive) |
| Kaopectate, Parepectolin | Diarrhea |
| Eye drops and artificial tears | Eye irritations |
| Antifungal preparations | Fungus |
| Hemorrhoid preparations | Hemorrhoids |
| | Pain and fever |
| Aspirin, acetaminophen, ibuprofen | in adults |
| Liquid acetaminophen, rectal suppositories of aspirin | in children |
| Syrup of ipecac | Poisoning (to induce vomiting) |
| Hydrocortisone cream | Skin rashes |
| Sodium bicarbonate (baking soda) | (soaking and soothing) |
| Elastic bandages | Sprains |
| Antacid (nonabsorbable) | Stomach, upset |
| Sunscreen agents | Sunburn (preventive) |
| Adhesive tape, bandages | Wounds (minor) |

## HALES INDEX

Percentage of patients who take prescription medicine as directed: 76

Percentage of heart attack patients who thought their chest pain would go away: 82

Percentage of heart attack patients who delayed seeking help for 2 hours or more: 50

Percentage of American women who examine their breasts monthly: 25

Percentage of patients who fail to fill their initial prescription: 20

Percentage of antihistamine takers who drive despite warnings not to: 61

Percentage of patients who discover a new problem during a routine physical: 10

Percentage of sexually active women who do not get regular Pap smears: 15 to 20

Amount Americans spend on prescription drugs every year: $22.6 billion

Number of prescriptions filled with generic drugs every year: 500 million

Amount spent on generic drugs every year: $1.9 billion

SOURCES: **1** Cramer, Joyce et al. "How Often Is Medication Taken as Prescribed?" *Journal of the American Medical Association*, vol. 261, no. 22, June 9, 1989. **2, 3** "Tick, Toc, Call the Doc," *American Health*, May 1989. **4** Centers for Disease Control. **5** American Association of Retired Persons. **6** Brody, Jane. "Personal Health," *New York Times*, March 22, 1990. **7** Henig, Robin Marantz. "Is the Pap Test Valid?" *New York Times Magazine*, May 28, 1989. **8** Carey, Benedict. "Do You Need a Physical?" *In Health*, March/April 1990. Avery, Caryl. **9, 10, 11** "Can You Trust Generic Drugs?" *American Health*, April 1990.

compounds that contain an antihistamine, which tends to dry sensitive tissues; check the ingredients on the label carefully or ask your pharmacist.

**Constipation** A high-fiber diet is the ideal treatment (see Chapter 4). Laxatives should be used only with caution. Best choices are milk of magnesia or psyllium (Metamucil, Effersyllium, Plova, Regulin) as a bulk laxative.

**Diarrhea** Occasional loose stools require no treatment. A clear liquid diet is recommended as a first choice for any diarrhea. Kaopectate, which has a gelling effect, helps form solid stools. If this fails, your doctor may recommend stronger agents containing drugs such as paregoric.

**Hemorrhoids** Zinc oxide powders and creams (such as Preparation H) soothe irritated tissue as the body heals. These should be applied after a bath so that no bacteria are trapped beneath them. In the long run, a change to a high-fiber diet to produce softer stools may help.

**Pain and Fever** Aspirin controls fever; eases inflammation; and relieves the pain of headaches, sore muscles, or menstrual cramps. No one brand of plain aspirin is better than any other. Frequent use may cause upset stomach or ringing in the ears.

Ibuprofen (Advil, Nuprin) is less irritating to the stomach than aspirin and particularly effective for menstrual cramps. Acetaminophen (Tylenol, Datril, Tempra, Liquiprin) is less irritating than either aspirin or ibuprofen and may be used for minor pain or fever. However, it does not reduce inflammation.

Use of any form of aspirin to relieve cold or flu symptoms in children or teenagers increases the risk of Reye's syndrome (a viral infection that can increase the pressure within the skull and cause coma, seizures, respiratory failure, mental retardation, movement disorders, and death). Acetaminophen is a safer alternative.

**Poisoning** Ipecac syrup induces vomiting and should be available wherever small children live. *Do not attempt to cause vomiting if the poison is petroleum-based or a strong acid or alkali.*

**Upset Stomach** Alka-Seltzer Gold, Rolaids, Tums, and other such products rely on sodium bicarbonate, which neutralizes acids—at least in test tubes on TV

SELF-SURVEY

## Can You Take Care of Yourself?

***Section 1: Home Pharmacy and Equipment***

Basic drugs and supplies should be kept at home to deal with common illnesses and injuries. Indicate with a yes or no which of the following items you might want to keep on hand.

| PREPARATIONS | YES OR NO |
|---|---|
| 1. Over-the-counter decongestant | _______ |
| 2. Over-the-counter combination cold medication | _______ |
| 3. Aspirin and/or acetaminophen | _______ |
| 4. Baking soda | _______ |
| 5. Calamine lotion | _______ |
| 6. Soap | _______ |
| 7. Hydrogen peroxide | _______ |
| 8. Mercurochrome | _______ |
| 9. Laxative in pill form | _______ |
| 10. Syrup of ipecac | _______ |
| 11. Sunscreen | _______ |
| 12. Antibiotics | _______ |

| EQUIPMENT | YES OR NO |
|---|---|
| 13. Rectal and oral thermometers | _______ |
| 14. Adhesive tape | _______ |
| 15. Cotton-gauze bandages | _______ |
| 16. Adhesive bandages | _______ |
| 17. Elastic bandage (3 in.) | _______ |
| 18. Ziploc plastic bag | _______ |
| 19. Stethoscope | _______ |
| 20. Sphygmomanometer (for blood pressure) | _______ |
| 21. Vaporizer | _______ |
| 22. Penlight | _______ |

***Section 2: Knowledge***

For each of the following statements, circle T if the statement is true or F if the statement is false:

1. Problems that can be treated at home include the common cold, flu, hay fever, and mononucleosis. T F
2. Medical treatment is generally required for strep throat and ear infections. T F
3. Most adults should consult a physician before beginning a serious exercise program. T F
4. A cough that produces mucus that is rusty green in color is most likely to be caused by bacterial infections. T F
5. A sore throat with a temperature of 101° Fahrenheit or greater and pus should be checked by a physician. T F
6. The old saying "Feed a cold; starve a fever" is a good rule to follow. T F
7. A second-degree burn that involves the face or hands should be seen by a physician. T F
8. A saline gargle should be used for a sore throat. T F
9. Antihistamines may decrease the nasal congestion accompanying a cold, but they also cause drowsiness. T F
10. Normal rectal temperature is the same as normal oral temperature. T F
11. You should use your thumb or forefinger to take a pulse. T F
12. Excess ear wax may be cleaned out at home. T F
13. Warm milk, exercise, and mental relaxation are aids to sleep. T F
14. A person's normal systolic blood pressure may change with age. T F
15. The first treatment to use for diarrhea is a regimen of clear liquids only for 24 hours. T F
16. Yearly screenings should include a blood-pressure check, a Pap smear for women, glaucoma screening, and stool testing. T F
17. Viral infections are best treated by antibiotics. T F
18. The normal resting pulse rate for adults is approximately 80 beats per minute. T F
19. Heat may be applied to sprains, but only after the first 24 hours. T F
20. For adults, tetanus booster shots are recommended approximately every five years. T F
21. Swimmer's ear may be treated at home, unless it persists beyond five days. T F
22. A boil appearing anywhere but on the face may be treated at home. T F

commercials. No one's certain whether this is true in the stomach, and the sodium may not be good for you. "Nonabsorbable" antacids (Maalox, Gelusil, Mylanta, Alugel, Digel, Riopan), which are not broken down in the stomach, are more effective and have no side effects.

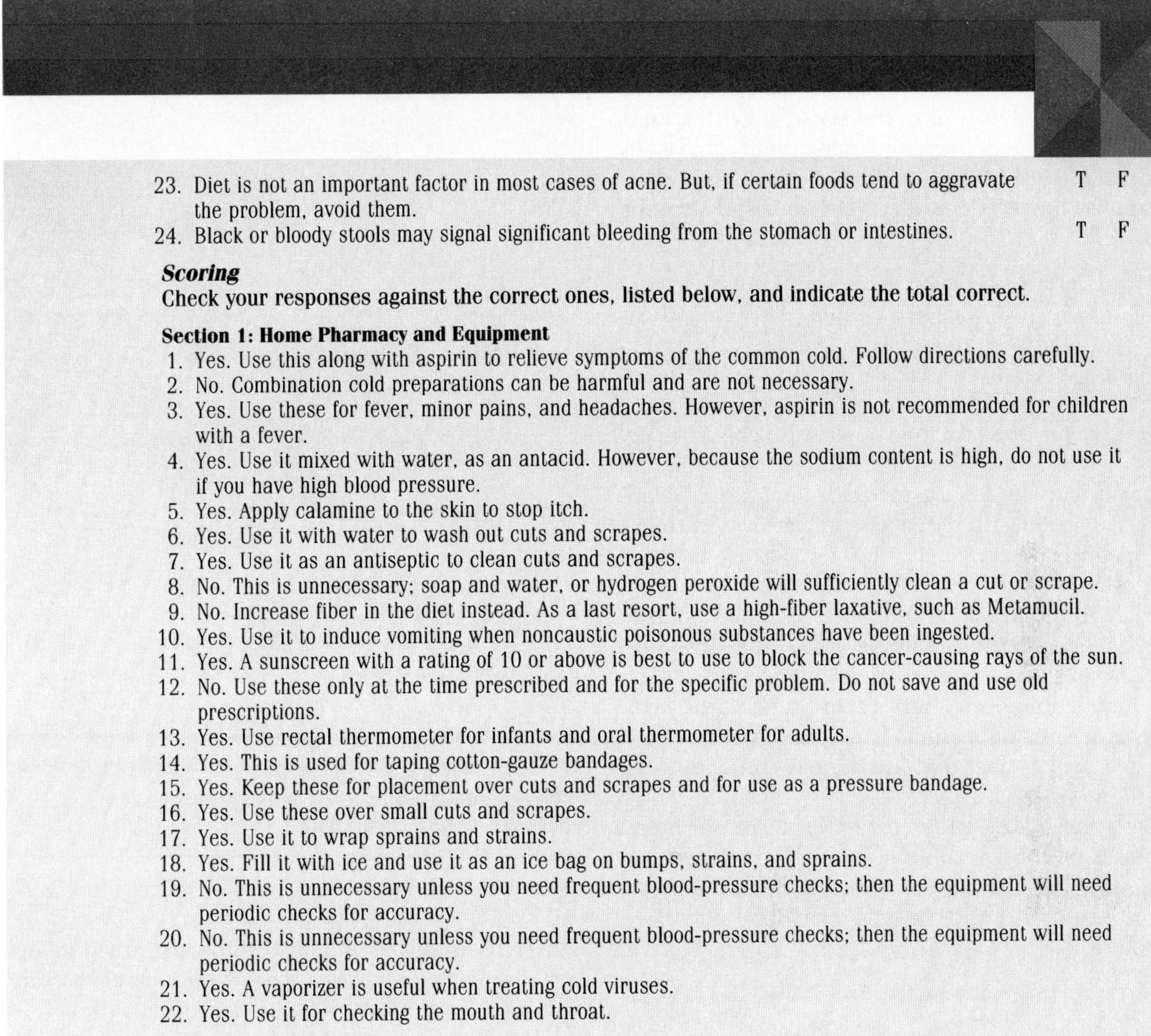
23. Diet is not an important factor in most cases of acne. But, if certain foods tend to aggravate the problem, avoid them. T F
24. Black or bloody stools may signal significant bleeding from the stomach or intestines. T F

***Scoring***

**Check your responses against the correct ones, listed below, and indicate the total correct.**

**Section 1: Home Pharmacy and Equipment**

1. Yes. Use this along with aspirin to relieve symptoms of the common cold. Follow directions carefully.
2. No. Combination cold preparations can be harmful and are not necessary.
3. Yes. Use these for fever, minor pains, and headaches. However, aspirin is not recommended for children with a fever.
4. Yes. Use it mixed with water, as an antacid. However, because the sodium content is high, do not use it if you have high blood pressure.
5. Yes. Apply calamine to the skin to stop itch.
6. Yes. Use it with water to wash out cuts and scrapes.
7. Yes. Use it as an antiseptic to clean cuts and scrapes.
8. No. This is unnecessary; soap and water, or hydrogen peroxide will sufficiently clean a cut or scrape.
9. No. Increase fiber in the diet instead. As a last resort, use a high-fiber laxative, such as Metamucil.
10. Yes. Use it to induce vomiting when noncaustic poisonous substances have been ingested.
11. Yes. A sunscreen with a rating of 10 or above is best to use to block the cancer-causing rays of the sun.
12. No. Use these only at the time prescribed and for the specific problem. Do not save and use old prescriptions.
13. Yes. Use rectal thermometer for infants and oral thermometer for adults.
14. Yes. This is used for taping cotton-gauze bandages.
15. Yes. Keep these for placement over cuts and scrapes and for use as a pressure bandage.
16. Yes. Use these over small cuts and scrapes.
17. Yes. Use it to wrap sprains and strains.
18. Yes. Fill it with ice and use it as an ice bag on bumps, strains, and sprains.
19. No. This is unnecessary unless you need frequent blood-pressure checks; then the equipment will need periodic checks for accuracy.
20. No. This is unnecessary unless you need frequent blood-pressure checks; then the equipment will need periodic checks for accuracy.
21. Yes. A vaporizer is useful when treating cold viruses.
22. Yes. Use it for checking the mouth and throat.

Number correct, Section 1: ______

**Section 2: Knowledge**

Give yourself 1 point for each correct response. All statements are true, except numbers 6, 10, 11, 16, and 17.

Number correct, Section 2: ______

| SCORE RANGE | INTERPRETATION |
|---|---|
| 35–46 | You have much of the knowledge and equipment required for good self-care. |
| 24–34 | You need to make some equipment and pharmacy purchases and to review self-care literature. |
| 0–23 | A good self-care class or talk with your physician is needed. |

SOURCE: Wellness RSVP.

**Wounds** Antiseptics remove dirt and kill germs. Hydrogen peroxide is an excellent cleansing agent and iodine a reasonably effective germ killer. Clean a wound thoroughly (even if it is painful) and apply an antiseptic. Small wounds often heal better if exposed to air, but bandages should be used to cover blisters, keep wounds clean, and hold the edges of a wound together.

### OTC Drugs

Like prescription drugs, nonprescription medications, or over-the-counter drugs (OTCs), can be misused and abused (see Chapter 9). You can become addicted to OTCs—not in the sense of getting high, but in the sense of becoming dependent, physically or psychologically, on a drug.

Among the OTCs most often misused are the following:

- *Nasal Sprays* —They work by shrinking blood vessels in the nose. If used too often or too long (three days is the recommended maximum), the blood vessels widen instead of contracting, and the surrounding tissues become swollen, causing more congestion. To make the vessels shrink again, many people use more spray more often. The result can be permanent damage to nasal membranes, bleeding, infection, and partial or complete loss of smell.
- *Laxatives* —Believing that they must have one bowel movement a day (a common myth), many people rely on laxatives. Brands that contain phenolphthalein irritate the lining of the intestines and cause muscles to contract or tighten, often making constipation worse rather than better. Bulk laxatives are less dangerous, but regular use is not advised. A high-fiber diet and more exercise are safer and more effective.
- *Eye Drops* —Like nasal sprays, they make the blood vessels of the eye contract. However, with overuse (several times a day for several weeks), the blood vessels expand, and the eye then looks redder than before.

### Home Tests

Increasingly, consumers are buying diagnostic equipment—from digital blood pressure cuffs that inflate automatically and print out the reading, date, and time to breath analyzers for estimating blood alcohol concentrations, ovulation predictors, and pregnancy tests. Home testing can be useful, but it's not a substitute for medical evaluation. An essential part of taking good care of yourself is knowing when to seek professional care. (See "Your Body's Warning Signals" in the appendix.)

## HOW TO FIND CARE

The time to think about the type of care you may need is when you're upright and healthy, rather than when you're horizontal and ill.

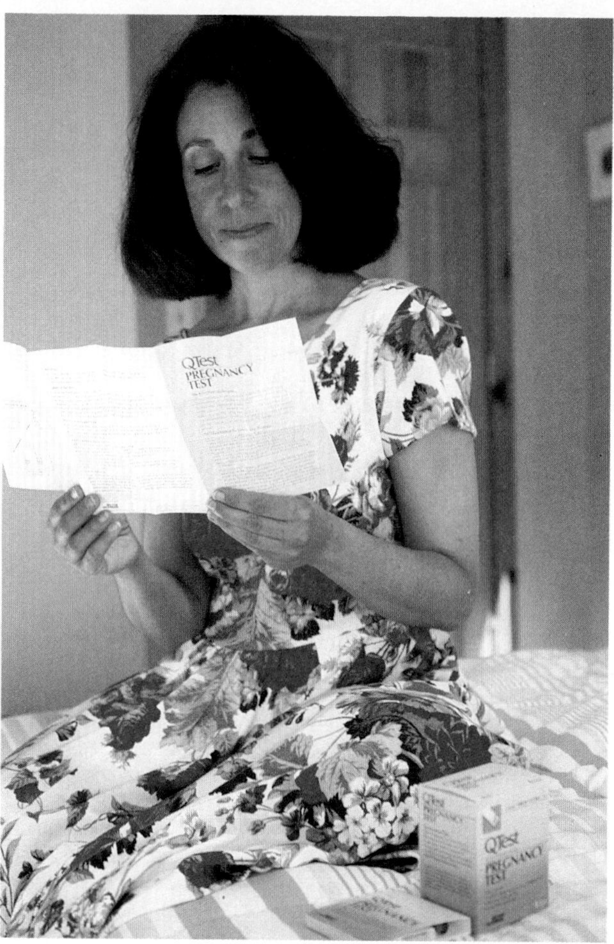


Home pregnancy tests are one of the most popular diagnostic devices on the market.

## Health-care Practitioners

Fewer than 10 percent of health-care practitioners are physicians; allied health professionals are assuming more important roles in delivering primary, or basic, health services. As a consumer, you should be aware of the range and special skills of the most common types of health-care providers.

### Nurses

A registered nurse (RN) graduates from a school of nursing approved by a state board and passes a state board examination. RNs today may specialize in certain areas, such as intensive care or nurse-midwifery. Nurse practitioners, RNs with advanced training and experience, may run community clinics, or provide screening and preventive care at group medical practices. Some have independent practices.

Practical nurses, also called licensed vocational nurses (LVNs), are licensed by the state. They graduate from state-approved schools of practical nursing and must take a state board exam. Practical nurses work under the supervision of RNs or licensed physicians.

Nursing aides and orderlies assist registered and practical nurses in providing services directly related to the comfort and well-being of hospitalized patients.

### Medical Paraprofessionals

More than sixty different types of health practitioners work with physicians and nurses in providing medical services. Some, like occupational therapists, have at least a bachelor's degree. Others, such as physician assistants, do not need college training.

### Dentists

Most dental students earn a bachelor's degree and then complete two more years of training in the basic sciences and two years of clinical work before graduating with a degree of DDS or DMD (Doctor of Dental Surgery or Doctor of Medical Dentistry). To qualify for a license, graduates must pass both a written and a clinical examination. Dentists may work in general practice or choose a specialty, such as orthodontics (straightening teeth).

### Dental Technicians

Dental hygienists provide such services as scaling and polishing teeth, processing X rays, and teaching patients about dental health. Dental assistants prepare the patient for treatment and help the dentist in caring for the patient. Dental lab technicians make dentures, bridgework, crowns, and other dental restorations.

### Specialized Health Professionals

Health professionals may specialize in a variety of fields. Clinical psychologists, for example, have doctoral degrees and provide a wide range of mental health services, but they do not prescribe medications. Optometrists, trained in special schools of optometry, diagnose visual abnormalities and prescribe lenses or visual aids; they do not prescribe drugs, diagnose or treat eye diseases, or perform surgery—functions performed by ophthalmologists. Podiatrists are specially trained, licensed health-care professionals who specialize in problems of the feet. Chiropractors believe that disease is caused by impaired nerve function caused by pressure, strain, or tension on the spinal cord and nervous system. Treatment relies on the manipulation of bones. State licenses are required; chiropractors cannot hospitalize patients or prescribe drugs.

### Physicians

Medical doctors (MDs) trained in American medical schools usually take at least three years of premedical college courses (with an emphasis on biology, chemistry, and physics) and then complete four (but sometimes three or five) years of medical school. The first two years of medical school are devoted to the study of human anatomy, embryology, pharmacology, and similar basic subjects. During the last two years, students work directly with doctors in hospitals. Medical students who pass a series of national board examinations then enter a one-year internship in a hospital, followed by another two to five years of residency, which leads to certification as a specialist. A **primary care** physician (one who provides "first-contact" care to patients who seek help directly, without referral by another doctor) may be a family practitioner or a specialist in internal medicine, pediatrics, or obstetrics-gynecology. Within the major specialties are subspecialties (see Figure 12-1). For example, specialists in internal medicine include cardiologists, who specialize in the heart; dermatologists, who specialize in the skin; and neurologists, who specialize in the brain and nervous system.

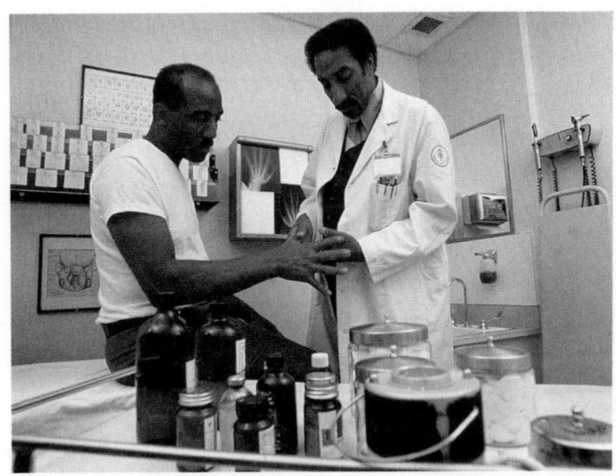

Primary-care physicians perform medical examinations and provide "first-contact" treatments to patients who seek help directly.

Osteopaths are doctors (ODs, not MDs) who emphasize the role of the musculoskeletal system. Trained in four-year programs in the basic medical, surgical, psychological, and pharmacological approaches of modern medicine, most now have the privileges once accorded only to MDs, including prescribing drugs.

**primary care** "First-contact" care provided by a health-care professional, usually in an office or clinic, without referral from a physician.

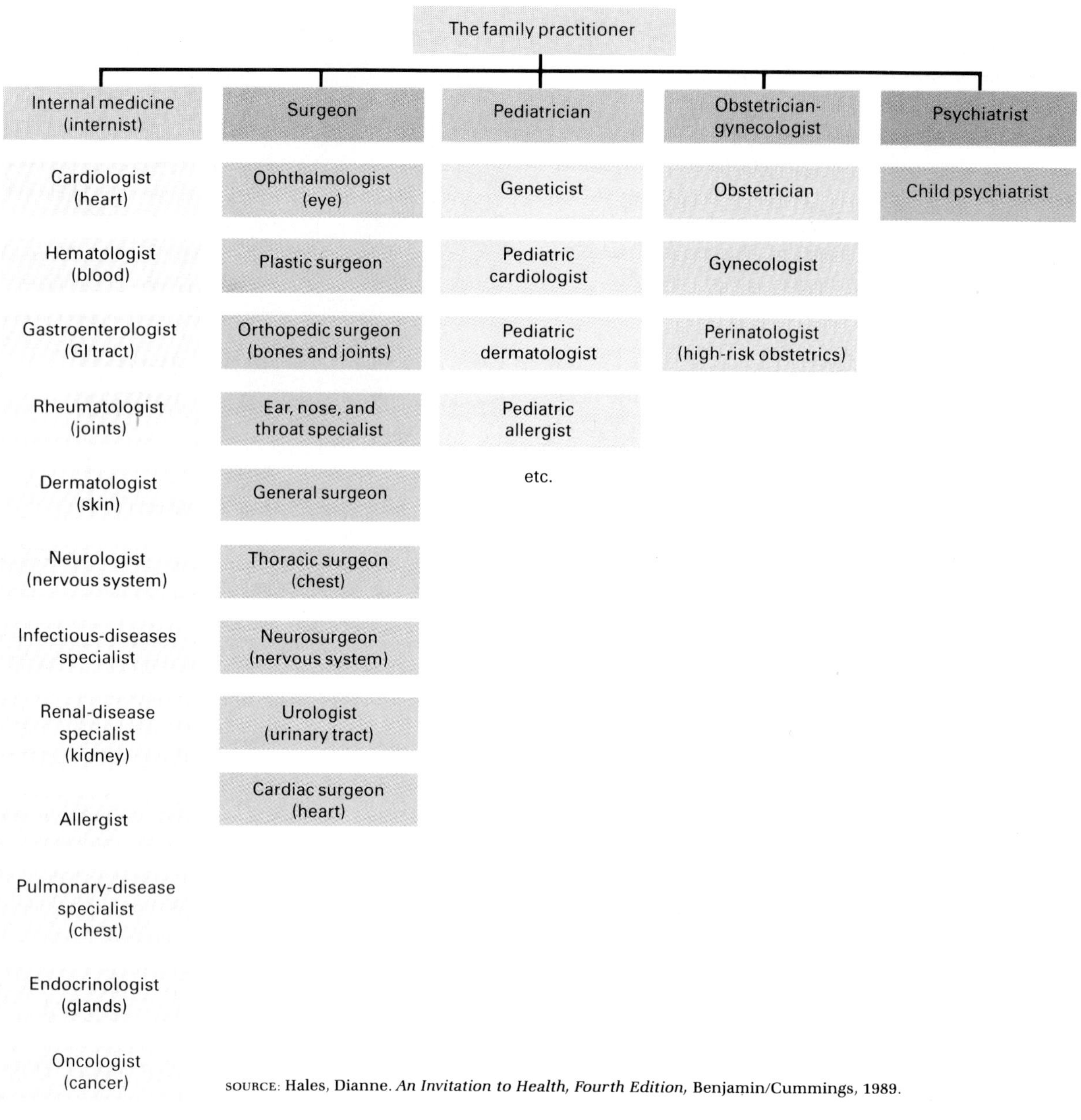


SOURCE: Hales, Dianne. *An Invitation to Health, Fourth Edition,* Benjamin/Cummings, 1989.

**Figure 12-1** Types of doctors. The five major specialties include many subspecialties. Radiology, clinical pathology, and anesthesiology are not listed here because the patient rarely goes directly to such physicians.

## Your Ideal Doctor

Most of us, most of the time, should deal with a primary care practitioner. Family physicians are trained in all aspects of primary care, including pediatrics and obstetrics. Internists get much more intensive training in the medical, as opposed to the surgical approaches, to disease.

To decide which type of physician you should see, think about your most common health needs. If you schedule appointments only for screening procedures and checkups every few years, choose a family practitioner or internist. If you have children, decide whether you want a doctor who specializes in their care or whether you want one doctor to care for the entire family.

If you're a woman and see a doctor primarily for birth control, you may choose to see a gynecologist. If he or she is the only doctor you see, make sure the gynecologist performs other tests, such as measuring your blood pressure, in addition to a vaginal exam.

STRATEGY FOR CHANGE

### Finding a Doctor and a Dentist

- Ask your friends about their doctors and dentists and what they think of the care they receive. Push for specific details.
- If you know any health professionals, ask whom they would choose for their own care.
- If there's a medical center nearby that teaches medical students and residents, call the appropriate department and ask for a list of the clinical faculty, the staff and affiliated physicians who see patients. You might also ask if the hospital has a primary care clinic. Generally, teaching hospitals have the most sophisticated facilities and provide the most advanced care.
- Find out to which hospitals the doctor admits patients. If you choose a physician who is affiliated only with a teaching hospital, you become "teaching material." If your problem is complex, the attention of many people—from medical students to specialists—guarantees you the most comprehensive diagnosis and care. However, you may find the attention intrusive. If you prefer to be seen only by your physician, choose a doctor affiliated with a community hospital and make your views clear.
- Call the doctor's secretary and inquire about the doctor's credentials, including medical school diploma and specialty certification.
- Ask if the doctor is in a solo or group practice. If you choose a doctor who practices alone, you'll see the same doctor on every scheduled appointment. Find out, however, who covers the practice on weekends, during the evening, and during the doctor's vacations. Group practices range from two-physician partnerships to huge corporations with more than one hundred physicians on staff. In some groups, you may not see the same physician on each visit.
- To find a dentist, call a local dental school, which may have a public clinic. Or, check with the county dental society. Ask for information regarding fees, hours, and after-hour emergencies.

### Evaluating Health Professionals

Evaluating medical care is tricky for consumers.[1] Some patients criticize a doctor who won't give them penicillin for their colds, even though the doctor is doing the right thing and not abusing antibiotics. Others feel relieved if a physician doesn't perform an awkward procedure, such as a rectal examination, even though the doctor could miss an early sign of cancer.

STRATEGY FOR CHANGE

### Giving Your Doctor a Checkup

- Does your doctor explain what he or she is doing?
- Do you feel free to ask questions?
- Does he or she give you straight answers?
- Does he or she listen to your complaints?
- Does your doctor reassure you when you're worried?
- Does he or she spend enough time with you?
- Did your doctor take a comprehensive history?
- Was your physical examination thorough?
- Were certain expensive services recommended almost too enthusiastically?
- Does every patient leave the office with an injection or a prescription?
- Does your doctor prescribe three or more medications at one time?
- Was your doctor unwilling to answer questions fully and clearly? Was your doctor unwilling to admit that he or she did not know the answers to some questions, and to suggest consultation with someone more knowledgeable?

Look back at your answers. If they make you feel at all uneasy, it's time have a talk with your doctor—or to find one who's better for you.

Finding a good dentist is also important. Your dentist should take a complete medical history from you and update it every six months, examine your mouth for signs of cancer, and thoroughly outline all treatment options. He or she should pay attention to your gums as well as to your teeth. Insist that everyone who works inside your mouth wear a mask and rubber gloves to prevent the spread of the virus that causes AIDS, herpes, hepatitis, and other diseases.

## WHEN TO SEEK CARE

You need to be able to judge when to seek help—in responding to emergencies and in managing your own preventive-care program.

### Emergencies

Life-threatening situations, such as car accidents or cardiac arrests, rarely happen more than once or twice in any person's life. At such times, never hesitate to get help: Many cities use the telephone code 911 to summon emergency care. If your community does not, keep the numbers of the ambulance service, the police and fire departments, the poison control center, and your doctor and neighbors handy. If you can't find a number quickly, call the operator.

Go to a hospital emergency room only in a true emergency. Learn to distinguish between an emergency and the normal onset of illness (see "Emergency!" in the appendix).

## Preventive Care

Preventive care can lower your risk of serious disease.

### Immunizations

Some diseases can be prevented altogether with **immunization,** treatment that helps the body resist specific illnesses. (See Chapter 15 for a complete guide to immunizations.) People living in the U.S. should have immunizations to prevent polio; diphtheria; tetanus; measles; and, for young children, pertussis (whooping cough). You should be aware of which immunizations you have had and when. For example, if you step on a nail, your doctor will want to know if you've had a tetanus shot in the last ten years.

### Checkups

Most physicians believe you don't need annual checkups if you are young and feel well.[2] However, certain types of screening tests should be performed periodically, particularly if you are age 45 or older or if you are at a higher-than-average risk of developing a particular disease (see Table 12-3).

**STRATEGY FOR CHANGE**

**When Should You Get a Checkup?**

Kaiser-Permanente, a giant health maintenance organization, recommends the following timetable for having complete checkups:

- between the ages of 18 and 35: every four years
- between the ages of 36 and 45: every three years
- between the ages of 46 and 55, every two years
- after age 55, yearly or as your doctor advises

### Screening for Major Health Risks

The most important preventive-care tests are blood-pressure readings, Pap smears, breast examinations, glaucoma tests, tuberculosis tests, and multiphasic laboratory tests.

**High Blood Pressure** Blood pressure is a result of the contractions of the heart muscle, which pumps blood through your body, and the resistance of the walls of the vessels through which the blood flows. Each time your heart beats, your blood pressure goes up and down within a certain range. It is highest when the heart contracts; this is called **systolic blood**

**immunization** The process of becoming immune; rendering someone immune.

**TABLE 12-3** When to Check Up on Yourself

For most healthy adults, the classic head-to-toe annual physical is a thing of the past. But there are certain tests you should have routinely, even if you have no symptoms. Your doctor will know if there are any special tests that you need in addition to these.

| TEST | AGE | | | |
|---|---|---|---|---|
| | 20–29 | 30–39 | 40–49 | 50 AND OVER |
| Blood Pressure | every 2 years* | every 2 years* | every 2 years* | every 2 years* |
| Cholesterol | — | once between ages 35 and 39 | every 4–5 years* | every 4–5 years to age 65* |
| Pap Smear | every 1–3 years** | every 1–3 years** | every 1–3 years** | every 1–3 years to age 70** |
| Breast Exam | every 2–3 years† | every 2–3 years† | every 2 years† | annually |
| Mammography | — | — | every 1–2 years | annually |
| Fecal Occult Blood | — | — | — | every 1–2 years |

*More often if person is overweight, a smoker, or has a family history of heart disease.
**More often if woman takes the pill, has been exposed to DES, has multiple sex partners, or has a family history of cervical cancer.
†More often if woman has a family history of breast cancer.
SOURCE: Carey, Benedict. *In Health,* March/April 1990.

**pressure.** It is lowest between contractions; this is called **diastolic blood pressure.** A blood-pressure reading consists of the systolic measurement "over" the diastolic measurement, recorded in millimeters of mercury (mmHG). (See Figure 12-2.)

About 15 percent of Americans have high blood pressure, or **hypertension.** Borderline hypertension ranges from 140/90 to 160/95; definite hypertension means a blood-pressure reading of 160/95 or above. The lower, or diastolic, number is used in categorizing high blood pressure, with a reading of 90 to 104 considered mild hypertension; 105 to 114, moderate; and 115 and over, severe. (See Chapter 13 for more on high blood pressure.)

Because hypertension is increasingly common among people in their twenties and thirties, it's important to have your blood pressure checked at least once a year. You can take your own blood pressure or have a reading done inexpensively or free at community health fairs or at your student health service.

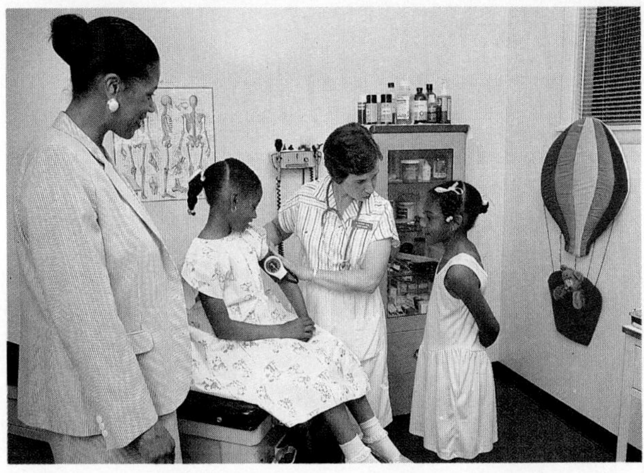

**Figure 12-2** To measure blood pressure, a sphygmomanometer (a cuff wrapped around the upper arm) is used. Air is pumped into the cuff until the blood flow is stopped. The air is slowly released from the cuff so that the blood can flow again. When a stethoscope placed on the inner arm transmits the first sounds of resumed blood flow, the pressure on the manometer indicates the systolic pressure. As the sounds become muffled and weaker, the manometer registers the diastolic pressure.

**Pap Smears** A **Pap smear** is a procedure in which cells are gently scraped from the cervix and examined under a microscope to determine if they are normal. Abnormal cells may indicate the presence of an infection or, more seriously, of cancer. Table 12-4 lists the five types of Pap smear results. Women should have a Pap smear every year to test for cervical cancer, a slow-growing cancer that is curable if detected early.

**Breast Self-examination** Careful self-examination can lead to early detection of breast tumors and, as a result, improved survival rates. Generally, a woman who is familiar with her breast tissue can easily detect any thickening or lumps. Follow the steps given in Chapter 14.

**Glaucoma** The treatable eye disease called glaucoma (a disorder characterized by increased pressure within the eye) can cause blindness if not detected early. After age 40, everyone should have his or her eyes checked for glaucoma every year, especially anyone at high risk because of glaucoma in the family.

**Tuberculosis** Tuberculosis (TB, a bacterial infection of the lungs) is a conquerable, not a conquered, disease (see Chapter 15). TB still kills more people than any acute infectious disease other than pneumonia.

If you know anyone who has TB, you may have been exposed to it and should be tested every two years. The test consists of an injection, just under the skin, of a small amount of material derived from dead tuberculosis bacteria. Swelling of the injection site within 48 hours indicates a positive reaction, which may mean that the tested person has an active infection. Further tests confirm the diagnosis.

**Multiphasic Screening** Multiphasic screening involves all the tests described in this section, as well as dozens more, including a urinalysis, X rays, and electrocardiograms. Although automation has re-

**TABLE 12-4** Pap Smear Results

| CLASS | NAME AND DESCRIPTION |
|---|---|
| I | Normal |
| II* | Atypical, some inflammation, occasional dysplasia |
| III | Suspicious, some precancerous cells |
| IV | Positive, many abnormal cells, high probability of cancer |
| V | Positive, definite cancer cells |

*Types II through V may require further evaluation and treatment.

SOURCE: Used by permission of the American Cancer Society, Inc.

**systolic blood pressure** The force exerted on the walls of a blood vessel by the blood during contraction of the heart.
**diastolic blood pressure** The force exerted on the walls of a blood vessel by the blood during relaxation and dilation of the heart, during which time the heart fills with blood.
**hypertension** High blood pressure.
**Pap smear** A test in which cells removed from the cervix are examined under a microscope for signs of cancer; also called a Pap test.

duced their costs, these tests are not recommended for healthy adults. A thorough physical exam every three to five years by a physician who knows your health history is far more effective.

**STRATEGY FOR CHANGE**

**Testing Medical Tests**

Many tests produce false positives, abnormal results that occur even though you are healthy. Before undergoing tests, discuss the following issues with your doctor:

- The reason for the test. Get a specific answer, not a "just in case" or "for your peace of mind."
- Ask how the test will help in diagnosis or treatment.
- If you've had the test before, could the earlier results be used? Would a follow-up exam be just as helpful?
- How often do false positives or negatives occur?
- What happens when the test indicates a problem: Is the test repeated? Is a different test performed?
- Does treatment begin immediately?
- What are the risks? Any invasive test—one that penetrates the body with a needle, tube, or viewing instrument—involves some risk of infection, bleeding, or tissue damage. Tests involving radiation also present risks. In addition, some people develop allergic reactions to the materials used in testing.
- Could any medications you're taking (including nonprescription drugs like aspirin) affect the testing procedures or results?
- How long will the test take?
- What will the test feel like?
- Are there specific things you should do before the test?
- Will you need help getting home afterward?

### Dental Checkups

Although most Americans say that they believe dental visits are important, many avoid visiting their dentist for years at a time. The principal reasons are that people think dental appointments result in pain or that they are not susceptible to dental disease. Routine checkups and cleanings once or twice a year are essential, however, to help control tooth decay and gum disease.

## GETTING THE MOST OUT OF MEDICAL CARE

Before you set off for the doctor's office, think over, and write down, the reasons for your visit. Do you have a specific complaint, such as a persistent fever? Do you need a screening test? Do you want advice on birth control? Organize your thoughts so you can convey them clearly.

### The History and Physical

If you have a specific symptom, such as lower back pain, the physician will want a **history**, an account of the events related to your problem. Focus on relevant details. If you are coming in with a sexual problem or if you are nervous, say so.

Your physician will also want a past medical and social history, including an account of major illnesses, surgery, and treatments. Report any allergies, particularly to drugs. Also tell the doctor about medications you take, including aspirin; antacids; sleeping pills; oral contraceptives; and "recreational" drugs, even if illegal. Your physician may also want to know about topics you consider private, such as a history of sexually transmitted disease. Remember that he or she is attempting to gather all the information needed to provide you comprehensive treatment. Note, too, that a physician must report certain information—for example, certain sexually transmitted diseases—to health authorities.

During the examination, point out any pains, lumps, or skin growths that you have noticed. If you feel pain when the physician palpates (feels) parts of your body, say so.

### Compliance

After the exam the physician will evaluate your health and symptoms, and advise you as to treatment. Write down any important instructions or information you're given. He or she may prescribe a medication; recommend an OTC drug, such as aspirin or an antihistamine; or want to give you an injection.

You then face another decision: Do you follow the advice? **Compliance** is a difficult issue for physicians and patients. If you don't follow through on the advised treatment, you've wasted your money and your and the doctor's time. You may also be risking actual harm if, for instance, you don't take the antibiotics prescribed for your strep throat or if you stop in midtreatment (strep throat can lead to heart damage).

---

**history** The health-related information collected during the interview of a client by a health-care professional.
**compliance** The act of carefully following treatment instructions.

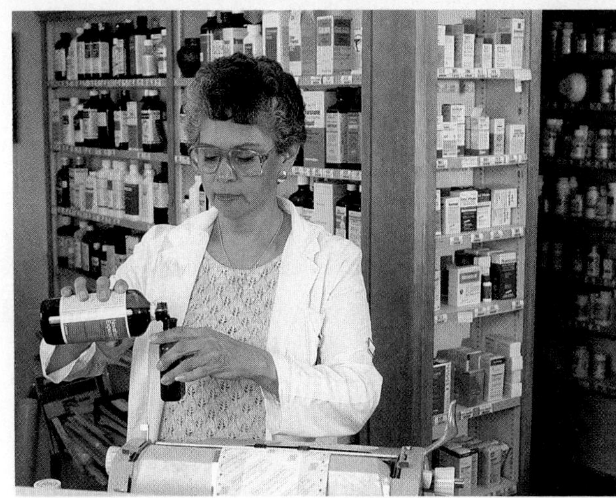

In some states, pharmacists can prescribe as well as dispense certain drugs.

## Prescription Drugs

In some states pharmacists have limited authority to write prescriptions. Several other states have adopted, or are considering, legislation allowing "write-and-pour" privileges for pharmacists. Just as pharmacists are doing more of what doctors alone once did, physicians may be doing more of what pharmacists alone once did: dispensing drugs. An increasing number of physicians dispense drugs to patients, often charging less than pharmacies.

No drug can help if it's not taken—and taken correctly. According to the Food and Drug Administration, 96 percent of patients with a new prescription do not ask any questions about the drug, and nearly 70 percent of physicians and pharmacists fail to tell patients about precautions and possible side effects.[3]

OTC and prescription drugs can interact in a variety of ways. For example, mixing some cold medications with tranquilizers can cause drowsiness and coordination problems, thus making driving dangerous.

## HEALTH HEADLINE

### New Role for MDs: More Talk, Fewer Tests

**Helping people change personal behavior should be the top priority for doctors in the future, according to a report from the U.S. Preventive Services Task Force, an independent group of twenty physicians and health experts. The group, sponsored by the U.S. Department of Health and Human Services, is urging doctors to think of themselves as consultants who should spend most of their time during checkups counseling patients about healthier life-styles rather than screening for possible problems. According to the experts, changing health behavior could do more to prevent the leading causes of death in the United States than expensive, invasive, and sometimes risky tests.**

SOURCES: U.S. Preventive Services Task Force, *Guide to Clinical Preventive Services*, Department of Health and Human Services, 1989. Zieglar, Jan. "Tomorrow's Checkup," *American Health*, January/February 1990.

## STRATEGY FOR CHANGE

### How to Avoid Problems When Taking Prescription Drugs

Before you leave the doctor's office with a prescription, you should tell the doctor about all other medications (including vitamins, laxatives, and home remedies) you are taking. Tell the doctor about any drug reactions you've had, and be sure to ask the following questions:

- What is the name of the drug?
- What is it supposed to do?
- How and when do I take it? For how long?
- What foods, drinks, other medications, or activities should I avoid while taking this drug?
- Are there any side effects? What do I do if they occur?
- What written information is available on this drug?

Once you get a prescription medication, be sure you use it correctly:

- If you have a complicated medication schedule to follow or if your memory is poor, devise a drug diary or calendar to help you remember what to take when. Check off each dose as you take it.
- Ask the pharmacist to write the name of each drug and the medication schedule and instructions on the container.
- Do not keep old medications around, and do not take drugs prescribed for someone else unless the doctor tells you to.
- Ask the pharmacist how best to store your prescriptions. (A hot, damp bathroom medicine chest is often the worst place.)

HEALTH SPOTLIGHT

## What to Expect in a Physical Exam

After the doctor has asked you questions about your complaints, medical history, and life-style, he or she will probably perform these tests:

- *Head.* Using a flashlight-like instrument called an ophthalmoscope, the doctor will look at the lens, retina, and blood vessels of the eye. He or she will also examine your ears for any signs of infection or perforations and your mouth, tongue, teeth, and gums for an idea as to your general health.
- *Neck.* Feeling around the neck, the doctor will check for enlarged lymph glands (a sign of infection), for lumps in the thyroid gland, and for warning signs of stroke in the neck arteries.
- *Chest.* With a stethoscope, the doctor will listen to the sounds made by your heart (to detect heart murmurs and irregular contractions) and by your lungs (to detect asthma or emphysema). By tapping on your chest and back with his or her fingers, the doctor can tell the size and shape of your heart, which may reveal some forms of heart disease and whether any fluid has collected in your lungs. The doctor will also check for abnormal lumps in women's breasts.
- *Abdomen.* Here the doctor uses his or her fingers to probe for tender spots and malformations of the liver and other organs, which may reveal signs of alcoholism, hepatitis, or hernias.
- *Rectum and genitals.* With a gloved hand, the doctor can feel in the rectum for growths and hemorrhoids. A rectal examination can also reveal enlargement of the male's prostate gland. The physician will check male testicles and spermatic cords for abnormalities.
- *Pelvic examination.* During a pelvic examination, a woman lies on her back, with her heels in stirrups at the end of the examining table and her legs spread out to the sides. The doctor inspects the labia, the clitoris, and the vaginal opening.

  A speculum is an instrument that is used to spread the walls of the vagina so that the inside may be seen. A Pap smear is taken to test for evidence of cervical cancer or other abnormalities.

  Using two gloved, lubricated fingers, the doctor will check for abnormalities in the vagina, uterus, tubes, and ovaries. Many physicians will also perform a rectal or rectovaginal (one finger in the rectum and one in the vagina) examination.

### Generic Drugs

The **generic** name is the chemical name for a drug. A specific drug may appear on the pharmacist's shelf under a variety of brand names, which may cost more than twice the generic equivalent. About 75 percent of all prescriptions specify a brand name, but pharmacists may—and in some states must—switch to a generic drug unless the doctor specifically tells them not to.[4–6] One-third of all prescriptions are filled with generic drugs.

The Food and Drug Administration (FDA) has found that not all generic drugs are safe and effective. As a result the FDA has taken more than 30 generics off the market. In some cases, manufacturers cheated in drug-approval tests or bribed FDA officials to consider their generics ahead of competitors. In a subse-

**generic** Refers to products without trade names that are equivalent to other products protected by trademark registration.

- *Extremities.* The doctor may check your knees for reflexes, which may indicate nerve disorders, and look for tremors in outstretched hands or in the face. The color, elasticity, and wetness or dryness of your skin may alert him or her to nutritional problems or indicate diabetes, skin cancer, and the like. Hair and nails may give indications of internal health, such as blood disorders. Swelling of the ankles can be an indication of heart, kidney, or liver disease.
- *Pulse and blood pressure.* Your doctor may check your pulse in various places, looking for signs of poor circulation. The rhythm and speed of the heart may also signal diseases of the heart or thyroid gland. High blood pressure can be an early warning sign of possible heart attack, stroke, or kidney damage.

Besides all the diagnostic tests listed, the doctor may also order you to undergo some laboratory and other tests:

- *Chest X ray.* A chest X ray can reveal abnormalities of the heart and lungs; if you're a smoker, the physician may insist on one.
- *Electrocardiogram.* The electrocardiogram is a test performed on you while at rest that records the electrical activity of your heart. It can show muscle damage, irregularities in heart rhythm, as well as hardening of the arteries.
- *Urinalysis.* Your urine may be analyzed by a medical laboratory. If sugar (glucose) is found in your urine, your doctor may order a separate blood test to check for diabetes. The presence of blood cells may indicate infection of the bladder or kidneys. Abnormal amounts of albumin (protein) in the urine may suggest kidney disease.
- *Blood-cell count.* The doctor or laboratory technician may draw blood to do a blood-cell count. An excess of white blood cells may be an indication of infection or, sometimes, leukemia. A deficiency of red blood cells may indicate anemia.
- *Blood chemistry.* A sample of your blood may also be analyzed to measure the levels of its various components. High levels of glucose possibly indicate diabetes, and high levels of uric acid may mean gout or kidney stones. A high cholesterol level may indicate cardiac risk.

quent analysis of 2,500 samples of the thirty most prescribed generic drugs, 1.1 percent failed to meet the agency's standards.[7]

Generic drugs have the same active ingredients as brand-name prescriptions, but their fillers and binders may be different. However, for some serious illnesses, the generics may not be as effective: Some experts recommend sticking with brand names for heart medications, psychotropics (mind-altering drugs), and anticonvulsant drugs (for epilepsy and other seizure disorders).

Generics can save consumers 30 to 70 percent of what they'd pay for brand-name drugs. To determine whether you should buy a generic, ask your physician the following questions at the time you get the prescription:[8]

- Does it matter whether I get a brand-name or generic drug for my condition?
- If so, did you specify a brand name?
- Could switching to a generic or from one generic to another harm my condition in any way?

## Second Opinions

As a consumer, you should base your decision about a specific treatment on information and professional advice. For nonemergency procedures, get more than one doctor's opinion. Find out the reasons why your doctor is recommending treatment or surgery, the alternatives, and their risks and benefits.

### STRATEGY FOR CHANGE

#### If Your Doctor Suggests Surgery

Whether you're getting a first, second, or third opinion, be sure to ask the following questions before going ahead with surgery:

- What will happen if I don't have the operation?
- If I don't have the operation now, how long can I delay it in order to try other treatments?
- What are the risks and side effects of the operation? How likely are they to occur?
- How do the risks change if I delay surgery?
- What nonsurgical treatments are available for this condition? What are their risks and side effects?
- Could I live comfortably without surgery? For how long?
- Can I speak to patients who've had the operation, as well as to others who've declined surgery?
- Tell me specific details: Exactly what will be done? How long will it take? Will the anesthesia be local (only the affected area is numbed, as in most dental procedures) or general (the patient is unconscious throughout the procedure)? How long will I be hospitalized? What kind of discomfort will I feel? For how long?
- When can I return to work?
- When will I feel like my normal self?
- How much will the operation cost?

Eight out of ten operations are elective, which means they're not life-and-death emergencies. If you schedule elective surgery, use the weeks between deciding to have surgery and entering the operating room to get in the best possible condition: Get plenty of rest; eat a well-balanced diet. Ask your doctor if you need any vitamin or mineral supplements (especially if you won't be able to take any food by mouth after the operation). Lose excess weight—but don't crash diet! Quit smoking. (Smoking reduces the amount of oxygen in the blood and can cause serious complications.) Have blood taken and stored in case a transfusion is necessary during your operation.

## Informed Consent

By law, a patient must give consent for hospitalization, surgery, and other major treatments. **Informed consent** is a right, not a privilege. Use this right to its fullest: Ask questions; seek other opinions. Make sure that your expectations are realistic and that you understand the potential risks as well as the possible benefits.

### STRATEGY FOR CHANGE

#### Surviving a Hospital Stay

In general, you're far better off staying out of hospitals. Always ask your doctor if there are any alternatives to hospitalization, such as an outpatient surgery center. However, when you must go, choose your hospital carefully and keep your wits about you. Your life may depend on it.

- Check out hospitals. Call the hospital your doctor recommended, and ask how many operations of the type you need were performed there in the last year and what the mortality rate was. You can compare that rate with the national rates given in the Med-

### HEALTH HEADLINE

#### Are Hospitals Hazardous to Health?

**Negligence kills thousands of people in New York hospitals and injures many more, according to a comprehensive study of medical malpractice by Harvard University researchers. In a one-year period, as many as 99,000 patients were harmed by hospital care. The "adverse events" ranged from falls to infections caused by surgery. Only a small percentage of injured patients ever file malpractice claims, the researchers noted.**

SOURCE: "Hospital Negligence—A Harvard Study," *San Francisco Chronicle*, March 1, 1990.

**informed consent** Permission given voluntarily, with full knowledge and understanding of the procedure or treatment, and its consequences.

icare report on almost 6,000 hospitals across the country.[9] (This report should be in most libraries.)

- Once admitted, make sure the name on your wristband is spelled correctly and clearly.
- Talk to everyone who brings you a pill or is to perform a test or procedure. Patient charts occasionally get mixed up, and you don't want to undergo a treatment meant for someone else.
- Know what medicines you're supposed to get and what they look like. If you're uncertain, ask for a double check.
- Make sure the people caring for you wash their hands. A polite reminder won't offend good professionals—and it could prevent infection.
- Be sure to bring along any recent test results or X rays that your doctor feels may be helpful. You may be able to avoid some repeat testing.
- If you're asked to sign a consent form, read it carefully. If you want more information, ask before signing. Don't feel pressured to sign if you want to discuss something with your doctor first.
- If you develop an emergency, such as sudden bleeding, and no one answers your calls or rings, use the bedside phone to call the hospital's main number. (Write it down next to your phone.)

### Alternatives to Hospitals

**Outpatient Surgery Centers** Outpatient surgery centers offer an alternative to the overnight hospital stay for patients in need of minor surgery. These centers can handle about 40 percent of all procedures, including cataract removal, tonsillectomy, breast biopsy, dilation and curettage (D&C), vasectomy, and face lifts.[10]

Without the high overhead costs of a hospital, outpatient-surgery costs run only about 30 to 50 percent of standard hospital fees. Today, 70 percent of hospitals do outpatient, or in-and-out, surgery. To cut health costs, insurance companies are encouraging, or in some cases requiring, their policyholders to choose outpatient surgery. However, operations requiring prolonged general anesthesia (such as abdominal surgery) or extensive postoperative care (such as heart surgery) must still be performed in hospitals.

**Freestanding Emergency Centers** Freestanding emergency centers (those not part of a hospital), which have spread across the country, claim that they deliver high-quality medical treatment with maximum convenience in minimal time. Critics dismiss them as impersonal and mechanized; they refer to them as "Big Mac" medicine.[11]

Yet customers seem to be pleased. Rather than going to crowded hospital emergency rooms when they slice a finger in the kitchen, the "walking wounded" can go to such emergency centers and get prompt attention and relief.

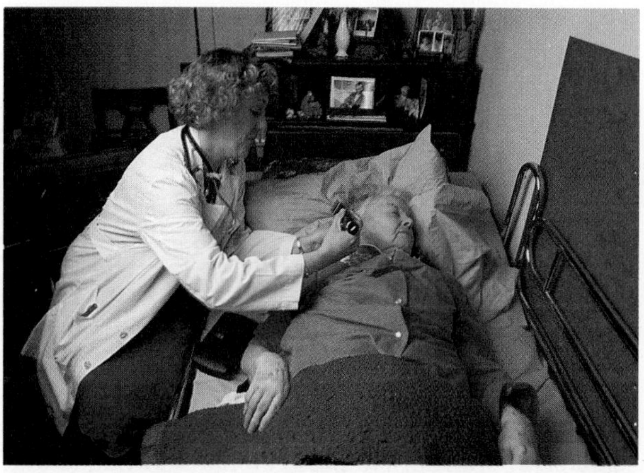

Home health nurses provide some services that once were available only in hospitals.

**Home Health Care** With hospitals discharging patients sooner, home care for patients has grown into a major industry that may grow to $25 billion by 1995. Advances in technology have also made it possible for treatments once administered only in hospitals, such as dialysis, chemotherapy, and traction, to be performed at home at a cost 60 to 90 percent lower than in hospitals.[12]

Hospital discharge planners usually arrange home health care for patients who've been hospitalized. Families can also contact health aides, nurses, and other needed professionals on their own. According to the Health Insurance Association of America, more than eight out of ten private insurance policies offer some coverage of these home health-care costs.

### Quality Control

At the federal level, the three agencies most involved in ensuring quality health care are the Food and Drug Administration, which approves the production and labeling of drugs; the Federal Trade Commission (FTC), which oversees advertising and prohibits deceptive or false claims; and the U.S. Postal Service, which prevents the use of the mails in defrauding the public.

An incentive for doctors to provide high-quality care has been the explosion of **malpractice** suits in the last decade. The essence of a malpractice suit is the claim that the doctor failed to meet the standard of care required of a reasonably skilled and careful physician. Although physicians do not have to guarantee good results to their patients and are not held liable for unavoidable errors, they are required to use the same care and judgment in treatment that would be used by other physicians in the same specialty under similar circumstances.

Most lawsuits are based on **negligence** and assert that a doctor failed to render diagnosis and treatment with appropriate professional knowledge and skill. Other cases are brought for failure to provide information, obtain consent, or respect a patient's confidentiality. To protect themselves financially, physicians—particularly those in surgical specialties, who are most likely to be sued—pay tens of thousands of dollars a year in malpractice-insurance premiums. Some of this cost is passed on to patients.

### Self-help Groups

More than 20 million Americans belong to the nation's 500,000 self-help groups—groups such as Emphysema Anonymous, HELP groups (fifty groups around the country for herpes victims), and the Stroke Club (for people recovering from strokes). (See the appendix of this book and the Yellow Pages in your telephone book.)

In self-help organizations, people with common problems share experiences, empathy, and solutions to their everyday difficulties. Most of these groups offer an accepting, nonthreatening atmosphere that helps people cope with serious mental and physical problems.

## PAYING FOR MEDICAL CARE

Americans spend more than $1 billion a day on health care. We see more doctors, get more tests, have more X rays, undergo more surgery, use more drugs, and spend more time in the hospital than do any other people in the world—and we pay dearly for it.

Fee-for-service medicine means that the physician or hospital performs treatment and presents you (or the insurance company) with a bill. Prepaid medicine means you pay for specified medical services ahead of time. The method of payment does not affect the quality of medical care, so far as anyone can determine, but it may affect the kind of treatment you get.

An estimated 37 million Americans do not have health insurance.[13] They face the very real risk of losing their cars, their homes, and all their financial assets should they require expensive medical care. The government pays a percentage of medical bills *only* for those over age 65 and those who have no resources of their own and cannot afford health care.

If you've always relied on your parents' or spouse's health insurance policy or if you've never required emergency or hospital care, you may never have concerned yourself with coverage. But if you broke your leg and went to the nearest emergency room or quick-care center, how would you pay for your treatment? What if your appendix ruptured or you developed pneumonia or another serious problem that required hospitalization? Are you sure you're covered by your own policy, a family member's, or an employee plan? What would you do if you had to pay out thousands of dollars to cover the costs of your care? The best time to check on insurance coverage is *before* you need to use it.

More than 1,700 commercial insurance carriers offer a wide range of health-coverage plans. If the payment doesn't fully cover the medical or hospital bill, the policyholder must come up with the balance. Supplemental health insurance is intended to complement regular health insurance, usually only if you are hospitalized. The best protection against being bankrupted by enormous medical bills is a major-medical policy, which picks up where basic hospital- and doctor-bill plans leave off.

Before purchasing insurance or selecting among options available through your employer, make sure you are dealing with a reputable company. Ask your friends if they are happy with their health-insurance programs. When considering a specific insurance plan, be sure to ask about the following:

- *Ambulatory Benefits* —Health-care benefits available to you when you are not confined to a hospital bed—benefits such as outpatient and home care
- *Deductible* —The part of the hospital or doctor bills you must pay before your policy's benefits begin
- *Major-Medical or Catastrophic Coverage* —Supplementary coverage of major-medical or hospital expenses exceeding basic benefits

---

**malpractice** The failure of a doctor or other health-care professionals to provide appropriate and skillful medical or surgical treatment.
**negligence** The failure to act in a way that a reasonable person would act.

- *Outpatient Benefits* —Benefits paid for hospital services, such as X rays, administered on an outpatient basis

STRATEGY FOR CHANGE

**How to Buy Health Insurance**

Here is a list of questions you should ask about your health insurance:

- What provisions have been made against a loss of personal income resulting from illness or accident?
- Exactly what costs will your insurance handle?
- Will it cover related hospital expenses, such as X rays and laboratory tests?
- Does it provide for physicians' services in and out of the hospital?
- What members of your family are covered?
- Does your policy provide convalescent-care coverage? What about extended-care coverage?
- What are the maximum benefits, in terms of amount of money and duration of payment?
- What are the waiting periods or exclusions specified in your policy?
- What is the deductible?
- In an individual policy, who has the right of renewal of coverage—the policyholder or the insurance company—and why?

### Health Maintenance Organizations

**Health maintenance organizations** (HMOs) are prepaid health-care groups that emphasize routine care and prevention by providing complete medical services in exchange for a predetermined monthly payment. Unlike fee-for-service hospitals and clinics, HMOs do not make their money by filling hospital beds. As a consequence, HMO members spend 65 percent less time in hospitals than the average for the nation's population as a whole. (HMO subscribers also tend to be slightly younger and healthier than the general population.)

STRATEGY FOR CHANGE

**Choosing a Prepaid Health-Care Program**

When choosing a health-care program, shop around. Every area offers different options. Here are some questions you should ask:

- How much will the plan cost?
- Are all dependents covered? To what age?
- Can I renew every year? Can my coverage be canceled?
- What happens if I leave my employer or the group through which my insurance was obtained?
- What if my spouse has the coverage and we get divorced?
- How can I be sure of being covered in an emergency?
- What happens if I'm out of town and need care?
- Can I select my doctor, or will one be assigned to me?
- What if I need a specialist? How difficult is it to get a referral?
- To which hospitals can I be admitted?
- Can I get a doctor on the phone when I need one?
- What about mental health services?

## ALTERNATIVE APPROACHES TO TRADITIONAL MEDICINE

Modern medicine, some people argue, is effective in injuries and illnesses that improve with drugs or surgery, but not as effective in dealing with life-style problems such as stress, drug addiction, and obesity. Alternative approaches, often referred to as holistic medicine, focus on the person as a whole. Among the assumptions of holistic therapies are the following:

- The mind and body are unified.
- The body can ward off disease or heal itself; it is basically a natural healing system intent on good health and able to right itself.
- Illness is not "the enemy" of the body; it is an important feedback message, which should be heard.
- Physicians serve to help the patient learn how stresses and misunderstandings—including environmental hazards, family and job stresses, and emotional upsets—interfere with health and healing.

Holistic health includes a variety of alternative health approaches, including the following.

### Homeopathy

Homeopathy is based on the principle that like cures like. By administering doses of animal, vegetable, or mineral substances to a large number of healthy people to see if all develop the same symptoms, homeo-

**health maintenance organization (HMO)** An organization that provides health services on a fixed-contract basis.

paths determine what substances may be given, in small quantities, to alleviate symptoms. (The concept of the microdose, or very small dose, is central to homeopathy.) Some of these substances are the same as those used in conventional medicine: nitroglycerin for certain heart conditions, for example.

### Creative Visualization

Creative visualization, or "imaging," uses positive thoughts and images to create a clear idea of that which you want to achieve. You repeatedly focus on a certain idea or mental picture, giving it positive energy, until you attain the desired result. You may relax, for example, by visualizing yourself lying on a beach in the sun.

### Herbal Medicine

Herbal medicine, or herbology, is an ancient form of treatment that uses herbs—substances derived from trees, flowers, ferns, seaweeds, or lichens—to treat disease. Many manufactured drugs are made from plants or are synthetic re-creations or modifications of naturally occurring substances. However, advocates of herbal medicine feel that herbs work differently on the body than do purified drugs. They believe herbal treatments have fewer side effects and promote faster healing. Herbal treatments have been developed for practically all known diseases—from corns and callouses to anemia and hypertension.

### Yoga

Yoga, an Indian-based philosophy that has evolved over 6,000 years, works on the premise that most illness is caused by wrong mental attitudes, diet, and posture. By combining a discipline of exercise, meditation, and diet, patients have learned to cope with such stress-induced conditions as hypertension, the desire to smoke, and obesity.

### Acupuncture

Acupuncture is a natural healing system based on the ancient Chinese belief in a life force circulating through the body along well-defined pathways called meridians. Pain or disease is the result of blockage of this life force by stress or injury. To restore balance, the physician inserts special needles into the proper meridians. Acupuncture tends to be most effective for pain relief in people who already believe in its powers.

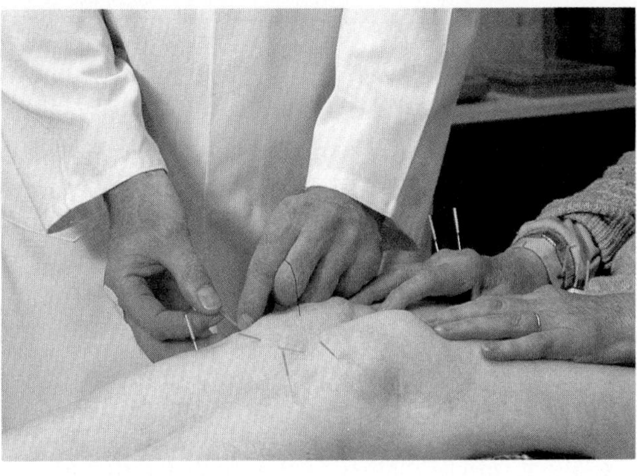

An acupuncturist applies needles to the knees of an elderly woman with painful arthritis.

### Faith Healing

Faith healing refers to a variety of practices, including the laying on of hands, that rely on a "higher power" to cure disease and restore well-being. Although for centuries reports of miracles have testified to the powers of belief, there is no scientific evidence that faith can heal any illness. Yet many people who turn to faith healers may feel better, at least temporarily, simply because they believe they've been helped.

**STRATEGY FOR CHANGE**

**Should You Try an Alternative Treatment?**

- Before you explore unconventional treatments, read up on what medical science has to offer and on what the alternatives claim.
- Avoid any practitioner who insists his brand of healing is the *only* effective approach.
- Check into credentials as carefully as possible. Some "doctors" in white coats have dubious degrees, often in fields not at all related to health.
- Remember that you are ultimately responsible for your well-being. Don't entrust it to anyone who doesn't deserve your trust.

## QUACKERY

Every year millions of Americans go searching for medical miracles that never happen. In all, they spend more than $10 billion on medical **quackery,** unproven health products and services.[14] Yet those who lose only money are the lucky ones. Many waste precious

**quackery** Medical fakery; unproven practices claiming to cure diseases or solve health problems.

time, during which their conditions worsen. Some suffer needless pain, along with crushed expectations. Far too many risk their lives on a false hope—and lose.

The peddlers of such false hopes are quacks, who, by definition, promote for profit worthless or unproven treatments. A quack's greatest skill is telling people what they want to hear. Quackery's most recent disguise has been in the form of megavitamins; macrobiotic diets; and other "natural" treatments for cancer, AIDS, and other life-threatening conditions. In a study of cancer patients who've tried such unorthodox treatments, researchers found that most had small, treatable tumors and excellent chances of recovery with conventional therapy.

**STRATEGY FOR CHANGE**

**Protecting Yourself Against Quackery**

- Arm yourself with up-to-date information about the disease from appropriate organizations, such as the American Cancer Society or the Arthritis Foundation, which keep track of unproven and ineffective methods of treatment.
- Ask for a written explanation of what the treatment does and why it works; evidence supporting all claims (not just testimonials); and published reports of the studies that have been done, including specifics on numbers treated, doses, and side effects.
- Don't part with your money quickly. Unlike legitimate researchers, quacks always charge for their care—and the patient winds up paying out of pocket because insurance companies won't reimburse for unproven therapies.
- Don't discontinue your current treatment without your physician's approval. Many doctors encourage "supportive" therapy—such as relaxation exercises, meditation, or visualization—in addition to standard treatments.
- Be wary of unorthodox diagnostic tests, including blood tests for food allergies and hair analysis. Hair analysis has been found meaningless, but unorthodox therapists still use it for "detecting" diseases and prescribing questionable treatments.

## MAKING THIS CHAPTER WORK FOR YOU

### Making Smart Health-care Decisions

**Self-care means learning about your body and what it takes to live as healthfully as possible, caring for minor illnesses, and taking responsibility for your health. Your home pharmacy should include such products as aspirin or acetaminophen to relieve minor pain or fever, ipecac for emergency use in some accidental poisonings, an antacid to relieve an upset stomach, and antiseptic and bandages for treating wounds. OTC drugs that are commonly misused include nasal sprays, laxatives, and eye drops. With**

## WHAT DO YOU THINK?

Rashid and Shanta are your new neighbors; they just moved from another city. They have asked you for information about your primary-care physician. What can you tell them about your doctor? Do you know if he or she is board-certified and in what specialty? What do you like about your doctor? What don't you like?

Imagine that you are in a car accident and suffer serious injuries requiring a long hospital stay and months of intensive rehabilitation therapy. Who would pay your bills? If you say your parents' insurance, what do you know about the policy? Would it cover only part of your care? Would their premiums go up? What if their policy's coverage expired on your eighteenth birthday?

Ray is 25 years old and feels healthy but knows that he has been infected with the virus that causes AIDS. Through a friend of a friend, he's heard about a therapist who uses multivitamins and herbal remedies to prevent the development of AIDS symptoms. The treatment program is expensive and wouldn't be covered by Ray's insurance. Also, the therapist discourages patients from continuing to see their regular doctors. Ray desperately wants to live as long as possible. What do you think he should do?

appropriate home tests, equipment, and knowledge about how to use them, you can identify any suspicious signs that require professional care.

As a consumer, you may turn to physicians, registered nurses, medical paraprofessionals, dentists and dental technicians; chiropractors and optometrists; podiatrists; and osteopaths. Preventive care includes immunizations for protection against diseases; physical examinations for assessment of general well-being; dental checkups; and periodic screening tests for hypertension, changes and abnormalities in the cervix, glaucoma, and tuberculosis.

Before a doctor begins a physical examination, he or she will take a history to gather all the details that may be relevant to the patient's problem. Lack of patient compliance with doctors' suggestions is a common problem. Getting a second opinion about surgical procedures and alternative therapies is a patient's way of exploring treatment options.

With the development of outpatient surgery centers and freestanding emergency centers and the growing acceptance of home health care, people now have convenient and less costly alternatives to hospital care. The responsibility for quality control of all health-care services lies with government agencies and peer-review organizations. A health professional can be sued for malpractice if a patient believes that the care received was substandard or that the physician was negligent.

There are two ways of paying for health care: fee-for-service care, in which the patient is presented with a bill for treatments as they are performed, and prepaid care, in which the patient pays for services ahead of time. Commercial health-insurance plans cover the costs of medical services rendered to those who purchase coverage by paying periodic premiums. Health maintenance organizations, or HMOs, are prepaid health-care groups that emphasize preventive health care.

Alternative, or holistic, approaches to conventional medicine include homeopathy, chiropractic, creative visualization, herbal medicine, yoga, acupuncture, and faith healing. Quackery involves worthless, fraudulent, or unproven treatments for incurable diseases, longer life, better health, or delayed aging.

The more you know about your body and your health, the better decisions you can make about health care. Here are a few simple steps you can take to form a partnership with the health-care professionals you see:

- Realize that what you have to say is worth the health expert's time.
- Think of each professional as a highly paid consultant who's there to perform a service for you.
- Be as specific as possible in describing symptoms.
- Ask questions whenever you're doubtful.
- Don't be intimidated if a health-care worker seems busy or restless. If you don't understand something, say something like "Tell me about the procedure again. I'm not sure I understood everything you said."
- Try not to be disagreeable. Doctors, nurses, dentists, and other health-care workers are human beings; just like the rest of us, they pull away from unpleasant people.
- Fill in your primary physician about what everyone else involved in your care—specialists, hospital nurses, physical therapists, and the like—is doing. Don't assume they're all in contact.
- Never leave a doctor's office uncertain about the diagnosis or recommended treatment. Ask about anything that's unclear and repeat the answers in your own words.
- If your doctor is unwilling to talk with you or incapable of communicating clearly, find another.

Your health is your most important asset. Consider the time and effort you spend learning about your body and caring for your health an investment in your future.

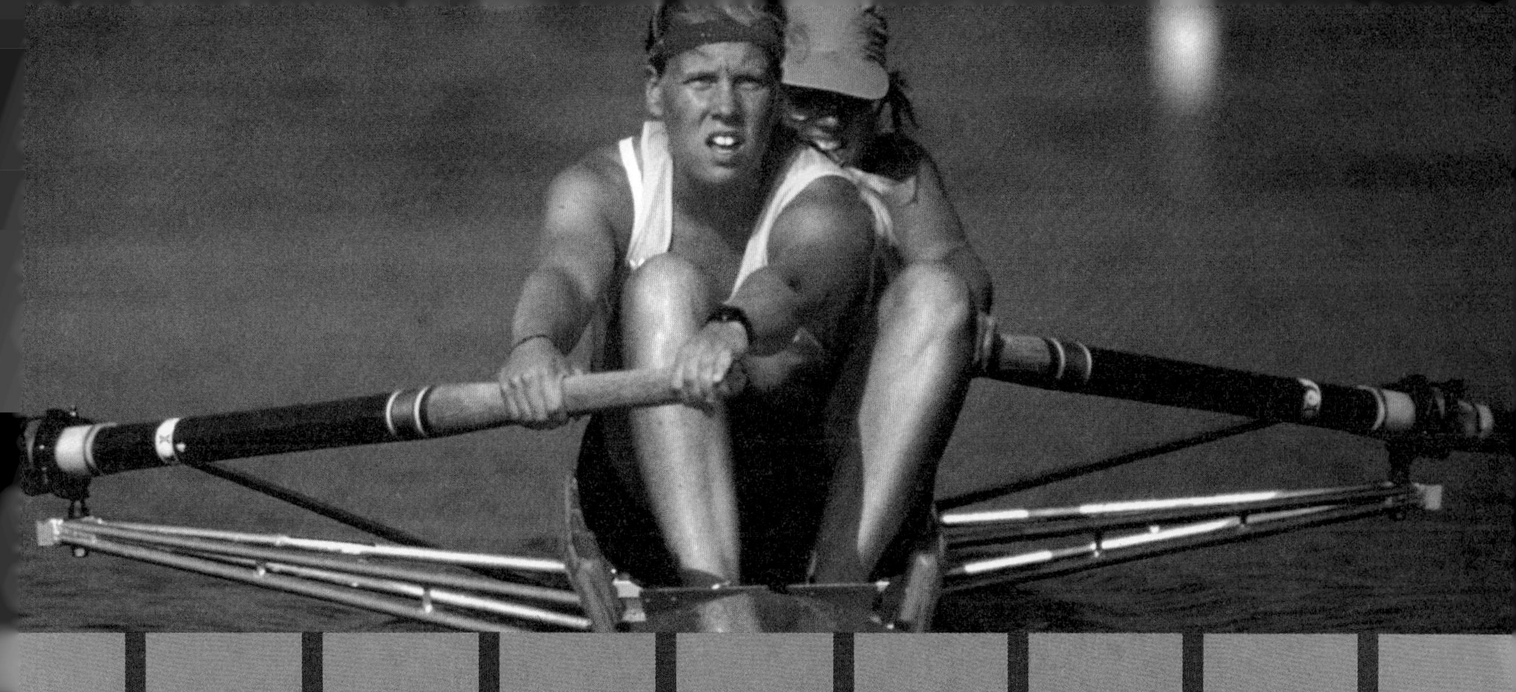

# 13 CARDIOVASCULAR DISEASE: BEATING THE NUMBER ONE KILLER

**In this chapter**

**The state of the heart**

**The silent killers**

**Crises of the heart**

**Heart savers**

**Stroke: Starving the brain**

**Making This Chapter Work for You: Keeping your heart healthy**

*As with every other aspect of your well-being, your heart's health depends to a great extent on you—the choices you make, the habits you create, and the life-style you adopt.* Prevention can save hearts and lives. In the last decade the death rate from diseases of the heart and blood vessels has fallen. A national campaign to treat high blood pressure, the main stepping-stone to heart disease and stroke, may be paying off. So are new ways of diagnosing and treating heart disease and better emergency systems for getting help where it's needed fast. Yet nearly one of every two Americans still dies of heart-related disorders.[1] This chapter will provide the information you need for a hardier heart and a healthier life.

## THE STATE OF THE HEART

The heart is a hollow, muscular organ with four chambers. The upper two, called **atria,** receive blood, which then flows through valves into the lower two chambers, called **ventricles,** which contract to pump blood out into the arteries through a second set of valves. A thick wall divides the right side of the heart from the left side. But even though the two sides are separated, they contract at almost the same time. Contraction of the heart is called **systole;** the period of relaxation between contractions is called **diastole.**

Your heart contracts (beats) between 60 and 80 times per minute, or about 100,000 times a day. With each beat, it pumps about 2-1/2 ounces of blood. This may not sound like much, but it adds up to nearly 5 quarts of blood pumped by the heart in 1 minute, or about 75 gallons per hour.

Blood circulates through the body, via the heart, as shown in Figures 13-1 and 13-2. The right ventricle (that is, the ventricle on your own right side) pumps blood, via the pulmonary arteries, to the lungs, where it picks up oxygen (a gas essential to the body's cells)

**atrium** (*plural:* **atria**) Either of the two upper chambers of the heart, which receive blood from the veins.
**ventricle** Either of the two lower chambers of the heart, which pump blood out of the heart and into the arteries.
**systole** The contraction phase of the cardiac cycle.
**diastole** The period between contractions in the cardiac cycle; when the heart relaxes and dilates as it fills with blood.

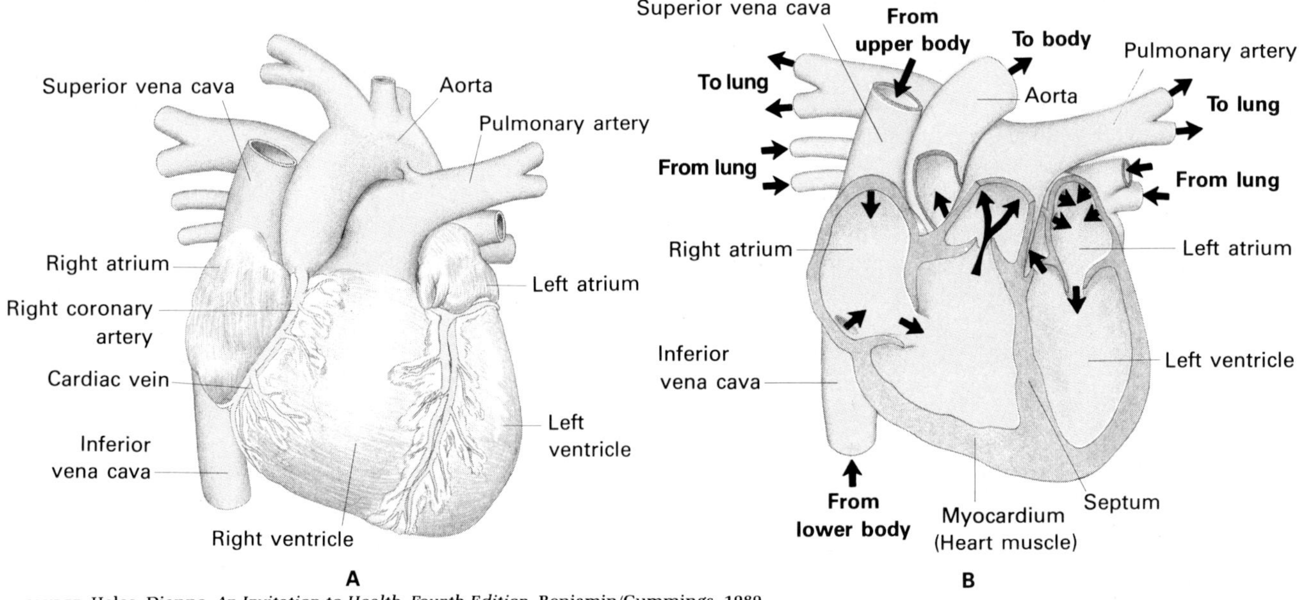


SOURCE: Hales, Dianne. *An Invitation to Health, Fourth Edition,* Benjamin/Cummings, 1989.

**FIGURE 13-1** The healthy heart. **(a)** Exterior view. The heart muscle is nourished by blood from the coronary arteries, which arise from the aorta. **(b)** Cross-section of the heart, showing the paths of blood flow. Blood returns from the body through the veins; enters the right atrium; and flows into the right ventricle, which pumps the blood through the pulmonary arteries and into the lungs.

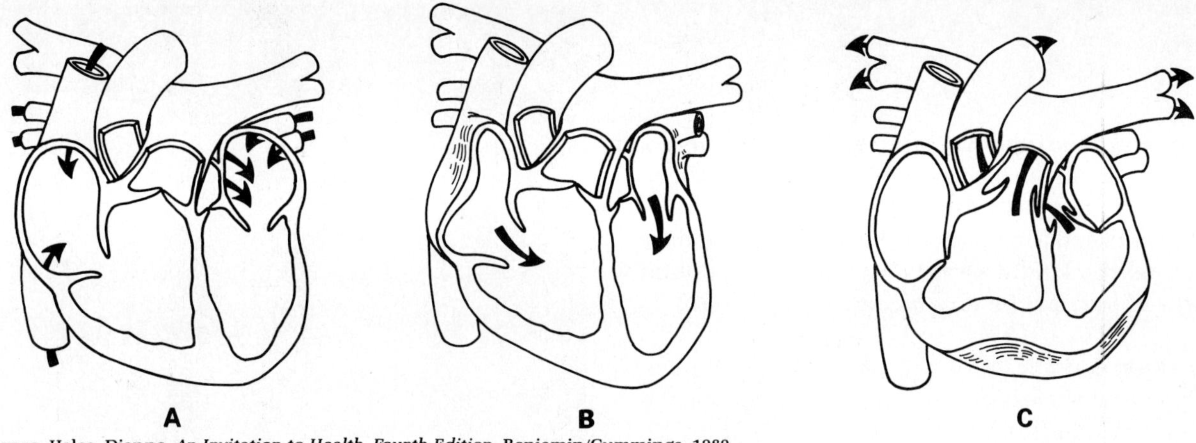


SOURCE: Hales, Dianne. *An Invitation to Health, Fourth Edition,* Benjamin/Cummings, 1989.

**FIGURE 13-2** The heart's pumping cycle. **(a)** Blood fills both atria and enters the ventricles (*diastole*). **(b)** The atria contract, squeezing blood into the ventricles. **(c)** The ventricles contract, pumping blood into the aorta and pulmonary arteries (*systole*).

and gives off carbon dioxide (a waste product of metabolism). The blood returns from the lungs to the left side of the heart, which pumps it, via the aorta, to the arteries in the rest of the body. The arteries divide into smaller and smaller branches and finally into **capillaries,** the smallest blood vessels of all (only slightly larger in diameter than a red blood cell). The blood within the capillaries supplies oxygen and nutrients to the cells of the tissues, and takes up various waste products. Blood returns to the right side of the heart via the veins.

## Hearts at Risk

**Cardiovascular disease**—disorders of the heart and blood vessels—occurs when one of three things happens:

- the flow of blood through the heart and to the rest of the body is blocked
- the flow of blood to the heart itself is blocked
- something goes wrong with the small bundle of highly specialized heart cells that generate electrical impulses that coordinate the heart's contractions

Following are the major risk factors in heart disease and stroke. The greater the number or severity of these risk factors, the greater your overall risk.

### Risks You Cannot Control

**Heredity** Although there is no hard evidence that cardiovascular disease is hereditary, it appears that a tendency toward such problems can be inherited. Abnormalities in the levels of blood fats (lipids) can be traced from generation to generation in vulnerable families.

**Sex** Men have a higher incidence of cardiovascular problems than do women, particularly in the first four decades of their lives. The rate of heart attacks in women before menopause is comparatively low, but heart disease is the number one killer of women over age 65.

**Race** Black Americans are twice as likely to develop high blood pressure as are whites. Also, blacks suffer strokes at an earlier age and of greater severity. Family history, life-style, diet, and stress may all play a role.

**Age** Almost four out of five people who die of heart attack are over age 65. However, the risk factors that are likely to cause heart disease later in life—including high cholesterol levels, high blood pressure, and Type-A personalities—can develop in childhood.

### Risks You Can Control

**Cigarette Smoking** The Surgeon General has declared that smoking is the most dangerous risk factor for heart disease. Smokers have 2 times the risk of heart attack and 2 to 4 times the risk of sudden cardiac death that nonsmokers have.[2] A smoker who has a heart attack is more likely to die from it than is a nonsmoker. Smoking is also the major risk factor for peripheral vascular disease, in which the blood vessels that carry blood to the leg and arm muscles narrow.

Cigarettes may damage the heart in three possible ways:

- The nicotine may overstimulate the heart.

**capillary** A tiny blood vessel that provides oxygen and nutrients to cells and takes away waste products.
**cardiovascular disease** Disorders of the blood and heart.

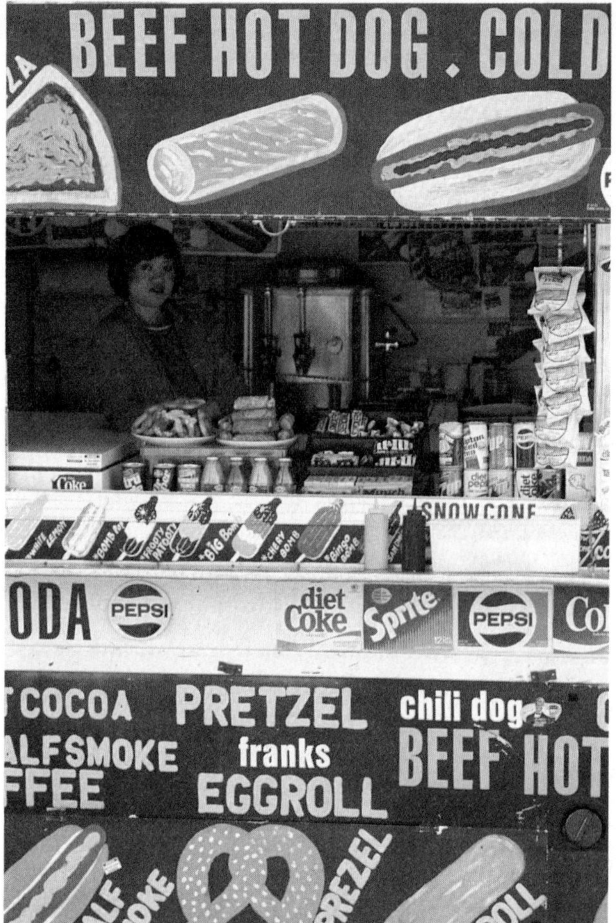


Fatty foods, such as hot dogs and burgers, are popular, but can increase the levels of cholesterol in the blood.

- Carbon monoxide may take the place of some of the oxygen in the blood, which reduces the oxygen supply to the heart muscle.
- The smoke may damage the lining of the coronary arteries, making it easier for cholesterol to build up and narrow the passageways.

**Cholesterol** Cholesterol is a type of fat. The measurement of cholesterol in the blood is one of the most reliable indicators of the formation of **plaque,** sludgelike deposits of cholesterol and other fats, fibrin (a clotting material), cell parts, and calcium that build up on the inner walls of the arteries. Lowering blood cholesterol can prevent heart attacks. For every 1 percent drop in blood cholesterol, studies show a 2 percent reduction in heart-attack risk.[3]

The National Heart, Lung and Blood Institute (NHLBI) recommends testing of cholesterol levels every 5 years for all Americans twenty years or older. Here are the NHLBI guidelines:

- Total cholesterol should be below 200 mg of total cholesterol per deciliter of blood (mg/dl).
- A reading of 201 to 239 mg/dl is considered borderline and presents a moderate to high risk for heart disease; individuals in this range should adopt a low-fat diet.
- Levels of 240 or more mg/dl are dangerously high and require strict dietary changes.

Adults with a cholesterol level of 220 mg/dl may be more than twice as likely to get heart disease as those with a level of 180 mg/dl; for those with levels of 300 mg/dl or higher, the risk is 4 times greater.[4,5] (Chapter 4 presents a more detailed discussion of cholesterol in daily diet.)

**Blood Fats** Compounds in the blood that are made up of proteins and fat (lipids) are **lipoproteins.** High-density lipoproteins (HDLs), which some cardiologists refer to as "the good guys," pick up excess cholesterol (a dangerous form of fat) in the blood and carry it back to the liver for removal from the body. The higher the level of HDL in the blood, the lower the risk of cardiovascular disease.

HDLs are most plentiful in the people least likely to get cardiovascular disease—people such as young women and athletes. The levels of the "bad," or low-density, lipoproteins (LDLs), which deposit cholesterol on the walls of the arteries, are lower in people who usually don't get heart disease. Thus, the higher the level of HDL and the higher the ratio of HDL to total cholesterol (HDL plus other blood fats), the lower the likelihood of heart disease seems to be (Figure 13-3). If the percentage of HDL in a man's cholesterol reading is less than 20 percent, he is at risk for coronary artery disease. A woman is at risk if her HDL is less than 25 percent of total cholesterol.[6]

**cholesterol** A type of fat.
**plaque** A substance composed of cholesterol and other materials that builds up in blood vessels.
**lipoprotein** A compound in the blood; made up of proteins and fat.

STRATEGY FOR CHANGE

### What You Need to Know About Cholesterol Testing

- Go to your own physician to have your cholesterol level checked. Although cholesterol tests at shopping malls can help identify people at risk, the analyzers often are not certified technicians. In addition, without a physician to counsel them, some people may be unnecessarily frightened by a high reading—or falsely reassured by a low one.

- Think about timing. For many people, the best testing time is during their routine physical. Cholesterol levels can rise 5 to 10 percent during periods of stress.
- Get real numbers. Don't settle for "normal" or "high," because laboratories can inaccurately label results. Find out exactly what your reading is.
- Get your HDL/LDL ratio. If your cholesterol level is up, have it retested and ask to find out HDL and LDL levels. The NHLBI says that LDL levels should be less than 130 mg/dl and that HDL levels below 35 mg/dl are considered "a major risk factor."[7]

If your cholesterol level is high, consult with your physician. The best way to lower cholesterol is by cutting down on high-fat foods, increasing exercise, and controlling your weight (see Chapter 4 for specific guidelines).

Anticholesterol medication can cut cholesterol levels by 40 percent, but because the long-term effects are not known, the NHBLI recommends drug therapy for patients only after dietary approaches and other medications have failed to bring cholesterol levels down.[8]

**Triglycerides** Triglycerides do not in themselves seem to increase the risk of heart disease, but they accompany other changes that do increase the risk. Therefore, high triglyceride levels are a concern.

Triglycerides are found in dietary fats, and their levels tend to be highest in those whose diets are high in calories, sugar, alcohol, and refined starches. Thus, triglycerides may contribute to heart disease by increasing the risk of obesity and diabetes.

According to the NHLBI, triglyceride levels should be between 30 and 150 mg/dl. Triglyceride levels in the range of 250 to 500 mg/dl are a danger signal of an increased risk of heart disease. Higher levels, especially over 1,000 mg/dl, increase the risk of pancreatitis, an inflammation of the pancreas requiring immediate medical attention.

**High Blood Pressure** High blood pressure, or hypertension, forces the heart to pump harder than is healthy. Because the heart must force blood into arteries offering increased resistance to blood flow, the left side of the heart often becomes enlarged. Overworked for long periods, the heart can go into congestive heart failure (which is discussed later in this chapter). Hypertension also increases the risk of stroke, heart attack, and kidney failure.

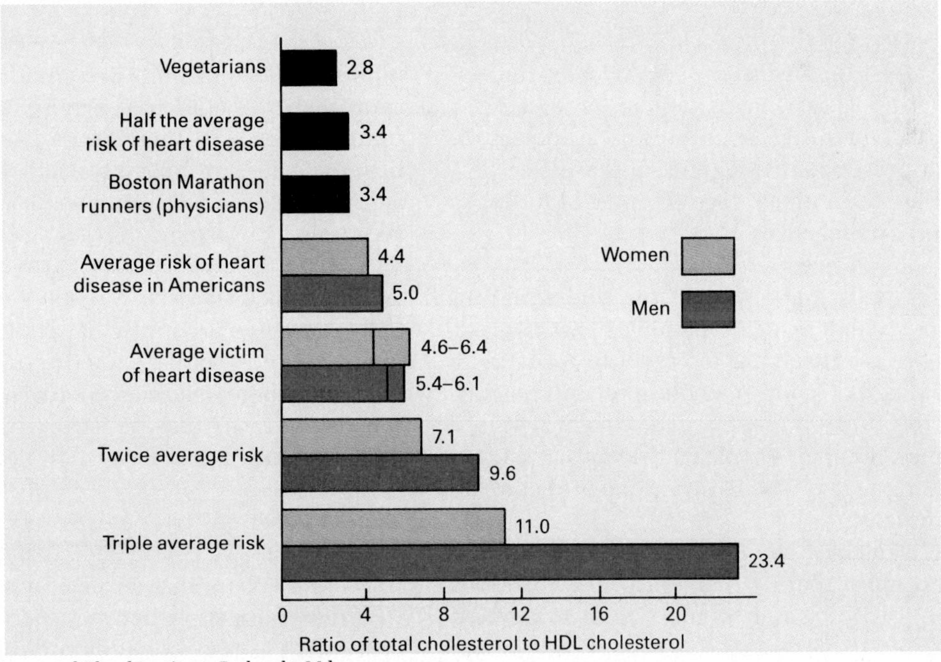


SOURCE: National Heart, Lung and Blood Institute, Bethesda, Md.

**FIGURE 13-3** The ratio of HDL to LDL is a good indicator of a person's risk of heart disease. The ratio is determined by dividing the total cholesterol in the blood by the level of HDL cholesterol.

## HALES INDEX

Number of Americans with some form of cardiovascular disease: 1 in 4

Number of children ages 5 through 8 with at least one heart-disease risk factor: 2 in 5

Frequency of inaccurate cholesterol readings: 1 in 4

Time most heart attack victims wait before seeking help: 3 hours

Number of Americans who suffer heart attacks every day: 4,100

Number of Americans who have heart attacks every year: 1,250,000

Number who die before they reach a hospital: 350,000

Number of women who die of heart disease each year: 250,000

Annual costs of heart problems in medical care and lost wages and productivity: $85.2 billion

People on waiting list for a heart transplant: 645

Cost of a heart transplant: $110,000

Americans living today who have had strokes: 2 million

SOURCES: **1** American Heart Association. **2** Williams, Lena. "Growing Up Flabby," *New York Times*, March 22, 1990. **3** "Flaws in Cholesterol Testing Found by 2 Research Teams," *New York Times*, March 2, 1990. **4, 5** National Heart, Blood and Lung Institute (NHBLI). **6** Kolata, Gina. "Report Urges Low-Fat Diet for Everyone," *New York Times*, February 28, 1990. **7** NHBLI **8** Ismach, Judith. "A Woman's Heart," *American Health*, January/February 1989. **9** Centers for Disease Control. **10, 11** James, Mary. "The Organ Transplant Catalog," *Hippocrates*, May/June 1988. **12** American Heart Association.

**Diabetes Mellitus** Diabetes, a disorder of the endocrine system, is associated with an increased risk of heart attack or stroke. A physician can detect diabetes and prescribe drugs, diets, and exercise programs to keep it in check. (See Chapter 14 for more information on diabetes.)

**Diet** Eating foods that are high in saturated fat increases your chances of developing heart disease. The risk of heart attack may be reduced by eating a nutritious diet that is low in cholesterol and polyunsaturated fats and by keeping your weight within a normal range. (Chapter 4 explains the whys and hows of eliminating excess fat from your diet and controlling your weight.)

All Americans over age 2 should eat a low-fat diet and get no more than 30 percent of their calories from fat in any form and no more than 10 percent from saturated fat.[9] The American Heart Association recommends limiting cholesterol intake to 300 mg a day—the amount in one large egg yolk.

**Lack of Exercise** Regular exercise reduces the risk of heart attack, helps maintain a desirable body weight, increases HDL levels, lowers blood pressure, and improves metabolism.[10] Even men who smoke or are overweight benefit from exercise. Women who don't exercise are three times more likely to have a fatal heart attack than their physically fit sisters. Regular aerobic exercise (see Chapter 5)—walking, cycling, swimming, or jogging—is best.

**Obesity** Fat, particularly, when stored in a big potbelly, may be as bad for the heart as smoking. According to a Swedish study of more than 2,000 men and women, a large belly may increase by five to tenfold the risk of heart disease, stroke, diabetes, and premature death.[11]

**Type A Personality** The definition and significance of Type A behavior have been debated for more than thirty years (see Chapter 3). Many experts now feel that the connection between personality, behavior, and health is more complex and individualized than had previously been thought. In a report in the *New England Journal of Medicine*, researchers found that Type A personalities—who may be more vulnerable to heart disease—are almost twice as likely to recover from heart attacks than more relaxed Type Bs. The authors observed that Type A survivors may respond

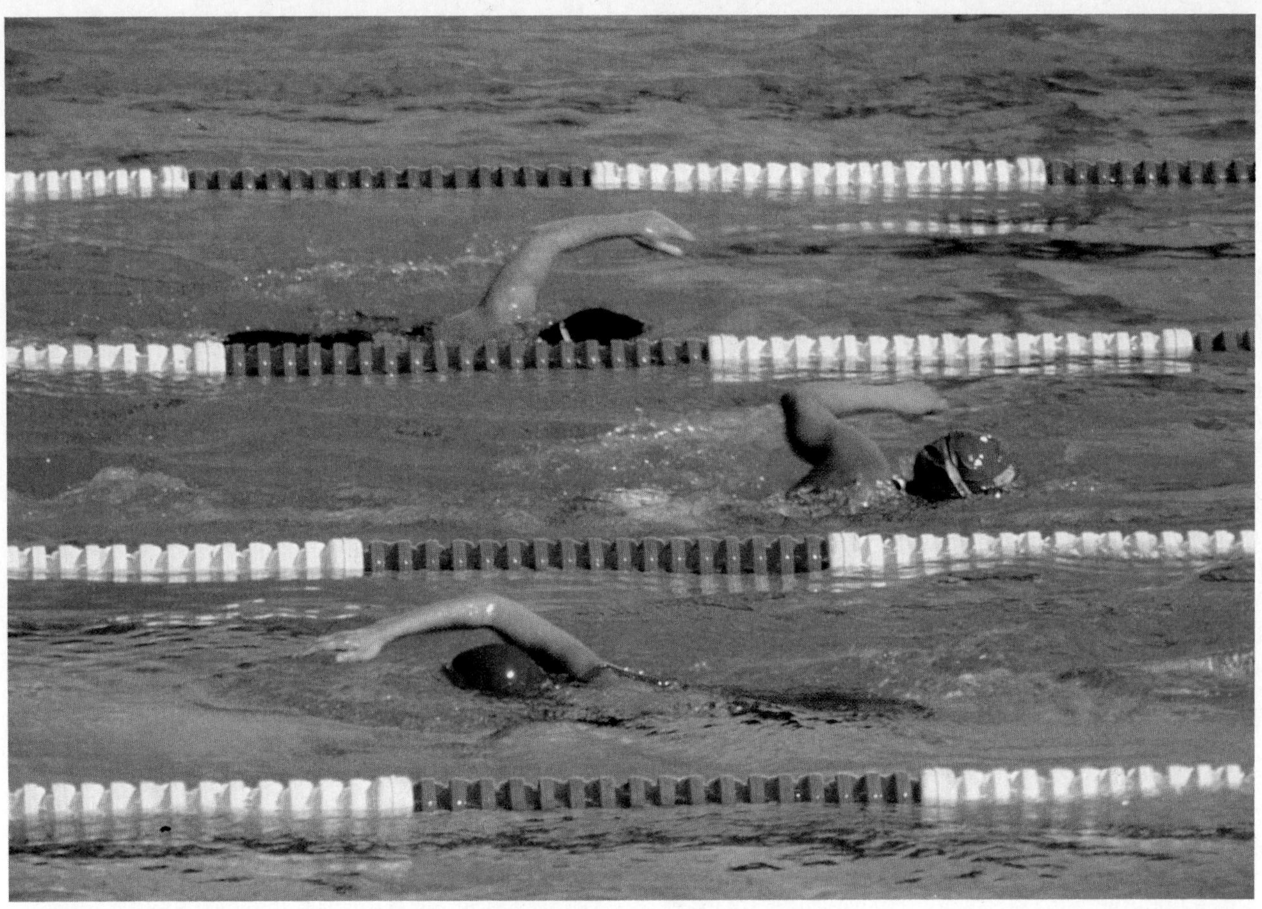

Swimming and other regular aerobic activities can lower the risk of heart disease.

more forcefully to heart disease, making more changes in their diets and life-style and taking charge of their medical situation.

## THE SILENT KILLERS

Heart disease starts slowly and silently. Years may pass before you notice any indication of something wrong. That's why it's important to be aware of the conditions that can weaken your heart without warning.

### Hypertension

High blood pressure, or hypertension, occurs when artery walls squeeze down excessively on the blood that flows by. Some 58 million Americans have high blood pressure that requires monitoring or treatment. More Americans are recognizing the dangers of hypertension, and three out of every four who need medical care are getting it.

Normal blood pressure in most young adults, when relaxed, is 120/80 (120 systolic pressure, 80 diastolic). As noted in Chapter 12, borderline hypertension is 140/90 to 160/95 and definite hypertension is 160/95 and above. The lower, or diastolic, number has increasingly been used in categorizing high blood pressure, with 90 to 104 indicating mild hypertension; 105 to 114, moderate; and 115 and over, severe. According to recent data, however, a high systolic reading indicates an increased risk of heart disease, even if the diastolic pressure is normal.

In most cases the cause of hypertension is unknown, although occasionally abnormalities of the kidneys or the blood vessels feeding them, or certain substances in the bloodstream may be at fault. Hypertension is dangerous because excessive pressure can wear out arteries, leading to serious cardiovascular diseases, vision problems, and kidney disease.

Once diagnosed, hypertension can be treated effectively. Sometimes diet and exercise alone can correct it. Other treatments include restriction of salt intake and medication. The drugs used to treat hypertension include diuretics, which increase urine output, and drugs that dilate the blood vessels, decrease cardiac output, relax the arteries, or prevent the release of hormones that boost blood pressure. The major problem in treating hypertension is that many patients who don't feel sick don't stick with their treatment plans.

## Atherosclerosis: Clogging the Arteries

Any impairment of blood flow through the blood vessels is called **arteriosclerosis,** often referred to as hardening of the arteries. The most common form is **atherosclerosis,** a disease of the lining of the arteries in which sludgelike plaque narrows the artery channels.

Atherosclerosis, which may begin in childhood, worsens with the continued buildup of plaque on the arterial lining (Figure 13-4). The arteries lose their ability to expand and contract. Blood moves with increasing difficulty through the narrowed channels, making it easier for a clot (**thrombus**) to form, perhaps blocking the channel and depriving vital organs of blood. When such a blockage (or **thrombosis**) is in a coronary artery, the result is coronary thrombosis, one form of heart attack. When the clot occurs in the brain, the result is cerebral thrombosis, one form of stroke.

Atherosclerosis is the underlying cause of most heart attacks and strokes. Early identification of risk factors—high blood pressure, high cholesterol levels, and smoking—and changing behavior and diet can prevent or slow its development.

# CRISES OF THE HEART

For many people the first sign of heart disease is pain, ranging from mild to excruciating. The primary causes of pain are **angina pectoris,** spasms of the coronary artery, and **myocardial infarction.**

## Angina Pectoris

Angina pectoris occurs when a temporary drop in the supply of blood to the heart tissue causes feelings of pain or discomfort in the chest. Some people suffer angina only when the demands on their hearts increase, such as during exercise or when under stress. Many people have angina for years and yet never suffer a heart attack; in some, the angina even disappears. However, angina should be considered a warning of danger if it becomes more severe or more frequent, occurs with less activity or exertion, begins to waken a person from a sound sleep at night, persists for more than 10 to 15 minutes, or causes unusual perspiration.

Angina is most commonly treated with nitroglycerin, a chemical (the same one used in explosives) that eases the load on the heart by selectively expanding the vessels to the heart and improving blood flow. Nitroglycerin is available in a controlled-release patch that attaches to the skin so patients don't have to worry about forgetting to take their medication.

**arteriosclerosis** Any of a number of chronic diseases characterized by degeneration of the arteries and hardening and thickening of arterial walls.
**atherosclerosis** A form of arteriosclerosis in which fatty substances are deposited on the inner walls of blood vessels.
**thrombus** A clot that is fixed or stuck to a vessel wall.
**thrombosis** Blood-clot formation within a blood vessel.
**angina pectoris** A severe, suffocating chest pain caused by a brief lack of oxygen to the heart.
**myocardial infarction (MI)** A condition characterized by dead-tissue areas in the myocardium; caused by interruption of the blood supply to those areas.

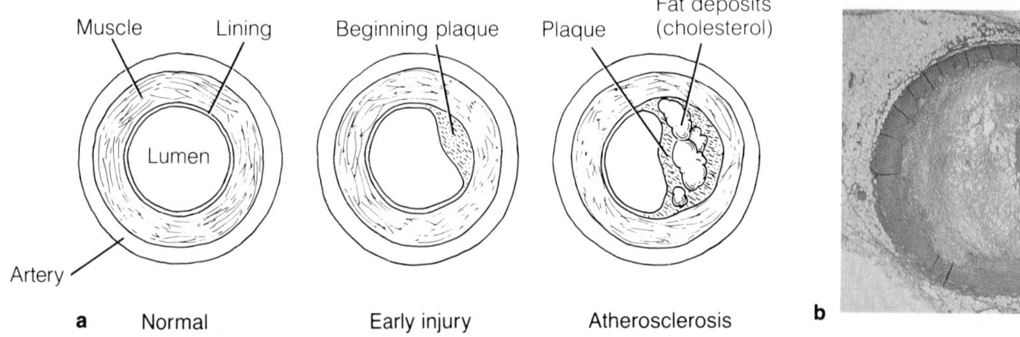


SOURCE: Christian, Janet L. and Janet L. Greger. *Nutrition for Living, Second Edition,* Benjamin/Cummings, 1988.

**FIGURE 13-4** The development of atherosclerosis. **(a)** The progression of atherosclerosis is shown in this cross-section of an artery. **(b)** This micrograph shows a human artery that is almost completely blocked.

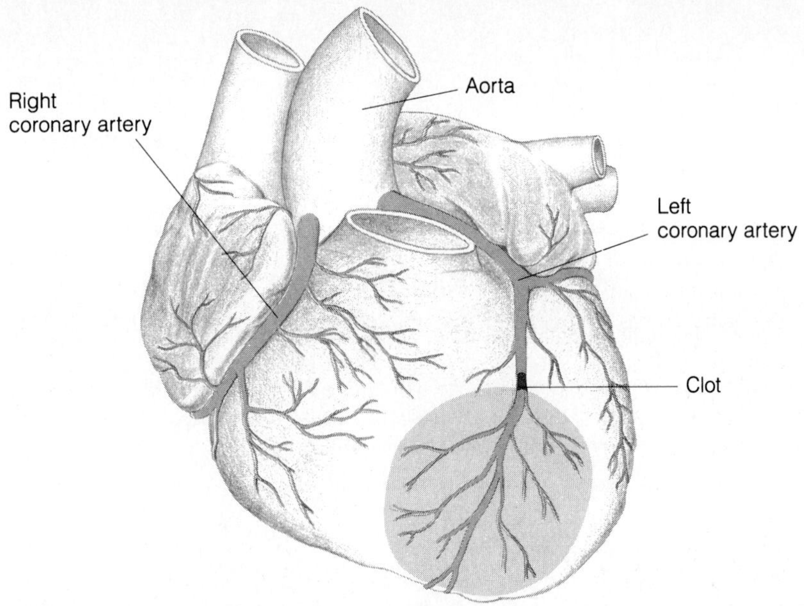


SOURCE: Hales, Dianne. *An Invitation to Health, Fourth Edition,* Benjamin/Cummings, 1989.

**FIGURE 13-5** A clot in one of the arteries that feeds the heart muscle (*myocardium*) can cut off the blood supply to part of the myocardium, causing cells in that area to die. This is a *myocardial infarction,* or heart attack.

## Coronary Artery Spasms

Sometimes the arteries tighten suddenly or go into a spasm, cutting off or reducing blood flow. Spasms can produce heart attacks and angina, and they can be fatal. Several factors may trigger spasms in the heart:

- *Clumping of Platelets* —When **platelets** (fragments of cells that float in the bloodstream and help in clotting) clump together, they can cause a blood vessel to narrow.
- *Smoking* —When some angina victims stop smoking, their chest pain declines or disappears.
- *Stress* —No one knows exactly how stress may lead to spasms, but many heart specialists feel it is a culprit.
- *Increased Calcium Flow* —Calcium regularly flows into smooth muscle cells; too much calcium may lead to a spasm. (This calcium flow has nothing to do with the calcium in the diet.)

## Myocardial Infarction

The medical name for a heart attack, or coronary, is myocardial infarction (MI). The **myocardium** is the muscle layer of the wall of the heart. It receives its blood supply, and thus its oxygen and other nutrients, from the coronary arteries. If an artery is blocked by a clot or by plaque, the myocardial cells do not get sufficient oxygen; the portion of the myocardium deprived of its blood supplies dies (see Figure 13-5). Although such an attack may seem sudden, usually it has been building up for years, particularly if the person has ignored risk factors and early warning signals.

According to the American Heart Association, as many as 1.5 million men and women have heart attacks each year; more than 540,000 die as a result. Almost 5 million Americans alive today have had a heart attack or chest pain, or both.[12]

**STRATEGY FOR CHANGE**

**Recognizing the Warning Signals of a Heart Attack**

Individuals should get immediate medical care if they experience the following symptoms:

- A heavy, squeezing pain or discomfort in the center of the chest, which may last for several minutes (sharp, stabbing pains usually don't mean heart disease)
- a pain that may radiate to the shoulder, arm, neck, or jaw
- additional symptoms, including anxiety, sweating, nausea and vomiting, shortness of breath, or dizziness or fainting

## Halting a Heart Attack

The hour immediately following myocardial infarction is the most crucial period. About 40 percent of those who suffer an MI die within this time. According to the American Heart Association, most patients

**platelet** A component of blood involved in clotting.
**myocardium** The cardiac muscle layer of the wall of the heart.

SELF-SURVEY

## Are You at Risk for Heart Disease?

Even though the number of deaths due to heart disease is declining, heart disease is still the number one cause of death in the United States. After years of research, scientists still cannot say with certainty what causes heart disease or who will have a heart attack. However, they have identified for the general population several risk factors associated with heart disease. The quiz that follows is designed to inform you about some of these risk factors.

1. Do you often eat foods high in fat or cholesterol, such as whole milk, hamburgers, or eggs? ______
2. Do you eat a lot of salty foods? ______
3. Are you overweight? ______
4. Is your blood cholesterol level greater than 200? ______
5. Is your blood pressure higher than 140/90? ______
6. Do you smoke? ______
7. Do you have diabetes or a family history of diabetes? ______
8. Do you have a family history or heart disease or stroke? ______
9. Do you engage in aerobic exercise fewer than three times a week? ______
10. Are you a woman using birth control pills? ______

***Scoring***
If you have answered yes to one or more questions, you may be at risk for developing heart disease. If you have not seen your physician in the past twelve months, it would be a good idea to get a complete physical soon.

wait 3 hours after the initial symptoms begin before seeking help. By that time, half of the affected heart muscle may be lost. New treatments that can halt a heart attack in progress make time even more critical in saving hearts—and lives.

### Clot-Busters

Clot-dissolving drugs called thrombolytic agents are the newest way of fighting back against a heart attack. They can be administered through a catheter (flexible tube) threaded through the arteries to the site of a blockage (the more effective method of delivery) or injected intravenously (the faster, cheaper delivery method).

Aspirin can help to prevent heart attacks in healthy men. In a study of more than 22,000 doctors who'd been taking a buffered aspirin every other day, the risk of a heart attack was cut by almost half in the aspirin takers. Aspirin can also prevent heart attacks in individuals with a condition called unstable angina, often a precursor of a heart attack.[13]

**cardiopulmonary resuscitation (CPR)** A method of artificial stimulation of the heart and lungs.

STRATEGY FOR CHANGE

### What to Do If a Heart Attack Strikes

- If you develop chest discomfort that lasts for 2 minutes or more, call the local emergency rescue service immediately. Or if you can get to a hospital faster by car, have someone drive you. If you are with someone who is having the "signals" and if they last for 2 minutes or more, act at once. Expect the person to deny the possibility of anything as serious as a heart attack, but insist on taking prompt action.
- Call the emergency rescue service, or get to the nearest hospital that offers 24-hour emergency cardiac care.
- Give **cardiopulmonary resuscitation (CPR),** a combination of mouth-to-mouth breathing and chest compression *if* it is necessary and *if* you are properly trained. CPR will keep oxygenated blood flowing to the brain and the rest of the body until advanced cardiac life support can be initiated. (See "Your Health Care and Survival Guide" in the appendix.)

After a heart attack the damaged heart muscle begins to heal. New small blood vessels form to carry more blood through the damaged area. This is called **collateral circulation,** the heart's own lifesaving method of taking over the functions of the blocked artery. (A collateral circulation system may begin to develop long before a heart attack, however, and may even prevent an attack.) With healing, scar tissue may replace part of the injured muscle.

Various medications can strengthen the heartbeat, control disturbances in heart rhythm, and relieve pain. Most people who have had a heart attack return to an active and productive life after two to three months of recuperation.

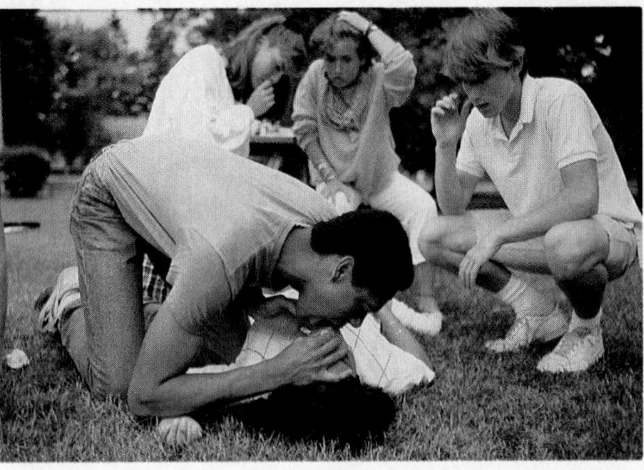

Cardiopulmonary respiration (CPR) can save lives, but requires proper training.

## Arrhythmias

The heart has its own electrical system, which produces an evenly timed, regular beat. When relaxed, most adults have a heart rate between 60 and 80 beats per minute, slower if they are in good physical condition. During strenuous activity or stress, the heart beats faster. Sometimes the heart seems to skip a beat or experience premature (or early) heartbeats. In many cases, these are no cause for alarm. But they can be dangerous in an MI victim.

A very fast heart rate (more than 100 beats per minute) is known as **tachycardia;** a very slow one (less than 60 beats per minute) is **bradycardia.** In **atrial fibrillation,** electrical impulses spread in all directions through the heart while the ventricle continues to beat. Various drugs are effective in correcting such irregularities, or **arrhythmia.**

For patients with a very slow heart that does not respond to drugs, implantation of an electrical **pacemaker** that causes contractions of the heart at a normal rate may be necessary. Such pacemakers, compact battery-powered systems, deliver a series of small electrical impulses to the heart muscle.

## Congestive Heart Failure

When the heart's pumping power is well below normal capacity, fluid begins to collect in the lungs, hands, and feet. The heart is then said to be in failure. Blood fluids accumulate in the lungs, causing shortness of breath. In other parts of the body, fluid seeps through the thin capillary walls and causes swelling (edema), especially in the ankles and legs.

Congestive heart failure can be the result of rheumatic fever, birth defects, myocardial infarctions, hypertension, or atherosclerosis. It is treated by reducing the work load on the heart, modifying salt

**HEALTH HEADLINE**

### Job Stress Harms Hearts

Work-related stress can cause both high blood pressure and potentially dangerous physical changes in the heart, according to a study of 215 men between the ages of 30 and 60. Job stress proved highest when workers faced high psychological demands without having much control over day-to-day decisions. Those experiencing such strain faced a 3 times greater risk of having high blood pressure. Men in their thirties in high-stress jobs also showed a significant thickening of part of the heart, a condition that often precedes heart disease and heart attacks.

SOURCE: Schnall, P. L. et al. "The Relationship Between 'Job Strain,' Workplace Diastolic Blood Pressure, and Left Ventricular Mass Index," *Journal of the American Medical Association,* vol. 263, no. 14, April 11, 1990.

**collateral circulation** The development of small blood vessels that detour blood through damaged heart-muscle tissue.
**tachycardia** An abnormally rapid heart rate, over 100 beats per minute.
**bradycardia** An abnormally slow heart rate, below 60 beats per minute.
**atrial fibrillation** A condition characterized by an irregular, abnormally rapid heartbeat.
**arrhythmia** Any irregularity in the rhythm of the heartbeat.
**pacemaker** Compact battery-powered system that delivers a series of small electrical impulses to the heart.

intake, administering drugs that rid the body of excess fluid, and using medications such as digitalis to improve the heart's pumping efficiency.

## Rheumatic Fever

Rheumatic fever, which strikes most often between the ages of 5 and 15, is a disease that causes painful, swollen joints; skin rashes; and heart damage in half its victims. It is always preceded by a streptococcal infection (see Chapter 15).

Although rheumatic fever and heart disease are preventable, incidence rates remain unnecessarily high in many parts of the country, particularly in rural areas. The first step to prevention is early identification of the streptococcal infection; the second is treatment with antibiotics.

## Congenital Defects

Approximately 8 of every 1,000 children born in the United States have congenital heart disease. The most common defects are holes in the ventricular septum, the wall dividing the lower chambers of the heart. Holes may also occur in the atrial septum, the wall between the upper chambers. Sometimes the arteries delivering blood to the body and lungs are transposed and attached to the wrong ventricles. Such babies have a bluish color because their blood is not carrying sufficient oxygen; the condition is known as **cyanosis,** and the babies are sometimes called blue babies. The chief cause of death from congenital heart disease is heart failure.

# HEART SAVERS

A generation ago physicians had no way of detecting problems before the symptoms of heart disease began; they could offer little more than bed rest as a therapy. The last decade has brought tremendous progress.

## Treatments

Most people with heart disease can be treated successfully with drugs. Other alternatives are balloon angioplasty, bypass surgery, and heart transplants.

### Drugs

Calcium-blockers can lower blood pressure, raise cardiac output in heart failure, relieve various forms of angina, and control arrhythmias. The drugs work by countering the flow of calcium into the heart muscle cells; calcium is believed to stimulate and contract heart muscle, occasionally causing a sudden spasm that can completely close an artery.

Beta-blockers lower the heart's demand for blood by slowing the rate and force of the heart's contractions. A variety of beta-blockers are widely used for medical problems, including migraines and high blood pressure, as well as heart disease.

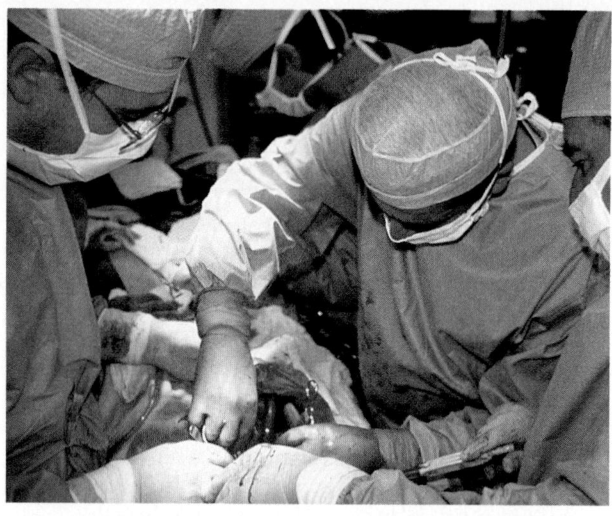

Coronary artery bypass is the most widely used operation for heart disease.

### Coronary Bypass

The most widely used operation for heart disease is a coronary bypass, a procedure in which a vein from the patient's leg is grafted onto a coronary artery to detour blood around a blocked area. Each year more than 200,000 bypasses are performed in the United States; each operation costs at least $20,000. About 1 to 2 percent of these patients die as a result of surgical complications. As many as 1 in 5 patients may suffer subtle, long-lasting impairment of mental performance, such as problems concentrating and learning.[14]

Bypasses do not extend life for individuals with mild to moderate angina unless the left main coronary artery is blocked. If drugs fail to control angina, a bypass can eliminate pain. In as many as 80 percent of bypass patients, the grafts themselves develop blockages within 10 years.

## Percutaneous Transluminal Coronary Angioplasty

Percutaneous transluminal coronary angioplasty (PTCA), or balloon angioplasty, is a method of un-

**cyanosis** A blueness of the skin due to an excess of reduced hemoglobin in the blood; caused by insufficient oxygen.

HEALTH SPOTLIGHT

## Unclogging Your Arteries

For years, heart specialists said it couldn't be done. However, recent research has shown that people can reverse the buildup of plaque inside their arteries. And that means that, rather than relying on expensive and risky treatments, more individuals may be able to help—and heal—themselves. But it's not easy.

In a small but significant study, 10 of 12 patients who followed a strict program of dietary and life-style change reversed the narrowing within their arteries over the course of a year. The key elements of their treatment were:

- a very low-fat, vegetarian diet, which included nonfat dairy products and egg whites, with fat making up less than 8 percent of total calories. Participants in the study ate no meat, poultry, fish, butter, cheese, ice cream, or any form of oil.
- moderate exercise, consisting of an hour of aerobic activity three times a week. Walking was the most popular choice. More rigorous exercise might be dangerous for heart patients, because of the increased risk of blood clots, irregular heartbeats, or coronary artery spasms during exertion.
- stress counseling. The patients learned how the body's stress response can cause a rapid heartbeat and narrowing of the arteries and how stress reduction can reduce cholesterol levels, even without dietary changes.
- an hour a day of yoga, meditation, breathing, and progressive relaxation. They also saw pictures of blocked arteries and visualized them opening up. One man's mental image was of "a tunneling machine, the type that digs into the earth and makes highway tunnels."

"The lifestyle changes are as important as the dietary ones," says Dr. Dean Ornish, director of the Preventive Medicine Research Institute in Sausalito, California, who conducted the research. All also quit smoking.

In the study, a control group of 17 men and women with clogged arteries were given standard medical counseling (quit smoking, lower blood pressure, exercise, cut fats and cholesterol), but their blood vessels continued to become more clogged. Ornish believes that a less strict version of his treatment program might help prevent arteries from becoming blocked in the first place.

SOURCES: Goleman, Daniel. "Lifestyle Shift Can Unclog Ailing Arteries, Study Finds," *New York Times*, February 1990. Grady, Denise. "Declogging Your Own Arteries," *American Health*, March 1989. Ornish, Dean. Director, Preventive Medicine Research Institute (Sausalito, Calif.), American Heart Association 1990 Annual Meeting, New Orleans, presentation.

clogging arteries that is less risky than coronary bypass. PTCA involves a precise, time-consuming technique called cardiac catheterization. A special dye that shows up on X rays is injected into the arteries and accumulates at the site of a blockage. A narrow tube, or catheter, with a tiny balloon at its tip is threaded through an artery to the blockage. By slowly inflating the balloon, physicians can break up the clog and widen the narrowed artery. When they deflate the balloon, circulation is restored.

Balloon angioplasties are not without risks. Approximately 5 percent of PTCA patients eventually need emergency bypass surgery; 1 to 3 percent die. PTCA is successful in 85 percent of patients, but 30 to 40 percent of balloon-opened arteries clog up.[15]

### Heart Transplants

For a variety of heart disorders, the only hope for patients is another heart. The survival rates for recipients have improved dramatically because of a drug called cyclosporine, which prevents rejection. More than 80 percent of heart recipients survive at least one year. More than 50 percent are alive after five years. About a third return to work; two-thirds are in good health.[16]

## STROKE: STARVING THE BRAIN

When the blood supply to the brain is blocked, a **cerebrovascular accident,** or **stroke,** occurs. About 500,000 people suffer strokes each year; strokes rank third, after heart disease and cancer, as a cause of death. Strokes kill more than 150,000 Americans a year.

One of the most common causes of stroke is blockage of a brain artery by a clot—**cerebral thrombosis**—that may form around deposits sticking out from the arterial wall. Sometimes a wandering blood clot (embolus) carried in the bloodstream becomes wedged in one of the cerebral arteries. Such a **cerebral embolism** can completely plug up a cerebral artery.

A stroke can also be caused by **cerebral hemorrhage,** the bursting of a diseased artery in the brain, or of an **aneurysm,** a blood-filled pouch that balloons out from a weak spot in the wall of an artery.

Brain tissue, like heart muscle, begins to die if deprived of oxygen. Tissue damage may cause loss of memory and difficulty in speaking and walking. Effects may be slight or severe, temporary or permanent, depending on how widespread the damage is and whether other areas of the brain can take over the function of the damaged area.

**STRATEGY FOR CHANGE**

**Recognizing the Warning Signs of Stroke**

The following symptoms should alert you to the possibility that you or someone with you has suffered a stroke:

- sudden temporary weakness or numbness of face, arm, or leg
- temporary loss of speech or difficulty in speaking or understanding speech
- temporary dimness or loss of vision, particularly in one eye
- double vision
- unexplained dizziness
- change in personality
- increase or change in usual pattern of headaches

### Transient Ischemic Attacks

Some people suffer transient ischemic attacks (TIAs), "little strokes" that cause minimal damage but serve as warning signals of a potentially more severe stroke. One of three people who suffer TIAs will have a stroke within five years if they do not get treatment.

Many TIAs are caused by a buildup of plaque in the carotid arteries of the neck. Aspirin and other drugs that make platelets less sticky and interfere with clotting are often effective. Physicians advise surgery to widen the carotid arteries in the neck only when this operation is clearly necessary.[17]

### Risk Factors

People who've experienced TIAs are at the highest risk for stroke. Other risk factors, like those for heart disease, include some that can't be changed (like sex and race) and some that can be controlled:[18]

- *Sex* —Men have a greater risk of stroke than do women. Women taking oral contraceptives are more

---

**cerebrovascular accident** A condition in which a cerebral blood vessel is blocked.
**stroke** See *cerebrovascular accident.*
**cerebral thrombosis** The formation of a blood clot in a blood vessel of the brain.
**cerebral embolism** A sudden obstruction of a blood vessel in the brain by an abnormal particle or clot.
**cerebral hemorrhage** The rupturing of a blood vessel in the brain.
**aneurysm** A localized, blood-filled sac in an artery wall; caused by dilation or weakening of the artery wall.

**HEALTH HEADLINE**

**Life-Style Changes Can Reduce the Risk of Heart Attack**

**Quitting smoking, lowering blood pressure, losing weight, and cutting cholesterol can indeed cut the risk of a heart attack, according to a ten-year study of more than 12,000 middle-aged men. The men who changed their life-styles for the sake of their hearts' health had a death rate from heart attacks 24 percent lower than did a control group of men who received only routine medical care.**

SOURCE: The Multiple Risk Factor Intervention Trial Research Group, "Mortality Rates after 10.5 Years for Participants in the Multiple Risk Factor Intervention Trial," *Journal of the American Medical Association,* vol. 263, no. 13, April 4, 1990.

## WHAT DO YOU THINK?

Marc, a 20-year-old college student, has scrambled eggs and sausage for breakfast, a cheeseburger for lunch, and steak for dinner. He exercises regularly, he's not overweight, and he feels fine. Should he worry about his diet? Is it a healthy one? Should he change it? Why? Which foods might be better for his heart?

One minute a talented college basketball star is playing at peak form; the next, he collapses and dies. Months earlier, doctors diagnosed an arrhythmia, a disorder of the heartbeat, but he may not have been taking his medication for fear it would harm his performance. Should he have taken such a risk? What would you do if you had the skill and ambition to be a professional athlete but found out you had a potentially fatal heart problem? Who should decide if an athlete at risk should play: the student, the school, the parents, the doctors?

Driving home late during an ice storm, Yuko smashes into a tree and dies instantly of a head injury. She does not have an organ donation card in her purse, and no one can track down her family. Should doctors assume that she or her family would want to donate her heart? How would you feel if someone you loved desperately needed a heart transplant? Have you filled out an organ-donor card?

likely to suffer strokes, especially if they are over age 35 and smoke, than are those who don't. A history of migraine headaches, combined with use of the pill, may also increase the danger.

- *Hypertension* —Detection and treatment of high blood pressure are the best means of prevention.
- *Race* —Black Americans have a much greater risk than do whites, possibly because blacks have a higher incidence of hypertension.
- *High Red Blood Cell Count* —A moderate to marked increase in the number of a person's red blood cells increases the danger of stroke.
- *Heart Disease* —Heart problems can interfere with the flow of blood to the brain; clots that form in the heart can travel to the brain, where they may clog an artery.
- *Diabetes Mellitus* —Diabetics have a higher incidence of stroke than do nondiabetics.

## MAKING THIS CHAPTER WORK FOR YOU

### Keeping Your Heart Healthy

**The heart is made of muscle tissue that pumps blood through the body by contracting many times a minute. The contraction of the heart is called systole. Between contractions, the heart relaxes and dilates; this stage is called diastole. The heart has four chambers—two atria and two ventricles. The atria receive blood from the veins; the ventricles receive blood from the atria and pump it into the arteries, through which it travels to other parts of the body.**

**Factors predisposing an individual to heart disease or stroke include a family history of heart disease, increasing age, cigarette smoking, obesity, high blood pressure, high cholesterol levels, diabetes mellitus, a Type A personality, and a sedentary life-style.**

**Although two types of lipids, cholesterol and triglyceride, have been linked to cardiovascular disease, cholesterol seems to be more dangerous. Individuals with high cholesterol levels are at risk for developing atherosclerosis and a heart attack. The ratio of high-density lipoproteins to low-density lipoproteins can indicate a person's risk of heart disease.**

**Hypertension occurs when the arteries' walls offer too much resistance to blood flow. Treatment includes diet modification, exercise, restriction of salt intake, and medication to widen the blood vessels or to decrease cardiac output.**

**The most common form of arteriosclerosis is atherosclerosis, in which blood flow is impaired because of plaque deposits inside the arteries. As plaque accumulates, the arteries narrow and lose their ability to dilate and contract. Thrombosis, or blockage of an artery by a thrombus, is the major danger of atherosclerosis because it can cause stroke or heart attack.**

Some people suffer from chest pains, or angina pectoris, caused by periodic and temporary inadequate blood flow to the heart. Chest pain may be a result of coronary artery spasms caused by the clumping of platelets. Such clumping results in narrowing of the blood vessel.

Myocardial infarction, or heart attack, occurs when heart muscle tissue in the myocardium begins to die because its supply of oxygen and other nutrients has been cut off by a blocked artery. The damage caused by a heart attack can be reduced with early treatment, including administering clot-dissolving drugs. As the heart heals, new blood vessels develop to carry additional blood.

Other heart problems include heartbeat irregularities, or arrhythmias; congestive heart failure, which occurs when the heart is unable to pump at its normal capacity; heart damage from rheumatic fever; and congenital heart defects.

Hypertension, heart failure, angina, and arrhythmias can be treated with drugs. Surgical treatments for heart disease include the coronary bypass operation, balloon angioplasty, pacemaker implantation, and heart transplants.

A stroke, or cerebrovascular accident, occurs when the blood supply to the brain is restricted or blocked. Cerebral thrombosis, cerebral embolism, or cerebral hemorrhage can cause a stroke. Transient ischemic attacks may precede a serious stroke.

In the last decade, deaths from stroke have fallen by 40 percent while heart disease deaths have dropped 25 percent. Much, if not most, of the credit belongs to us, the American people. We are smoking less, exercising more, and avoiding fatty foods. As a result, we are helping to protect our own hearts and to save our own lives.

To join in the fight, follow these guidelines from the American Heart Association:

- Do not smoke
- Maintain a desirable body weight
- Eat a diet low in saturated fats and cholesterol. This could prevent high blood cholesterol levels, obesity, and heart disease.
- Engage in regular physical activity. Get your body moving, and keep it moving 30 minutes at a time, three times a week.
- If you're a woman using oral contraceptives, have yearly tests of blood pressure and triglyceride and glucose levels.
- If you respond intensely to stress, try the relaxation techniques described in Chapter 3.

The payoffs of such preventive care can be great. If heart disease mortality rates keep falling, 1 million more Americans may be alive to welcome the twenty-first century.

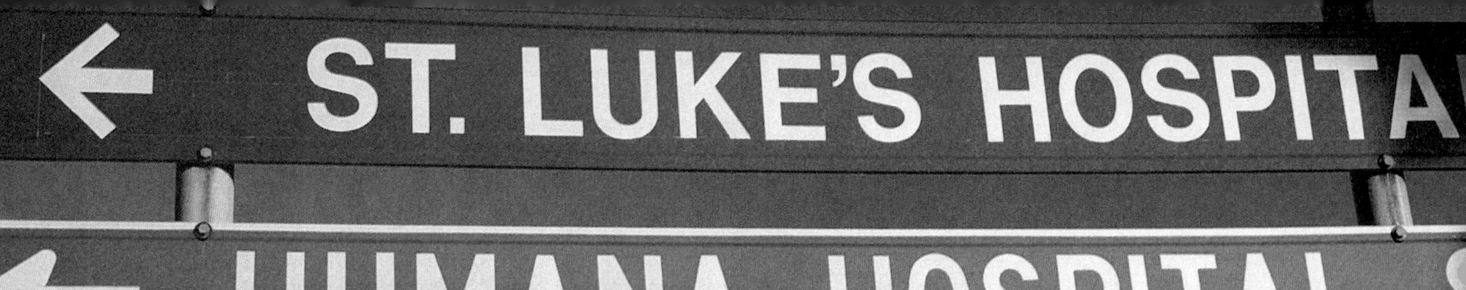


# 14 CANCER, MAJOR ILLNESSES, AND ACCIDENTS: BEATING THE ODDS

In this chapter

Cancer: What you need to know

Other major diseases

Accidents: Saving your own life

Making This Chapter Work for You: Staying alive and healthy

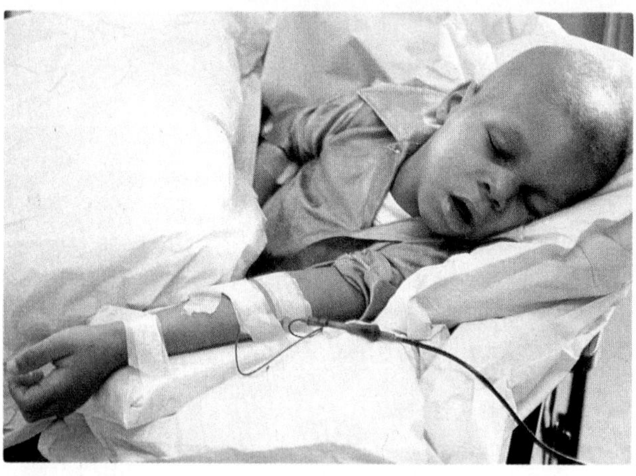

Cancer can strike at any age, but early detection and treatment could save thousands of lives.

*Our bodies are extremely durable.* By their very nature, however, they break down. Illness and injury are inevitable some of the time, but you can prevent many diseases and delay others for years, even decades. This chapter—which covers accidents and the most common noninfectious diseases, including cancer—shows how to postpone or prevent illness. The key is taking responsibility for yourself by doing everything possible to avoid major health threats, detect them early, and overcome them.

## CANCER: WHAT YOU NEED TO KNOW

**Cancer** is a disease we all dread. About three out of every ten Americans now living will eventually get cancer; one out of every five will die of it. Anyone, at any age, can develop cancer. It kills more children than any other disease, and it strikes more frequently with advancing age. The human toll, in pain and loss, is beyond measure.

A diagnosis of cancer is not a death sentence, however. According to the American Cancer Society, more than 5 million Americans alive today have a history of cancer; 3 million were diagnosed five or more years ago. About half of all cancer patients survive at least five years after diagnosis.[1] Most are considered "cured" if they've had no evidence of cancer for five years. These cancer survivors have the same life expectancy as a person who has never had cancer. Others survive in **remission** (a state in which patients have no symptoms and the spread of cancerous cells is assumed to be temporarily stopped).

If more cancers were diagnosed earlier, as many as two-thirds of those who develop cancers could be saved. The others would die because the types of cancer they have cannot yet be controlled. The key to survival is early detection and state-of-the-art treatment. National Cancer Institute officials believe we could cut the overall cancer mortality rate by 50 percent by the year 2000 through prevention, early detection, and proper treatment.[2]

### What Is Cancer?

Cancer is not a single, simple disease, but a group of about 110 different diseases, all caused by the uncontrolled growth and spread of abnormal cells. Normal cells follow the code of instructions embedded in DNA (the body's genetic material); cancer cells do not.

Think of the DNA within the nucleus of a cell as a computer program that controls the cell's functioning. Cancer interferes with this program or its operation, and so the cell goes out of control. The nucleus no longer regulates growth. The abnormal cell divides to form other abnormal cells, which again divide, eventually forming **neoplasms** (new formations), or tumors.

Tumors can be either **benign** (collections of cells that are only slightly abnormal and are not considered life-threatening) or **malignant** (cancerous). The only way to determine whether a tumor is benign is by microscopic examination of its cells.

Without treatment, cancer cells continue to grow, crowding out and replacing healthy cells. This process is called **infiltration,** or invasion. They may also **metastasize,** or spread to other parts of the body via the bloodstream or lymph system (see Figure 14-1). Although all cancers have similar characteristics, each is distinct. Some cancers are relatively simple to cure, whereas others are more threatening and mysterious. The earlier any cancer is found, the easier it is to treat and the better the patient's chances are of beating the disease.

**cancer** A disease in which a malignant cellular tumor that is capable of spreading to other parts of the body develops.
**remission** A period during which a former victim of cancer or another disease shows no recurring symptoms.
**neoplasm** Any tumor, whether benign or malignant.
**benign** Harmless; not malignant.
**malignant** Harmful; life-threatening.
**infiltration** A gradual penetration or invasion.
**metastasis** The spread of cancer cells beyond their site of origin in the body.

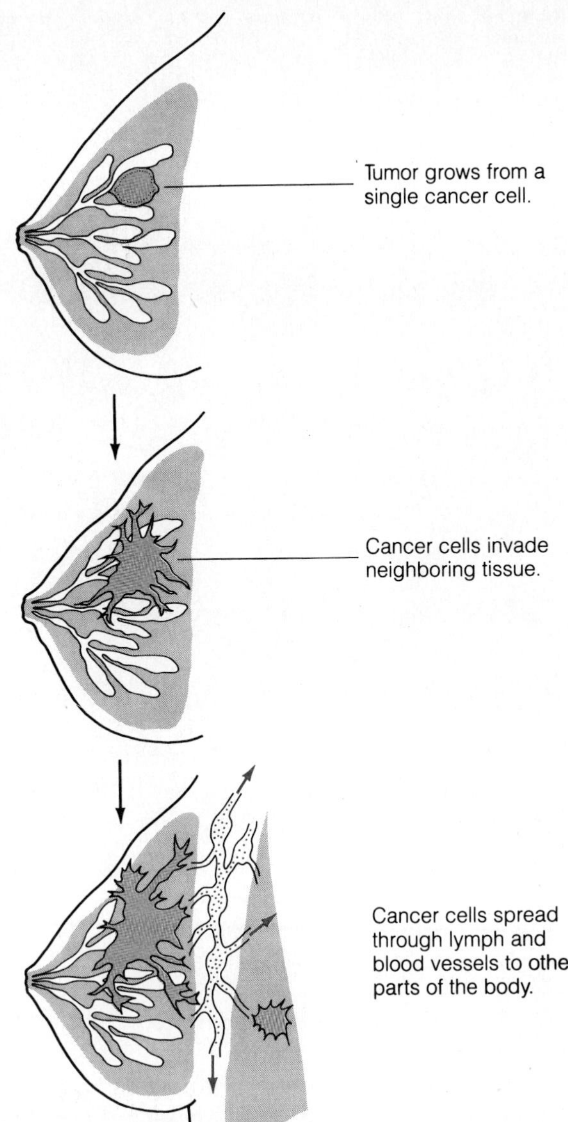


**FIGURE 14-1** Growth and metastasis of a malignant tumor of the breast.

## What Causes Cancer?

No one knows exactly how a normal cell turns into a cancer cell. Researchers believe that most cancers have no single cause. A combination of factors—genetic, viral, chemical, and physical—may play a role, as does the response of each person's immune system (see Table 14-1). Some **oncologists** (cancer specialists) think that isolated cancer cells appear in many, if not all, persons and that only those people with inadequate immune responses develop cancer.

### Heredity

Heredity may make certain families cancer-prone. Scientists have identified more than 100 hereditary cancers, including colon, breast, ovarian, and pancreatic cancer. Eventually, genetic clues could lead to improved diagnosis and treatment.

### Race

The cancer rate among blacks is higher than that among whites, and blacks also have a higher cancer death rate. Over a thirty-year period, cancer death rates among blacks rose almost 50 percent, compared to a 10 percent increase for whites. The reason may be that cancers of whites are more likely to be detected at an early, more treatable stage.[3]

### Viruses

Viruses may play a role in certain leukemias (cancers of the blood system) and lymphomas (cancers of the lymph system); cancers of the nose; liver cancer; and cervical cancer. Human immunodeficiency virus (HIV), which causes AIDS, can lead to certain lymphomas and leukemias and to a type of cancer called Kaposi's sarcoma (see Chapter 15).

### Occupational Carcinogens

Many chemicals used in industry are **carcinogens,** substances that may start a cancer. People living near a factory that creates smoke, dust, or gases are at risk, as are employees inside the plant (see Chapter 16).

**oncologist** A physician specializing in the treatment of cancer.
**carcinogen** A substance that may cause cancer.

**TABLE 14-1** Some Risk Factors and Their Associated Cancers

| RISK FACTOR | TYPE OF CANCER |
|---|---|
| Exposure to carcinogens | |
| Tobacco | Lung, throat, oral, bladder, and pancreas |
| Alcohol | Liver, larynx, throat, esophagus, and breast |
| Ultraviolet light | Skin |
| Radiation | Leukemia |
| Asbestos | Lung |
| Family history | Ovary, colon, uterine, breast, and retinoblastoma |
| Hepatitis B | Liver |
| Cirrhosis of the liver | Liver |
| AIDS | Kaposi's sarcoma, leukemia, and lymphoma |

### Tobacco

Cigarette smoking is the single greatest cause of cancer deaths in the United States. People who smoke two or more packs of cigarettes a day are 15 to 25 times more likely to die of cancer than are nonsmokers. Cigarettes cause most cases of lung cancer and increase the risk of cancer of the mouth, throat, larynx, esophagus, pancreas, and bladder. Pipes, cigars, and smokeless tobacco increase the danger of cancers of the mouth and throat.

### Ultraviolet Light

Whether it's from the sun or from artificial tanning lights, **ultraviolet radiation** increases the risk of skin cancer, the most frequent form of cancer. The sun's rays are strongest and most dangerous at midday, but you should wear a sunscreen or protective clothing whenever you're outdoors for an extended period. Using tanning salons or sun lamps also increases the risk of skin cancer, because they produce ultraviolet radiation. Contrary to advertising claims, machines are no safer than sunshine.[4,5]

**STRATEGY FOR CHANGE**

**Saving Your Skin**

- Stay out of the sun between 10:00 A.M. and 2:00 P.M., when ultraviolet rays are strongest.
- Be especially cautious about sun exposure if you have been using a synthetic preparation derived from vitamin A (Retin A) as an acne treatment; it can increase your susceptibility.
- Limit use of sun lamps or tanning salons. Always follow manufacturers' directions.
- Experiment with lotions, creams, and sprays until you find one that doesn't irritate your skin. Make sure any sunscreen you buy has a sun protection factor (SPF) of at least 15, which gives 85 to 90 percent of maximum protection. Higher SPFs offer slightly more protection and should be used by fair-skinned sun lovers.
- Scan your skin regularly. Watch for changes in the size, color, number, and thickness of moles.
- Once a year, stand in front of a full-length mirror to check for funny-looking moles that are irregularly shaped or bigger than a pencil eraser. With your arms raised, examine your front and back and your left and right sides. Check the backs of your legs, the tops and soles of your feet, and the surfaces between your toes. Using a hand mirror, check the back of your neck, behind your ears, and your scalp.

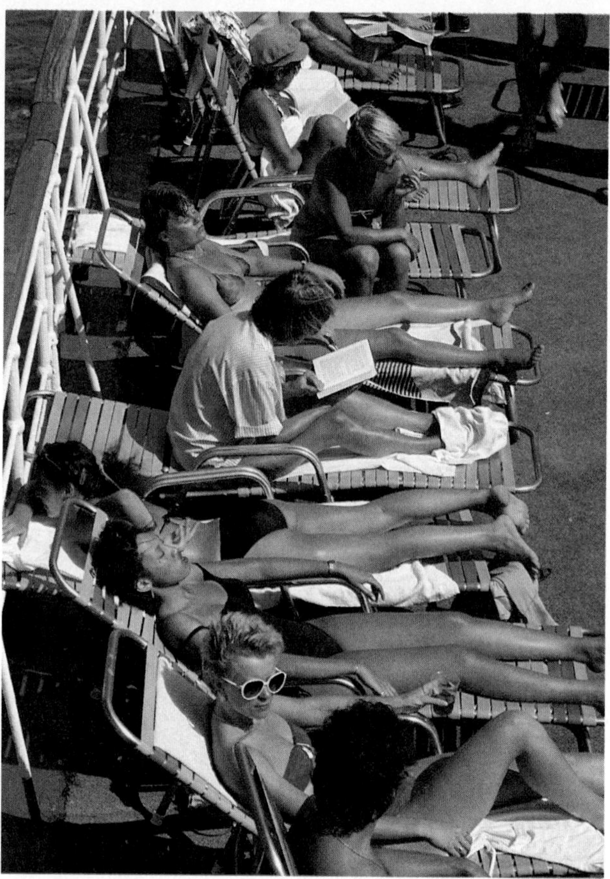

Sun-worshipers should use sunscreens and avoid the mid-day sun to lessen their risk of skin cancer.

### Radiation

Clinical studies, particularly of survivors of the atomic bombings of Hiroshima and Nagasaki, have shown that a long time may pass before a radiation-induced cancer appears (usually a minimum of five years). The higher the dose of radiation, the greater the risk of cancer. The most common form of postradiation cancer is myelogenous leukemia, a blood cancer. Most susceptible are infants, children, and pregnant women.

### Alcohol

Compared to those who drink little or no alcohol, heavy drinkers are more likely to develop oral cancer and cancers of the larynx, throat, esophagus, liver, and breast. Those who drink and smoke are particularly vulnerable. Women who drink, even moderately, may be at greater risk of developing breast cancer. Women who consume as few as three drinks a week may have a 30 percent greater chance of developing

**ultraviolet radiation** The light rays of a specific wavelength emitted by the sun; most is screened out by the ozone layer in the upper atmosphere.

## HALES INDEX

Number of families affected by cancer: 3 in 4

Annual cost of cancer, including medical bills and lost earnings: $70 billion

Number of cases of cancer that could be prevented each year by simple changes in the way we eat, drink, and live: 20 million

Overall risk of developing melanoma in 1980: 1 to 250

Projected overall risk of developing melanoma in 2000: 1 in 90

Number of diabetics in the United States: 10 million

Number who require insulin therapy: 1 in 10

Number of Americans who will suffer a digestive problem at some time: 1 in 2

Number of Americans who die from injuries each year: 150,000

Number one cause of death and disability for Americans under age 44: Head injury

Number of head injuries suffered in traffic accidents: 1 in 2

Peak time for single-car accidents: 1:00 to 4:00 A.M.

Number of bicyclists killed in accidents every year: 1,300

SOURCES: **1, 2, 3** American Cancer Society. **4, 5** "Factors Said to Predict Skin Cancer," *New York Times*, March 27, 1990. **6, 7** Yulsman, Tom. "Sweet News on the Sugar Disease," *American Health*, April 1987. **8** National Digestive Diseases Advisory Board. **9** Will, George. "The Trauma in Trauma Care," *Newsweek*, March 12, 1990. **10** Hales, Dianne and Robert Hales. "Coming Back from Head Injury," *American Health*, November 1989. **11** "Facts on Head Injury," New Medico Head Injury System, 1989. **12** Mitler, Merrill et al. "Catastrophes, Sleep, and Public Policy," *Sleep*, February 1988. **13** Thompson, RS et al. "A Case-Control Study of the Effectiveness of Bicycle Safety Helmets," *New England Journal of Medicine*, vol. 320, no. 21, May 25, 1989.

breast cancer than do those who seldom or never drink.

### Foods

The National Academy of Sciences has stated that diet may play a role in as many as 60 percent of the cancers in women and 40 percent of the cancers in men. Although some foods, particularly fats, increase the risk of cancer, others lower it. (Chapter 4 provides guidelines for an anticancer diet.)

Obesity increases the risks of colon, breast, and uterine cancer. A high-fat diet, which can lead to obesity, contributes to breast, colon, and prostate cancers. Salt-cured, smoked, and nitrite-cured foods have been linked to cancers of the esophagus and stomach.

Among the primary cancer fighters in foods are vitamins A and C and selenium, a trace metal. A low intake of vitamin A has been linked to cancers of the breast, bladder, lung, skin, mouth, and cervix. Foods rich in vitamin C may protect against cancers of the stomach, esophagus, lung, skin, colon, and rectum. A small amount of selenium, a mineral that makes its way into food and water from soil, may protect us from liver, colon, and breast cancers.

**STRATEGY FOR CHANGE**

**Take Five to Fight Cancer**

Five fruits or vegetables a day may keep cancer away. Here's some advice on taking five from California's Nutrition and Cancer Prevention Program:[6]

- Eat five servings of fruits and vegetables a day.
- Eat at least one that's rich in vitamin A: cantaloupe, carrots, spinach, sweet potatoes.
- Eat at least one that's high in vitamin C: grapefruit, oranges, cauliflower, green peppers.
- Eat at least one high-fiber selection: winter squash, corn, figs, apples.
- Eat cabbage-family (cruciferous) vegetables several times a week.

## The War Against Cancer

Are we winning the war against cancer? Fifty percent of cancer patients now survive for five years after diagnosis, compared to only about 33 percent who survived that long in the 1950s (Figure 14-2). Survival rates for cancer improved dramatically throughout the 1980s, and American Cancer Society officials be-

**FIGURE 14-2** Five-year cancer survival rates for selected cancers. If the cancerous cells are confined to one tumor or growth, the cancer is localized. If cancerous cells have spread to the nearest lymph glands, the cancer is considered regional. If cancerous cells have traveled to other organs of the body (such as colon cancer cells that have spread to the liver), the cancer is distant.

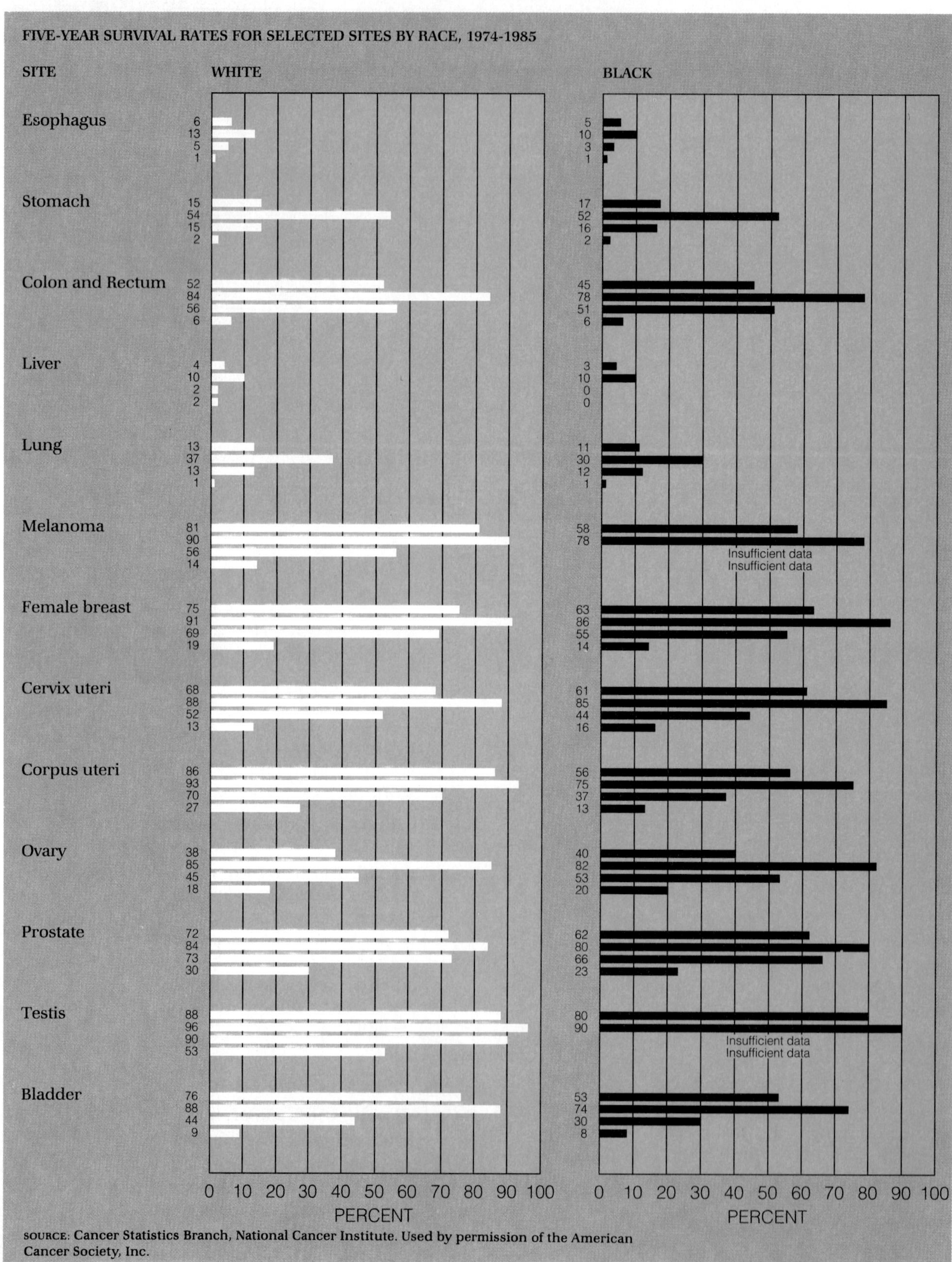


SOURCE: Cancer Statistics Branch, National Cancer Institute. Used by permission of the American Cancer Society, Inc.

lieve that by applying today's state-of-the-art treatments they could increase the rate by another 10 to 15 percent in the 1990s.[7]

The more you know about different types of cancer, the risks, and the symptoms, the more likely you are to stay healthy (see Table 14-2). Prevention could save many lives. Smoking alone kills about 145,000 people in the United States each year, far more than the estimated 5,000 to 10,000 lives saved through chemotherapy.[8] The risk of lung cancer drops almost to that of nonsmokers within ten years after a smoker puts out his or her last cigarette.

Cancer can strike virtually any area of the body. Early detection is critical. More than 10,000 of the 41,000 annual U.S. breast-cancer deaths might be prevented if all women over age 50 examined their own breasts regularly (see Figure 14-3) and underwent regular breast examinations and mammograms (diagnostic X rays). Regular mammograms can also prevent deaths in women in their forties. According to the National Cancer Institute, regular mammograms for women over age 40 might reduce the national death rate for breast cancer by 46 percent.[9,10] Men should perform regular testicular self-exams (see Figure 14-4).

**STRATEGY FOR CHANGE**

**What Women Should Know About Mammography**

Mammograms can pick up a cancer two to three years before a woman or her doctor feel a lump[11] (see Figure 14-5). Yet many women hesitate to undergo this simple test. Here is what you need to know:

- Today's low-dose techniques pose very slight risks, if any, for women. Before scheduling a mammogram, make sure the test will be done with "dedicated" equipment (equipment designed only for mammography).
- For the test, always go to a person experienced in doing mammograms. Your doctor can refer you.
- Don't wear underarm deodorant or powder on the day of the test. It could create suspicious-looking specks on the film.
- The test is not painful, but you may feel a brief moment of discomfort if your breasts are large or tender.
- Avoid scheduling a mammogram just before your period if your breasts become tender then.

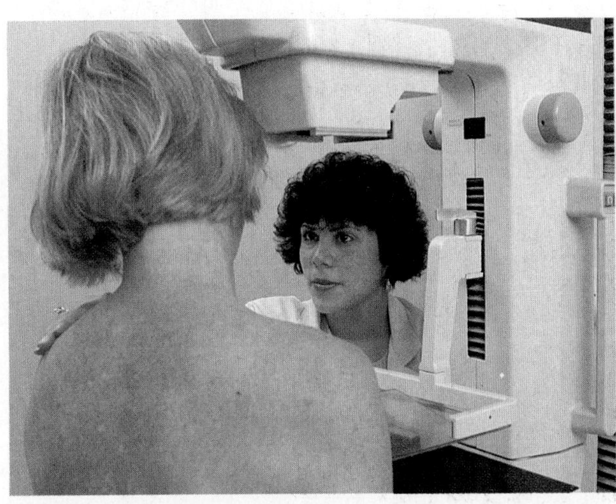

A mammogram can detect cancer two to three years before a woman or her doctor feels a lump.

## Scheduling Cancer Checkups

People with no symptoms should have regular checkups for cancer (Table 14-3), including the following tests:

- *Mammograms*—One baseline X ray between the ages of 35 and 39, then every one to two years from age 40 to age 49, and yearly for women over 50
- *Pap Test*—Every year from the time a young woman becomes sexually active
- *Digital Rectal Exam*—Yearly after age 40
- *Proctosigmoidoscopy* (insertion of a fiber-optic tube for visual inspection of the colon and rectum)—Every three to five years after age 50
- *Stool Blood Tests*—Every year after age 50

**STRATEGY FOR CHANGE**

**Recognizing the Seven Warning Signs of Cancer**

When cancer strikes, its early symptoms often resemble those of other diseases. If you note any of the following, immediately schedule an appointment with your doctor:

- a change in bowel or bladder habits
- a sore that doesn't heal
- unusual bleeding or discharge
- a thickening or lump in the breast or elsewhere
- frequent indigestion or difficulty swallowing
- an obvious change in a wart or mole
- a nagging cough or hoarseness

**TABLE 14-2** Most Common Cancers, Their Risk Factors, Warning Signals, and Treatments

| | RISK FACTORS | WARNING SIGNALS | EARLY DETECTION | TREATMENT | 5-YEAR SURVIVAL WITH TREATMENT |
|---|---|---|---|---|---|
| **Lung cancer** (157,000 cases a year | Cigarette smoking for 20 or more years; exposure to certain industrial substances, particularly asbestos; passive smoking; radiation | Persistent cough, sputum streaked with blood, chest pain, recurring bronchitis or pneumonia | Difficult to detect early. Diagnosis based on chest X ray, sputum cytology (cell) testing, fiber-optic bronchoscopy (direct examination of the lungs by means of a specially lighted tube). | Surgery, radiation therapy, chemotherapy. | 13% |
| **Breast cancer** (150,900 new cases a year; affects 1 of 10 women) | Over age 50, personal or family history of breast cancer, not having children, having first child after age 30, dense breast tissue, obesity, high fat intake, alcohol | Breast changes: lumps; thickening; swelling; puckering; dimpling; skin irritation; nipple distortion, scaliness, discharge, pain | Monthly breast self-examination. Professional breast exam every 3 years for women ages 20–40 and every year over age 40. Yearly mammography for all women over 50, every 1 or 2 years for women 40–49; and a baseline mammogram for those 35–39. Tissue biopsy confirms diagnosis. | Surgery, from lumpectomy (local removal of tumor) to a modified radical mastectomy (removal of breast and lymph glands, leaving underlying muscle intact); radiation; chemotherapy; or all three. | Almost 100% if no spread, 90% if diagnosed stage; 40% if cancer has metastasized |
| **Uterine and cervical cancer** (48,500 new cases a year) | For cervical cancer: early age of first intercourse, multiple sex partners, genital herpes, human papilloma virus infection For uterine cancer: infertility, failure to ovulate, prolonged estrogen therapy, obesity | Unusual vaginal bleeding or discharge | Pap smear once every 3 years after 2 initial negative tests 1 year apart. | Surgery, radiation, or a combination of the two. In precancerous stages, cervical cells may be destroyed by extreme cold or intense heat. Precancerous endometrial changes are treated with the hormone progesterone. | For cervical cancer, 66%; for uterine cancer, 83%. If detected early, 80–90% for cervical and almost 100% for endometrial. |
| **Colon and rectum cancer** (155,000 new cases each year) | Personal or family history of colon and rectal cancer or polyps (growths) in the colon or rectum; inflammatory bowel disease; high-fat, low-fiber diet | Unusual bleeding from rectum, blood in stool, a change in bowel habits | Digital rectal exam by physician (once a year after age 40); stool-blood slide test that detects blood in feces (every year after age 50); proctosigmoidoscopy, inspecting rectum by using a hollow, lighted tube (every 3–5 years after age 50, following 2 consecutive normal annual exams). Diagnosis may require a colonoscopy (viewing of the entire colon) or a barium enema. | Surgery, sometimes in combination with chemotherapy or radiation. | 86% for colon cancer, 77% for rectal cancer, if detected early; below 50% once cancer has spread. |

## Cancer Therapy

The three traditional forms of treatment for cancer are: (1) surgery to remove a tumor and surrounding cells; (2) radiation therapy, which exposes the involved area of the body to powerful radiation; and (3) chemotherapy, which uses powerful drugs to interfere with reproduction of the fast-multiplying cancer cells.

All these treatments affect normal, healthy cells as well as cancerous cells. Most vulnerable to radiation

**TABLE 14-2** Most Common Cancers, Their Risk Factors, Warning Signals, and Treatments *(Continued)*

| | RISK FACTORS | WARNING SIGNALS | EARLY DETECTION | TREATMENT | 5-YEAR SURVIVAL WITH TREATMENT |
|---|---|---|---|---|---|
| **Melanoma** (600,000 people a year) Malignant melanoma is the deadliest form of skin cancer. | Excessive exposure to the sun, fair complexion, occupational exposure to carcinogens | Unusual skin condition, especially a change in the size or color of a mole; appearance of darkly pigmented growth or spot; oozing, scaliness, bleeding; appearance of a bump; change in sensation, itchiness, tenderness, or pain | Examine moles on your skin once a month, using the ABCD rule: A is for asymmetry (one half of a mole does not match the other), B is for border irregularity (edges are ragged, notched, or blurred), C is for color (pigmentation is not uniform), and D is for a diameter greater than 6 mm. | Surgery, radiation, electrodesiccation (tissue destruction by heat), cryosurgery (tissue destruction by cold), or a combination of therapies. | 89% if the cancer is localized; 46% if the cancer has spread. |
| **Oral cancer** (can affect any part of the lip, tongue, mouth, or throat; 30,500 new cases each year) | Heavy smoking of cigarettes, cigars, pipes; excessive drinking; use of chewing tobacco | A sore that bleeds easily and doesn't heal; a lump or thickening; a reddish or whitish patch; difficulty in chewing, swallowing, or moving the tongue or jaws | Regular exams by your dentist or primary-care physician. | Surgery and radiation. | 51% overall |
| **Leukemia** (cancer of the blood-producing organs; 27,800 new cases each year) | Down's syndrome and other inherited abnormalities; excessive exposure to radiation and to certain chemicals, such as benzene | | Difficult to detect early because its symptoms are often similar to those of less serious conditions, such as the flu. Diagnosis is based on blood tests and a biopsy of bone marrow. | Chemotherapy, drugs, blood transfusions, and antibiotics; transplants of bone marrow. | 32% for white patients; 27% for black patients. For children, as high as 75%. |
| **Testicular cancer** (5,900 new cases a year) | Young men under age 35 | | Testicular self-examinations. | Surgical removal of the diseased testis, radiation therapy, chemotherapy, removal of nearby lymph nodes. | 96% if the cancer is localized; 89% overall. |
| **Prostate cancer** (106,000 cases each year) | Risk increases with age | Frequent urination, difficulty urinating, blood in the urine, lower back pain | Rectal exam. | Surgical removal of prostate, conventional radiation, implanting "seeds" of radioactive iodine in the prostate. | 70% overall; 83% if cancer hasn't spread. |

SOURCE: Used by permission of the American Cancer Society, Inc.

and chemotherapy are the fastest-growing body cells: hair cells; cells of the gastrointestinal tract; cells in the reproductive organs; and cells of the blood-producing tissue, the bone marrow. Oncologists often combine various treatments for the best possible results.

## Life after Cancer

For cancer survivors, getting on with the rest of their lives can be difficult. Many lose their jobs or have problems getting new jobs because of their experience with cancer. Sometimes they miss out on bo-

**FIGURE 14-3** Breast self-exam. The best time to examine your breasts is after your menstrual period.

**Looking**

Stand in front of a mirror with your upper body unclothed. Look for changes in the shape and size of the breast, and for dimpling of the skin or "pulling in" of the nipples. Any changes in the breast may be made more noticeable by a change in position of the body or arms. Look for any of the above signs or for changes in shape from one breast to the other.

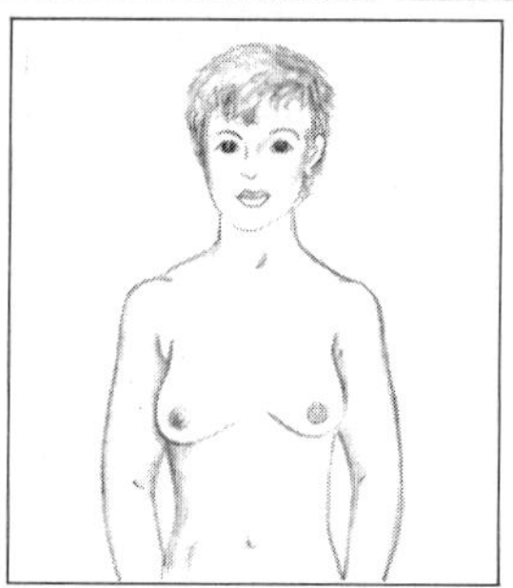

1. Stand with your arms down.

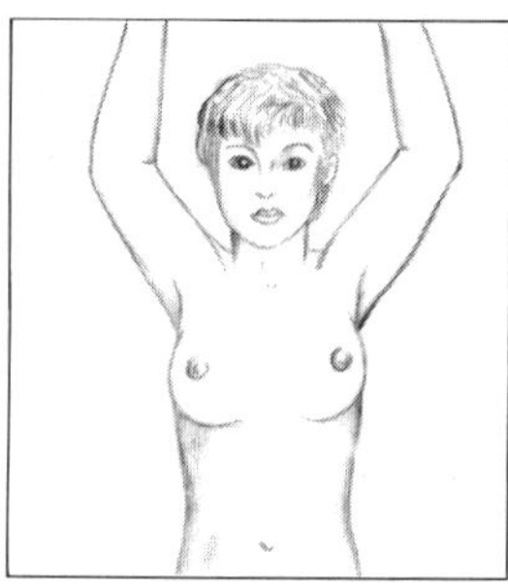

2. Raise your arms overhead.

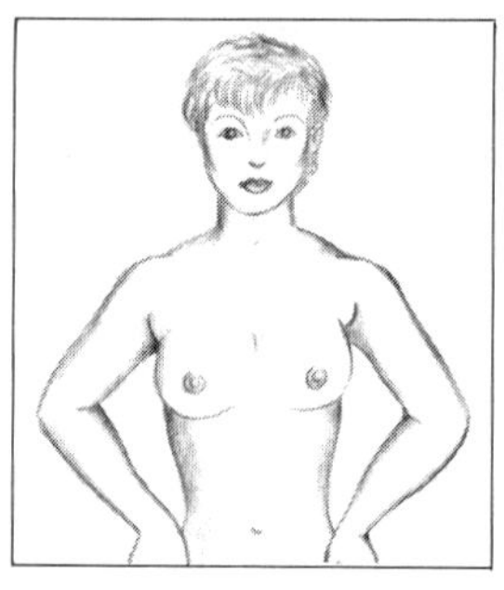

3. Place your hands on your hips and tighten your chest and arm muscles by pressing firmly.

**Feeling**

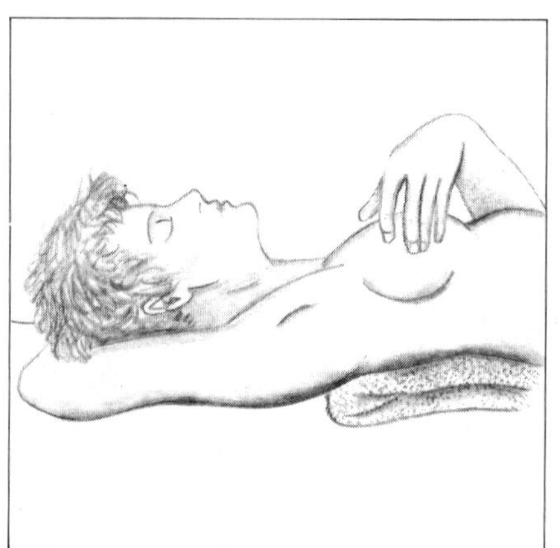

1. Lie flat on your back. Place a pillow or towel under your left shoulder, and raise your left arm over your head. With the hand slightly cupped, feel with flattened fingertips for lumps or any change in the texture of the breast or skin. Feel gently, firmly, carefully, and thoroughly. Do not pinch your breast between thumb and fingers. This may give the impression of a lump that is not actually there.

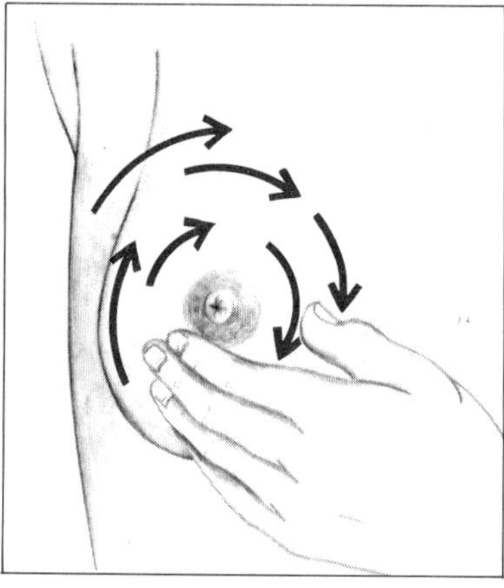

2. With your right hand, pressing gently in a circular motion, begin at the outermost top of your left breast and move in a circle around the outermost part of your breast. Pay special attention to the area between your breast and armpit. Then move inward toward the nipple an inch and circle again. Continue this procedure until you have examined every part of your breast, including the nipple. Repeat this same process for your right breast.

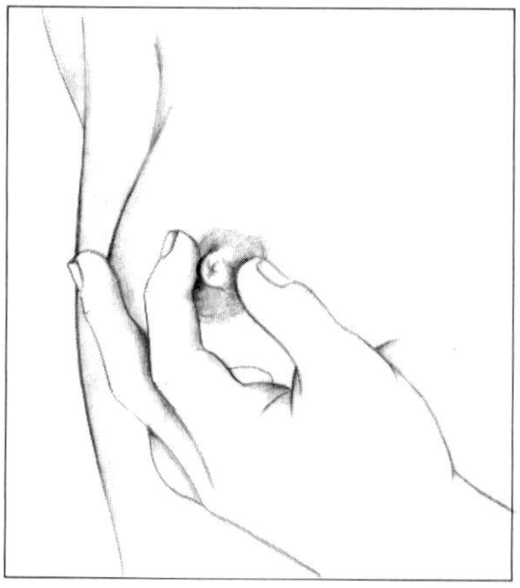

3. Gently squeeze the nipple of each breast between your thumb and index finger. Any discharge, clear or bloody, should be reported to your doctor immediately.

**FIGURE 14-4** Testicular self-exam. The best time to examine your testicles is after a hot bath or shower, when the scrotum is most relaxed. Place your index and middle fingers under each testicle and the thumb on top, and roll the testicle between the thumb and fingers. If you feel a small, hard, usually painless lump or swelling or anything unusual, consult a urologist.

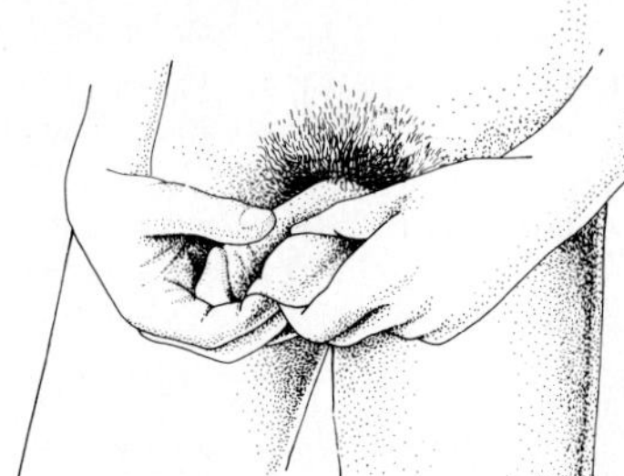

SOURCE: Hales, Dianne. *An Invitation to Health, Fourth Edition,* Benjamin/Cummings, 1989.

**FIGURE 14-5** Comparison of cancer sizes found by various detection methods for breast cancer.

Average–size lump found by women practicing occasional breast self–exam.

1.7 cm (11/16 in)

Smallest size cancer which can be felt by physician's palpitation exam.

1 cm (4/10 in)

Average–size lump found by women practicing frequent breast self–exam.

0.8 cm (5/16 in)

Average–size lump found by mammogram.

0.4 cm (5/32 in)

Cancer calcifications of this size and smaller can be seen on mammograms.

0.1 cm

SOURCE: DuPont Co.

nuses, full health benefits, or new group health insurance. Another problem for cancer survivors is money. Even people with comprehensive insurance end up paying huge amounts of money for services that are not covered. If they don't have adequate insurance, they may find it impossible to get further coverage.[12]

## OTHER MAJOR DISEASES

Most of the illnesses discussed in this section can be avoided or controlled, depending on the responsibility you take for your own body.

### Diabetes Mellitus

**Diabetes mellitus** occurs when the body either stops producing **insulin** or does not produce sufficient insulin to meet the body's needs. Normally, insulin regulates the amount of sugar in the body, either converting it into energy or storing it for future use. Diabetes mellitus interferes with insulin production; in severe cases, the body produces virtually no insulin at all. The lack of insulin means that glucose, the body's basic fuel, is not available as a source of energy and a condition similar to starvation develops, no matter how much food a person eats.

Every year, 30,000 Americans die from the disease itself; another 300,000 die from its complications, which include coma, blindness, kidney disease, blood-vessel damage, infection, heart disease, nerve damage, high blood pressure, and stroke.

#### Risk Factors

Approximately half of all Americans with diabetes have not been diagnosed. Those at highest risk include relatives of diabetics (whose risk is 2 1/2 times that of others); obese persons (85 percent of diabetics are or were obese); older persons (four out of five diabetics are over age 45); and mothers of large babies, because this is an indication of maternal prediabetes.

Diabetes can be either insulin-dependent (Type I) and require daily doses of insulin via injections, an insulin infusion pump, or oral medication; or insulin-independent (Type II), which can be regulated by a well-balanced diet, exercise, and weight control.

**diabetes mellitus** A disease in which the inadequate production of insulin leads to failure of the body tissues to break down carbohydrates at a normal rate.
**insulin** A pancreatic hormone that is necessary for the metabolism of carbohydrates.

**TABLE 14-3** American Cancer Society Recommendations for Cancer Detection

| DETECTION PROCEDURE | CANCER | WHO | WHEN |
|---|---|---|---|
| Health counseling and cancer checkup | Thyroid, testes, prostate, ovary, lymph node, mouth, and skin | Everyone over age 20 | Every 3 years between ages 20–40; yearly after age 40 |
| Breast self-examination | Breast | Women over age 20 | Every month |
| Breast physical examination | Breast | All women over age 20 | Every 3 years for women age 40 and under; yearly thereafter |
| Mammography (breast X ray) | Breast | All women over age 35 | Baseline between ages 35–40; every 1 to 2 years between ages 40–49; yearly thereafter |
| Pelvic examination | Reproductive system cancers in women | All women over age 20 | Every 3 years for women age 40 and under; yearly thereafter |
| Pap test (microscopic examination of cells) | Cervical | Women ages 20–65; younger women who are sexually active | After two negative exams 1 year apart, perform at least every 3 years* |
| Endometrial (uterine) tissue sample | Uterine | Women at high risk** | At menopause |
| Test for blood in stools | Colo-rectal | Everyone over age 50 | Annually |
| Digital rectal examination | Rectal | Everyone over age 40 | Annually |
| Sigmoidoscopy (examination of colon/rectum) | Colo-rectal | Everyone over age 50 | After two negative exams 1 year apart, perform every 3–5 years |

*The American College of Obstetrics and Gynecology recommends a yearly Pap test.
**High-risk women have histories of infertility, obesity, failure to ovulate, abnormal uterine bleeding, or estrogen therapy.
SOURCE: Used by permission of the American Cancer Society, Inc.

About 90 percent of the diabetics in the United States are Type II and do not require insulin.

The early signs of diabetes are frequent urination, excessive thirst, a craving for sweets and starches, and weakness. Diagnosis is based on a variety of tests of the level of sugar in the blood.

### Treatment

There is no cure for diabetes. The best option, according to the latest research, is to keep blood-sugar levels as stable as possible to prevent complications. Home glucose monitoring allows diabetics to check their own blood-sugar levels and adjust their diet or insulin doses.

All diabetics should eat a diet of complex carbohydrates (bread and other starches) and high-fiber foods and little sodium and fat. Weight control is essential. Weight loss alone can sometimes decrease or eliminate the need for insulin or oral drugs.

## Asthma

Periodic attacks of wheezing, difficulty in breathing, shortness of breath, and coughing are characteristic of **asthma.** The attacks range from mild to so severe

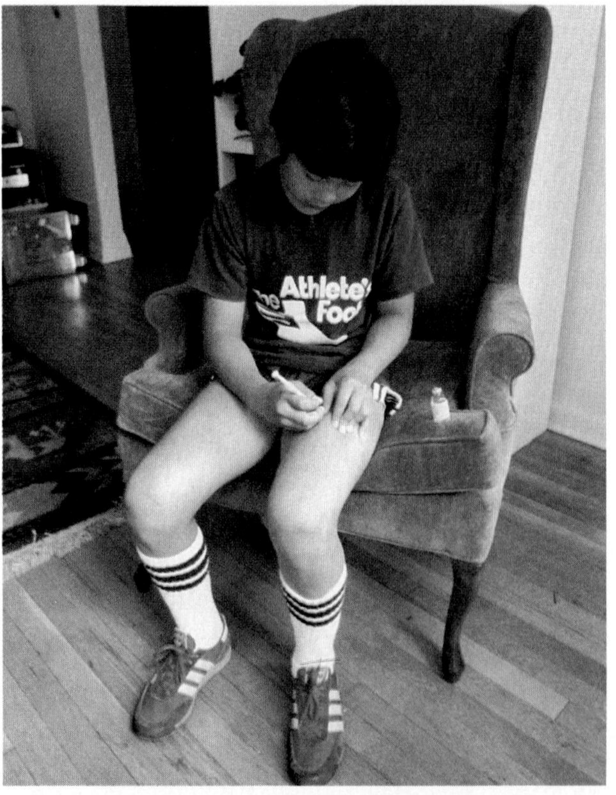

About 10 percent of diabetics require regular injections of insulin to control their blood sugar levels.

**asthma** A disease or allergic response characterized by bronchial spasms and difficult breathing.

that medical treatment is needed to prevent death. Between attacks, patients are relatively free of symptoms. In about half the cases, asthma begins before age 10, striking twice as many boys as girls. Many children outgrow the condition; however, symptoms may recur at midlife.

Three main factors may trigger an attack in an asthma-prone person: allergy to external irritants such as dust or pollen, respiratory infections, and stress. During an attack, the bronchioles, small tubes inside the lungs, contract as a result of a swelling of their lining, a spasm or constriction, or mucus blockage.

Treating infections and eliminating allergens (substances that trigger an immune response in certain individuals, such as ragweed pollen) can prevent attacks. If emotional stress seems to be the primary cause of the attacks, relaxation methods can be effective (see Chapter 3). More potent drugs can also provide relief.

## Epilepsy and Seizure Disorders

Between 0.5 percent and 1 percent of all Americans suffer from **epilepsy,** a brain-function disorder characterized by recurring, sudden attacks (seizures) of violent muscle contractions and unconsciousness. Epilepsy is rarely fatal; the primary danger to life is to suffer an attack while driving or swimming.

Seizures can be major, or grand mal; minor, or petit mal; or psychomotor. In a grand-mal seizure, the person loses consciousness, falls to the ground, and experiences convulsive body movements. Petit-mal seizures are brief and are characterized by a loss of consciousness for 10 to 30 seconds, by eye or muscle flutterings, and occasionally by a loss of muscle tone. A psychomotor seizure involves both mental processes and muscular movements, such as confusion accompanying a physical activity.

Ninety percent of epileptics have grand-mal seizures; about 40 percent suffer both petit-mal and grand-mal seizures. The frequency of attacks defines the severity of the epilepsy. After half of all cases of epilepsy have no known cause; others stem from conditions that affect the brain, such as trauma, tumors, or congenital malformations.

Seizure disorders do not reflect or affect intellectual or psychological soundness; persons who suffer from them are of normal intelligence. Therapy with anticonvulsant drugs can control seizures. Once seizures are under control, epileptics can live full, normal lives by continuing to take their medications.

## Ulcers

An **ulcer** is an open sore, often more than an inch wide, develops in the lining of the stomach or the duodenum (the first part of the small intestine). Ulcers are caused by acidic digestive juices. The major symptom is a burning pain felt throughout the upper abdomen. The pain may come and go, lasting up to 3 hours. It may begin right after eating or several hours later.

Risk factors include heavy smoking or drinking, large amounts of painkillers that contain aspirin, manual work, and advanced age. Treatment includes self-help measures, such as avoiding aspirin; eating small, frequent meals rather than three large meals a day; tak-

**epilepsy** A neurological disorder characterized by severe convulsions.
**ulcer** A lesion in, or an erosion of, the mucous membrane of an organ.

## HEALTH HEADLINE

### Predicting the Risk of Skin Cancer

People with one or more of six characteristics run a risk of getting melanoma, the most deadly form of skin cancer. The six risk factors are:

- blond or red hair
- marked freckling of the upper back
- rough red bumps on the skin called actinic keratoses
- family history of melanoma
- three or more blistering sunburns in the teenage years
- three or more years at an outdoor summer job as a teenager.

Any one or two of these factors increases a person's risk of melanoma 3 or 4 times. A combination of three or more factors increases the risk 20 to 25 times. The overall risk of getting melanoma for Americans is about one in 120. If detected early, melanoma is highly curable.

SOURCE: Rigel, Darrell. Presentation, American Cancer Society conference, March 25, 1990.

HEALTH SPOTLIGHT

## Helping Cancer Patients Live Longer

Psychological treatment can affect not only the quality, but the quantity of life for cancer patients. In one landmark study that followed advanced breast cancer patients for ten years, supportive group therapy *doubled* survival times.

The women, who all had metastatic breast cancer, received standard cancer care. About 60 percent were assigned to two weekly support groups that dealt with the psychological impact of their disease, doctor-patient issues, and pain control. At the end of a year, this treatment group reported less depression, anxiety, fatigue, and pain and greater self-esteem than the control group.

"We clearly showed that psychosocial interventions can improve psychological functioning, but we never thought about extending survival," says David Spiegel, M.D., an associate professor at Stanford University, who initially found the startling results of his ten-year follow-up hard to believe: "I nearly fell out of my chair when I saw the differences in survival. We're not talking weeks, but an average of a year and a half."

The support groups—led by a therapist and a counselor with breast cancer in remission—used no visualization or positive thinking techniques. The emphasis was on facing often-grim realities. "Even though certain things about dying are frightening, the nothingness of death was less terrifying to the women than pain and physical helplessness at the end of their lives," says Spiegel. "They learned that there were things they could do, that they could keep making choices even as their disease advanced. Watching and reaching out to members whose condition deteriorated helped the women see the process of dying as something endurable, rather than overwhelming."

Also, the women gained a greater sense of control over the time they had left. "They had to give up and grieve for the things they couldn't do, but they learned to focus on life projects that

ing antacids; and not smoking or drinking alcohol. Drugs such as cimetidine, ranitidine, and sucralfate can reduce the amount of acid produced by the stomach.[13]

## Disorders of the Muscles, Joints, and Bones

Because they are constantly being used, muscles, joints, and bones are more susceptible to damage from injury than are most other parts of the body.

### Arthritis

More than 17 million people suffer from some form of **arthritis,** an inflammatory disease of the joints that takes over one hundred forms. Degenerative arthritis, or osteoarthritis, found generally in the aged, is characterized by changes in bone tissue and cartilage (primarily at the joints), and seems to be the result of normal wear and tear. Rheumatoid arthritis is an autoimmune disease in which the body attacks its own connective tissue; it is fairly common among younger people. Women are generally affected by arthritis 3 times more often than are men until the seventh or eighth decade of life. Drugs can relieve pain and reduce inflammation; surgical treatments, including total joint replacement, and physical therapy are also used to maintain motion and strength.

### Hernias

A **hernia** is a bulge of soft tissue that forces its way through or between strained or weakened muscles. Hernias can occur in many parts of the body, but they're most common in the abdominal wall. A surgeon can push the protruding tissue back into place, and tighten or sew together the loose muscles. Regular exercise decreases the risk of getting an abdominal hernia.

**arthritis** An inflammation of the joints.
**hernia** The abnormal protrusion of an organ or body part through the tissues of the walls containing it.

were doable," says Spiegel. A frustrated writer published two small books of poetry before her death. Another woman devoted herself to imparting her life values to her young children. An unhappy wife decided to write off a bad relationship with a spouse rather than waste more energy on it. "The women emerged with a wisdom in living," Spiegel notes.

In their 90-minute sessions, the women provided encouragement and shared strategies for better communication and relationships with their physicians. Group members also phoned each other, sent cards and letters, and visited each other in the hospital. "They all felt that their relationships with friends and family had changed, and the group may have provided replacements for bonds that had been broken," says Spiegel. "They came to care deeply about one another."

Within four years of the study's beginning, all the women in the control group were dead, while 30 percent of support group participants were still alive. Average survival time for support group members was 36.6 months, compared to 18.9 months for the controls. Three women—all group members—remain alive, with their cancer in remission.

"There's no magic here; we didn't make the cancer go away," says Spiegel, "but something happened. We don't know what. Maybe the women's general health improved because they had less pain and fatigue and could be more active. Maybe their doctors perceived they were ready to fight and treated them more aggressively. Maybe there were changes in their immune systems. Whatever happened, it was remarkable."

SOURCES: Spiegel, David. Personal interview. Goleman, Daniel. "Cancer Patients Benefit from Therapy Groups," *New York Times*, November 23, 1989. Hales, Dianne. "Helping Cancer Patients Survive Longer," *Psychology Today*, January 1990.

### Backaches

One serious back problem is a prolapsed, or slipped, disc in the spinal cord. Each disc in the spinal cord is made up of a fibrous outer layer surrounding a jellylike substance. As people age or strain their backs, pressure may squeeze some of the softer central material through a weak point in the harder outer layer. The result is a loss of the disc's cushioning effect and painful pressure on a nerve at the squeezed-out portion of the disc. The discs of the lower back are most susceptible. Self-help measures include simple painkillers or antiinflammatory medications, heat treatments, and lying flat on one's back on a firm bed for two weeks. In some cases, surgery may be necessary to remove the damaged portion of the disc.

## ACCIDENTS: SAVING YOUR OWN LIFE

Among persons between the ages of 15 and 24, accidents are responsible for more deaths than all other causes combined. Motor vehicle accidents, falls, drownings, fires and burns, and poisoning are the primary accidental causes of death (see Figure 14-6).

### Cars and Motorcycles

The basic rules of safe driving are as follows:

- Don't let feelings of competition and frustration cloud your judgment.
- Be alert and anticipate possible accident situations.
- Don't drive while under the influence of alcohol or other drugs. Drugs and alcohol are involved in as many as half of all automobile fatalities.
- Always wear seat belts, which reduce accidental injury by 60 percent and accidental death by 50 percent.[14]

Mile for mile, motorcycling is far more risky than automobile driving. Because the most common motorcycle injury is to the head, helmets are required in most states; head injuries are 3 times more frequent for nonhelmeted cyclists.

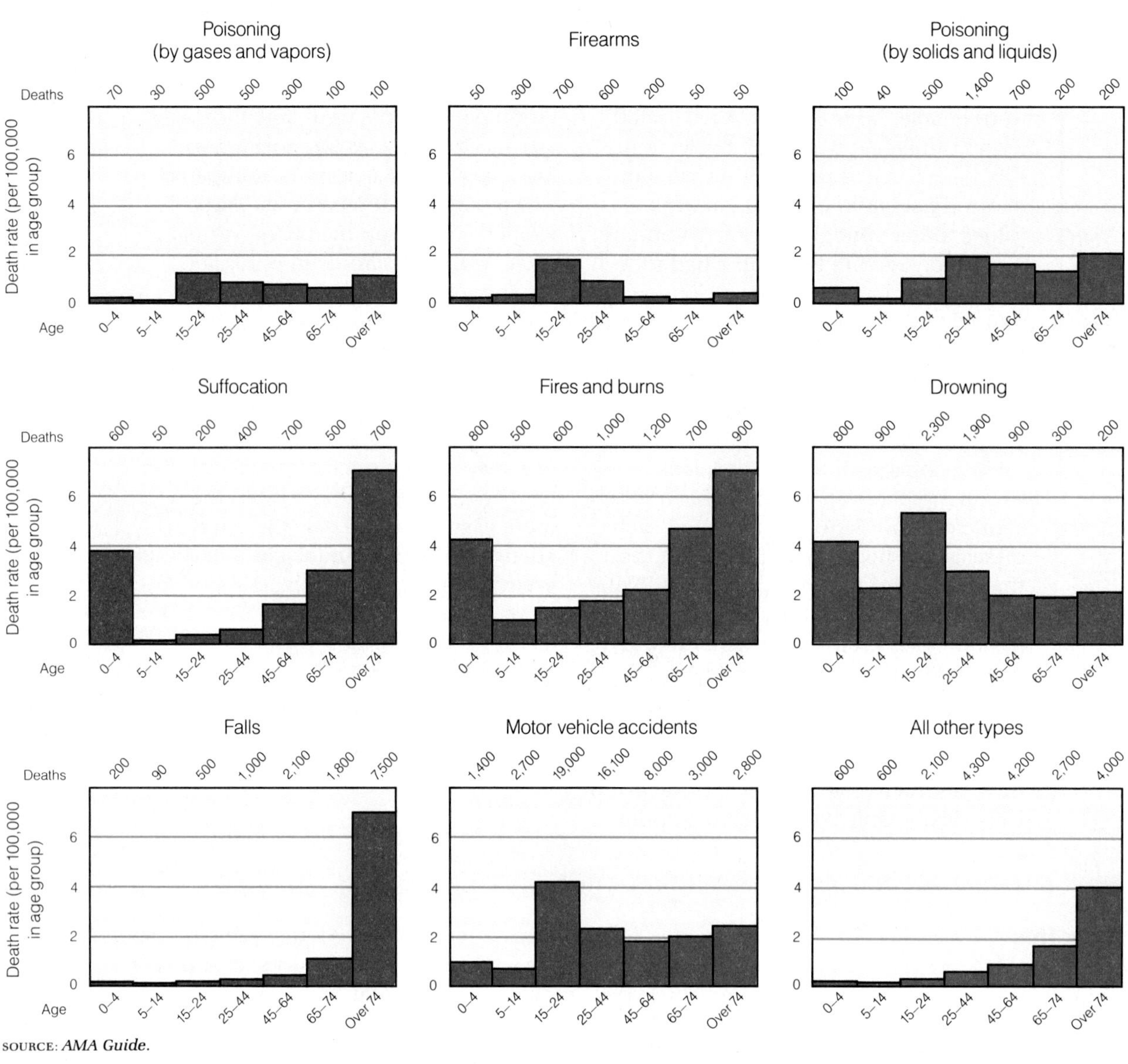


**FIGURE 14-6** Accidental deaths by age.

**STRATEGY FOR CHANGE**

**How to Drive Safely**

- Don't get too comfortable. Alertness matters.
- Use the rearview mirror often.
- If someone cuts you off, back off to a safe distance.
- When you can, drive so that you have space around you. If something unexpected happens, you'll be able to move.

## Falls

Over 20 percent of all accidental deaths are the result of falls; of all home-accident deaths, over 50 percent result from falls. Falls can be the result of wearing high heels or worn footgear, poor lighting, slippery or uneven walkways, broken stairs and handrails, loose or worn rugs, or objects left where people walk.

## Drowning

Drowning is the third most common cause of accidental death in the United States, according to the National Safety Council. About 85 percent of drowning victims are teenage boys. Many drowned persons were strong swimmers. In one study, half the people age 15 or older who had drowned had high blood-alcohol levels. Most drownings (80 percent) occur at

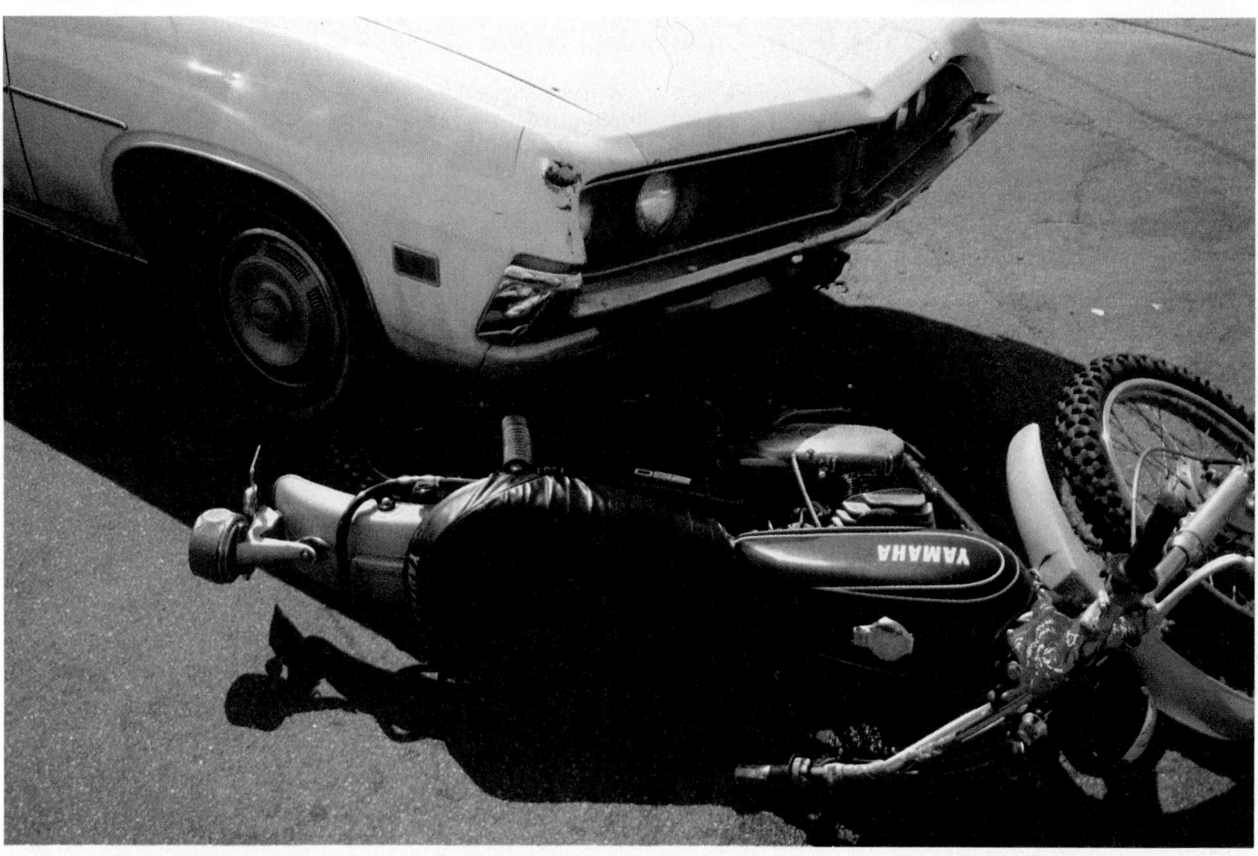


Mile for mile, motorcycling is far more risky than automobile driving.

unorganized facilities, such as ponds or pools with no lifeguards present.

The causes of drowning, in order of frequency, are exhaustion, being swept into deep water, losing support, becoming trapped or entangled, having a cramp or other attack, and striking an underwater object after diving into shallow water.

## Burns and Shocks

Approximately 8,000 people are killed each year by fires and burns, a fourth of them children under age 14. Cigarette-ignited fires kill an estimated 2,000 Americans and injure another 3,000 every year.

Burns are of three degrees: A first-degree burn is a superficial reddening of the skin, such as from a sunburn or a mild scald. A second-degree burn involves damage to deeper layers of the skin and causes deep reddening and blistering; it might be the result of a severe sunburn or scalding with hot water. A third-degree burn involves all layers of the skin and perhaps deeper tissues. The skin shows charring and, initially, does not feel painful because nerve endings have been destroyed.

## HEALTH HEADLINE

### Seat Belts Pay Off

**Seat belts not only save lives, but also reduce the severity of injuries and save money. In a study of 1,364 accident victims in the Chicago area, seat belts reduced the extent of injuries by 60 percent, hospital admissions by 64.6 percent, and hospital charges by 66.3 percent. None of those killed in car accidents was wearing a seat belt. As a whole, seat-belt wearers tended to be slightly older and more often women than men.**

SOURCE: Dean, Cory. "Seat Belt Study Assesses Savings in Medical Costs and Injuries," *New York Times*, November 12, 1989.

SELF-SURVEY

## Are You Doing Enough to Prevent Accidents?

Accidents frequently result in serious injury, and accidents cause a large number of deaths. The following questions are designed to test how well you protect yourself and your family from accidental injury. The first group of questions concentrates on guarding against possible hazards in and around your house or apartment. The second group deals with safety measures that should be taken against accidents that might happen to you or your family on the road, whether in a vehicle or as pedestrians. The third group is mainly concerned with safety on vacations, when unfamiliar surroundings and activities present special hazards.

***Group 1: Safety at Home***

Answer yes or no to the following questions:

1. Do you make it a point never to smoke in bed? ______
2. When cooking, do you guard against accidental tipping by positioning pan handles so that they do not extend outwards? ______
3. If you own a gun, do you keep it unloaded, separate from the ammunition, and locked away? ______
4. Are your carpets firmly fixed, with no ragged spots or edges, and are loose rugs placed to minimize the risk of sliding or tripping? ______
5. Are your stairs, halls, and other passages well lit (brightly enough to read a newspaper)? ______
6. Is it a rule in your house that nothing is left on the stairs? ______
7. If you spill or drop something on the floor that might be slippery, do you always clean it up right away? ______
8. Do you keep nonslip mats both in and alongside the bath or shower? ______

***Group 2: Safety on the Road***

Answer yes or no to the following questions:

9. When walking in streets or open roads at twilight or in the dark, do all members of your family carry a light, or wear a markedly visible outer garment such as a white or luminous jacket? ______
10. Do you always drive within the speed limit and drive defensively? ______
11. Are you always careful to drink very little alcohol or none at all if you are going to drive a car soon afterward? ______

STRATEGY FOR CHANGE

### Preventing Fires

- Keep the following away from pilot lights, heaters, and other sources of heat: gasoline, paint, oily rags, newspapers, plastics, glues, and lightweight materials.
- Clean up grease on stoves.
- Don't overload electrical circuits, use worn wiring, or use portable heaters that have no cutoff feature if they tip over.
- Use common sense about children. Don't leave food unattended. Keep matches out of a child's reach.
- Don't smoke in bed or use gasoline to start fires.
- To avoid shocks, be careful about anything that involves electricity and water: Avoid using power tools in the rain, be careful about electric heaters in the bathroom, and use tools with nonconducting handles.

## Poisons

Half a million children will swallow poisonous materials this year; nine-tenths of them will be under age 5. Adults may also be poisoned by mistakenly taking someone else's prescription drugs or reaching for medicines in the dark and taking the wrong one. In most cities, you can call a poison control center for advice.

12. Do you avoid driving when you feel unusually tired or ill or if you are taking drugs (such as antihistamines) that are known to impair alertness? ______
13. Do you have your car fully serviced—including lights, tires, windshield washer and wipers, brakes, and steering—either every 6,000 miles or at least every six months? ______
14. Do you check at least once a week to make sure that your car windows, lights, mirrors, and reflectors are clean? ______
15. When driving, do you always try to keep a gap between your car and the one in front of you of at least a meter (a yard) for each mile per hour of speed you're traveling? ______
16. Do you always make sure that you and all passengers in your car use available seat belts? ______

***Group 3: Safety on Vacations***

Answer yes or no to the following questions:

17. Can you swim? ______
18. Do you test the depth of the water and go in feet first? ______
19. In a boat, do you always wear a life jacket? ______
20. If you do any skiing, hiking, or climbing, do you always go properly prepared with the right clothing and equipment? ______
21. When going on an excursion for a day or longer, do you tell someone what your route is and when you expect to be back? ______
22. Do you and your family take full safety precautions and have the proper equipment when you engage in contact and other possibly dangerous sports? ______
23. Before taking up a new and potentially dangerous activity such as hang-gliding, do you make sure you get proper instruction? ______
24. During a vacation, do you make sure you get adequate rest and relaxation? ______

***Evaluation***

A no answer to any of the above questions indicates that you are not doing all you can to minimize your risk of accidents. You can and should take all the protective steps suggested in the questions.

SOURCE: Kunz, Jeffrey and Asher Finkel (eds.). *The A.M.A. Family Medical Guide.* New York: Random House, 1987.

## MAKING THIS CHAPTER WORK FOR YOU

### Staying Alive and Healthy

You can do a great deal to prevent or delay many serious illnesses, including the one we fear most: cancer. In all types of cancer, normal cells turn into abnormal cells and multiply. Genetic, viral, chemical, and physical factors can cause malignant, or cancerous, tumors.

Foods containing vitamin A, vitamin C, and selenium may reduce the risk of developing cancer; foods linked to cancer include fats, those preserved with nitrites, those that have been browned, and burned food. You can also help in the fight against cancer by avoiding dangerous behaviors, such as smoking, having regular cancer checkups, and knowing the warning signs of cancer.

The most common cancers include lung cancer, which most often is the result of heavy cigarette smoking and exposure to asbestos and other industrial substances; breast cancer, which can be detected early if a woman routinely examines her breasts and undergoes mammography; cancer of the cervix and uterus, which can be detected by Pap smears; cancer of the colon and rectum, which is most likely to occur in certain families, and those who eat too much fat and too little fiber; skin cancer, which most often is caused by excessive exposure to ultraviolet radiation; oral cancer, which may be the result of the heavy use of alcohol and all forms of tobacco; leukemia, which can affect children and adults; testicular cancer, which strikes men under age 35; and

## WHAT DO YOU THINK?

Your grandmother and aunt died of colon cancer, and you know that your mother, who is in her fifties, hasn't been to the doctor for years. She confesses that she's afraid of a cancer checkup and would rather not know about something that the doctors might not be able to do anything about anyway. What could you tell her to persuade her to have a thorough exam? What about your own potential risk? What do you think you can do to protect yourself?

Imagine that you are the parent of a desperately ill child. Without a transplanted organ, your youngster will certainly die. Doctors inform you that the best—and perhaps only—hope is removing a healthy organ—or part of it—from your body and transplanting it to your child. However, the operation involves serious, possibly life-threatening risks to you. What would you do? Who do you think should make such decisions: the parents, a hospital ethics committee, or the doctors?

Newall brags about "living on the edge." He drives fast; never wears seat belts; and loves the thrill of hang-gliding, surfing, and motorcycle racing. What do you think of this attitude? Have there been situations in which you have avoided or ignored safety measures because you didn't want to play it safe? Were others at risk because of your actions? Can you engage in adventurous activities safely?

---

prostate cancer, which usually strikes older men. Early diagnosis and treatment—including surgery, chemotherapy, and radiation therapy—are helping more people win their fight against cancer than ever before.

Other major illnesses include diabetes mellitus, in which the body produces an insufficient amount of insulin, a hormone that is required by the body's cells to convert sugar into energy. Treatment for mild cases is a carefully controlled diet; for more severe cases, insulin.

Reactions to allergens, respiratory infections, and stress may trigger asthma, which is characterized by wheezing, difficulty in breathing, and other symptoms. The symptoms of chronic bronchitis, a common disorder among smokers, include a persistent cough, shortness of breath, and wheezing. Other major diseases include epilepsy; ulcers; and disorders of the muscles, joints, and bones.

The most common causes of accidental death are motor-vehicle injuries, falls, drownings, fires and burns, and poisonings. Wearing seat and shoulder belts can reduce by 90 percent the risk of injury in an automobile accident.

Diseases and accidents may seem to be a matter of odds. Genetic tendencies, environmental factors, and luck do seem to affect your chances of having to deal with these health threats. However, *you* have more control over such risks than anyone or anything else in your life:

Don't smoke, and you all but eliminate the threat of lung cancer—and brighten your heart's future, too. Eat right, and you not only look good, but also keep your arteries free of fat, lower your blood pressure, and avoid diabetes. Exercise regularly, and you not only tone muscles, but also strengthen your cardiovascular system. Have regular screening tests, and you cut off some life-threatening diseases before they get an edge on you. Proceed with caution on land and water, and you head off accidents.

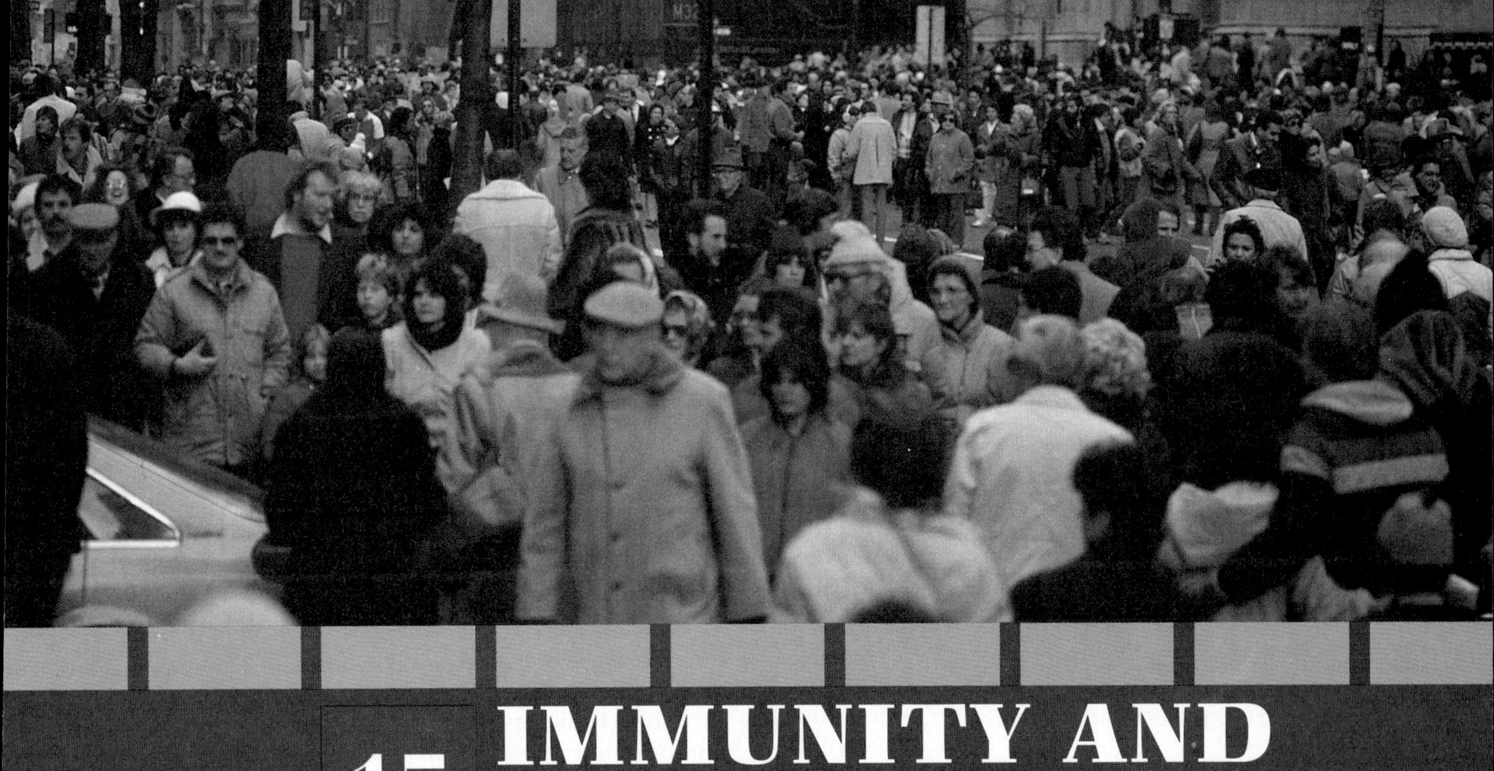

# 15 IMMUNITY AND INFECTIOUS DISEASES:

*Modern science has won many victories against the agents of infection.* Yet some—primarily the tiniest killers of all, the viruses—have resisted every drug. In this country the most threatening infections today are sexually transmitted diseases (STDs). Their incidence has skyrocketed in recent years. But they cannot be halted or prevented in the laboratory. Only you, by your behavior, can prevent and control them. This chapter is a lesson in self-defense against infection. The information it provides can help you recognize and avoid dangers.

# INFECTIONS

Infection is a complex process, triggered by various disease-causing organisms called **pathogens** and countered by the body's own defenders.

## Agents of Infection

Among the various pathogens that can cause infection are viruses, bacteria, fungi, protozoa, and parasitic worms (see Figure 15-1).

### Viruses

The tiniest and toughest pathogens are **viruses.** Consisting simply of a bit of genetic material (DNA or RNA—the basic building blocks of life—but never both) within a protein coat, they are the most primitive form of life. Unable to reproduce on its own, a virus takes over a body cell's reproductive machinery and instructs it to produce new viral particles, which eventually are released to enter other cells.

The problem in fighting viruses is that it is difficult to find drugs that harm the virus and not the cell it has commandeered. **Antibiotics,** drugs that inhibit or kill bacteria, have no effect on viruses. Table 15-1 lists the most common viruses.

### Bacteria

Bacteria, simple one-celled organisms, are the most plentiful pathogens. However, most kinds of bacteria do not cause disease; some, like the *Escherichia coli (E. coli)* of the digestive tract, play important roles within our bodies. Even friendly bacteria, though, can get out of hand and cause acne, urinary tract infections, vaginal infections, and other internal problems.

Bacteria harm the body by releasing chemicals that digest body cells, or toxins (poisons) that produce the specific effects of such diseases as diphtheria or tetanus.

Streptococcus bacteria are particularly hazardous. If untreated, a strep throat can lead to potentially fatal problems, including infections of the blood or rheumatic fever (see Chapter 13). Analysis of a sampling of the microorganisms in the throat (a throat culture) indicates whether medication is necessary to prevent these complications.

Because bacteria are sufficiently different from the cells that make up our bodies, antibiotics can kill them without harming our cells. Tuberculosis, tetanus, gonorrhea, scarlet fever, and diphtheria are examples of bacterial diseases.

### Fungi

Fungi are single-celled or multicelled organisms that

**pathogen** A microorganism that produces disease.
**virus** A tiny pathogen consisting of either DNA or RNA surrounded by a protein coat.
**antibiotic** A substance produced by one type of microorganism that is toxic to other types of microorganisms; in dilute solutions, used to treat infectious diseases.

**TABLE 15-1** Common Viruses

*Rhinovirus and Adenovirus*—Get into your mucous membranes and cause upper respiratory-tract infections and the common cold.
*Influenza*—Can change their outer protein coats so dramatically that individuals resistant to one strain cannot fight off a new one.
*Herpesviruses*—Take up permanent residence in the cells and flare up periodically. Seven different human herpesviruses have been identified.
*Papillomavirus*—Causes few symptoms in women and almost none in men, but may be responsible, at least in part, for a rise in the rate of cervical cancer among younger women.
*Hepatitis*—Causes several forms of liver infection (hepatitis A, B, C), diseases that range from mild to potentially life-threatening.
*Slow Viruses*—Give no early indication of their presence but produce rare, fatal illnesses within a few years.
*Retroviruses*—Named for their backward ("retro") sequence of genetic replication compared to other viruses. The two that infect humans are HTLV, which causes a rare form of cancer called lymphoma, and HIV, or human immunodeficiency virus, which causes AIDS. Scientists have identified different types of HIV.

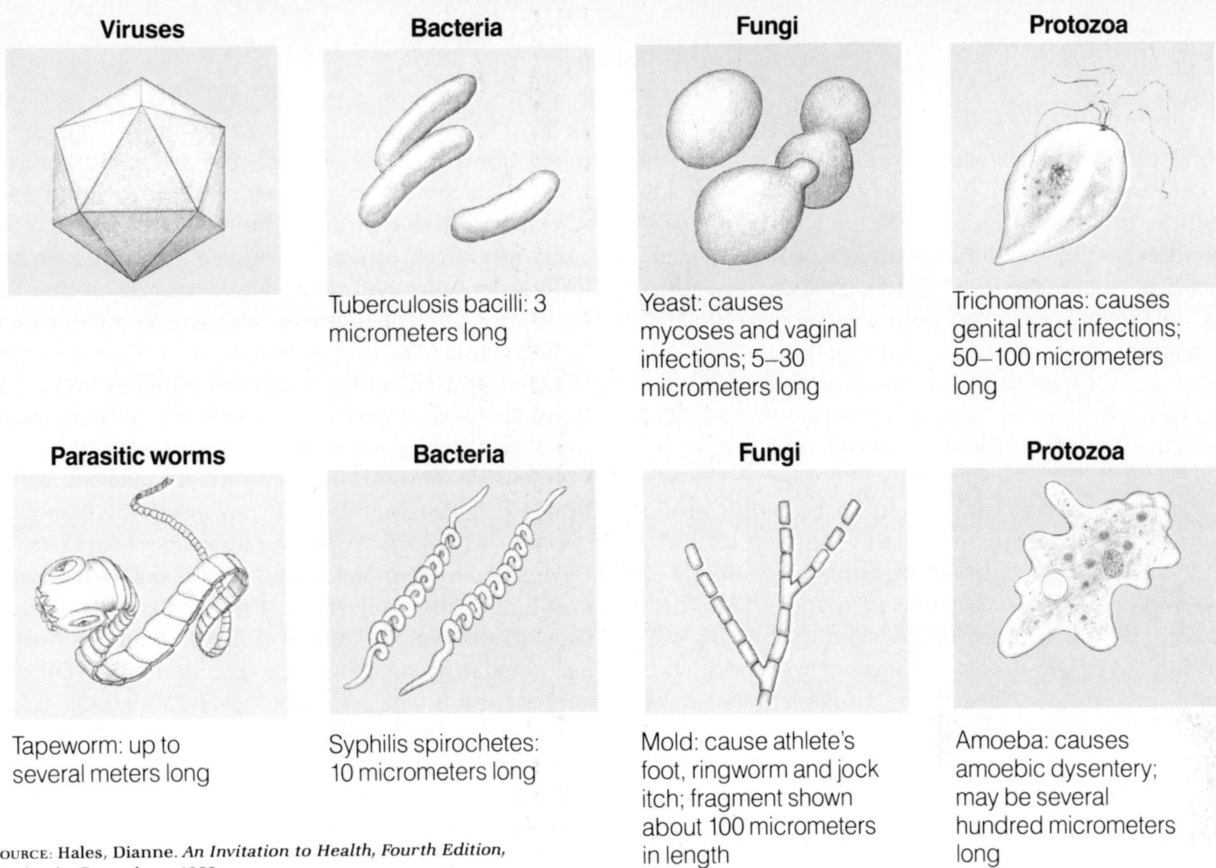


SOURCE: Hales, Dianne. *An Invitation to Health, Fourth Edition,* Benjamin/Cummings, 1989.

**FIGURE 15-1** Viruses, bacteria, fungi, protozoa, and parasites form the major categories of organisms that cause disease in humans. Except for the parasitic worms, which can be very long, pathogens are microorganisms, which means they can be seen only with the aid of a microscope.

consist of threadlike fibers and reproductive spores. They are plants that must obtain their food from organic material, which may include human tissue. Fungi release chemicals that digest cells and are most likely to attack hair-covered areas of the body, such as the scalp, beard, groin, and external ear canals. They also cause athlete's foot. Treatment consists of antifungal drugs.

### Protozoa

Protozoa are single-celled, microscopic animals that release chemicals and toxins that destroy cells or interfere with their function. Diseases caused by protozoa are not a major health problem in this country, primarily because of public health measures. Examples of protozoal diseases are malaria, African sleeping sickness, and amoebic dysentery. Treatment consists of general medical care to relieve the symptoms, replacement of lost blood or fluids, and drugs that kill the specific protozoa.

### Parasites

Round or flat, parasites are multicellular animals that attack specific tissues or organs; they compete with the host for nutrients. The most common parasitic disease in the United States is giardiasis, which is caused by a protozoa that lives in the intestine and multiplies by splitting in two. Hard to diagnose and even more difficult to overcome, this parasite causes severe diarrhea and intestinal distress. Children in day-care centers, travelers, and those using contaminated water supplies are at high risk. Treatment consists of drug therapy.

## Transmission

The four major means of transmission of infectious disease are animals, food, water, and person-to-person contact.

Insects can carry various diseases. The housefly may spread dysentery, diarrhea, typhoid fever, tuberculosis, or trachoma (an eye disease rare in the United States but common in Africa). Other insects—including mosquitoes, ticks, mites, fleas, and lice—can transmit malaria, yellow fever, encephalitis, and Lyme disease (discussed later in this chapter).

Still other illnesses are food-borne. The larvae of the parasitic roundworm, *Trichina spiralis,* can be found in uncooked meat (particularly pork) and cause trichinosis. This infection—which causes nausea, vomiting, diarrhea, fever, thirst, profuse sweating, muscular weakness, and pain—can be avoided by thoroughly cooking meat. Salmonella bacteria are common in the intestines of chickens (and other fowl) and cause disease in humans who have eaten chicken that was not thoroughly cooked or properly refrigerated. A deadly food disease, botulism, is caused by certain bacteria that grow in improperly canned foods. Although botulism is rare in commercial products, it is a danger in home canning.

Waterborne diseases, such as typhoid fever and cholera, have been rare in this country but are still widespread in less-developed areas of the world. They can be transmitted directly in drinking water or by food (such as lettuce) that has been watered or washed with contaminated water.

The people you're closest to also can transmit pathogens by coughing, sneezing, kissing, or sharing food or dishes with you. To avoid infection, stay out of range of anyone who's coughing, sniffling, or sneezing. Carefully wash your dishes, utensils, and hands—and don't hesitate to ask a sexual partner about a blister or lesion or to avoid contact if you think you might catch a sexually transmitted disease (see the section on STDs in this chapter).

## HOW YOUR BODY PROTECTS ITSELF

Various parts of your body protect you against infectious diseases. Your skin, when unbroken, keeps out most potential invaders. Your tears, sweat, skin oils, saliva, and mucus contain chemicals that can kill bacteria. Mucus traps inhaled bacteria, viruses, dust, and foreign matter. Cilia, tiny hairs, move the mucus to the back of the throat, where it is swallowed. The digestive system then destroys the invaders.

### The Immune System

When these protective mechanisms cannot keep you infection-free, your body's **immune system** swings into action. Like a sixth sense on constant alert for foreign substances that might threaten the body, the immune system includes more than a dozen defensive weapons concentrated in the spleen, thymus gland, and lymph nodes.

Two of the most important defensive weapons in the immune system are complement and lymphocytes. Complement is a group of proteins that burns through bacterial membranes, causing bacterial cells to explode. These proteins can also kill viruses.

Lymphocytes, or white blood cells, react to toxins, foreign proteins, and microorganisms. (These foreign substances are called **antigens.**) Lymphocytes called B-cells mature in the bone marrow and produce **antibodies**—proteins that bind with antigens and make them harmless. Lymphocytes called T-cells are manufactured in the bone marrow and carried to the thymus for maturation. Some T-cells activate other immune cells, some help in antibody-mediated responses, and some suppress lymphocyte activity.

Attacked by pathogens, the body musters its forces and fights. Together, the immune cells work like an internal police force. Some cells, such as the T-cells, are constantly on patrol for troublemakers. Others, such as the B-cells, serve as precinct stations at key locations in the body. Also busy at surveillance are natural killer cells that, like the elite forces of a SWAT team, seek out and destroy viruses and cancer cells. When an antigen enters the body, the T-cells engage in hand-to-hand combat with the invader. Meanwhile, the B-cells churn out antibodies, which rush to the scene and join the fray.

The **lymph nodes,** or glands, are small tissue masses where some protective cells are stored. If pathogens invade your body, many of them are carried to the lymph nodes, where they are destroyed. That's why the lymph nodes in your neck often feel swollen when you have a cold or flu.

If the pathogens establish a foothold, the blood supply to the area increases, bringing oxygen and nutrients to the fighting cells. Tissue fluids, as well as antibacterial and antitoxic proteins, accumulate. You may develop redness, swelling, local warmth, and pain—the signs of **inflammation.** As more tissue is destroyed, a cavity, or **abscess,** forms and fills with fluid, battling cells, and dead white cells (pus).

---

**immune system** The internal organs, tissues, cells, and mechanisms that protect the body against disease by producing antibodies against foreign bodies (antigens).

**antigen** Any of a number of substances—including toxins, foreign proteins, and microorganisms—which, when introduced to the body, cause antibody formation.

**antibody** A specialized protein produced by the body; combines with a specific antigen to play the central role in immunity to specific pathogens.

**lymph nodes** Storage sites for lymphocytes and macrophages.

**inflammation** A localized response by the body to tissue injury; characterized by swelling and the dilation of blood vessels.

**abscess** A localized accumulation of pus and disintegrating tissue.

## HALES INDEX

Number of minutes a flu virus can survive on human skin: 5

Number of days a flu virus can survive on a kitchen countertop: 1.5

Number of adults who get immunized against diseases that could jeopardize their lives: 1 in 5

Number of new cases of Lyme disease reported every year: 5,000

Number of people who think most people with AIDS have only themselves to blame: 1 in 2

Number of people who believe employers should be able to dismiss employees who test positive for HIV: 1 in 4

Number of Americans who catch an STD every year: 13 million

Percentage of people with STDs who are under age 24: 63

Risk of a college student's getting chlamydia or HPV: 1 in 10

How often an American contracts syphilis or gonorrhea: Every 14 seconds

Economic cost of STDs in United States each year: $4 billion

SOURCES: **1, 2** "Vital Statistics," *Hippocrates*, September/October 1989. **3** Brody, Jane. "Resurgence of Measles Across the Nation Prompts New Recommendations on Vaccinations," *New York Times*, January 11, 1990. **4** Schmitz, Anthony. "After the Bite," *Hippocrates*, May/June 1989. **5, 6** "Vital Statistics," Hippocrates, November/December 1988. **7, 8** American Social Health Association. **9** Johnson, Dirk. "At Colleges, AIDS Alarms Muffle Older Dangers," *New York Times*, March 8, 1990. **10** Centers for Disease Control. **11** "Boom in STDs Setting Off Alarms," *Medical World News*, August 22, 1988.

If the invaders are not killed or inactivated, the pathogens are able to spread into the bloodstream and cause what is known as **systemic disease.** The toxins released by the pathogens cause fever, and the infection becomes more dangerous.

## Immunity

Once the body produces antibodies against a specific antigen—mumps, for instance—you're usually protected against that antigen for life. If you're again exposed to mumps, the antibodies already in your system rush to your rescue and prevent another episode. This type of long-lasting immunity is called **active immunity.**

However, you don't have to suffer through an illness to be protected against many infectious diseases: You can be inoculated with a **vaccine,** which contains inactive or weakened antigens that stimulate the immune system to create antibodies so you're no longer susceptible to infection. However, a vaccine is effective against only one strain and cannot prevent other infections. (See Table 15-2 for the latest vaccination recommendations.)

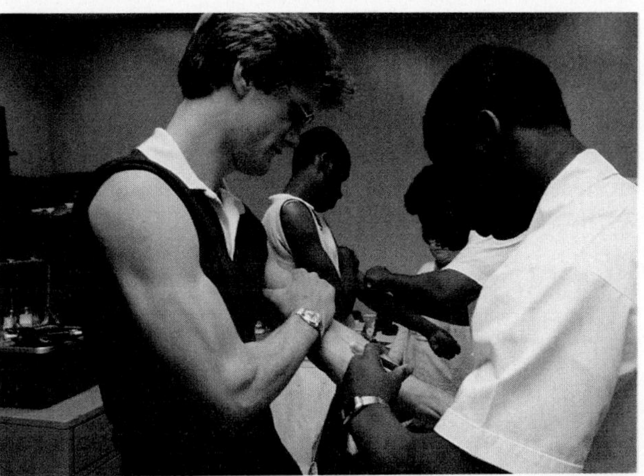

Vaccinations can protect adults as well as children from many infectious illnesses.

**systemic disease** A pathologic condition that spreads throughout the body.
**active immunity** Immunity resulting from the body's production of antibodies in response to a pathogen or a vaccine.
**vaccine** A treatment containing weakened or inactive antigens; given to stimulate production of antibodies.

**TABLE 15-2** Immunization Schedule and Recommendations

| IMMUNIZATION | CHILDREN | ADULTS |
|---|---|---|
| Diphtheria/pertussis/tetanus combination | At 2, 4, 6, and 18 months and at 4–6 years (before or at school entry) | |
| Dipthera/tetanus booster | At 14–16 years of age | Every 10 years |
| Polio | At 2, 4, and 18 months and at 4–6 years | Those who might be exposed (e.g., those in health and sanitation occupations, travelers) |
| Measles/mumps/rubella combination | At 15 months and just before entering school<br>Any child over 6 | Adults under 32 who received only one measles shot at one year of age or after<br>Adults whose initial dose was given along with immune globulin–as routinely occurred from 1963–1975—should get 2 doses at least 1 month apart. |
| Influenza | | Yearly, because of the changeability of viral strains |
| Tuberculosis | Those exposed to individuals with active tuberculosis | Those exposed to individuals with active tuberculosis (e.g., health workers) |
| Cholera, yellow fever, typhoid fever | For travelers and others who may be exposed | For travelers and others who may be exposed |
| Hepatitis B | Those exposed to infected individuals or to contaminated food and water | For those who may be exposed (e.g., health workers, who ingested contaminated food/$H_2O$, travelers) |

Annual flu vaccinations are recommended for those most endangered by a bout with the flu: the elderly; those with chronic diseases; and those in high-risk professions, such as nursing and medicine. However, an increasing number of health officials are urging everyone to get annual flu shots. Officials at the federal Centers for Disease Control estimate that 70 to 90 percent of healthy young adults who get flu shots will avoid infection.[1] Since the body takes 12 to 20 days to produce protective antibodies, it's best to get flu shots in the fall, before the flu season hits. Side effects are minimal.

Another way to hold off disease is through **passive immunity,** immunity received from antibodies already created by another person or animal. Resistance is temporary, but passive immunity may prevent illness during a critical time, for example, if you have just come down with a disease like infectious hepatitis and do not have time to develop antibodies of your own. Infants who breast-feed receive passive immunity to some diseases from their mother's milk, though they become susceptible to them once they are weaned.

**passive immunity** Temporary immunity acquired from the injection of antibodies produced by another person or animal.

**STRATEGY FOR CHANGE**

### Natural Ways to Bolster Immunity

- Get the recommended daily allowances of essential vitamins. Severe deficiencies in vitamins $B_6$, $B_{12}$, and folic acid can cause significant immune impairments. Too little vitamin C also increases susceptibility.
- Keep up your iron and zinc intake. Iron influences the number and vigor of certain immune cells. Zinc is crucial for cell repair.
- Avoid fatty foods. A low-fat diet can increase the activity of immune cells that hunt down and knock out cells infected with viruses.
- Get enough sleep. Most people need at least 6 to 8 hours a night. Without adequate rest, your immune system cannot maintain and renew itself.

- Exercise three or four times a week for a minimum of 20 to 30 minutes. Aerobic exercise stimulates production of an immune-system booster called interleukin 2.
- Don't smoke. Chronic smoking decreases the levels of some immune cells.
- Watch your alcohol intake. Heavy drinking interferes with normal immune responses and lowers the number of defender cells.[2]

## COMMON INFECTIOUS DISEASES

Although infections can be unavoidable at times, the more you know about the process of infection and specific infectious diseases, the more you can do to protect yourself.

### The Process of Infection

If someone with a cold sits next to you on a bus, tiny viral particles may travel into your nose and mouth. Immediately the virus finds or creates an opening in the wall of a cell, and the process of infection begins.

During the incubation period, the time between invasion and the first symptom, you're unaware of the pathogen multiplying inside you. In some diseases, incubation may go on for months, even years. But for most, it's a matter of days or weeks.

The early stage of the battle between your body and the invaders is called the prodromal period. As infected cells die, they release chemicals that help block the invasion. Other chemicals, such as histamines, cause blood vessels to dilate, thus allowing more blood to reach the battleground. During all of this, you feel mild, generalized symptoms: headache, irritability, discomfort. You're also highly contagious. At the height of the battle—the typical illness period—you cough, sneeze, sniffle, ache, feel feverish, and lose your appetite. Recovery begins when the body's forces gain the advantage and destroy the last of the invaders.

### The Common Cold

There are more than 110 viruses that cause colds. So, although in a single season you may develop a temporary immunity to one or two cold viruses, you may then be infected by a third form.

The only way to avoid cold viruses is to avoid people. Trouble often starts with a handshake. Nasal mucus has the highest concentration of the cold virus, which travels to the hands in the process of wiping one's nose. As you shake hands with a cold sufferer, you pick up the virus from his or her hand, and carry it to whatever you touch, including your own eyes and nose. To avoid infection, wash your hands frequently and don't put your fingers in your mouth.

In 1990 scientists developed a substance that prevented major cold viruses from infecting cells in test tubes—a possible first step toward a cure for the common cold. Existing antiviral drugs act only after cells have been infected. The new approach might be able to stop infection from taking hold but will require years of testing.[3]

**STRATEGY FOR CHANGE**

**Coping with a Cold**

There is no cure for the common cold, but you can make yourself more comfortable:

- Adults can take two 325-mg tablets of aspirin or acetaminophen (an aspirin-equivalent, such as Tylenol or Ibuteron) every 4 hours for fever and muscular aches. (Children and teenagers should *never* take aspirin for a cold, flu, or other viral infections, because of the danger of Reye's syndrome.)
- If you have a sore throat, gargle with warm salty water.
- If you have a dry, hacking cough, cough suppressants may help you sleep through the night.
- If you have a stuffy head, try nasal sprays or drops. Take these decongestants only as directed and for no more than three days.
- Check the label of any cold remedy for antihistamines, common ingredients that turn off nonstop drips and sneezes, but may thicken the mucus in your lungs, increasing the risk of complications in the lungs. Ask the pharmacist if you are not sure whether the remedy is right for you.
- Ask your doctor about trying zinc. According to preliminary studies, the compound zinc gluconate seems to cut a week off recovery if a cold has already taken hold and stops a cold in its tracks if it's just starting.[4]
- Drink plenty of liquids (except alcohol) to liquefy mucus, replace lost fluids, and prevent complications such as ear infections and bronchitis.

### Influenza

**Influenzas** (flus) are a lot like colds, only with more severe symptoms that last longer. Flu victims typi-

**influenza** A fairly common, highly contagious viral disease.

cally develop fever (up to 103 degrees Fahrenheit in adults, higher in children), all-over muscle pain, nausea, vomiting, and headache. Most flu viruses are one of three strains: A, B, or C. But viruses change genetically over time, resurfacing in different forms every few years. In 1990 an epidemic of a particularly nasty A virus, called Shanghai flu, struck 50 to 60 million Americans and killed more than 8,100 people, most of them elderly.[5,6]

Flu viruses—transmitted by coughs, sneezes, laughs, and even normal conversation—are extraordinarily contagious, particularly in the first three days of the disease. The usual incubation period is two days, but symptoms can hit hard and fast.

Children and teenagers should *never* take aspirin for colds or flus. The CDC has traced a potentially fatal complication, Reye's syndrome, to a combination of a viral illness, especially flu or chicken pox, and aspirin. The antiviral drugs amantadine and rimantadine can reduce flu symptoms in people of all ages, but sufferers must start taking them in the first 48 hours after exposure.

## Measles

Measles, a potentially deadly infection, has become a serious health threat among high school and college students and inner-city preschool children. From 1987 to 1989, the number of cases tripled, with many outbreaks occurring on college campuses.[7] Though measles can be a mild disease in healthy children, the risk of severe complications, including permanent damage and death, increases with age.

Symptoms include a rash on the face and body, runny nose, high fever, cough, eye inflammation, and fatigue. From 10 to 15 percent of measles patients develop serious complications, such as ear infections, diarrhea, or pneumonia. One of every 1,000 develops encephalomyelitis, an inflammation of the brain that can be fatal or lead to mental retardation or movement, behavioral, or neurological disorders.

CDC officials estimate that 5 to 15 percent of college students are susceptible to measles.[8] At highest risk are men and women born between 1957 and 1967, when the measles vaccine was introduced. Many were vaccinated too early or were given antibodies that interfered with the vaccine's effectiveness. Many colleges are requiring students to submit proof of immunization before allowing them to enroll.

### STRATEGY FOR CHANGE

### Protecting Yourself from Measles

In 1990 the federal Centers for Disease Control issued new vaccination recommendations for measles:

- Every child should get two doses of measles vaccine, the first at 15 months and the second just before entering kindergarten or first grade.
- If a child lives in a high-risk area, where five or more cases a year have been reported in the last five years, the first dose should be given at 12 months.
- Any child over 6 and adults under 32 who received only one measles shot at one year of age or after should consider getting a second dose.
- If the initial dose was given along with immune globulin—as routinely occurred from 1963 to 1975–that person should get two doses at least one month apart.

## Pneumonia

An inflammation of the lungs, **pneumonia** fills the fine, spongy networks of the lungs' tiny air chambers with fluid. Pneumonia can be caused by bacteria, viruses (including flu), or foreign material (such as smoke) in the lungs. The symptoms of classic bacterial pneumonia are fever, shortness of breath, and general weakness. Pneumonia can be fatal.

Antibiotics can control bacterial pneumonia, but only certain types of viral pneumonia respond to drugs. Recovery from the other types depends on rest and the body's ability to heal itself.

## Tuberculosis

Once the nation's leading killer, **tuberculosis (TB)** is not yet a disease of the past, although it is rare. Transmitted from person to person by coughing, sneezing, or spitting, the bacteria can enter the body without causing an active case of tuberculosis. A simple skin test can determine whether you have been infected. If the skin test is positive, indicating that TB is present, you'll be monitored with yearly chest X rays or you may require treatment.

**pneumonia** An inflammation of the lungs; caused by infection or irritants.

**tuberculosis (TB)** A highly infectious disease that primarily affects the lungs and is often fatal; caused by bacteria.

## Mononucleosis

Yes, you can get **mononucleosis** by kissing—or by any other form of close contact. "Mono" is a viral disease that is most common among persons 15 to 24 years old; its symptoms include a sore throat, headache, fever, nausea, and prolonged weakness. The spleen is swollen and the lymph nodes are enlarged. You may also develop jaundice or a skin rash similar to German measles.

The major symptoms usually disappear within 2 to 3 weeks, but weakness, fatigue, and depression may linger for at least 2 more weeks. The greatest danger is from physical activity that might rupture the spleen, resulting in internal bleeding. The liver may also become inflamed. A blood test can determine whether you have mono. There is no special treatment, other than rest.

### STRATEGY FOR CHANGE

#### Recovering from Mono

- Drink plenty of water and fruit juice, especially while you have a fever.
- Stay indoors for as long as your fever persists.
- For discomfort or pain, take the medication your doctor recommends. (If you're in your teens, do *not* take aspirin.)
- Get as much rest as possible. Don't even try to return to your daily routine for at least a month.
- Although you need not avoid people, avoid exposure to other illnesses, because your resistance is low.

## Chronic Epstein-Barr Virus

The Epstein-Barr virus (EBV) that causes mononucleosis is a permanent resident in more than 90 percent of American adults, though it is usually inactive. However, it can spring to life—sometimes after a recent bout with mono—and cause an active infection. Patients may report sore throats, swollen lymph glands, low-grade fevers, headaches, confusion, memory problems, nausea, diarrhea, chest pain, shortness of breath, irregular heartbeats, sleep problems, numbness, and heat and cold sensitivities. In some people with high EBV levels, researchers have found that depression causes or contributes to many of their symptoms.[9]

## Hepatitis

The various forms of **hepatitis** are all viral infections of the liver. Hepatitis A, a less serious form, is generally transmitted by fecal contamination of food or water. Hepatitis B—a potentially fatal disease transmitted through the blood and other body fluids, including semen and saliva—infects an estimated 200,000 Americans each year. Once spread by contaminated tattoo needles, needles shared by drug addicts, or transfusions of contaminated blood, hepatitis B is now transmitted most frequently through sexual contact. Male homosexuals who have many sexual partners are at particularly high risk.

Symptoms of hepatitis include fever, chills, aches, nausea, vomiting, and diarrhea. The liver becomes enlarged and tender to the touch; sometimes the yellowish tinge of jaundice develops. Treatment consists of rest and a high-protein diet until the disease runs its course.

**mononucleosis** An infectious viral disease characterized by an excess of white blood cells in the blood, fever, bodily discomfort, a sore throat, and kidney-liver complications.
**hepatitis** An inflammation and/or infection of the liver; caused by a virus; often accompanied by jaundice.

### HEALTH HEADLINE

#### Measles Menace for College Students

Men and women born since 1957 may have to be revaccinated because they were vaccinated too soon, according to the federal Centers for Disease Control. They are at particularly high risk of becoming severely ill and developing serious complications from measles, because most were vaccinated at 12 months, rather than the currently recommended 15 months, and their bodies did not develop immunity. In addition, many were given immune globulin, a form of antibodies, to reduce the risk of reactions to the vaccine; however, the immune globulin also reduced the vaccine's effectiveness.

SOURCES: American Academy of Pediatrics Advisory, January 1990. Brody, Jane. "Resurgence of Measles Across the Nation Prompts New Recommendations on Vaccinations," *New York Times*, January 11, 1990.

Though a safe, effective vaccine against hepatitis B is available, only one in every nine Americans at high risk of developing the disease—health-care workers, intravenous drug abusers, sexually active gay men, and kidney dialysis patients—has received the vaccine. (The new vaccine is synthetic and cannot carry HIV.)

If a person with the symptoms of hepatitis tests negative for both A and B forms, the diagnosis traditionally was non-A, non-B hepatitis. Scientists have identified a third virus that produces hepatitis and dubbed it type C. This virus may account for most cases of non-A, non-B hepatitis, which is most likely to occur after a transfusion. Scientists, however, are still looking for other types that may be responsible for the remaining cases.[10]

Hepatitis C may afflict an estimated 150,000 Americans each year. It is spread primarily by sexual activity and through contaminated blood on dirty needles or in transfusions. In a report in the *New England Journal of Medicine* in 1990, two separate teams of scientists reported that treatment with the drug interferon halted destruction of liver cells in about half the patients with hepatitis C.[11]

## Toxic Shock Syndrome

Bacteria cause **toxic shock syndrome** (**TSS**), also discussed in Chapter 7, a potentially deadly disease associated with the use of tampons, particularly high-absorbency types. Toxins (poisonous waste products) released in the bloodstream can cause a high fever; a rash that leads to peeling of the skin on the fingers, toes, palms, and soles; dizziness; dangerously low blood pressure; and abnormalities in several organ systems (the digestive tract, kidneys, muscles, and blood). Victims can enter the state of life-threatening crisis called shock (a state in which blood flow throughout the body is inadequate to sustain life). Treatment consists of immediate hospitalization, intravenous fluids, medications to raise blood pressure, and powerful antibiotics.

In addition to women using high-absorbency tampons, those who have given birth within the preceding 6 to 8 weeks are at greater risk. Children (including newborns), men, and postmenopausal women have also developed TSS, which usually has been traced to bacteria in skin abscesses, boils, cuts, or postsurgical wounds.

Without prompt treatment, TSS can cause severe and permanent damage, including muscle weakness, partial paralysis, amnesia, disorientation, an inability to concentrate, and impaired lung and kidney function. Sometimes toxic shock weakens the blood vessels, increasing the risk of heart problems.

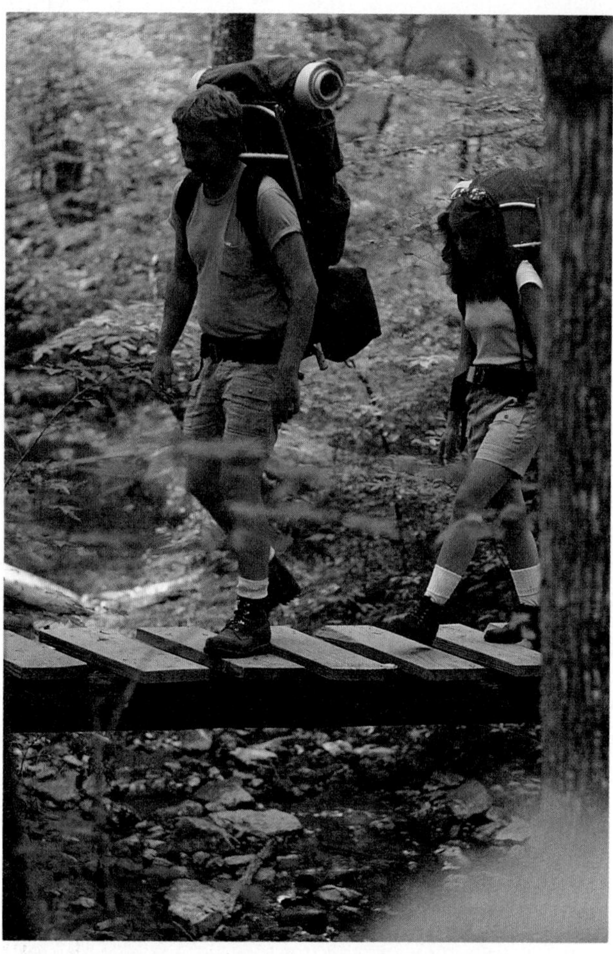

Hikers should protect themselves against Lyme disease, a bacterial infection spread by ticks.

## Lyme Disease

An increasing health threat, spread by ticks, is Lyme disease, a bacterial infection that produces various serious symptoms, including joint inflammation, heart arrhythmias, blinding headaches, and memory lapses. The first telltale sign is often a rash that looks like a bull's eye, which erupts from two days to five weeks after a tick bite. Antibiotics are usually effective, particularly if the disease is diagnosed early.[12]

**toxic shock syndrome** (**TSS**) A disease characterized by fever, vomiting, diarrhea, and often shock; caused by bacteria that release toxic waste products into the bloodstream.

**STRATEGY FOR CHANGE**

**Preventing Lyme Disease**

- When walking through woods or fields of high grass, wear long pants rather than shorts, and tuck your pants into your socks. You may be able to spot ticks easier on light-colored clothing.
- In tick-infested areas, use a repellant containing DEET, which washes off in sweat or water, or Permanone, which repels ticks from treated clothing (do not use Permanone on skin).
- If you spot a tick on your body, remove it as soon as possible so it doesn't become too embedded. The best way to remove it is to grab the tick as close to your skin as possible, using tweezers or your fingers (wear rubber gloves or use a paper towel). Pull back steadily. Don't squeeze the tick's body.
- Don't handle or crush the tick once it's removed.
- If any parts remain in your skin, remove them as you would a splinter. Disinfect the bite with Betadine (an over-the-counter disinfectant), and wash your hands.

### Preventable Infections

Every year 70,000 Americans die of infectious diseases that can be prevented by vaccination. Hundreds of thousands suffer through the illnesses needlessly. The problem is that, too often, adults think of immunizations as only for children. As Table 15-2 shows, however, vaccines are not just for kids, although children undeniably need the greatest protection.

Immunization is most essential for polio, a viral infection that attacks the nerves that control the muscles; tetanus, a potentially fatal disease caused by certain bacteria that live in the soil and can invade the body through a wound from a nail, thorn, or other sharp object; diphtheria, a dangerous bacterial infection that causes fever and interferes with breathing; and measles. Infants should also be immunized against pertussis (whooping cough), which can develop into pneumonia and is potentially fatal.

In addition to these essential immunizations, vaccines are also available against mumps and **rubella** (German measles), which resembles measles. About 85 percent of adults are immune to rubella, even if they have no history of the disease. The most serious result of this otherwise mild disease is the destructive effect it has on an unborn baby following infection of the mother in early pregnancy. All children should be immunized against rubella at one year of age or later.

Adults who are not immune may be immunized at any age, but women should not receive the vaccine during pregnancy or during the 2 to 3 months immediately preceding pregnancy. All unimmunized children in a pregnant woman's household should be immunized against rubella, because they are the most likely potential carriers.

**Mumps** is usually a mild childhood disease with almost no serious symptoms except discomfort. Deafness in one ear is a rare complication. In adult males mumps may cause painful swelling of the testicles, but fear of sterility is rarely justified. There are no special risks for women contracting mumps and little risk to an unborn child if the mother is infected during pregnancy.

## IMMUNE SYSTEM DISORDERS

Sometimes our immune system overreacts to certain substances or mistakes the body's own tissues for enemies or doesn't react adequately. The result is an immune disorder.

An **allergy** is a hypersensitivity to a substance in the environment or the diet. An estimated 35 to 40 million Americans have allergies. Their immune systems overreact to some substance and cause rashes, wheezing, or irritation of the respiratory and digestive systems. Some people with allergies to insect stings or drugs such as penicillin develop a life-threatening reaction that quickly leads to breathing problems, low blood pressure, rapid pulse, and collapse. If the exact substance causing the reaction—the allergen—is identified, the immune system can sometimes be deactivated through a series of minute injections of the allergen.

**Autoimmune disorders** result when the immune system fails to recognize body tissue as self and attacks it. Many of these severely disabling diseases—such as myasthenia gravis, rheumatoid arthritis, and

**rubella** A disease similar to, but milder than, typical measles; also known as German measles.

**mumps** A usually mild disease occurring most frequently in childhood.

**allergy** A hypersensitivity to a particular substance or to an environmental condition.

**autoimmune disorder** Any of several disabling conditions in which the immune system attacks body tissues, causing progressively worse degeneration.

lupus erythematosus—primarily strike healthy women in the childbearing years. These diseases, which worsen with time, are treated with drugs that suppress the immune system, but this treatment leaves the person highly vulnerable to infections.

Some people have an **immune deficiency.** The most dramatic instances are the very few children born without an effective immune system, who must live in sterile environments; any infection is likely to be fatal to them. The deficiency may be caused by a genetic defect, radiation, or certain drugs.

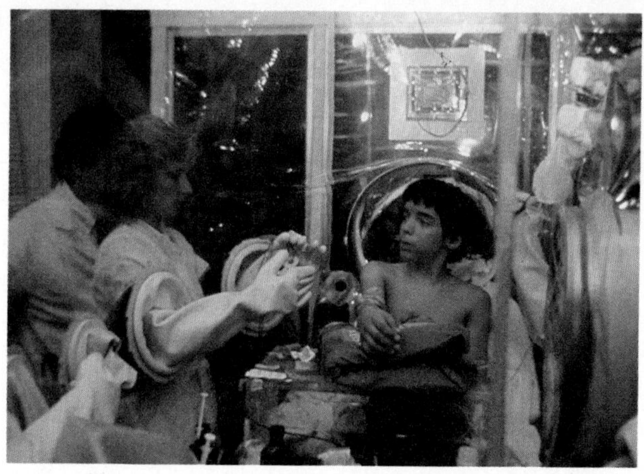

Children born without an effective immune system must live in a sterile environment because any infection could be fatal.

## ACQUIRED IMMUNE DEFICIENCY SYNDROME

**Acquired immune deficiency syndrome (AIDS)** is a disease, caused by a virus, in which some of the body's white blood cells are destroyed, impairing the body's natural defense system and making the person more susceptible to certain infections and diseases. The virus that causes AIDS is a retrovirus called the human immunodeficiency virus, or HIV, which destroys one type of lymphocyte known as the T-4, or helper, cell (see Figure 15-2). Because of this immune deficiency, infected individuals can develop lung infections, such as the pneumonia caused by *Pneumocystis carinii,* and various cancers, most commonly a once rare cancer known as Kaposi's sarcoma.

About 80,000 Americans are infected with HIV every year. The Public Health Service estimates that a total of 800,000 to 1.2 million Americans have been infected with, and carry antibodies to, HIV. Since the rate of infection has slowed, scientists predict that the AIDS epidemic may reach its peak in the mid-1990s. The rate of infection among homosexual and bisexual men has dropped, but AIDS continues to increase among drug users, some minorities, and heterosexuals.[13]

### The History of AIDS

Most epidemiologists believe that HIV first infected humans in a remote area of Africa, possibly in Zaire. As more Africans moved from their villages to cities, where they had many more sexual contacts than in the past, HIV spread quickly. Haitians, recruited to Zaire as civil servants, may have carried the virus back to their native land.

Epidemiologists speculate that HIV carriers may have been among the sailors who came to New York (where AIDS first appeared in this country) from fifty-five nations for the bicentennial in 1976. Others have traced AIDS cases to a male Canadian flight attendant (called Patient Zero) who had as many as 250 homosexual contacts a year in different countries. He developed Kaposi's sarcoma in 1980 (before AIDS had been identified) and continued to be sexually active until his death in 1984.[14] AIDS has since spread

**immune deficiency** Partial or complete inability of the immune system to respond to pathogens.

**acquired immune deficiency syndrome (AIDS)** A fatal disease caused by a virus that destroys the ability of the immune system to fight disease.

**HEALTH HEADLINE**

**Longer Life Before AIDS Strikes**

**The period of time between infection with the AIDS virus and development of AIDS symptoms is getting longer. In 1990, half of those with AIDS infection developed the disease in less than eleven years; half took longer. "We anticipate the incubation period will become even longer as a result of earlier intervention with new treatment," the researchers noted. In the 1980s, the mean time between infection and development of AIDS was seven years.**

SOURCE: Lemp, G. F. et al. "Projection of AIDS Morbidity and Mortality in San Francisco," *Journal of the American Medical Association,* vol. 263, no. 11, March 16, 1990.

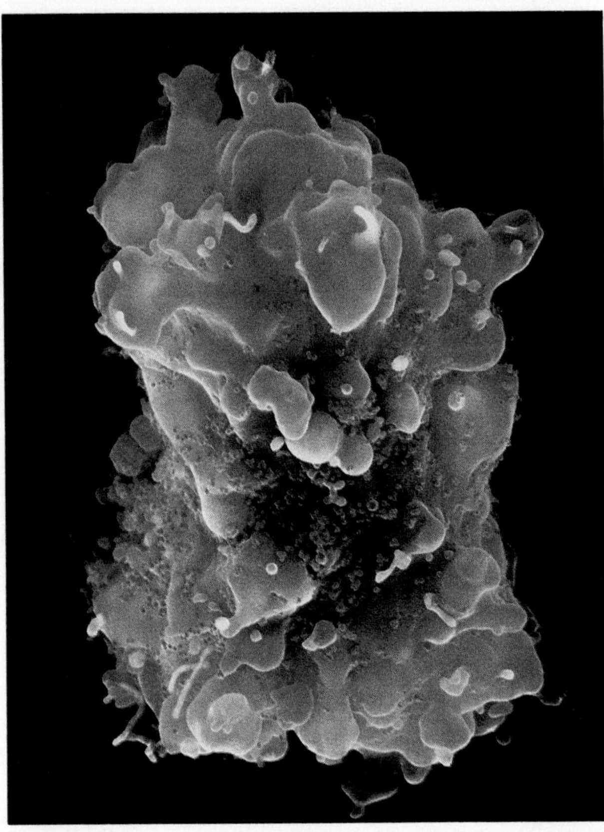

**FIGURE 15-2** The AIDS virus, HIV.

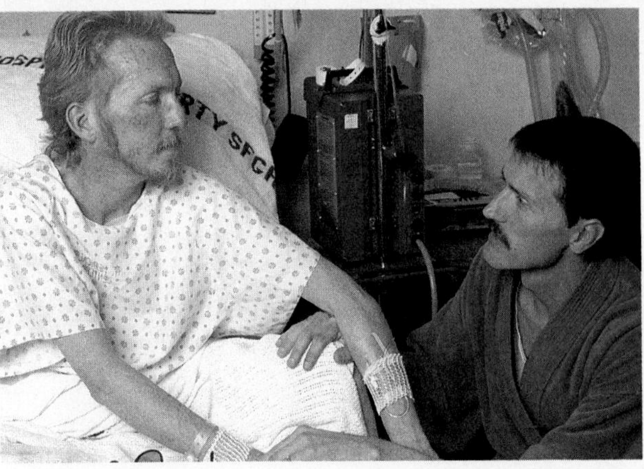

Friends can help AIDS patients struggling against this deadly disease feel less isolated.

throughout North America, South America, Europe, and Asia.

## Transmission

HIV can live only in blood, semen, vaginal fluids, breast milk, and other bodily fluids, such as tears. Many chemicals—including household bleach, alcohol, and hydrogen peroxide—can inactivate it. The means of transmission of HIV are the following:

- *Exchange of bodily fluids (semen or vaginal fluids) during sexual activity.* HIV can be spread by anal, vaginal, and possibly oral sexual contact between heterosexuals, bisexuals, or homosexuals. (See Chapter 7 for detailed information.)
- *IV drug use with shared needles or sex with an IV drug user who shares needles.* IV drug use has been the number one source of AIDS in heterosexual men; sex with IV drug users has been the number one cause of AIDS in women. (Chapter 9 discusses IV drug use.) Approximately 25 percent of all AIDS cases in this country have occurred in persons who use IV drugs; 17 percent, in individuals for whom IV drug use is the only risk factor.[15] The use of crack cocaine, especially among the poor, may have contributed to the rise in AIDS among IV drug users. IV drug users represent the largest pool of HIV-infected heterosexuals in both the United States and Europe.
- *Transfusions of blood or blood products between 1978, when HIV spread to America, and 1985, when testing to identify contaminated blood became routine.* About 9 million Americans received transfusions during those years; the CDC estimates that 12,000—only 0.0013 percent—may have thereby been infected with HIV. At greatest risk are those who received multiple transfusions in areas with a high incidence of AIDS in 1984 and 1985, when the disease was much more widespread than it had been before. Since the late spring of 1985, all blood donations have been screened for antibodies to HIV; donors are also screened for risk factors. Every unit of donated blood with a positive test result is discarded. To protect hemophiliacs who require a blood-clotting substance called Factor VIII, manufacturers use a heat treatment to inactivate any HIV present.
- *Mother-to-child transmission.* Approximately 80 percent of all children with HIV infection have a parent with the disease or in a high-risk category for HIV infection. Infants whose mothers have AIDS or are HIV-positive have a 30 percent risk of being infected.[16] The virus can be transmitted to the infant in three possible ways: (1) before birth, through the mother's circulation; (2) during labor and delivery; or (3) after birth, through infected breast milk.
- *Accidental contact with HIV-contaminated blood or body fluids.* A small number of health workers have tested positive for HIV after accidentally sticking themselves with needles containing HIV-positive blood or after being splashed with blood because

SELF-SURVEY

## Do You Know Enough About STDs?

***Purpose***

Because sexually transmitted diseases (STDs) represent an intimately personal health issue affecting the entire community, your decision to help control this problem is crucial. This quiz will help you identify what you know, feel, and do about STDs.

***Directions***

The quiz consists of four parts; Part I through Part III refer to STDs generally: (1) knowledge, (2) attitude, and (3) behavior. Part IV deals with AIDS specifically.

***Part I: Knowledge***

Select one answer per question:

1. For good hygiene and prevention of sexually transmitted diseases, women should:
   a. use a vaginal spray regularly
   b. take a medicinal douche regularly, especially after intercourse
   c. ignore bad smells that come from her genitals
   d. wash the vulva with soap and warm water during a bath or shower
   e. use external pads during menstrual periods
2. Changes in methods of choice in birth-control practice have been credited with part of the rise in STD rates. Which of the following is thought to be most responsible for this?
   a. use of IUDs, which may be expelled
   b. so many women using the pill
   c. marked reduction in condom use
   d. the use of spermicidal jellies and foams
   e. use of a diaphragm
3. The most common STD is:
   a. syphilis
   b. pelvic inflammatory disease
   c. herpes simplex
   d. nongonococcal urethritis
   e. gonorrhea
4. The first syphilis symptom in males is:
   a. a body rash
   b. pus and pain when urinating
   c. the chancre
   d. intolerable itching
   e. blisters on the sex organs
5. Herpes simplex makes a woman susceptible to:
   a. diabetes
   b. cervical cancer
   c. heart disease
   d. cirrhosis of the liver
   e. influenza
6. The incubation period (that is, the time between infection and appearance of symptoms) in persons with symptomatic syphilis is about:
   a. 3 to 4 days
   b. 25 days
   c. 10 to 90 days
   d. 3 to 4 weeks
   e. 1 to 4 months

7. Diagnosis of nongonococcal urethritis includes:
   a. appearance of discharge
   b. pain on urination
   c. history of sexual exposure
   d. examination of sexual partners
   e. all of the above

***Part II: Attitude***

1. What do you feel is the major cause of the currently high rate of STDs?
   a. drug/alcohol use
   b. changing sexual values
   c. improved birth control methods
   d. lack of education
   e. promiscuity and irresponsibility
   f. breakdown in morals
   g. other
2. STD education is the responsibility of:
   a. the immediate family
   b. the private physician
   c. the public and private schools
   d. public health agencies
   e. mass media (radio, television)
   f. no one—not really needed
   g. other
3. The most effective single method of reducing STDs would be to:
   a. reduce sexual promiscuity
   b. promote protection methods (develop vaccine, use of condoms, and so on)
   c. increase education
   d. pass stricter pornography laws
   e. control prostitution
   f. establish more free clinics
   g. other
4. People who get STDs can best be described as:
   a. victimized
   b. self-centered
   c. indiscriminate (promiscuous)
   d. oversexed
   e. lower class
   f. ignorant
   g. other
5. Some public agencies diagnose and treat STDs in youths (under age 18) without parents' knowledge or permission. This is:
   a. an infringement of parents' rights
   b. illegal (or should be)
   c. prompting youths to risk getting STDs
   d. probably a way to help control STDs
   e. a very good way to help youth
   f. supporting sexual activity in youth
   g. other

## SELF-SURVEY

6. If schools are going to teach about STDs, the best place for it is:
   a. K–3
   b. 4–6
   c. 7–12
   d. 10–12
   e. all grade levels
   f. college level
   g. other
7. The agencies or groups that have an essential role if we are to solve the STD problem are:
   a. churches
   b. schools
   c. public health agencies
   d. medical profession
   e. susceptible families
   f. general hospitals
   g. other

***Part III: Behavior***

1. Your lover informs you that he or she has gonorrhea. What do you do?
   a. become furiously angry
   b. end the relationship
   c. thank the person for his or her honesty
   d. talk about real issues facing the relationship
   e. experience shock
   f. seek diagnosis and treatment
   g. other
2. Given your choice, if you thought you had gonorrhea, where would you go for treatment?
   a. personal physician
   b. emergency room at hospital
   c. public health clinic
   d. free medical clinic
   e. drug store
   f. school nurse
   g. other
3. A free STD clinic is being proposed for your neighborhood. Both residents and nonresidents will be eligible for diagnosis and treatment. You will most likely take the position:
   a. we need one
   b. put it someplace else
   c. leave treating STDs to hospitals and private doctors
   d. limit to residents over age 18
   e. would not bother to take a position
   f. we need one, but charge fees
   g. other
4. Not knowing your bedpartner, you insist on:
   a. contraception before STD prevention
   b. STD prevention before contraception
   c. both contraception and STD prevention
   d. male's using a condom
   e. only sexual intercourse (that is, no oral or anal intercourse)
   f. a physical examination of his or her sexual organs prior to sex
   g. other

5. Today you have been treated for gonorrhea; what do you now do?
   a. tell your lover
   b. have sex with someone new
   c. abstain from sex until after three separate culture tests are negative
   d. pay the clinic, never to return
   e. tell your lover after intercourse
   f. not know what to do
   g. other
6. You have discovered crabs on your pubic hair. Now what?
   a. wash all bathroom toilets
   b. apply a drug called gamma benzene hexachloride, known as Kwell
   c. purposely infect innocent victims
   d. do nothing but scratch
   e. do not wear clothing that has been worn within 24 hours
   f. warn all possible contacts
   g. other
7. You have herpes simplex. What will you tell your partner?
   a. condom should be used until desiring children
   b. both should accept fact of equal exposure
   c. nothing
   d. that, together, you should seek professional advice
   e. that the disease will go away
   f. that it's too late to worry
   g. other
8. Knowing about STDs, will you:
   a. have many sex partners
   b. be selective in your sex partners
   c. reduce your sexual activities to a few partners
   d. maintain a monogamous relationship
   e. have sex only for reproductive purposes
   f. abstain
   g. other
9. Learning about STDs will affect your behavior. How so?
   a. to be more open about STD-related problems with lover
   b. to not be promiscuous
   c. to use a condom at all times
   d. will not have an effect
   e. will continue the pickup scene
   f. to help others learn
   g. other

***Scoring***

By answering the preceding questions, you have discovered new observations about yourself in regard to STDs. Because this quiz does not cover more than an ice cube on the top of the iceberg, you should refer to your text and other materials for a complete STD discussion. In North America, prevalent STDs include gonorrhea, syphilis, nongonococcal urethritis, vaginitis, urinary tract infections, chancroid, genital warts, herpes simplex, and crabs.

***Part I: Knowledge***

The correct answers are: (1) d, (2) c, (3) e, (4) c, (5) b, (6) d, (7) c.

***Part II: Attitude***

There are no correct answers, only opinions and viewpoints. Share your answers with others and possibly you will arrive at a group consensus.

## SELF-SURVEY

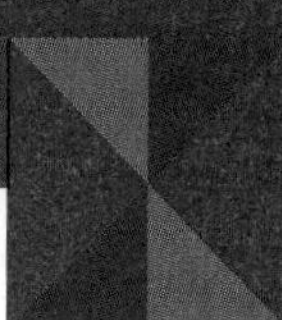

***Part III: Behavior***
Some of the answers are better than others, from a public-health viewpoint. So, while there are no correct answers in the sense of right and wrong, the list below identifies the preferred behavior: (1) c, d, f; (2) c, d; (3) a, f; (4) c, d, f; (5) a, c; (6) b, e, f; (7) b, d; (8) none; (9) a, f.

And remember, letter *g* may have been your best answer throughout these nine questions. Again, share your answers with others.

***Part IV: Do You Know Enough to Talk About AIDS?***
It's important for each of us to share what we know about AIDS with family members and others we love. Knowledge and understanding are the best weapons we have against the disease.

| | True | False |
|---|---|---|
| 1. If you are not in a "high risk group," you still need to be concerned about AIDS. | _______ | _______ |
| 2. Condoms are an effective, but not foolproof, way to prevent the spread of HIV. | _______ | _______ |
| 3. You can't tell by looking that someone is HIV-positive. | _______ | _______ |
| 4. If you think you've been exposed to HIV, you should get an HIV antibody test. | _______ | _______ |
| 5. People who provide help for someone with AIDS are not personally at risk for getting the disease. | _______ | _______ |

6. HIV is not spread through:
   a. insect bites
   b. casual contact
   c. sharing drug needles
   d. sexual intercourse

***Part IV: AIDS***

1. True. It's risky behavior that puts you at risk for HIV infection, regardless of the group you belong to.
2. True. However, the most effective preventive measure against AIDS is not having sex or shooting drugs.
3. True. You cannot tell by looking if someone is infected. The virus by itself is completely invisible. Symptoms may first appear years after someone has been infected.
4. True. You should be counseled about getting an HIV antibody test if you have been engaging in risky behavior or think you have been exposed to the virus. There is no reason to be tested if you don't engage in this behavior.
5. True. You won't get HIV infection by helping someone who has the disease.
6. a and b. HIV is not spread by insects, kissing, tears, or casual contact.

SOURCE, parts I–III: Cox et al. *Wellness RSVP.* 1986.
SOURCE, part IV: *Understanding AIDS: A Message from the Surgeon General.* Department of Health and Human Services, 1989.

of faulty equipment or test tubes. Some workers had open wounds and were not wearing protective gloves. According to the CDC, health-care workers who accidentally stick themselves with HIV-contaminated needles have less than a 1 percent chance of contracting HIV.

**STRATEGY FOR CHANGE**

**What Doesn't Cause AIDS**

According to the U.S. Surgeon General, you do not have to worry about getting AIDS in any of the following ways:[17]

- You won't get HIV through everyday contact

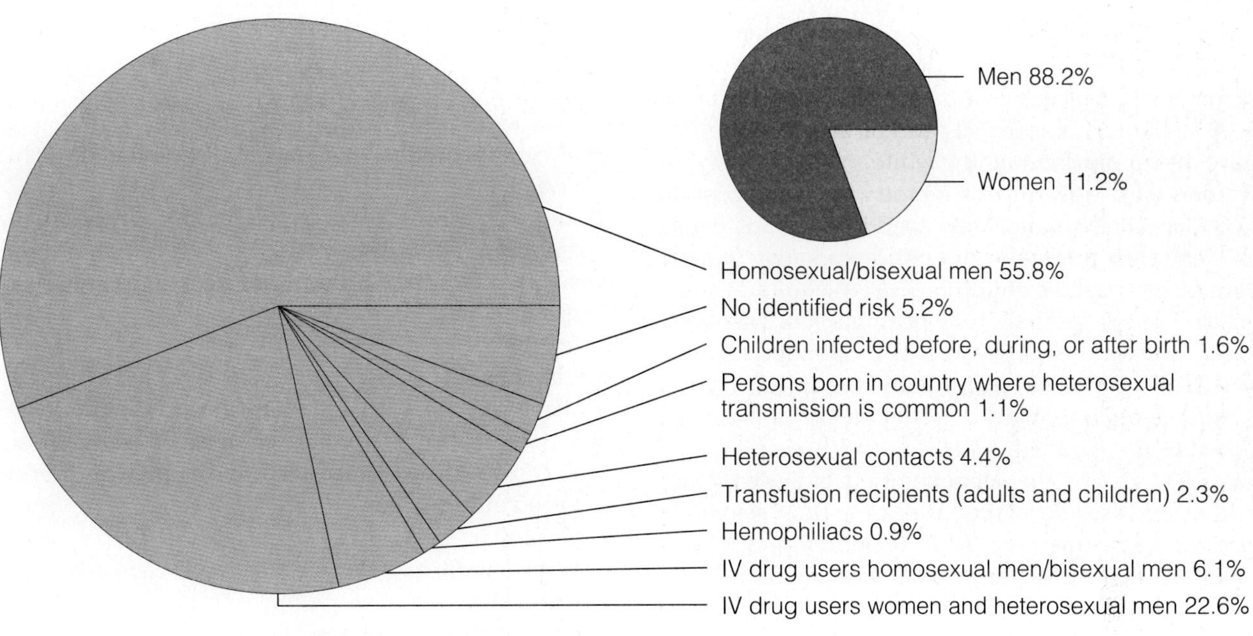


SOURCE: Centers for Disease Control, Morbidity and Mortality Weekly Report, March 2, 1990.

**FIGURE 15-3** Who has AIDS?

with the people around you in school, in the workplace, at parties, child care centers, or stores.

- You won't get it by swimming in a pool, even if someone in the pool is infected with HIV.
- Students attending school with someone infected with HIV are not in danger from casual contact.
- You won't get HIV from a mosquito bite. HIV is not transmitted through a mosquito's salivary glands as are other diseases such as malaria or yellow fever. You won't get it from bedbugs, lice, flies, or other insects, either.
- You won't get HIV from saliva, sweat, tears, urine or a bowel movement. You won't get HIV from a kiss.
- You won't get HIV from clothes, a telephone, or from a toilet seat. It can't be passed by using a glass or eating utensils that someone infected with HIV has used.
- You won't get the virus by being on a bus, train, or crowded elevator with a person who is infected with HIV or who has AIDS.

SOURCE: "Understanding AIDS: A Message from the Surgeon General."

## Who Gets AIDS?

The groups at risk for AIDS vary geographically. As Figure 15-3 shows, most AIDS patients in the United States fit into the following categories:

- homosexual and bisexual men (or men who have had sex with another man since the mid-1970s)
- people who inject illegal IV drugs or have done so in the past
- homosexuals and bisexuals who are also IV drug abusers
- people who received blood transfusions between 1978 and 1985
- hemophiliacs who have received blood-clotting products before 1985
- sexual partners of people infected with the AIDS virus
- infants of high-risk or infected mothers

About 5 percent of all AIDS patients do not fit into any of these groups, nor will everyone in the listed categories who is exposed to the virus be infected. Some people seem more genetically resistant to infection. A history of genital infections, particularly past exposure to hepatitis B virus, may increase susceptibility. HIV carriers may become more infectious—and, therefore, more likely to transmit the virus—the longer they have the infection.

AIDS has taken a devastating toll on some economically disadvantaged minorities. AIDS patients with a history of IV drug use have been predominantly black and Hispanic; homosexuals and bisexuals with AIDS have been predominantly white. The majority of women with AIDS in this country are young, poor, and black or Hispanic. Most used intravenous drugs or slept with men who did. Approximately 90 percent of HIV-positive children who've acquired the virus from their mothers have been black or Hispanic.

Not everyone infected with HIV develops AIDS or **pre-AIDS** (also called **AIDS-related complex,** or **ARC**). Scientists once thought only 10 percent of those exposed to HIV would ever develop the disease, but the virus has an average latency period of eleven years and more cases developed over time than scientists expected. Treatment with AZT (azidothymidine) can delay the onset of AIDS. In 1990 federal officials approved the use of AZT for individuals who test positive for HIV, have no symptoms, and show specific changes in their immune cells.[18]

**STRATEGY FOR CHANGE**

**Reducing Your Risk**

You can take practical steps to minimize your risk of HIV infection and AIDS:

- Always practice safer-sex measures, such as using condoms. (See Chapter 7 for other specific guidelines.)
- If you're scheduled for surgery, donate your own blood prior to the operation to eliminate the need for donor transfusions.
- If your job may put you in jeopardy because of possible contact with the blood of HIV-positive individuals, follow safety precautions to avoid contamination.
- Avoid casual, multiple sexual contacts.
- Don't share toothbrushes, razors, or other implements that could be contaminated with the blood of anyone who might be infected with HIV.
- If you use intravenous drugs, do not share needles.

## Pre-AIDS or Symptomatic HIV Infection

Symptoms of pre-AIDS, or ARC, include a loss of appetite and weight; diarrhea; night sweats; and swollen lymph nodes in the neck, armpits, or groin. Anyone with one or more of these symptoms for more than two weeks should see a doctor. In rare cases patients with pre-AIDS return to normal health. However, most people with pre-AIDS eventually develop a full-blown case of AIDS.

## AIDS As an Illness

The symptoms of AIDS are similar to those of pre-AIDS:

- fevers of more than 100 degrees Fahrenheit or night sweats
- for no apparent reason, a weight loss of more than 10 pounds in two months
- swollen lymph glands in the neck, underarm, or groin
- fatigue
- diarrhea
- white spots or unusual blemishes in the mouth
- a herpes sore that won't go away or purplish or dark red lumps that may appear anywhere and keep getting larger
- weakness
- a dry cough
- headaches
- coordination problems
- weakness in the arms or legs
- confusion
- infections of the skin and chest

In addition to these symptoms, AIDS patients develop life-threatening infections (such as pneumocystis pneumonia), cancer (such as Kaposi's sarcoma), wasting syndrome, and other diseases, because their immune systems are so severely weakened. AIDS also causes serious damage to the brain and nervous system.

A loss of mental function may appear long before other symptoms. Tests conducted on infected but apparently healthy men have revealed impaired coordination, problems in thinking, or abnormal brain scans. The majority of people with AIDS eventually develop symptoms such as memory loss, an impaired ability to speak and think, and dementia (confusion and impaired thinking).

### The HIV Antibody Test

The HIV antibody does not detect HIV itself, but antibodies that the body forms in response to exposure to HIV. A negative result indicates no exposure to HIV 3 to 6 months prior to testing: It can take that long for the body to produce the telltale antibodies.

The standard blood tests used to detect infection by HIV are the *enzyme immunoassay* (ELISA, or EIA)

**pre-AIDS** A group of symptoms that develop in some individuals exposed to the AIDS virus.
**AIDS-related complex (ARC)** See *pre-AIDS*.

HEALTH SPOTLIGHT

## A Message About AIDS

These are excerpts from a videotaped talk from James Hurley, a real-estate lawyer from Bloomfield, Connecticut, who was dying of AIDS:

"I caught AIDS, so to speak, out of ignorance; and I caught it at a time when no one else knew about it. It galls me when I hear one of these reporters mention that the babies who contract AIDS through their mothers are the *innocent* victims of AIDS, as though the rest of us are somehow *guilty* victims. There's no such thing as an innocent or guilty victim of AIDS. Either you have AIDS or you don't have AIDS. It doesn't make any difference how it was contracted.

"To have it is to have a disease that will end your life. That *anyone* has AIDS is a tragedy; but we live in a society that very much wanted to believe that this was a gay disease—and somehow if it's a gay disease, and gay people are just going to kill themselves off, it won't affect the rest of us, or what the *New York Times* would call "the general population." It hurts me very deeply to read that I'm not part of the general population. It hurts me very deeply to read that it's not important that I have AIDS, because it's not affecting most people. . . .

"Many *good* things have happened to me because of having contracted AIDS. . . . AIDS has opened me to a lot of the power of living. . . . There isn't time for cross words. There is a preciousness that comes into life, once one begins to grab every day as it comes along. There's a sadness, too; there are times when I just stop and I cry, and I can't believe how good life is today, and it's going to end—uh—in the foreseeable future. . . .

"I hope that one thing that you take from this is the sense that every human life is of value. The statistics about AIDS are irrelevant. Whether it's 30,000 here, or 600 in England, or one in Japan, it's all irrelevant. Whether a person who has AIDS is an IV drug user, or contracted it in the womb, or is a mother who contracted it from a husband, or is a gay man doesn't matter. That we make this matter tells us something about ourselves, not about the person suffering from AIDS—and we will, I hope, be mindful of the kind of compassion that's needed for anyone who is suffering.

"The issues are such simple issues, once you have AIDS, and once you experience blood transfusions on a regular basis and chemotherapy and oxygen tanks in the bedroom in case you can't breathe. Monday morning, I got up; and I couldn't walk for 2 hours. The pain in my bones was so great that I just couldn't be on my feet—and once you begin to deal with these symptoms on a daily basis, it all looks crazy that people want to sit around and discuss what we should do about AIDS. It's too late. These are arguments that we should have had a few years ago. There's no doubt about how AIDS is passed. There's no doubt in my mind about how it was passed to me. What we should be doing is educating people.

"I'm going to stop here, but I want to close by just saying: I have AIDS, and AIDS is not my problem any longer. AIDS is *your* problem, and I hope you'll do something about it."

Ten days later, Hurley died. He was 33 years old.

SOURCE: "I'm Dying—AIDS Is Your Problem Now," *Newsweek*, August 10, 1987.

and the Western Blot. The ELISA detects protein antibodies produced against particles of HIV by an infected individual's immune system. The *Western Blot* is a more accurate and expensive test than the ELISA, and it is done to confirm the results of a positive ELISA.

When perfectly performed, both tests can detect antibodies in 99.6 percent of infected persons and can correctly give negative results in uninfected persons at least 99 percent of the time. However, actual percentages of false readings are higher.

Laboratories testing for HIV can have such a high error rate that, in some low-risk groups, nine out of ten positive findings are wrong, according to the congressional Office of Technology Assessment. The labs may also report false negatives for as many as 10 percent of individuals infected with the virus.[19] Most centers repeat the test if the initial results are positive. Experienced counselors can refer men and women with two positive readings to physicians who specialize in AIDS-related problems.

Health officials recommend HIV testing for those in the following groups:

- men who have had sex with a man in the last ten years
- anyone who uses IV drugs and has shared needles or has had sex with someone who has done so
- anyone who has had sex with prostitutes in the last ten years
- women who've had sex with bisexual men
- anyone who's had sex with someone from a country with a high incidence of AIDS (for example, Haiti or central Africa)
- individuals who've had multiple anonymous sex partners and are worried about being infected
- anyone who received blood transfusions between 1978 and 1985 (Their sexual partners or, if they are new mothers, their infants may also be at risk.)

### Treatment

Within twenty-one months of the discovery of HIV, the first drug that could prolong AIDS patients' survival, AZT, went from initial testing to final approval; the usual time for this process is 8.8 years. AZT has helped prolong the lives and improve the quality of life of AIDS patients. More than half of those treated with AZT regain lost weight, feel more energetic, and can think clearly again. AZT is not a cure, however. Over time its serious side effects, including anemia and bone marrow damage, can force many patients to stop using it.

In the past, AZT was reserved for desperately ill patients. However, since early treatment might improve chances for thousands of HIV-positive individuals, the FDA has approved the use of AZT to persons who test positive for HIV and have failing immune systems but no other signs of disease.

Research has led to other promising approaches, including still experimental medications such as Compound Q and therapies such as bone marrow transplants. New compounds, still undergoing testing, have proven effective in stopping HIV from multiplying in test tubes. Scientists also are more hopeful of developing a vaccine against HIV.

### The Invisible Impact of AIDS

Parents, potential sex partners, teachers, and hospital workers all have one thing in common—fear. Even though there is no evidence that HIV can be spread by casual contact, many people want to avoid all persons at risk. AIDS patients, struggling against a deadly disease with no known cure, often feel terribly isolated because friends and family are afraid to visit. Even the necessary precautions of doctors and nurses add to their feelings of being "untouchable."

**STRATEGY FOR CHANGE**

**When a Friend Has AIDS**

In our society AIDS has become so widespread among people in the prime of life that almost everyone knows someone at risk or infected by the disease. While you may feel helpless or inadequate when a friend is seriously ill, you can offer comfort:[20]

- Touch your friend. A simple squeeze of the hand or a hug can let him or her know that you care.
- Respond to your friend's emotions. Weep with your friend when he or she weeps. Laugh when your friend laughs. It's healthy to share these intimate experiences.
- Offer to help answer any letters that may be giving your friend some difficulty or that your friend may be avoiding.
- Check in with your friend's partner or roommate, who may need a break from time to time. Offer to care for the person with AIDS so the loved ones have some free time.
- It's okay to ask about the illness, but be sensitive to whether your friend wants to discuss it. You can find out by asking, "Would you like to talk about how you're feeling?" However, don't pressure.
- Bring a positive attitude. It's catching!

SOURCE: San Francisco Community Partnership on AIDS.

## SEXUALLY TRANSMITTED DISEASES

Venereal diseases (from the Latin *venus*, meaning love or lust) are more accurately called **sexually trans-**

**mitted diseases** (**STDs**). STDs are the major cause of preventable sterility in America. They have tripled the rate of ectopic (out-of-the-womb) pregnancies in women.[21] These pregnancies require surgery to remove the misplaced fetus and can be fatal to the mother if not detected early. STD complications—including miscarriage, premature delivery, and uterine infections after delivery—affect more than 100,000 women annually.

STDs strike both sexes, all classes, and all ages. However, cases occurring in teenagers between the ages of 15 and 19 outnumber the total for other groups 2 to 1. By age 25, as many as half of all young people may develop an STD.[22,23] The incidence of STDs among homosexuals is particularly high. In some cities 50 to 75 percent of the cases of syphilis are in homosexuals, particularly gay men. Other victims of STDs have never been sexually active: These are the unborn and newborn children who catch STDs in the womb or during birth.

Although each STD is a distinct disease, all STD pathogens like dark, warm, moist body surfaces, particularly the mucous membranes that line the reproductive organs. They hate light, cold, and dryness. It is possible to catch or have more than one STD at a time. Curing one doesn't necessarily cure another; none of the treatments even prevents another bout with the same STD. Table 15-3 presents a list of common STDs and their symptoms and treatments.

**STRATEGY FOR CHANGE**

**Avoiding STDs**

- Talk to every prospective partner directly about STDs.
- Look before you leap into bed. Any obvious sore, growth, or indication of discharge should be a warning signal of a problem your partner might not have recognized.
- Urinate a few minutes after sex to wash away germs. Soap and water have a similar effect; douching is not advised.
- Always use a latex condom or insist that your partner use one.[24] After taking off the condom, wash the penis immediately.
- Use spermicidal creams and jellies containing nonoxynol-9.

## Gonorrhea

One of the most common and dangerous sexually transmitted diseases in the United States is **gonorrhea.** Sexual contact is the primary means of transmission. Figure 15-4 shows the gonococcus microbe (microorganism), which can survive for up to eight hours outside the body and is hardier than the syphilis bacterium. An increasingly common form of transmission of gonorrhea is oral-genital contact.

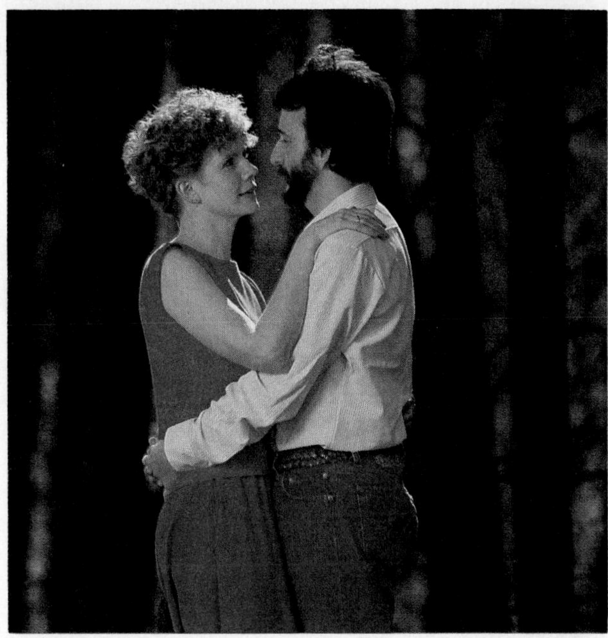

Talking about STDs is one way in which two people can show that they truly care about each other.

### Symptoms

Most men who have gonorrhea know it. Thick, yellow-white pus oozes from the penis; urination causes a burning sensation. These symptoms usually develop 2 to 9 days after sexual contact. Men have a good reason to seek help: It hurts too much not to.

Women may also experience discharge and burning on urination. However, as many as nine out of ten infected women have no symptoms at all. The gonococcus can live in the vagina, cervix, and fallopian tubes for months, even years, and continue to infect the woman's sexual partners. Approximately 5 percent of sexually active American women have positive gonorrhea cultures and are unaware that they are silent carriers and victims.

### Complications

If left untreated in men or women, gonorrhea spreads through the urinary-genital tract. In women, the inflammation travels from the vagina and cervix, through the uterus, and to the fallopian tubes and ovaries. The pain and fever are similar to those caused by

**sexually transmitted disease (STD)** Any of a number of diseases that are acquired through sexual contact.
**gonorrhea** A sexually transmitted disease caused by the bacteria *Neisseria gonorrhea;* symptoms in men include discharge from the penis; women may be asymptomatic.

**TABLE 15-3** Common STDs: Mode of Transmission, Symptoms, and Treatment

| STD | TRANSMISSION | SYMPTOMS | TREATMENT |
|---|---|---|---|
| Candidiasis (yeast infection) | The *Candida albicans* fungus may accelerate growth when the chemical balance of the vagina is disturbed; it may also be transmitted through sexual interaction. | White, "cheesy" discharge; irritation of vaginal and vulvar tissue. | Vaginal suppositories or cream, such as clotrimazole, nystatin, and miconazole |
| Trichomoniasis | The protozoan parasite *Trichomonas vaginalis* is passed through genital sexual contact or less frequently by towels, toilet seats, or bathtubs used by an infected person. | White or yellow vaginal discharge with an unpleasant odor; vulva is sore and irritated. | Metronidazole (Flagyl), effective for both sexes |
| Chlamydial infection | The *Chlamydia trachomatis* bacterium is transmitted primarily through sexual contact. It may also be spread by fingers from one body site to another. | In men, chlamydial infection of the urethra may cause a discharge and burning during urination. *Chlamydia*-caused epididymitis may produce a sense of heaviness in the affected testicle(s), inflammation of the scrotal skin, and painful swelling at the bottom of the testicle. In women, PID caused by *Chlamydia* may include disrupted menstrual periods, abdominal pain, elevated temperature, nausea, vomiting, and headache. | Tetracycline, doxycycline, erythromycin, or trimethoprim-sulfamethoxazole |
| Gonorrhea ("clap") | The *Neisseria gonorrhoeae* bacterium ("gonococcus") is spread through genital, oral-genital, or genital-anal contact. | Most common symptoms in men are a cloudy discharge from the penis and burning sensations during urination. If disease is untreated, complications may include inflammation of scrotal skin and swelling at base of the testicle. In women, some green or yellowish discharge is produced but commonly remains undetected. At a later stage, PID may develop. | Tetracycline or doxycycline is usually effective |
| Syphilis | The *Treponema pallidum* bacterium ("spirochete") is transmitted from open lesions during genital, oral-genital, or genital-anal contact. | *Primary stage:* A painless chancre appears at the site where the spirochetes entered the body. *Secondary stage:* The chancre disappears and a generalized skin rash develops. *Latent stage:* There may be no observable symptoms. *Tertiary stage:* Heart failure, blindness, mental disturbance, and many other symptoms may occur. Death may result. | Benzathine penicillin, tetracycline, or erythromycin |

**TABLE 15-3** Common STDs: Mode of Transmission, Symptoms, and Treatment *(continued)*

| STD | TRANSMISSION | SYMPTOMS | TREATMENT |
|---|---|---|---|
| Pubic lice ("crabs") | *Phthirus pubis,* the pubic louse, is spread easily through body contact or through shared clothing or bedding. | Persistent itching. Lice are visible and may often be located in pubic hair or other body hair. | Preparations such as A-200 pyrinate or Kwell (gamma benzene hexachloride) |
| Nongonococcal urethritis (NGU) | Primary causes are believed to be the bacteria *Chlamydia trachomatis* and *Ureaplasma urealyticum,* most commonly transmitted in coitus. Some NGU may result from allergic reactions or from *Trichomonas* infection. | Inflammation of the urethral tube. A man has a discharge from the penis and irritation during urination. A woman may have a mild discharge of pus from the vagina but often shows no symptoms. | Tetracycline, doxycycline, or erythromycin |
| Herpes | The genital herpes virus (HSV-2) appears to be transmitted primarily by vaginal, oral-genital, or anal sexual intercourse. The oral herpes virus (HSV-1) is transmitted primarily by kissing. | Small, red, painful bumps (papules) appear in the region of the genitals (genital herpes) or mouth (oral herpes). The papules become painful blisters that eventually rupture to form wet, open sores. | No known cure; a variety of treatments may reduce symptoms; oral acyclovir (Zovirax) promotes healing and suppresses recurrent outbreaks |
| Viral hepatitis | The hepatitis B virus may be transmitted by blood, semen, vaginal secretions, and saliva. Manual, oral, or penile stimulation of the anus are strongly associated with the spread of this virus. Hepatitis A seems to be primarily spread via the fecal-oral route. Oral-anal sexual contact is a common mode for transmission of hepatitis A. | Vary from nonexistent to mild, flulike symptoms to an incapacitating illness characterized by high fever, vomiting, and severe abdominal pain. | No specific therapy; treatment generally consists of bed rest and adequate fluid intake |
| Human papilloma virus (genital warts) | HPV is spread primarily through genital, anal, or oral-genital interaction. | Warts are hard and yellow-gray on dry skin areas; soft pinkish red, and cauliflowerlike on moist areas. | Topical agents like podophylln, cauterization, freezing, surgical removal, or vaporization by carbon dioxide laser |
| Acquired immunodeficiency syndrome (AIDS) | Blood and semen are the major vehicles for transmitting HIV, which attacks the immune system. It appears to be passed primarily through sexual contact or by needle sharing among IV drug abusers. | Vary with the type of cancer or opportunistic infections that afflict a person with HIV. Common symptoms include fevers, night sweats, weight loss, loss of appetite, fatigue, swollen lymph nodes, diarrhea and/or bloody stools, atypical bruising or bleeding, skin rashes, headache, chronic cough, a whitish coating on the tongue or throat. | At present, therapy focuses on specific treatment(s) of opportunistic infections and tumors: some antiviral drugs, such as AZT, slow progression of AIDS and extend patients' lives |

SOURCE: Crooks, Robert and Karla Bauer. *Our Sexuality, Fourth Edition,* Benjamin/Cummings, 1990.

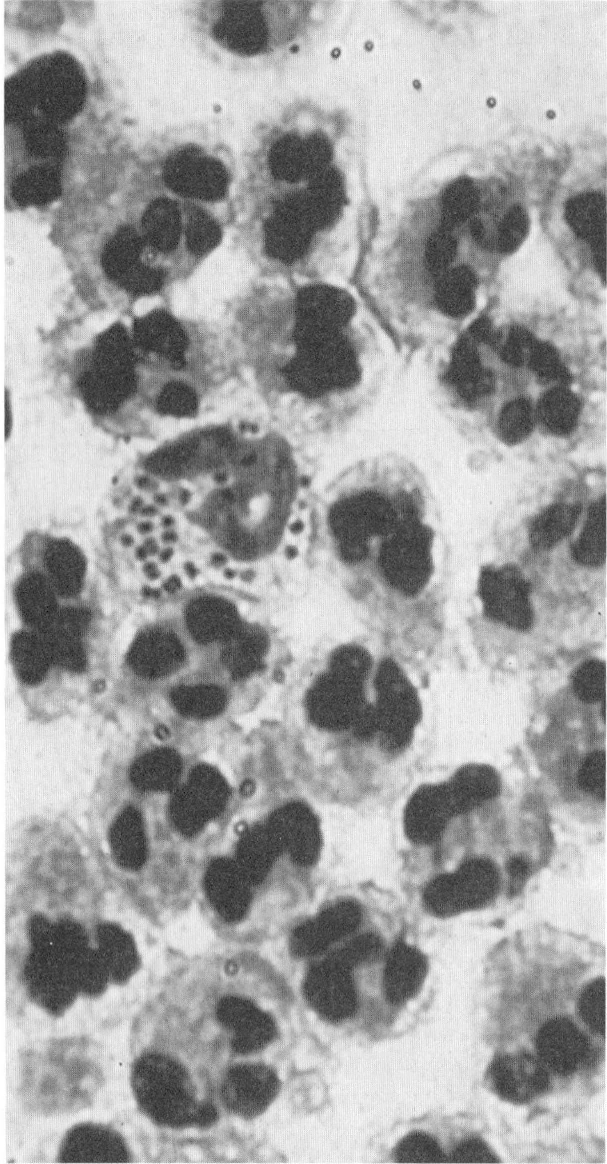

**FIGURE 15-4** The bacteria that cause gonorrhea, *Neisseria gonorrhea,* usually occur in pairs, as shown here.

stomach upset, and a woman may dismiss the symptoms. Eventually these symptoms diminish, even though the disease spreads to the entire pelvis. Pus may ooze from the fallopian tubes or ovaries and into the peritoneum (the lining of the abdominal cavity), sometimes causing serious inflammation. However, this, too, can subside in a few weeks.

Gonorrhea can eventually cause a chronic pelvic infection that lasts for years and damages the reproductive organs. Gonorrhea is the leading cause of sterility in women. **Pelvic inflammatory disease (PID),** a massive infection of the abdomen and pelvis, is also a serious complication of gonorrhea.

For women with gonorrhea who become pregnant, gonorrhea is a threat to the newborn. It can infect the infant's external genitals and cause a serious form of conjunctivitis, an inflammation of the eye that may lead to blindness. As a preventive step, newborns may have silver nitrate or penicillin dropped into their eyes at birth.

In men, untreated gonorrhea spreads to the prostate gland, testicles, bladder, and kidneys. Among the serious complications are urinary obstruction, sterility caused by blockage of the vas deferens, and a painful downward curvature of the penis during erection.

In both sexes, gonorrhea can develop into a serious, even fatal, systemic, blood-borne infection that can cause arthritis in the joints, attack the heart muscle and lining, cause a brain disease called meningitis, and attack the skin and other organs.

### Diagnosis and Treatment

Although a blood test has been developed for gonorrhea, the tried-and-true method of diagnosis is still a microscopic study and analysis of cultures from the male's urethra, the female's cervix, and the throat and anus of both sexes. Penicillin is the most common treatment. Because of their dose or type, antibiotics taken for other reasons may not affect or cure gonorrhea. You cannot develop immunity to gonorrhea; within days of recovering from one case, you can catch another.

A grave and increasing problem is the spread of penicillin-resistant gonorrhea. Following reports that the number of cases had risen sharply, the CDC has recommended routine tests to detect this dangerous gonorrhea.

## Syphilis

**Syphilis** is caused by a corkscrew-shaped, spiral bacterium (spirochete) called *Treponema pallidum,* a frail microorganism that dies in seconds if dried or chilled (see Figure 15-5). However, it grows quickly in the warm, moist tissues of the body, particularly in the mucous membranes of the genital tract. Entering the

**pelvic inflammatory disease (PID)** An inflammation of the internal female genital tract; characterized by abdominal pain, fever, and tenderness of the cervix.

**syphilis** A sexually transmitted disease caused by the bacteria *Treponema pallidum* and characterized by early sores, a latent period, and a final period of life-threatening symptoms, including brain damage and heart failure.

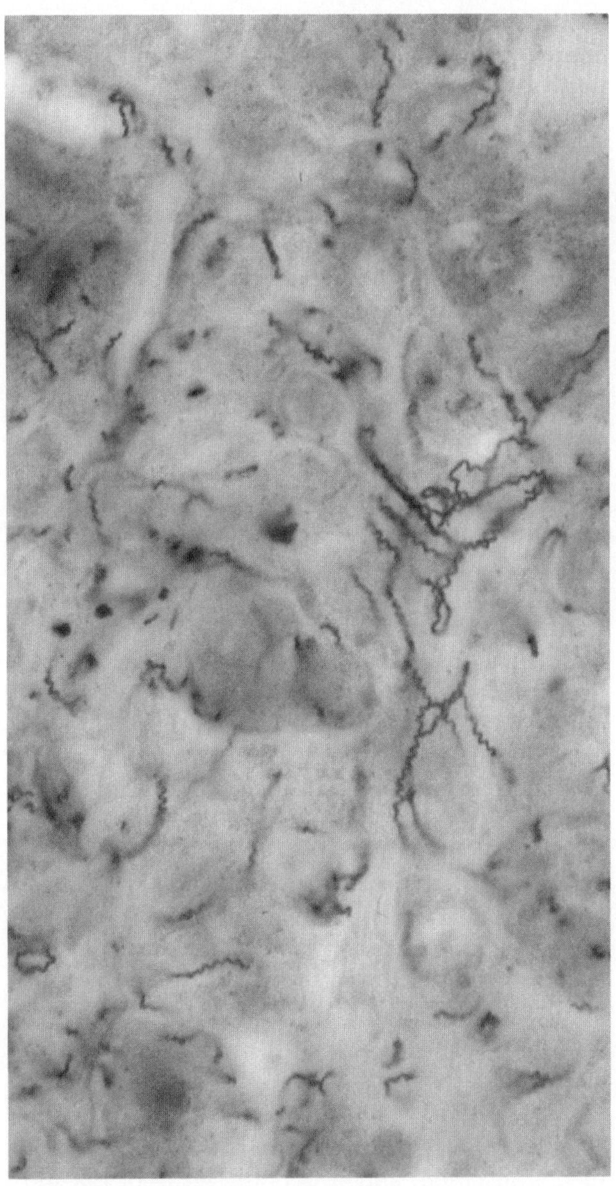

**FIGURE 15-5** A single corkscrew-shaped cell of *Treponema pallidum*, the causative bacteria of syphilis.

body through any tiny break in the skin, the microbe burrows its way to the bloodstream. Kissing, oral-genital contact, and intercourse are virtually the only means of transmission.[25]

### Stages

There are four clearly identifiable stages of syphilis.

**Primary Syphilis** The first sign of syphilis is a lesion, or **chancre** (pronounced "shank-er"), an open lump or crater the size of a dime or smaller, filled with spirochetes. The incubation period before its appearance ranges from 10 to 90 days; 3 to 4 weeks is average. The chancre appears exactly where the spirochete entered the body: in the mouth or throat or vagina or rectum or penis. Any contact with it is likely to result in infection.

**Secondary Syphilis** Anywhere from 1 to 12 months after the chancre's appearance, secondary-stage symptoms may appear. Some people have no symptoms. Some develop a skin rash or a small, flat rash in moist regions on the skin; whitish patches on the mucous membranes of the mouth or throat; temporary baldness; low-grade fever; headache; swollen glands; or large, moist sores around the mouth and genitals. These are loaded with spirochetes; contact with them, through kissing or intercourse, may transmit the infection. Symptoms may last for several days or several months. Even without treatment, they eventually disappear as the syphilis microbes go into hiding.

**Latent Syphilis** Although there are no signs or symptoms, no sores or rashes at this stage, the spirochetes are invading various organs inside the body, including the heart and brain. For 2 to 4 years, there may be recurring infectious and highly contagious lesions of the skin or mucous membranes. However, syphilis loses its infectiousness as it progresses: After the first two years, a person rarely transmits syphilis through intercourse.

After four years, even congenital syphilis is rarely transmitted. Until this stage of the disease, however, a pregnant woman can pass syphilis to her unborn child. If the fetus is infected in its fourth month, it may die or may be deformed. If infected late in pregnancy, the child may show no signs of infection for months or years after birth, but he or she may then become disabled with the symptoms of late syphilis.

**Late Syphilis** From 10 to 20 years after the beginning of the latent period, the most serious symptoms of syphilis emerge, generally in the organs in which the spirochetes settled during latency. Victims of late syphilis may die of a ruptured aorta or of other heart damage or may have progressive brain or spinal cord damage, eventually leading to blindness, insanity, or paralysis. Because of modern treatment, syphilis that has progressed to this stage has become increasingly rare.

**chancre** A sore or ulcer at the entry point of a pathogen; the first sign of syphilis.

### Diagnosis and Treatment

Early diagnosis can lead to a complete cure. The best diagnostic technique is a blood test called a VDRL. However, it may be positive only during the secondary stage of the disease, when the spirochetes have reached the bloodstream. The earlier treatment begins, the more effective it is.

Penicillin is the drug of choice for treatment; larger doses are required than for gonorrhea. It has become common practice to check gonorrhea victims for syphilis, to make sure that the dose of penicillin prescribed is strong enough to wipe out both.

## Chlamydia and Nongonococcal Urethritis

The most common sexually transmitted bacteria among college students is **chlamydia.** Chlamydia causes up to half of all cases of **nongonococcal urethritis** (**NGU**), inflammation of the urethra not caused by gonorrhea. Public health officials fear that chlamydia may be even more common than estimated—and spreading. Those in the following groups are at highest risk:

- those 24 years of age or younger—chlamydia is widespread in young adults
- individuals who have engaged in sex with one or more new partners within the preceding two months
- users of birth control pills or other nonbarrier methods

### Symptoms

Men with chlamydia may experience pain during urination and a clear, watery, mucoid discharge from the penis. In the past, these symptoms usually indicated gonorrhea; now chlamydia is the more common culprit. Men with NGU develop symptoms similar to those of gonorrhea, including discharge from the penis and mild burning during urination.

In women, chlamydia causes about half of all cases of cervicitis (infection of the cervix). From 3 to 5 percent of all young, healthy women have chlamydia in their cervices, as do 5 to 10 percent of pregnant women and 25 percent of women seeking treatment at STD clinics. Chlamydia is hard to detect because most women experience no symptoms.

Women with NGU are generally unaware of the disease until informed that their sexual partners have it, because women usually experience no symptoms. (Occasionally they develop some itching, vaginal discharge, or burning on urination.)

### Complications

In men, untreated chlamydia can cause an infection of the epididymis, the tube that leads out of the testicle, or rectal infection as a result of anal intercourse. In women, chlamydia is most likely to travel up into the uterus. From 60 to 70 percent of infected mothers pass the organism to their babies during birth, resulting in eye infections and chlamydial pneumonia, which affects 30,000 newborns every year.

Chlamydia, which can travel into the fallopian tubes or ovaries, may account for 250,000 to 500,000 cases of PID each year. Because the symptoms, even in men, are relatively mild, victims often forgo treatment. The infection often bounces back and forth, or "ping-pongs," between sexual partners.

### Diagnosis and Treatment

Rapid diagnostic tests, newly available around the country, can detect chlamydia much more quickly and accurately than in the past. The new techniques "tag" the bacteria so they can be detected by looking at a slide under a special microscope. Many physicians recommend testing for any woman who has more than one partner.

Antibiotics such as tetracycline and erythromycin are the primary treatments for chlamydia. For NGU, the usual antibiotics are tetracycline, doxycycline, or erythromycin. If untreated, NGU can spread to the prostate and epididymis in men, and to the cervix and fallopian tubes in women.

## Herpes Simplex

The word *herpes* comes from the Greek word that means to creep, and it denotes some of the most common viral infections in man. Characteristically, **herpes simplex** causes blisters on the skin or mucous membranes. Once a person has contracted herpes, it doesn't ever go away completely, although it may go into long latent periods. Attacks diminish in frequency and severity over time.

---

**chlamydia** A sexually transmitted disease caused by *Chlamydia trachomatis,* which is often asymptomatic in women but sometimes characterized by urinary pain; if undetected and untreated, may result in pelvic inflammatory disease.
**nongonococcal urethritis** (**NGU**) Inflammation of the urethra; caused by organisms other than the gonorrhea bacteria.
**herpes simplex** A condition caused by one of the herpes viruses and characterized by lesions of the skin or mucous membranes; herpes virus Type 2 is sexually transmitted and causes genital blisters or sores.

Herpes simplex comes in two varieties: Generally, Type 1 herpes causes cold sores and fever blisters. Type 2 herpes causes genital lesions. Each year half a million Americans develop the itching genital blisters that are characteristic of the disease sometimes dubbed lovers' leprosy, joining an estimated 20 million who already have herpes. As recently as ten years ago, doctors estimated that 5 percent of the sexually active population had been exposed to herpes; now 30 percent have been exposed. In 1990, University of Washington researchers reported in the *Journal of the American Medical Association* that—contrary to what they had believed—women with genital herpes can spread the virus even when they have no obvious signs of the disease.[26]

Women with Type 2 herpes are 8 times more likely to develop cervical cancer than are uninfected women and should have a Pap smear twice a year. Each year 250 to 500 babies in the U.S. develop severe herpes infection as a result of exposure before or at birth. One of four dies or suffers a severe deformity. Obstetricians generally recommend cesarean delivery for women with herpes infections that are active when the women go into labor.

### Symptoms

Type 2 herpes has been described as cold sores of the genitals. It appears as a series of very painful blisters on the penis or inside the vagina or cervix. The blisters may also appear in the pubic area, on the buttocks, or on the thighs. With the increase of oral-genital sex, some doctors report finding Type 2 lesions in the mouth and throat. The first blisters persist for 2 to 4 weeks and then disappear.

The virus that causes herpes never entirely goes away; it retreats to nerves near the lower spinal cord, where it remains for the life of the victim. The sores can return without warning weeks, months, or even years after the first occurrence, often during menstruation or times of stress or with sudden changes in body temperature. Herpes has a strong psychological effect; many victims feel shame, guilt, and even depression.

### Treatment

What can you do for herpes? For relief of symptoms, apply a mild anesthetic cream or a compress of cold water, skim milk, or warm salt water. Avoid heat, including that produced by hot baths and nylon underwear. In recent years physicians have tried a host of treatments, including topical ointments, various vaccines, exposure to light, and ultrasonic waves—all with little success. Some have used laser therapy to vaporize the lesions. Acyclovir (ACV), a prescription drug, has proven effective in treating and controlling herpes, but it does not kill the virus.

Because active sores mean a definite risk of transmission, it's always a good idea to refrain from intercourse when they're present. Unfortunately, people with herpes may become infectious before a recurring sore becomes visible. Usually there are warning or prodromal signs, such as a slight tingling or itchy feeling a day or two before a flare-up. People with herpes should watch for these early signals to prevent transmitting the disease to others.

## Human Papilloma Virus

Infection with human papilloma virus (HPV), a pathogen that causes genital warts and increases the risk of cervical cancer, is spreading so rapidly that some epidemiologists have dubbed it "*the* STD of the '90s." In some cities, transmission of HPV is outpacing the spread of herpes, chlamydia, syphilis, and gonorrhea.

More than half of HPV-infected individuals do not develop any symptoms. However, genital warts may appear several months after contact with an infected individual. They are treated by freezing, cauterization, chemicals, or surgical removal.

Five of the fifty-six papilloma viruses known to cause warts have been linked to cervical cancer. HPV infection greatly increases a woman's risk of developing a precancerous condition called cervical intraepithelial neoplasia and cervical cancers. HPV transmission may be the reason why women are five times as likely to get cervical cancer if their steady sexual partner has had twenty or more lovers.[27]

The Pap smear, the standard diagnostic test for cervical cancer, does not pick up HPV infection. A newer, more specific test can identify HPV soon after it enters the body. Women who test positive should undergo checkups for cervical changes every 6 to 12 months. If precancerous cells develop, surgery or laser treatment can prevent further growth.

HPV, which is carried in lesions on the penis or cervix, can also cause genital warts in a woman's sex partner and increase his risk of cancer of the penis. HPV-infected men, who may not develop any symptoms, can spread the infection to other partners.

## Chancroid

A **chancroid** is a soft, painful sore or localized infection usually acquired through sexual contact. Half

**chanchroid** A soft, painful sore or localized infection usually acquired through sexual contact.

heal by themselves. The other half spread to the lymph glands near the ulcer, where large amounts of pus can accumulate and destroy much of the local tissue. Chancroids, which are treated with antibiotics, can be prevented by keeping the genitals clean and washing with soap and water if you suspect exposure. The rate of this STD is rapidly increasing.[28,29]

**STRATEGY FOR CHANGE**

**What to Do If You Have an STD**

If you suspect that you have an STD, don't feel too embarrassed to get help. Treatment relieves discomfort and prevents complications.

- Get prompt treatment by your own physician or through a clinic. Take oral medication (which may be given instead of or in addition to shots) exactly as prescribed.
- Try to figure out from who you got the STD. Be sure to inform that person, who may not be aware of the problem.
- If you have an STD, never deceive a prospective partner about it. Tell the truth—simply and clearly.
- Be sure your partner understands exactly what you have and what the risks are. Discuss the subject *before* you make love. Quiet, private settings are often best.

### Crab Lice and Scabies

Crab lice are usually found in pubic hairs, although they may migrate to any hairy areas of the body. Lice lay eggs called nits that attach to the base of the hair shaft. Irritation from lice may produce intense itching. Scratching to relieve the itching can produce sores. Scabies is caused by a mite that burrows under the skin and lays eggs that hatch and undergo many changes in the course of their life cycle. The mites cause great discomfort, including intense itching.

Lice and scabies, which are sometimes, but not always, transmitted sexually, are treated with applications of Kwell (or A-200) shampoo, which kills the adult lice but not always the nits. You must repeat treatment in seven days to kill any newly developed adults. Wash and dry or dry-clean clothing, sheets, and blankets.

## INFECTIONS OF THE REPRODUCTIVE AND URINARY SYSTEMS

Some of the most common urinary and reproductive tract infections are not spread exclusively by sexual contact.

### Yeast Infection

A yeast called *Candida albicans*, a normal inhabitant of the mouth, digestive tract, and vagina, is usually held in check. Under certain conditions, such as poor nutrition or use of antibiotics, the microbes multiply, causing burning, itching, and a whitish discharge. Common sites for the infection, which is also called moniliasis, are the vagina, vulva, penis, and mouth. Prescribed vaginal or oral medications provide effective treatment. Although yeast infections are not

**WHAT DO YOU THINK?**

How would you react if a good friend or coworker told you he or she was HIV-positive? What if you found out that your child's schoolmate—a hemophiliac—had AIDS? What if your work—perhaps as a dentist or a nurse—put you into direct physical contact with people who might be HIV-positive? What do you think would be the right response?

James is a gay college student who has had several sexual relationships in the last five years. His sister has urged him to undergo testing for exposure to HIV, but he keeps putting it off. What would you say if James asked your advice about testing? What are the pros and cons of finding out whether he has been exposed?

Melissa has just found out that she has chlamydia, a treatable STD. She feels angry and betrayed by the two men she'd slept with in the last year. One has moved to another city. The other broke up with her to date one of her friends. She hates the thought of contacting either one, especially about something that embarrasses her. What do you think she should do? How would you handle the situation?

usually sexually transmitted, male sexual partners may be advised to wear condoms. Women should keep the genital area dry and wear cotton underwear.

### Trichomoniasis

Trichomoniasis is caused by *Trichomonas vaginalis* protozoa that live in the vagina. These protozoa can multiply rapidly, causing itching, burning, and discharge. Usually, male carriers have no symptoms, although some may develop urethritis, or inflammation of the prostate and seminal vesicles. All sexual partners must be treated with oral medication, even if they have no symptoms.

### Cystitis

Cystitis is an inflammation of the bladder and is caused by bacteria. Symptoms include frequent burning, painful urination, chills, fever, fatigue, and blood in the urine. Cystitis is more common in women, perhaps because the urethra is shorter and bacteria can more easily reach the bladder. If not treated with antibiotics, these infections can spread to the kidneys.

## MAKING THIS CHAPTER WORK FOR YOU

### Overcoming Infectious Diseases

Infectious diseases threaten everyone's health, but—as with many other illnesses—you can do a great deal to lessen your odds of becoming a victim. Cleanliness is an important first step. The liberal use of soap and hot water kills pathogens. Colds and flus are occasionally unavoidable, but preventive measures, like avoiding obvious carriers, can help.

Among the pathogens that cause infectious disease are viruses, which invade a body cell and take over its reproductive processes; bacteria, one-celled organisms that release disease-causing toxins; fungi, microscopic plants that feed on human tissue; protozoa, one-celled organisms that release substances that destroy or damage cells; and parasitic worms that invade body tissue. Infections may be transmitted by animals, people, contaminated food, or contaminated water.

The body's defenses against pathogens include the skin; antibacterial substances in tears, sweat, skin oils, saliva, and mucus; and the immune system, which includes many different types of defenders. The B-cells produce antibodies, which fight off harmful antigens. Once a person has produced antibodies to a pathogen, he or she has developed active immunity and is usually protected from that disease for life. Immunizations are our best defense against infectious diseases such as polio, tetanus, diphtheria, rubella, measles, and mumps.

The process of infection begins with an incubation period, when the pathogen is multiplying. In the prodromal period, symptoms appear; during active infection, symptoms are most intense; during recovery, symptoms subside. Antibacterial drugs, sulfa drugs, and antibiotics treat diseases caused by bacteria but have no effect on viruses or other pathogens. Antiviral drugs can damage cells invaded by viruses.

Common infectious diseases caused by viruses include the common cold, influenza, measles, viral pneumonia, mononucleosis, and hepatitis; bacterial diseases include tuberculosis, bacterial pneumonia, and toxic shock syndrome. Hepatitis A is generally transmitted by contaminated food or water; hepatitis B, through sexual contact, contaminated blood transfusions, and needles shared by drug users. A recently recognized hepatitis virus, type C, can also be spread through sex and tainted blood or needles.

Immune system disorders include allergies, autoimmune disorders, and immune deficiency. AIDS, or acquired immune deficiency syndrome, is a fatal disease caused by a retrovirus known as human immunodeficiency virus, or HIV, that damages the immune system. This disease is transmitted through contaminated sexual contact, blood transfusions, and needles of drug users. Some people exposed to HIV develop pre-AIDS, or AIDS-related complex (ARC). Because of their severely weakened immune systems, AIDS patients can develop neurologic (nervous system) symptoms, life-threatening infections (such as pneumonia), cancer (such as Kaposi's sarcoma), wasting syndrome, and other diseases.

The incidence of sexually transmitted diseases (STDs) is increasing, and two populations at particular risk are young adults and homosexual men. Gonorrhea, caused by the gonococcus bacteria, can be diagnosed with a blood test or a culture, and is treated with ampicillin or penicillin. Syphilis, diagnosed by a blood test called the VDRL, is treated with penicillin. Chlamydia, caused by a bacteria, often produces no symptoms but can be diagnosed by a culture analysis and treated with antibiotics other than penicillin. Nongonococcal urethritis, often caused by the organism that causes chlamydia, is also treated with antibiotics.

Herpes simplex, caused by a virus, comes in two forms (Type 1 and Type 2) and appears as painful blisters during flare-ups. There is no cure for herpes, only symptom relief. Human papilloma virus and chancroid infections are spreading rapidly. Moniliasis (yeast infection) and trichomoniasis are common vaginal infections not usually transmitted sexually.

Sexually transmitted diseases are a particularly personal responsibility. You owe it to yourself, to those you love, and to the children you might conceive to be aware of the signs, symptoms, and stages of STDs and to avoid exposure. If you fear that you have been exposed, don't wait for serious symptoms. Self-treatment doesn't work for STDs; you need a doctor's help.

Prevention is always the wisest course. If you are sexually active, wear or have your partner wear a condom and use spermicide. This barrier provides some protection, although it carries no guarantee. Ultimately, you have to take responsibility for deciding about the possible risks of any sexual encounter.

SECTION VI

# YOUR FUTURE

Our world may sometimes seem large and impersonal; it may be only among our family and friends that we feel important and necessary. But we are all vitally necessary to the health of our world. By taking care of our environment, we are taking care of ourselves. How we treat our planet and how we treat each other make a community livable and worth living in.

The understanding that caring for others is a way of caring for ourselves comes with age. Maturity and wisdom may accompany age along with wrinkles and thinning hair, but unlike wrinkles, we must work at acquiring wisdom. We can't stop the aging process, but we can use our aging to acquire a deeper appreciation of life and its richness. This section will show you how your beliefs and actions affect your community, your maturity, and your mortality.

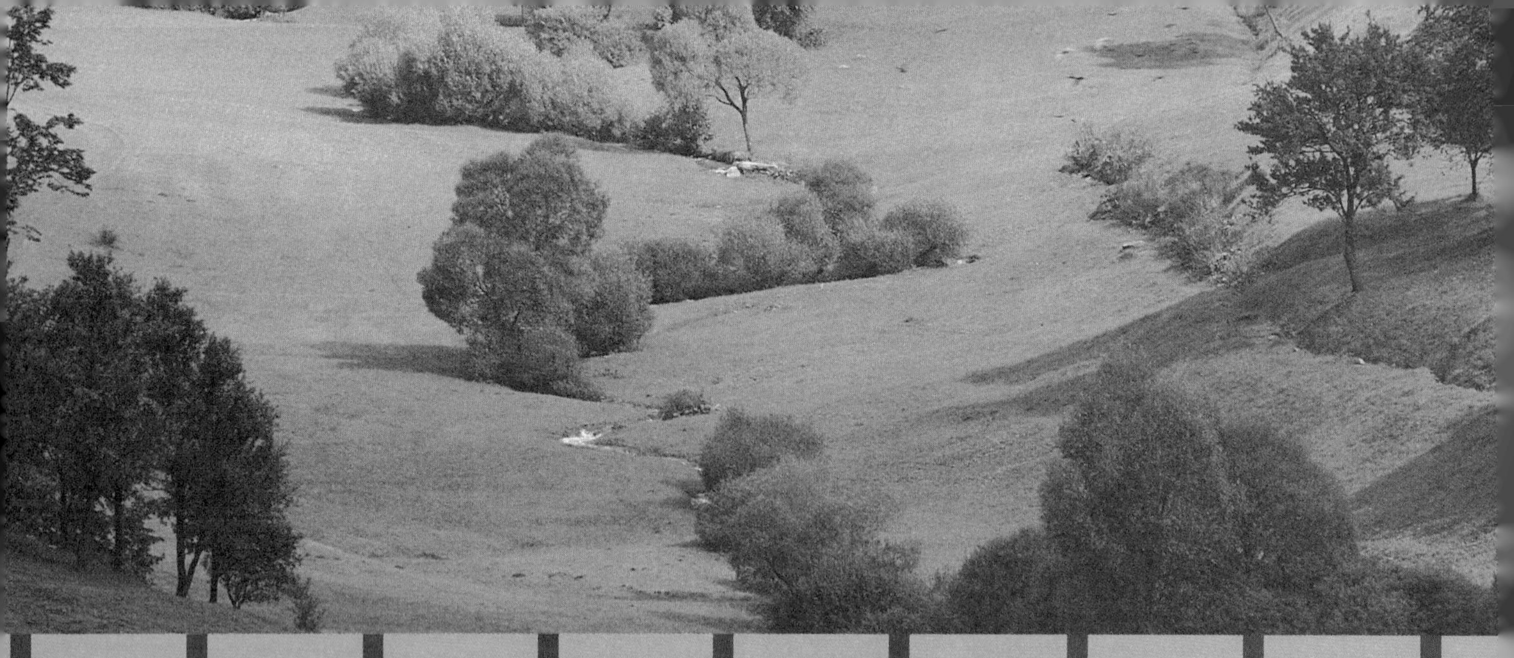

# 16 THE ENVIRONMENT'S IMPACT

In this chapter

Understanding enviromental hazards

Air pollution

Indoor pollution

Water pollution

Chemical pollution

Noise pollution

Radiation and radioactivity

Overpopulation

Violence

Making this chapter work for you: Creating a healthier environment

*Everything in your environment—from the air you breathe to the water you drink to the chemicals in the products you buy—has an impact on your well-being.* In turn, your decisions and actions—the car you choose, the products you use, the waste you create—have an impact on your environment. The problems discussed in this chapter, which affect both you and your environment, may seem so overwhelming that you may think that one individual can't make a difference in solving them. But if you don't become part of the solution, you end up as part of the problem. And the fact is that, both on your own and with others, you *can* find solutions. The first step is realizing that your planet's health, like your own, is your personal responsibility.

## UNDERSTANDING ENVIRONMENTAL HAZARDS

**Pollution** refers to any change in the air, water, or soil that could reduce its ability to support life. Some pollution is caused by natural events, like smoke from fires triggered by lightning, but usually it's a by-product of human activities.

The effects of pollution depend on the concentration (amount per unit of air, water, or soil) of the **pollutant,** how long it remains in the environment, and its chemical nature. An acute effect is a severe immediate reaction, usually after a single large exposure. For example, pesticide poisoning can cause nausea and dizziness. A chronic effect, which may not appear for many years, is a recurrent or constant reaction after repeated small exposures.

We can absorb toxic substances in three ways: (1) through the skin, (2) through the digestive system, and (3) through the lungs. The combined interaction of two or more hazards can produce an effect greater than that of one alone. Toxins can affect an organ or organ system directly or indirectly and can produce the following health effects:

- headaches and dizziness
- eye irritation and impaired vision
- nasal discharge
- cough, shortness of breath, and sore throat
- constricted airways

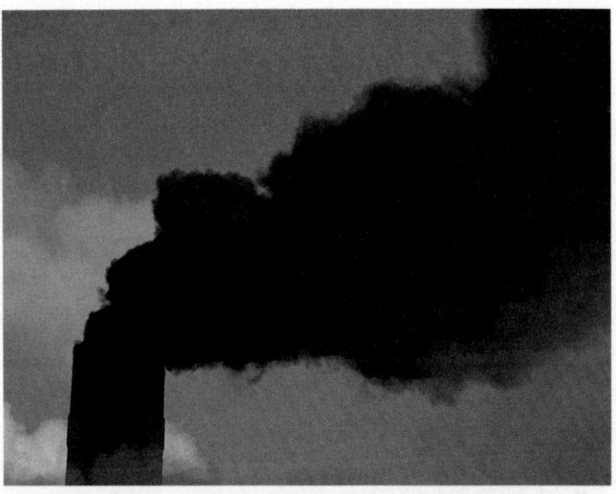

More than half of all Americans live in areas where pollution has made breathing hazardous to their health.

- chest pains; aggravation of symptoms of colds, pneumonia, bronchial asthma, emphysema, chronic bronchitis, lung cancer, and other respiratory problems
- nausea and vomiting
- stomach cancer

Environmental agents that trigger changes, or **mutations,** in the genetic material, the DNA, of living cells are called **mutagens.** The changes can lead to the development of cancer. (As discussed in previous chapters, a substance or agent that causes cancer is a carcinogen: All carcinogens are mutagens; most mutagens are carcinogens.) Further, when a mutagen affects an egg or a sperm cell, its effects can be passed on to future generations. Agents that can cross the placenta of a pregnant woman and cause a spontaneous abortion or birth defects in the fetus are called **teratogens.**

Pollution also affects us in indirect ways. One of the most serious is the **greenhouse effect.** According to some scientists, we have already burned enough

**pollution** The presence of pollutants in the environment.
**pollutant** A substance or agent that is the by-product of human industry or activity and that is injurious to human, animal, or plant life.
**mutation** A change in genetic material that can be transmitted to future generations and that is brought about by radiation, mutagenic chemicals, or natural causes.
**mutagen** An agent that causes alterations in the genetic material of living cells.
**teratogen** Any agent that causes defects or malformations in a fetus.
**greenhouse effect** The warming of the earth's surface and atmosphere; caused by an accumulation of carbon dioxide.

carbon (fossil) fuels like oil and gas to add 1 to 2.5 degrees Fahrenheit to the world's average temperature.[1] The 1980s were the hottest decade on record, though scientists debate whether the high temperatures represent a permanent climate change.[2] No one knows exactly what effects a continuing temperature rise may have, but some experts have predicted severe drought and a rise of 2 to 20 feet in ocean levels—conditions that would affect everyone on earth by devastating agriculture and flooding low-lying communities.[3]

## AIR POLLUTION

If you live in a city of over 50,000 people, you are breathing polluted air, according to the U.S. Public Health Service. Besides natural air pollutants, such as dust and smoke from forest fires, man-made pollutants, such as automobile exhaust and coal soot, can make breathing a hazard to health.[4]

### Smog

Chemical vapors from auto exhaust and industrial and commercial pollutants that react with sunlight form **smog,** a combination of smoke and fog. More than 100 major American cities exceed the maximum permissible smog levels at some point during the year.

Gray-air, or sulfur-dioxide smog, is often seen in Europe and much of the eastern United States. Gray-air is produced by burning oil of high sulfur content. Among the cities that must deal with gray-air smog are Chicago, Baltimore, Detroit, Philadelphia, and Birmingham. Like cigarette smoking (see Chapter 11), gray-air smog affects the cilia in the respiratory passages; so the lungs are unable to expel particulates, such as soot, ash, and dust, which remain and irritate the tissues. This condition is hazardous to persons with the chronic respiratory problems described in Chapter 14.

Brown-air, or photochemical smog—which occurs in Los Angeles, Salt Lake City, Denver, Mexico City, and Tokyo—results principally from nitric oxide in car exhaust reacting with oxygen in the air. The result is nitrogen dioxide, which produces a brownish haze and, when exposed to sunlight, other pollutants. One of these, **ozone,** can impair the body's immune system and cause long-term lung damage. Current "safe" levels may be set far too high, and scientists at the Environmental Protection Agency (EPA) are urging that the acceptable limit for ozone emissions be cut by 50 percent.

Automobiles also produce carbon monoxide, a colorless and odorless gas that impairs the ability of red blood cells to carry oxygen. The resulting oxygen deficiency can impair breathing, hearing, and vision.

Though it is impossible to establish direct links between specific pollutants and specific diseases, air pollution may cause or contribute to many diseases. Emphysema may develop or worsen because pollutants constrict the bronchial tubes and destroy the air sacs (alveoli). As a result, breathing becomes more difficult. As pollutants destroy the hairlike cilia that remove irritants from the lungs, individuals may suffer chronic bronchitis, characterized by excessive mucus flow and continuous coughing. Air pollution may also be partly responsible for increased rates of lung cancer, stomach cancer, and heart disease in industrialized countries.

### The Shrinking Ozone Layer

**Chlorofluorocarbons (CFCs)**—gases used in hairspray and deodorant cans, fire extinguishers, refrigerators, and air-conditioning units—rise into the atmosphere, where they damage a protective layer of ozone many miles above the earth. This **ozone layer** is a region of the upper atmosphere where ozone, created by the energy of sunlight acting upon ordinary oxygen, traps the most dangerous ultraviolet radiations.

Scientists estimate that as much as 7 percent of the ozone belt has already been destroyed.[5] Every 1 percent loss may lead to a 2 percent increase in skin cancer, particularly melanoma, the most deadly. In 1982 the average person's risk of melanoma was 1 in 250. By the year 2000, it will be less than 1 in 100.[6]

Twenty-four industrialized nations have agreed to cut in half their production and use of ozone-destroying chemicals by 1999. However, developing nations are allowed to increase their use of CFCs for a decade so they can advance in basic technologies like refrigeration. The net effect will be a 35 percent reduction in total CFCs by the year 2000—not enough to protect the ozone that protects us, say many concerned scientists.[7]

---

**smog** A grayish or brownish fog caused by the presence of smoke and/or chemical pollutants in the air.

**ozone** A form of oxygen ($O_3$) naturally present in the upper atmosphere, sometimes present in the lower atmosphere as a component of air pollution.

**chlorofluorocarbons (CFCs)** A group of gases that, when emitted into the atmosphere, may damage the ozone layer.

**ozone layer** An upper layer of the earth's atmosphere that protects the earth from harmful ultraviolet radiation from the sun.

## HALES INDEX

Amount of garbage the average American household throws away each week: 87.5 gallons

Amount it throws away each year: 4,550 gallons

Amount of plastic Americans throw away each year: 11.5 million tons

Time it takes for a plastic six-pack ring to decompose: 450 years

Number of Americans living in an area where breathing is a health hazard: 3 in 5

Annual costs of dirty air in health bills, disability, and lost income: $40 billion

Number of Americans who consider themselves environmentalists: 3 of 4

Estimated amount of radioactive nuclear waste by the year 2000: 40,000 tons

Number of Americans whose hearing may have been harmed by noise: 20 million

Number of people who die worldwide of starvation or malnutrition every day: 1,400

Number of children who die as a consequence of hunger every minute: 18

Acts of violence average American child sees on TV by age 16: 200,000

Number of college students victimized by crime every year: 1 in 3

SOURCES: **1, 2** Beck, Melinda. "Buried Alive," *Newsweek*, November 27, 1989. **3, 4** "Breaking Down," *Everyone's Backyard*, January-February 1990. **5, 6** Seabrook, Charles. "Breathing: The Latest Hazard to Nation's Health," in *Ill Winds: The Earth's Endangered Atmosphere*. Atlanta: Atlanta Journal & Constitution, 1989. **7** Sancton, Thomas. "The Fight to Save the Planet," *Time*, December 18, 1989. **8** Perlman, David. "The Waste Nobody Wants," *San Francisco Chronicle*, February 18, 1990. **9** Leary, Warren. "Risk of Hearing Loss Is Growing, Panel Says," *New York Times*, January 25, 1990. **10, 11** Worldwatch Institute. **12** Toufexis, Alexandra. "Our Violent Kids," *Time*, June 12, 1989. **13** Congressional hearings on crime on campus, March 12, 1990.

### Acid Rain

Rain, sleet, snow, mist, fog, and clouds containing sulfuric acid and nitric acid—called **acid rain**—are produced by the burning of fossil fuels, such as oil and gas. The pollutants are carried through the atmosphere and fall to earth when it rains. Acid rain may be contributing to the destruction of forests in several regions of the country. Ozone and other pollutants, however, may play more significant roles. In cities acid rain erodes buildings, monuments, and other structures.

According to a 1990 report by the federal National Acid Precipitation Assessment Program, acid rain threatens a much greater area than had been thought, including parts of the Northeast, East, Midwest, Northern Florida, and New Jersey.[8] Although the overall effect on the nation's water seems less than once was feared, about 4 percent of lakes in areas affected by acid rain have been fully acidified and cannot support life. Another 5 percent are acidic enough to threaten some forms of water life.[9]

**acid rain** Rain with a high concentration of acids produced by air pollutants emitted during the combustion of fossil fuels; damages plant and animal life and buildings.

### Electromagnetic Fields

Electromagnetic fields produced by everything from household appliances to overhead power lines are one of the newest environmental concerns because such things as radio, radar, and television signals may cause biological changes. One study found a higher incidence of brain tumors in workers whose occupations were associated with electricity or electromagnetic fields. Others indicate that electromagnetic radiation may alter the release of calcium in the brain and other tissues, including the bone and pancreas.[10,11]

## INDOOR POLLUTION

The air in today's houses and offices, which are often sealed as tight as a plastic sandwich bag, may be more polluted than the air outside. Unlike outdoor contaminants from exhaust pipes or smokestacks, indoor pollutants come from the very materials the buildings are made of and from the appliances in them.

## Formaldehyde

Commonly used in building materials, carpet backing, furniture, foam insulation, plywood, and particleboard, formaldehyde is a chemical irritant that can cause nausea, dizziness, headaches, palpitations, stinging eyes, and burning lungs. Most manufacturers have voluntarily stopped using it, but many homes contain materials made with formaldehyde.

## Asbestos

The mineral **asbestos,** widely used in building insulation, has been linked to lung and gastrointestinal cancer among asbestos workers and their families, although it may take 20 to 30 years for such cancer to develop. If fibers from asbestos insulation or fireproofing in a home become airborne, they can cause progressive deadly lung diseases, including cancer. However, a 1990 report by University of Vermont researchers in *Science* found that the danger to the general public is low and noted that the risk of dying from smoking or airplane crashes is 100 to 1,000 times greater than the risk of dying from asbestos exposure.[12]

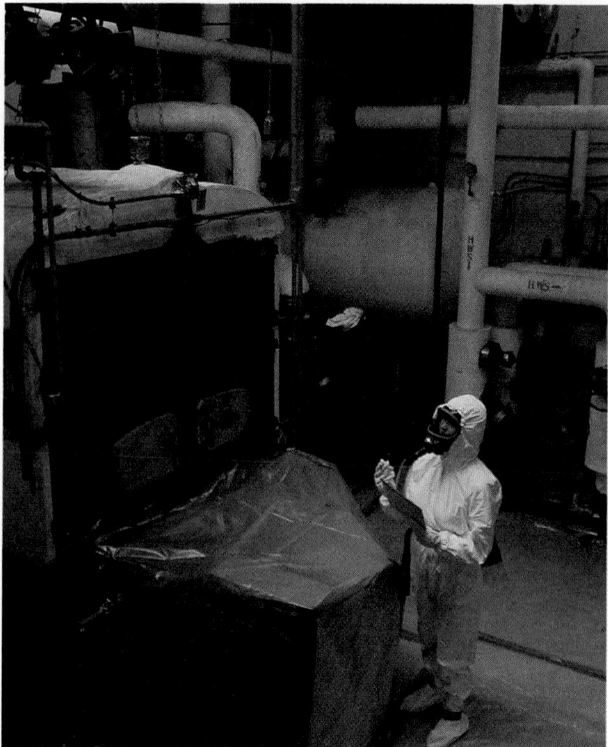

At elementary schools like this one, workers wear protective gear to remove hazardous insulation materials containing asbestos.

## Lead

Lead is a danger inside and outside the home. We all breathe lead that's in the atmosphere, 98 percent of which comes from the burning of leaded gasoline. We're exposed also to the lead used to make batteries, solder, and other metal products and to lead that's settled on the food we eat, particularly fruits and vegetables grown near highways. (Although lead can be washed off, the washing done is often too superficial.)

The main source of lead poisoning in American children is lead-based paint, which flakes from ceilings or walls. According to the EPA, 3 million American children suffer permanent neurologic damage because of lead poisoning.[13] The effects include impaired concentration, reduced short-term memory, slower reaction times, and learning disabilities. Workers exposed to lead may become sterile or suffer irreversible kidney disease, anemia, damage to the central nervous system, or stillbirths or miscarriages. Infants of exposed mothers can die or suffer mental retardation.

## Carbon Monoxide

Tasteless, odorless, colorless, and nonirritating, carbon-monoxide (CO) gas is also deadly. Produced by the incomplete combustion of fuel in space heaters, furnaces, water heaters, and engines, it reduces the delivery of oxygen in the blood. Every year an estimated 10,000 Americans seek treatment for CO inhalation.

Typical symptoms of CO poisoning are headache, nausea, vomiting, fatigue, and dizziness. A blood test can measure CO levels; inhaling pure oxygen speeds removal of the gas from the body. Most people who do not lose consciousness as a result of CO poisoning recover completely.

**STRATEGY FOR CHANGE**

**Preventing Carbon-Monoxide Poisoning**

- Provide adequate ventilation when using wood-burning stoves, space heaters, and fireplaces.
- Ensure that all flame-burning appliances are properly installed, adjusted, and operated.
- Don't use ovens or gas ranges to heat your home. Don't operate gasoline-powered engines in confined spaces, such as garages or basements.
- Never burn charcoal inside a home, cabin, recreational vehicle, or tent, whether it's in a grill, hibachi, or fireplace.
- Make sure your furnace has adequate air intake.

**asbestos** A mineral widely used for building insulation; has been linked to lung and gastrointestinal cancer.

### Radon

Radioactive radon diffuses from brick and concrete building materials and produces a gas that clings to dust particles, which often lodge in the lungs. According to the National Council on Radiation Protection and Measurements, this naturally occurring radioactive gas may cause 9,000 lung cancer deaths each year as it seeps from soil and bedrock into up to 1 million homes. Radon levels tend to be highest in areas with granite and black shale topped with porous soil. If you live in a high-radon area, don't panic. Your hypothetical risk of dying from radon-caused lung cancer is about equal to the known risk of dying in a home fire or fall.[14]

If you're in a danger zone, check with the geology department at the nearest university or with the state health department to find out if the organization has performed radon tests. If they indicate possible danger, you can buy a radon detector. In most homes, the readings turn out to be low. If not, your state health department can provide guidelines for bringing them down.

**STRATEGY FOR CHANGE**

**Protecting Yourself from Indoor Air Pollution**

- Limit your use of cleaners and aerosols that fill the air with chemicals. Ventilate your house immediately afterward.
- Make sure all gas ovens are vented to the outside.
- Contact local health officials for advice on sealing materials containing formaldehyde or radon.
- Air your room, apartment, or house daily or as often as possible—particularly in the winter, when pollutants build up inside because of closed doors and windows.
- If you live in a formaldehyde-insulated home, keep heat and humidity down because vapors increase in hot, humid weather. Air-conditioning and dehumidifiers reduce emissions.
- Before doing any renovations, inspect pipe and furnace coverings and insulation in attics and crawl spaces for signs of cracking or flaking.
- Don't touch any loose asbestos.
- Don't waste money testing your air for asbestos. The results of such tests are meaningless. To check a building material for asbestos, put three small pieces in a film canister and send it to an EPA-approved laboratory. The cost is usually \$25 to \$75 a sample.

## WATER POLLUTION

According to various EPA reports, as many as 37 percent of public water-supply systems contain measurable quantities of man-made chemicals. Some make water look or taste funny. Others have lethal effects. Some contaminants enter the water as a result of natural processes, such as the decay of vegetation. Others are the result of urban growth, industrial activity, and agricultural runoff.

### Fluoride

About half (53 percent) of Americans drink water containing fluoride, an additive to water and toothpaste that helps teeth resist decay. According to the American Dental Association, tooth decay is 50 to 70 percent lower in areas with fluoridated water. But fluoride may carry risks as well as benefits.

**HEALTH HEADLINE**

**The State of the World**

**Everyone senses that Planet Earth is in bad shape, but just how bad is a matter of heated debate. Consider some statistics about environmental changes that occurred in just one year (1989):**

- **The earth's population rose by 87.5 million to a record 5.2 billion.**
- **The burning of fossil fuels released at least 19 billion tons of carbon dioxide into the atmosphere.**
- **Some 28 million acres of tropical forest were destroyed.**
- **The United States, with 5 percent of the world's population, used 26 percent of the world's oil, released 26 percent of the world's nitrogen oxides, produced 22 percent of the world's carbon dioxide emissions, and disposed of 290 million tons of toxic waste.**

SOURCES: Sancton, Thomas. "The Fight to Save the Planet," *Time*, December 18, 1989. Worldwatch Institute.

SELF-SURVEY

## Assessment of Environmental Sensitivity

***Purpose***

The purpose of this assessment is to promote personal responsibility for environmental conditions by identifying specific environmental problems that are susceptible to individual influence.

***Directions***

Check the items that are true.

1. I smoke cigarettes. ______
2. I sometimes litter. ______
3. I sometimes waste electricity. ______
4. I sometimes use phosphate detergents. ______
5. I sometimes like to play music as loud as possible. ______
6. I buy only blemish-free farm produce. ______
7. I sometimes use spray cans. ______
8. I throw away aluminum cans and returnable bottles. ______
9. I sometimes burn leaves or trash. ______
10. I sometimes idle my automobile needlessly. ______
11. I use colored toilet tissues, paper, and/or napkins. ______
12. I waste water by taking lengthy showers. ______
13. I purchase liquids sold in opaque, white-plastic containers. ______
14. I use paper products instead of cloth handkerchiefs, napkins, and towels. ______

***Scoring***

If you checked any of these items, you should consider how your behavior might be modified to improve the environment around you.

1. The inhalation of smoke increases your risk of lung disease, and also pollutes the air.
2. Litter may be classified as either solid waste or visual blight. Only through individual effort can this form of pollution be managed. Recycling is an important approach to its containment.

The federal National Toxicology Program reported in 1990 that laboratory rats given fluoridated water had a higher rate of a rare type of bone cancer called osteosarcoma. The more fluoride they drank in their water, the more likely they were to develop cancer. However, scientists noted that osteosarcoma is extremely rare in humans. The lifetime risk of getting this cancer for any individual who drinks fluoridated water is less than one in 5,000.[15,16]

### Chlorine

Three-quarters of the American population drink water that has undergone bacteria-killing chlorine treatment. The Council on Environmental Quality has warned that people drinking chlorinated water have a 53 percent greater risk of getting colon and bladder cancer and a 13 to 93 percent greater risk of getting rectal cancer than those not drinking chlorinated water.

## CHEMICAL POLLUTION

Each year, a thousand new chemicals join the 50,000 to 75,000 already in common use. In most cases, little is known about their potential ill effects.

### Pesticides

Each year 1.09 million pounds of pesticides, 1 billion pounds of wood preservative, and 0.40 billion pounds of disinfectants are used in America.[17] **Pesticides** are used to destroy unwanted insects, plants, and fungi,

3. Electric consumption affects the thermal-water-pollution loads at electricity-generating plants. One simple way to lower your electricity consumption is to switch to bulbs of lower wattage any light bulbs not used for reading.
4. A great deal of pollution comes from detergent phosphates. The new biodegradable detergents still contain phosphates, which fertilize algae and, in turn, reduce the supply of oxygen necessary to support life in streams, lakes, and oceans.
5. Learn to enjoy music at lower volumes. Excessively loud noises over a period of time may lead to irreversible hearing losses.
6. The use of pesticides merely saves the appearance, and not the food value, of farm produce. The long-term effects of these pesticides on human health are unclear.
7. Fluorocarbon propellants are depleting the ozone layer, which absorbs the solar ultraviolet rays known to cause skin cancer. Variations in weather, food supply, and disease will be inevitable if use of these propellants continues.
8. Most communities have recycling centers for both aluminum cans and glass. Use them.
9. Rather than burning leaves, start your own compost pile to return the nutrients in leaves to the soil. Trash is solid waste which should be handled through the sanitary landfill.
10. The automobile is the single greatest source of air pollution. If you will be waiting more than 1 minute, shut off your car.
11. When colored paper products enter the water system, dyes are released. Dyes pollute water visually and biologically.
12. North America currently has the best freshwater supply in the world, but future generations may be forced to restrict personal consumption. To conserve water, take shorter showers, use drought-resistant landscaping, and conserve rinse water during dishwashing.
13. Opaque, white-plastic containers consist of polyvinyl chloride. It is a hazardous substance; when burned it can destroy nearby vegetation, the insides of incinerators, and the lining of your lungs.
14. Excessive use of paper products places an unusual burden upon our national forests. Take the time to use cloth handkerchiefs, napkins, and towels.

SOURCE: *Wellness* R.S.V.P.

and these chemicals save billions of dollars of valuable crops from pests. But at the same time, they may endanger human health and life. Recent National Cancer Institute studies suggest that at least one herbicide widely used in agricultural and lawn spraying—2,4-D—may cause cancer in humans.

Other high-risk substances that have been restricted or banned because they may cause cancer, birth defects, neurological disorders, and damage to wildlife and the environment are DDT, kepone, and chlordane. Organic phosphates—including chemicals such as malathion—can cause cramps, confusion, diarrhea, vomiting, headaches, and breathing difficulties;

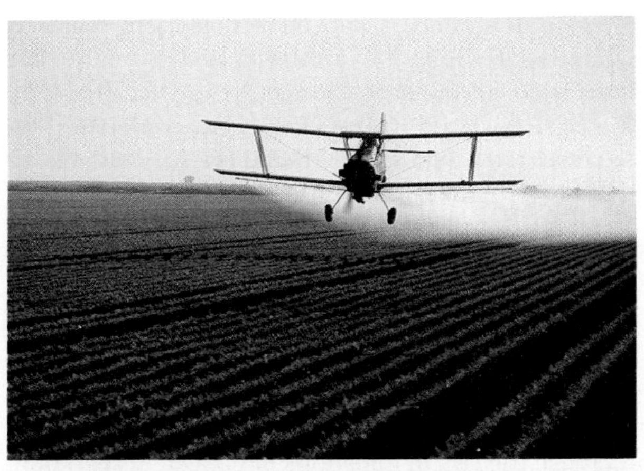

Pesticides protect crops from insects, plants and fungi but may endanger human health and life.

**pesticide** Any toxic substance used to kill pests; types include insecticides, herbicides, fungicides, and others.

higher doses can lead to convulsions, paralysis, coma, and death.

**STRATEGY FOR CHANGE**

**Using Pesticides Safely**

- Before using any pesticide or household chemical, read the label carefully. Make sure you understand the directions for use, precautions, and first-aid instructions.
- Store these products in a locked place, out of the reach of children.
- Don't measure chemicals with food-preparation utensils.
- Don't mix chemicals with each other unless the label tells you to do so.
- Wear rubber gloves.
- Store chemicals in the manufacturer's container only.
- If you have your house commercially fumigated for termites, hire licensed exterminators. Make sure they don't use chlordane or spray into heating or cooling vents. Find out which chemicals the exterminators use. To check safety of fumigants, call the EPA's hot line. Keep everyone out of the house while the exterminators are working. If possible, sleep elsewhere for a few days after a full-scale fumigation.

## Dioxin

The family of seventy-five chemicals called **dioxins** has been widely used in paper and plastic products as well as in agriculture and industry. The most infamous dioxin is Agent Orange, which was used to clear vegetation during the Vietnam war. Some studies have found no birth defects in children whose fathers served in Vietnam. Others found a higher incidence of stillbirths and birth defects in children whose fathers fought in areas where they might have been exposed to Agent Orange. A five-year report by the CDC, released in 1990, found "no evidence" that Agent Orange had harmed soldiers in Vietnam, although Vietnam veterans are more likely to get a rare, fatal cancer called non-Hodgkin's lymphoma.[18]

In sunlight, dioxin breaks down fairly quickly into less-toxic compounds. However, when it gets into the upper layers of the soil, it retains its original structure. Long-term exposure to dioxin—a chemical already linked to birth defects, tumors, and skin problems—may damage the body's immune system and increase the risk of infections or cancer. Researchers have found dioxin in human breast milk and estimate that nursing for one year may expose babies to 27 times the recommended *lifetime* limit for exposure to cancer-causing dioxins. Critics of the research charge that these controversial findings were based on overstated estimates of risk.

## PCBs

**PCBs** (polychlorinated biphenyls) belong to a family of 209 chemical compounds widely used as coolants and lubricants in electrical equipment; in insulating fluids; and in the manufacture of common products such as plastics, adhesives, paints, and varnishes. PCBs made their way into the environment when industries discharged PCB-laden wastes into rivers and streams or disposed of them in open landfills. A possible human carcinogen, PCBs are no longer commercially produced in the United States, but high levels of PCB remain in certain parts of the country, and in eggs, poultry, and fish.[19]

## Cadmium and Beryllium

In the United States, exposure to the heavy metal **cadmium** results mainly from inhaling cigarette smoke or city air. Cadmium may be linked to high blood pressure, which is linked to heart disease.[20] The use of **beryllium,** a metal with many industrial uses (fluorescent-bulb manufacture, for example), has increased 500 percent over the past 25 years. According to the EPA, beryllium can cause severe respiratory problems, including bronchitis and lung cancer.

## Dumps and Landfills

Before the environmental laws of the last two decades, industry dumped most of its waste into open pits, abandoned mines, or nearby rivers. The EPA's Superfund program has identified 1,219 dumps, pits, ponds, lagoons, and landfills as clearly hazardous and another 32,000 as potentially dangerous (see Figure 16-1). Many of these are industrial waste sites, but even a town dump can be a danger if it contains toxic materials.[21]

---

**dioxins** A family of chemicals widely used in industry and as a defoliant; some forms are believed to be extremely toxic.

**PCB** Polychlorinated biphenyls; compounds—ranging from light, oily fluids to greasy or waxy substances—that have been widely used as industrial coolants and lubricants and in the manufacture of plastics, paints, and varnishes.

**cadmium** A toxic metallic element common in industrial waste and as a component of environmental pollution; used industrially in electroplating and in atomic fusion.

**beryllium** A toxic metallic element that forms hard alloys with other metals and is a good electrical conductor; considered a dangerous pollutant.

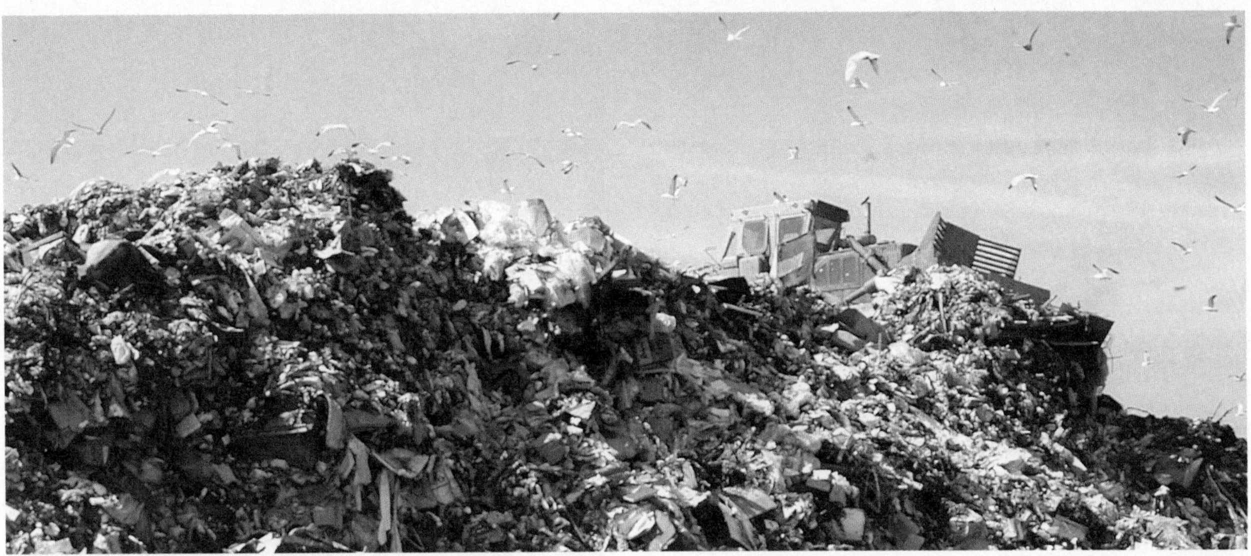

Thousands of local and industrial dumps contain toxic materials that are potential threats to surrounding communities.

Industrial waste is extremely resistant to breakdown: It is not easily **biodegradable.** Most organic materials are broken down by sunlight; heat; and, mostly, by bacteria. The results of this decomposition are carbon dioxide and nutrients that enrich the soil. However, many synthetic products remain in their original state for decades (or longer), resisting degradation and contributing to the heaps of trash we see along the highways and in our communities. Dis-

**biodegradable** Capable of being broken down into harmless components, especially by the action of bacteria, sunlight, and heat.

**FIGURE 16-1** Each dot represents a hazardous waste dump on the government's priority list for cleanup. But thousands of other sites in the United States also pose serious threats to life.

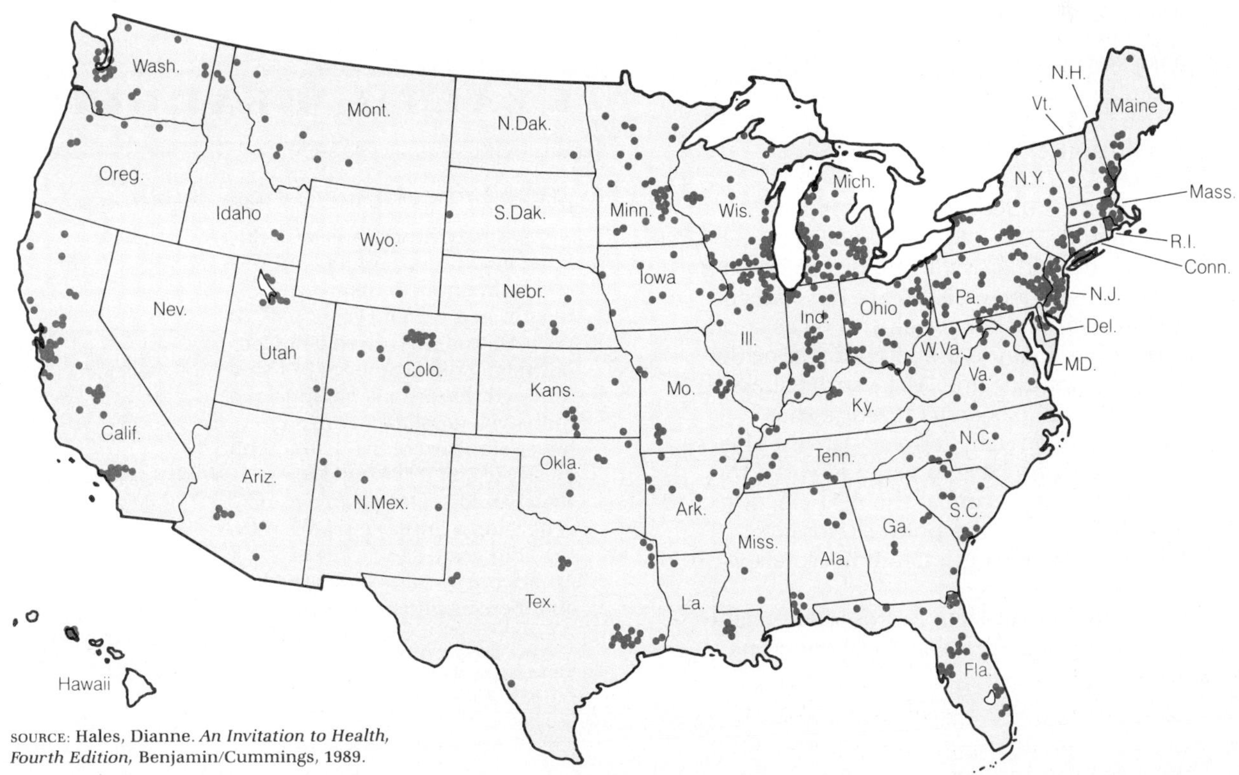


SOURCE: Hales, Dianne. *An Invitation to Health, Fourth Edition,* Benjamin/Cummings, 1989.

carded chemicals, including pesticides, pose the added risk of remaining active poisons that may contaminate our water supply and infiltrate the food chain for years to come.

### Incinerators

In the United States the burning of garbage and industrial wastes in the 450 municipal and 121 toxic waste incinerators has created a new problem: emissions containing dangerous pollutants, including lead and dioxins.

### Leaking Underground Storage Tanks

More than 2 million tanks containing gasoline, petroleum, or other chemicals are buried underground at gas stations, factories, and other sites around the country. The EPA estimates that the contents of 10 to 30 percent of them may be leaking into the water supply.

**STRATEGY FOR CHANGE**

**Speaking Out for a Safer World**

One of the simplest, most effective actions you can take is to write to your congressional representatives and senators—the people who vote on pollution controls, budgets for the enforcement of safety regulations, and the preservation of forests and wildlife. Here's how to make the most of your right to write:

- Make sure you have the right addresses:
  Hon. ____________
  House Office Building
  Washington, D.C. 20515 or
  Senator ____________
  Senate Office Building
  Washington, D.C. 20510
- Identify the bill or issue you are discussing. Because more than 20,000 are introduced during each session, it helps to be as specific as possible. Include the bill number or describe its popular title. Make sure you write before the bill has come up for a vote.
- Concentrate on your representatives. They're the people who have to listen to you if they want to win your vote at the next election.
- Be as brief and to the point as possible.
- If you can, type your letter. If not, make sure it's legible.
- Also write to your state representatives and senators, especially about local concerns.

## NOISE POLLUTION

Experts called together by the National Institutes of Health in 1990 reported that more than 20 million Americans may suffer hearing loss because of exposure to loud noise at home, on the job, and during recreation. The damage noise causes in the ear cannot be reversed. Two warning signs of potential harm are ringing in the ears (tinnitus) and a muffling of the sounds you hear.[22,23]

Sensitivity to noise varies greatly from person to person. Beginning in their teens, men, who tend to have greater exposure to loud noise, have poorer hearing than women. Damage to the ear is cumulative and gets worse over time.

### How Loud Is Too Loud?

Loudness is measured in **decibels (dB)**. A whisper is 20 decibels; a conversation in a living room is about 50 decibels (see Figure 16-2). On this scale, 50 is not 2-1/2 times louder than 20, but 1,000 times louder: Each 10-decibel rise in the scale represents a tenfold increase in the intensity of the sound.

High-intensity noise damages the delicate hair cells that serve as sound receptors in the inner ear. Pro-

**decibel (dB)** A unit for measuring noise levels.

**HEALTH HEADLINE**

**More Concern for Mother Earth**

**Increasingly, Americans are realizing how important a healthy environment is to their own health. In a recent Harris poll, 84 percent said that, given a choice between a high standard of living (but with hazardous building and industrial development) and a lower standard of living (but with clean air and drinking water), they would prefer clean air and water and a lower standard of living. Ten years ago far fewer Americans were as concerned about environmental dangers.**

SOURCE: "Health over Money: The New Environmental Consciousness," *Psychology Today,* November 1989.

**FIGURE 16-2** Decibel levels for various noises. On this scale, each 10-decibel rise in the scale represents a tenfold increase in the intensity of the sound.

SOUND LEVELS AND HUMAN RESPONSE

| COMMON SOUNDS | NOISE LEVEL (dB) | EFFECT |
|---|---|---|
| Boom car | 145 | Beyond threshold of pain (125 dB) |
| Jet engine (near) | 140 | |
| Shotgun firing | 130 | |
| Jet takeoff (100–200 ft.) | 130 | |
| Rock concert | 110–140 | |
| Oxygen torch | 121 | |
| Symphony orchestra | 110 | |
| Boom box | 120 | Threshold of sensation (120 dB) |
| Thundercap (near) | 120 | |
| Stereo (over 100 watts) | 110–125 | |
| Chain saw | 110 | Regular exposure of more than 1 min. risks permanent hearing loss (over 100 dB) |
| Jackhammer | 110 | |
| Snowmobile | 105 | |
| Jet flyover (1,000 feet) | 103 | |
| Electric furnace area | 100 | No more than 15 min. unprotected exposure recommended (90–100 dB) |
| Garbage truck/cement mixer | 100 | |
| Farm tractor | 98 | |
| Newspaper press | 97 | |
| Subway, motorcycle (25 ft.) | 90 | Very annoying, hearing damage begins after 8 hrs. |
| Lawnmower, food blender | 85–90 | |
| Recreational vehicle, TV | 70–90 | |
| Diesel truck (40 mph, 50 ft.) | 84 | |
| Washing machine | 78 | |
| Dishwasher | 75 | |
| Average city traffic noise | 80 | Annoying, interferes with conversation, constant exposure may cause damage |
| Garbage disposal | 80 | |
| Vacuum cleaner, hair dryer | 70 | Intrusive, interferes with telephone use |
| Inside a car (loud engine) | | |
| Garbage disposals | 50–60 | |
| Normal conversation | 50–65 | Comfortable (under 60 dB) |
| Quiet office | 50–60 | |
| Refrigerator humming | 40 | |
| Whisper | 30 | Very quiet |
| Rustling leaves | 20 | |
| Normal breathing | 10 | Just audible |

longed exposure to any sound over 85 decibels (the equivalent of a power mower or food blender) or brief exposure to louder sounds can harm hearing. Rock concerts often have sound levels of more than 100 decibels; personal stereos can blast sounds of up to 115 decibels. Extremely loud car stereo systems known as boom cars can produce an ear-splitting 145 decibels—louder than a jackhammer, jet engine, or thunderclap.

## The Impact of Noise

High-volume sound has been linked to high blood pressure and other stress-related problems that can lead to heart disease, insomnia, anxiety, headaches, colitis, and ulcers. Noise frays the nerves; people tend to be more anxious, irritable, and angry when their ears are constantly barraged with sound. Even unborn babies respond to sounds; some researchers speculate that noise, particularly if it stresses the mother, may be hazardous to them.[24]

**STRATEGY FOR CHANGE**

**Protecting Your Ears**

- If you must live or work in a noisy area, wear hearing protectors to prevent exposure to blasts of very loud noise.
- Limit exposures to loud noise. Several brief periods of noise seem less damaging than one long exposure.
- Be careful if you wear Walkman-type stereos. The volume is too high if you can feel the vibrations.
- Don't think cotton or facial tissue stuck in your ears can protect you. Foam or soft plastic earplugs are more effective.
- Keep your home quiet. Whenever you buy an appliance, ask how quiet it is. (Some are labeled with decibel levels.) Foam pads under countertop appliances will cut their sound. Padded carpeting cushions background sounds.
- Have your hearing checked if you are at all concerned about hearing loss.

## RADIATION AND RADIOACTIVITY

We are surrounded by low-level radiation every day. Most comes from cosmic rays and radioactive minerals, which vary according to geography. (Denver has more than Atlanta, for instance, because of Denver's altitude.) Man-made sources—including medical and dental X rays, color television sets, radar, video screens for computers, and microwaves—account for 18 percent of the average person's lifetime exposure. Nuclear power plants account for less than 0.5 percent of average exposure.

Is low-level radiation harmful to health? According to the most recent report of the National Research Council, it is. The risk of getting cancer is 4 times what had been previously estimated, and there is much greater danger of mental retardation among babies exposed to low-level radiation in the womb from 8 to 15 weeks after conception.[25]

Most people are not exposed to enough radiation to exceed safe limits. But high amounts of radiation can damage the genetic material in human reproductive cells, producing mutations in future generations that may lead to miscarriages, infant deaths, physical and mental deformities, several kinds of cancer (of blood, bone, lungs, thyroid, and the central nervous system), cataracts, and a shortened life span.

### Diagnostic X Rays

Both the Environmental Protection Agency and Ralph Nader's health research group have estimated that 30 to 50 percent of the 700 million X rays taken every year in the United States are unnecessary. However, doctors sometimes prescribe X rays to protect themselves from malpractice suits, and hospitals benefit financially from the heavy use of X-ray equipment.

**STRATEGY FOR CHANGE**

**Avoiding Unnecessary X Rays**

- Always ask why the X ray is being ordered. Do not give your consent unless there is a clear need.
- Keep a record of the date and location of every X-ray exam. These X rays may someday provide information that will make more X-rays unnecessary.
- Ask the radiologist to explain specifically how much radiation you will be exposed to.
- Don't refuse a needed medical X ray just because you're afraid of the radiation exposure. The risk of dying from even relatively high-dose X rays is much smaller than that of riding in a car for a few hundred miles.

### Video Display Terminals

Chances are there's a video display terminal (VDT) in your life—at the school library, at the office where you work, or maybe in your home. Is it a health hazard? In terms of radiation exposure, the answer seems to be no—so far. Although VDTs have been blamed for increases in reproductive problems and cataracts, repeated measurements of radiation from VDTs have shown that leakage is well below present standards for safe occupational exposure. Some health officials, however, have recommended that pregnant women be allowed to shift from operating VDTs to other types of work.

### Microwaves

Microwaves are a form of radiation that generates heat. There is no evidence that existing levels of microwave radiation encountered in the environment pose a health risk to people, and all home microwave ovens must meet safety standards for leakage.

### Frequent Flying

In 1990 the Department of Transportation identified a new radiation risk: air travel. The occasional traveler faces slight danger, but the radiation that penetrates the thin metal skins of airplanes can increase the risk of cancer in airline crews and very frequent fliers.

HEALTH SPOTLIGHT

## Saving Your Planet

What can one person do to overcome such global threats as air pollution, the shrinking ozone layer, the greenhouse effect, and toxic wastes? Here are some suggestions for what you can do every day to protect your environment:

- Recycle paper and glass products.
- Use public transportation whenever possible.
- Drive a high-mileage, low-emission car. Have it tuned and inspected regularly.
- Fix any leaks in your car's air conditioner, which may be leaking harmful chlorofluorocarbons (CFCs).
- Plant a tree, which when mature, can absorb about 13 pounds of carbon dioxide a year.
- Don't litter.
- Before discarding plastic six-pack holders, snip each circle with scissors so birds and small animals are not trapped in them.
- Buy the product with the simplest packaging.
- Avoid "squeezable" plastic containers, which are not biodegradable.
- Look for a logo on products indicating that recycled paper was used in the packaging.
- Buy items in bulk to avoid excessive packaging.
- Ask for paper rather than plastic bags at grocery stores.
- Use paper picnic plates, cups, and bowls instead of Styrofoam plastic products made with CFCs.
- Buy milk in paper rather than plastic cartons.
- Use both sides of scrap paper.
- Use newspapers as packing material.
- Share magazines and newspapers.
- Use low-wattage fluorescent light bulbs, which require 75 percent less energy than incandescents.
- Turn out lights when you leave a room.
- Don't let water faucets drip or leak.
- Use a water-efficient shower head.
- To save water, shut off the faucet as you brush your teeth; take showers rather than baths.
- Don't use aerosol sprays.
- When buying appliances, buy the most energy-efficient models.
- Buy clothes that do not require dry cleaning, which uses toxic solvents.
- If you're cold, put on a sweater rather than turning up the thermostat.
- Buy rechargeable batteries.
- Don't buy disposable razors, flashlights, lighters, or the like.
- Use sponges and rags rather than paper towels for cleaning.
- Use cloth napkins and handkerchiefs rather than paper products.
- Choose products in reusable glass jars and bottles.
- Carry a cloth or string bag when you go shopping.
- When you do use toxic products, make sure you read the label and dispose of them properly.
- Don't turn your radio or stereo up to ear-splitting volumes.
- Take action. Use your rights as a citizen. Petition, protest, and write your congressional representatives.

SOURCES: Begley, Sharon. "Life in 2010," *Family Circle*, February 1, 1990. Dold, Catherine. "Green to Go," *American Health*, April 1990. EarthWorks Group. *50 Simple Things You Can Do to Save the Earth*, Berkeley: EarthWorks Press, 1989. Garelik, Glenn. "It's Not Easy Being Green," *Time*, December 18, 1989. MacEachern, Diane. *Save Our Planet: 750 Everyday Ways You Can Help Clean Up the Earth*. New York: Dell, 1989. Sancton, Thomas. "The Fight to Save the Planet," *Time*, December 18, 1989.

Those flying at high altitudes and over the earth's north or south poles are at greater risk. If 100,000 crew members spent 20 years aloft on the high-risk routes, radiation could cause 1,000 "premature cancer deaths." Pregnant women crew members may face a slightly increased risk of birth defects, especially from the 8th to 15th week after conception.[26]

## Irradiated Foods

The process of **irradiation** uses radiation, either from radioactive substances or from devices that produce X rays, on food. It does not make the food radioactive. Its primary benefit is to prolong the useful life of food. Like the heat in canning, irradiation can kill all the microorganisms that might grow in a food. The sterilized food can then be stored without spoiling for years in sealed containers at room temperature. In addition, low-dose irradiation can inhibit the sprouting of vegetables (potatoes and onions, for example) and delay the ripening of others (bananas, mangoes, tomatoes, pears, and avocados). Therefore, irradiation can produce cost-saving benefits of great appeal to the food industry.[27]

Are irradiated foods safe to eat? The best available answer is a qualified yes, because we don't have complete data yet. Most of the research has focused on low-dose irradiation to delay ripening and to destroy insects.

## Radioactive Wastes

More than 23,000 tons of highly radioactive waste materials have accumulated around the 111 operating nuclear plants in the United States. Some radioactive by-products must be stored for periods of 10 to 20 times their half-lives. (A half-life is the time it takes radioactivity to reduce to one-half the original amount.) Therefore, some by-products must be stored for tens of thousands of years before their radioactivity reaches safe levels. Most nuclear waste is stored temporarily in a cooling water bath at the reactor site. This is only a short-term solution; no permanent way has yet been found to store radioactive waste safely.

## Nuclear Reactors

In the United States nuclear power has not become the major energy source some had predicted. One reason is the fear of a catastrophic accident, such as those that occurred at Three Mile Island in Pennsylvania and at Chernobyl in the Soviet Union.

At Three Mile Island—as a result of operator mistakes, design flaws, and mechanical failures (a stuck valve, in particular)—the nuclear reactor destroyed itself by overheating to 2,500 degrees Fahrenheit. Radioactivity leaked out. Children and pregnant women living nearby were evacuated. Eight similarly designed plants throughout the United States were shut down, and a nationwide furor over the danger of nuclear power stalled other nuclear projects.

At Chernobyl, operators testing the plant's turbines to examine how they might be used in an emergency deactivated several safety systems. During the test, the reactor's temperature soared to 5,000 degrees Fahrenheit, and an enormous steam explosion blew the roof off the building. The radioactive uranium core melted, giving off radioactivity that eventually circled the globe.

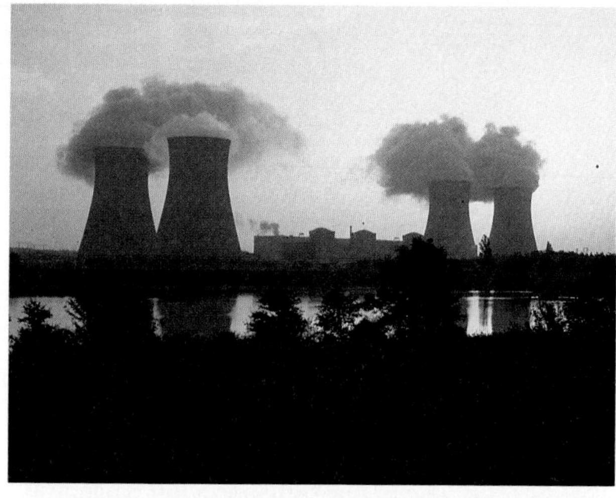

The fear of catastrophic accidents has limited the construction of nuclear power plants in the U.S.

Even if no accidents occur, a nuclear plant is expected to be safe for only about 30 years. After that, parts of the reactor mechanism are so weakened by radioactivity that they must be removed and the plant shut down.

## OVERPOPULATION

Many of the environmental problems facing us now and in the future stem from overpopulation. By the year 2025, there may be more than 8 billion people on the earth. Although the rate of population growth is slowing, the number of people in the world will continue to increase for some time.[28]

In the United States in the year 2025, if current trends continue, we may reach what is known as **zero population growth,** the point at which the number of births equals the number of deaths. But in that year, 7 billion of the earth's 8.3 billion people will be residents of underdeveloped countries. What will happen when other countries grow in population and reach out for energy and other resources? The answer is sure to affect us.

**irradiation** The exposure to or treatment by some form of radiation.

**zero population growth** The point at which the number of births equals the number of deaths.

An increasingly serious problem is hunger and starvation, which affect 50 million people around the world. Most of the malnourished live in Africa, India, Bangladesh, Pakistan, Indonesia, and Latin America. Only half the world's people live in countries capable of growing or buying enough food for their populations. More people have died as a result of hunger in the last decade than in all the wars, revolutions, and murders of the last 150 years.

## VIOLENCE

You may not think of the threat of crime as an environmental health issue, but it is. Violence is the leading killer of young people in the United States. Accidents, homicides, and suicides account for 77 percent of all deaths among adolescents. According to the Federal Bureau of Investigation (FBI), the murder rate among 15- to 24-year-olds tripled from 1950 to 1990.[29]

People of every age have grown not just more fearful about crime, but more frustrated with our slow and overburdened criminal justice system. Growing numbers of would-be victims are fighting back with unexpected fury. Thousands of neighborhood citizen-patrol organizations have sprung up across the country. Local communities have voted more money for police. The trend across the country is toward longer prison sentences, particularly for repeat offenders. According to the Justice Department, the nation's prison population doubled from the 1970s to the 1980s.

While officials are getting tough on criminals, more agencies are paying attention to their victims. More than 400 victims' advocacy groups have been set up across the country to advise those hurt by crime. In some cases, victims have won cash settlements for lost income from work, medical treatment, and the burial costs for murder victims.

### Domestic Violence

Domestic violence—spouse beating, child and elder abuse, and incest—is emerging from decades of silence and shame as a major problem in our society. One-third of all murders occur within the family. The FBI estimates that a woman is physically abused every 18 seconds, and that women have a 50 percent chance of being hit at least once by their husbands or lovers.

The primary factors contributing to wife abuse are the frustration and stress the husband is under, his use of alcohol (alcohol is involved in up to 60 percent of battering cases), and whether he was raised in an abusive home. Only one in twenty men who beat their wives are violent outside the home; nine in ten refuse to admit that they have a problem. The National Council on Child Abuse and Neglect estimates that in homes where the wife is beaten, 30 to 70 percent of the children are also abused.[30]

Abused wives and children are often trapped in terror. Wives may stay with abusive husbands because of love, financial dependence, shame, guilt, fear of being harmed or killed, or a sense of responsibility to the children. In the last decade hundreds of shelters for battered wives and their children have been set up across the country. They offer physical and psychological treatment and a haven where women can begin to rebuild their shattered self-esteem as well as their daily lives.[31]

### Child Abuse

Child abuse is another common and deadly hazard in American homes. The number of reported cases is on the rise, but no one knows whether the problem is growing or simply receiving greater recognition. Almost without exception, abusive parents were themselves either abused or neglected as children.

Among the psychological traits most often associated with child abusers are immaturity and dependency, extremely low self-esteem, a sense of incompetence, difficulty in seeking pleasure and finding satisfaction in the adult world, social isolation, a reluctance to seek help, fear of spoiling children, a strong belief in the value of punishment, unreasonable expectations of children, and a serious lack of ability to empathize with a child's needs. When a crisis occurs, some parents and caregivers, pushed beyond their ability to cope, end up abusing their children.

**STRATEGY FOR CHANGE**

**How to Help Victims of Violence**

Sometimes well-intentioned friends and relatives make victims feel worse. Here's how to offer comfort, without implying criticism:

- Don't blame the victim. Any second-guessing adds to the burden of blame and shame.
- Don't try to deny that it happened. Denial makes victims question themselves at a time when they crave reassurance.
- Don't force the victim to talk—or not to talk. Some individuals need to go over every detail of what happened, again and again, until they work out their feelings of outrage. Others find going into details too humiliating.
- Don't try to rush the victim on to the next stage. Recovery takes time, and only the victim knows the appropriate pace.

## WHAT DO YOU THINK?

Some radical environmentalists have torn down power lines, sunk whaling ships, and destroyed oil-exploration gear—and gone to jail for these illegal acts against the polluters they call greedheads and eco-thugs. Are their actions justified? Are they going too far by breaking the law? What alternatives would you suggest?

Some people who live near some chemical plants have had abnormally high rates of miscarriages, birth defects, and cancers. Should they be able to sue the factories? Should the government pay for their legal suits or their medical expenses because it failed to protect them adequately? What if affected residents cannot prove chemical plants directly responsible for their medical problems? What are an industry's responsibilities to nearby residents?

In some communities, teenagers have been murdered and robbed by other teens for their expensive athletic shoes or jackets. Arrests of those under 18 for murder and aggravated assault have been climbing every year. Some experts blame drugs; others trace teen violence to excessive violence on TV and in movies and records. Why do you think more young people are committing acts of violence? What can our society do about its violent youth?

## MAKING THIS CHAPTER WORK FOR YOU

### Creating a Healthier Environment

The overall effect of all forms of pollution is to reduce the earth's ability to support life. Toxic substances, such as pollutants in the air and water, can be absorbed through the skin, digestive system, and lungs and can produce acute or chronic effects.

Air pollution may be caused by natural events, such as dust storms or forest fires. Or it may be human-made, as is smog, which may cause or worsen emphysema, chronic bronchitis, lung and stomach cancer, and heart disease. Certain pollutants are dangerous to the health of the planet as well as individual health. These include chlorofluorocarbons, (found in spray cans, fire extinguishers, refrigerators, and air conditioners), which may damage the ozone layer, and acid rain, which is threatening plant and animal life in some regions. Electromagnetic fields may cause biological changes in body tissues in humans and animals.

The air inside the buildings where we live and work may also be hazardous. Indoor air pollutants include formaldehyde, asbestos, and radon from building materials and carbon monoxide from gas stoves and heaters. The water that we drink may also be dangerous because of additives like fluoride and chlorine and contamination by toxic chemicals. Chemical threats to health include industrial wastes, pesticides, lead, dioxin, PCBs, cadmium, and beryllium.

Another environmental threat is radiation, which can come from natural and man-made sources. Even low levels of radiation can damage the genetic material in the body's cells and result in cancer and birth defects. We are exposed to radiation from X rays, irradiated food, airplanes, computer terminals, microwaves, and radioactive wastes.

One environmental threat we can often avoid or prevent is noise. Sounds above 85 decibels can damage sound receptors in the inner ear, resulting in hearing problems. Rock concerts and powerful stereos can produce sounds as loud as—and sometimes louder than—jackhammers and jet planes.

As the world's population continues to grow, the result may be increased hunger, malnutrition, and starvation and the depletion of energy, mineral, and food resources. But chemicals, radiation and overpopulation are not the only reason why people can be dangerous to health. Violence has become the leading cause of death of young people in the United States. Domestic crime, including spouse and child abuse, is no longer a hidden form of violence but a sad, ugly part of daily life for millions of Americans.

Problems like crime, overpopulation, nuclear waste, industrial pollution, and the greenhouse effect can seem so complex that you may think you can do little about them. That's not the case. The environment *can* be made better instead of worse. The job won't be easy, and every one of us will have to do our part. Just as many diseases of the previous century have been eradicated, so, in time, may we be able to remove many of the environmental threats. Our future—and our planet's future—may depend on it.

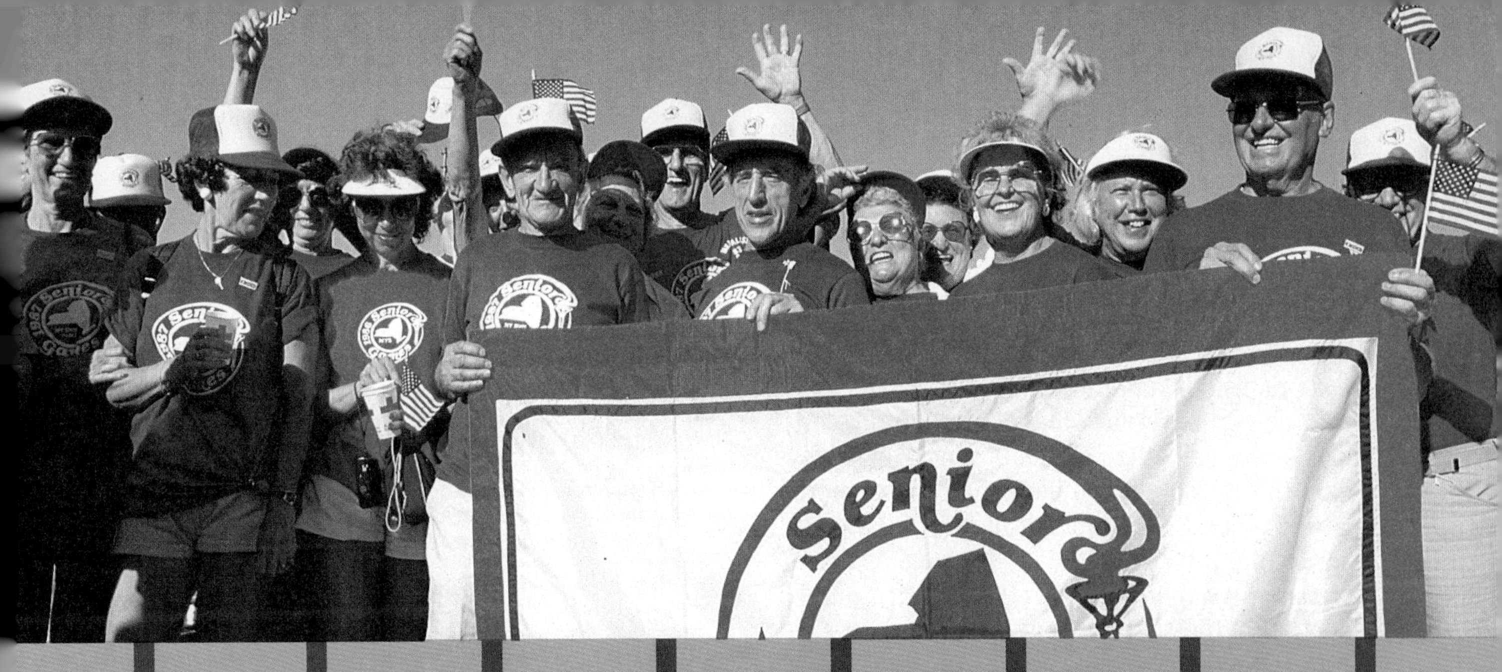


# 17 GROWING OLDER AND FEELING BETTER

## In this chapter

A look into the future

The good news about getting older

Problems of the elderly

How long can you live?

Living in an aging society

Making this chapter work for you: Getting older and better

*Aging doesn't start at age 65.* Every day you make decisions and take actions that affect the way you feel now and will feel in the future. At any age, at any stage of life, at any level of physical fitness, you can get better instead of merely getting older. This chapter will give you a preview of the future—of the changes age brings as well as ways you can age better and make the most of all the years of your life.

## A LOOK INTO THE FUTURE

Aging isn't what it used to be. The 30 million Americans over age 65 today are healthier than their parents and grandparents who survived to that age. The average 65-year-old can expect to live at least two decades more (see Figure 17-1). Seniors over age 85 are the fastest-growing segment of our society.[1] The keys to a vital and healthy old age are healthful behaviors throughout life.

**STRATEGY FOR CHANGE**

**Staying Younger Longer**

- Watch your weight. Animals live longer if they're underweight. And as humans we definitely need less food as we age.
- Eat a low-fat, balanced diet. Most physicians feel the elderly do not need special supplements—unless they're not eating a healthful mix of fruits, vegetables, low-fat dairy products, and low-fat meat.
- Don't smoke. Heavy smokers have the lung capacity of persons about 10 years older than they are. On the average a nonsmoker lives more than eight years longer than a smoker.
- Get regular medical checkups. Keep high blood pressure and other chronic problems under control. Try to avoid accidents, the fourth leading killer of Americans.
- Stay away from antiaging gimmicks. None of the products on the market today has any scientific proof behind the claims.
- Work out a good balance of work and play in your life. Try to keep stress within enjoyable limits, and remember that quality of life will always matter more than quantity.

**FIGURE 17-1** The life expectancy of adults today is longer than ever before. The average 40 year old has at least thirty more years to which to look forward. Even the average 65 year old has more than ten years to live.

PROJECTED LIFE EXPECTANCY

Boys born in 1990 can expect to live 76.1 years, and girls to the age of 83.4. The trick is to stay alive; life expectancy increases with age.

| If you are now... | Your life expectancy at birth... | | Your life expectancy today is... | |
|---|---|---|---|---|
| | Men | Women | Men | Women |
| 25 | 72.7 | 80.6 | 76.2 | 83.1 |
| 45 | 70.4 | 77.9 | 77.3 | 82.8 |
| 65 | 64.1 | 71.9 | 80.6 | 84.9 |
| 85 | 54.0 | 61.4 | 90.5 | 91.9 |

SOURCE: Office of the Actuary, Social Security Administration.

### As Time Goes By: The Impact of Age

From a purely physical standpoint, the body's finest years come in youth when lung capacity is greatest, grip firmest, motor responses quickest, and physical endurance longest. After age 30, the body's powers gradually decline, although decades pass before you notice any great differences.

Many of the changes time brings have more to do with the way you look than with the way you feel. At age 30, you'll have a few lines on your forehead. At age 40, you'll find crows'-feet (from squinting) at the corners of your eyes and arcs linking your nostrils to the sides of your mouth (from smiling). At age 50, the lines will look more pronounced, and the skin at your cheeks may sag; at age 60, excess skin and fat deposits may form bags under your eyes. At age 70, your skin will be rougher, and your face will be wrinkled. And your earlobes will droop about a quarter-inch lower than they did at age 20.[2]

#### Cardiovascular Changes

After age 30, the heart's ability to pump blood decreases about 1 percent each year. At age 30, your heart pumps 3.6 quarts of blood per minute; at age 70, 2.6 quarts per minute. Blood pressure rises; circulation slows. These changes simply mean that the average 70-year-old can't compete with a 30-year-old in wrestling or running, but the 70-year-old still has sufficient energy and stamina for day-to-day functioning.[3]

## HALES INDEX

Median age of population of the United States in 1790: 16

Median age in 1980: 30

Median age in 2000: 35

Median age in 2030: 40

Americans living in nursing homes: 1.7 million

Average cost of nursing-home care per year: $25,000

Percentage of nursing-home costs paid by private insurance: 1.4

Percentage of people over age 71 who need eyeglasses: 32

Percentage who need hearing aids: 39

Percentage of people over age 65 with Alzheimer's disease: 10

Percentage of people over age 85 with Alzheimer's: 47

Percentage of people over 65 who suffer from depression: 16.7

SOURCES: **1, 2, 3, 4, 5** Beck, Melinda. "Be Nice to Your Kids," *Newsweek*, March 12, 1990. **6** Gelman, David. "The Brain Killer," *Newsweek*, December 18, 1989. **7** Beck, Melinda. "Be Nice to Your Kids," *Newsweek*, March 12, 1990. **8, 9** "Living Well . . . Into the 21st Century," *HealthSpan*, Winter 1990. **10, 11** Purvis, Andrew. "Alzheimer's Rise," *Time*, November 20, 1989. **12** Blazer, Dan. "Epidemiology of Late-Life Depression and Dementia: A Comparative Study, in *Review of Psychiatry*. Washington, D.C.: American Psychiatric Press, 1990.

### Respiratory Changes

Aerobic capacity, the amount of oxygen the body can use and the best measure of ability to do work, declines with age. By age 75, a man's aerobic capacity is less than half of what it was at age 17; a woman's is about a third of the capacity of her twenties.

### Muscular and Skeletal Changes

Strength diminishes very slowly. By age 60, men have lost 10 to 20 percent of their maximum muscular power, whereas women have lost somewhat more. Each decade after age 25, men and women lose 3 to 5 percent of their muscle mass, which often is replaced by fatty tissue.

As you get older, bones lose minerals and become softer and shorter. Your muscles weaken and your back slumps. The disks between the bones of the spine deteriorate, moving those bones closer together. As a result, both sexes shrink by as much as 1/2 inch in total height with each decade.

### Metabolic Changes

Basal metabolism, the fundamental chemical process of living, slows because the aging body requires less upkeep. The rate at which the body turns food into energy declines by about 3 percent every ten years.

### Nervous System Changes

As we age, the brain becomes smaller, but mental abilities do not diminish. Aging nerve cells, however, result in slower reaction time and movement, and we process information more slowly. A grandfather playing a computer game with his 14-year-old grandson will lose every time. (Instead of responding in 1/5 second, he needs 2/5 second.) However, on tests that involve real-life experience and acquired knowledge, he has the edge.

## THE GOOD NEWS ABOUT GETTING OLDER

As many as half of the losses linked to age may be the result, not of time's passage, but of disuse. In other words, what you *don't* do may matter more than what you do.

## Heredity's Role

From conception throughout life, your genetic legacy continues to have an impact. Studies of identical twins in Sweden—some separated at birth, some reared together—found that some individuals seem born with genes that make them "fast agers." However, healthful behaviors can modify the impact of these genes.

## Exercise's Effects

Staying in bed for twenty-one days has the same effect as aging thirty years. At any age, the unexercised body—though free of the symptoms of illness—will rust out long before it ever could wear out. Inactivity can make anyone old before his or her time.

Just as inactivity accelerates aging, activity slows it down. In one study, a group of sedentary middle-aged adults who began exercising regularly almost literally stopped the clock: Their hearts and lungs became almost as powerful as in their youth, and their weight and blood pressure decreased.[4] The effects of ongoing activity are so profound that some specialists in aging refer to exercise as "the closest thing to an antiaging pill."

**STRATEGY FOR CHANGE**

**Staying Fit After Fifty**

- Always undergo a thorough medical examination before starting an exercise program.
- Be sure to stretch and warm up properly.
- Gradually work up to 20 to 30 minutes of aerobic exercise three times a week.
- Remember that the best exercise for most elderly is walking. For increased benefit, walk vigorously uphill.
- Some good alternatives to walking include jogging (if you have no joint problems), swimming, riding a stationary or moving bicycle, and dancing.
- Avoid quick movements, sudden bursts of intense exercise, or situations where you may fall.

## The Aging Brain

Ten years ago, scientists thought that the aging brain, once worn out, could never be fixed. They've since learned that the brain can and does repair itself. When brain cells (neurons) die, the surrounding cells develop "fingers" to fill the gaps and establish new connections, or synapses, between surviving neurons. Although self-repair occurs more quickly in young brains, the process continues in older brains.

Even in victims of Alzheimer's disease, the most devastating form of senility, there are enough healthy cells in the diseased brain to regrow synapses. Scientists hope to develop drugs that someday may help the brain repair itself.

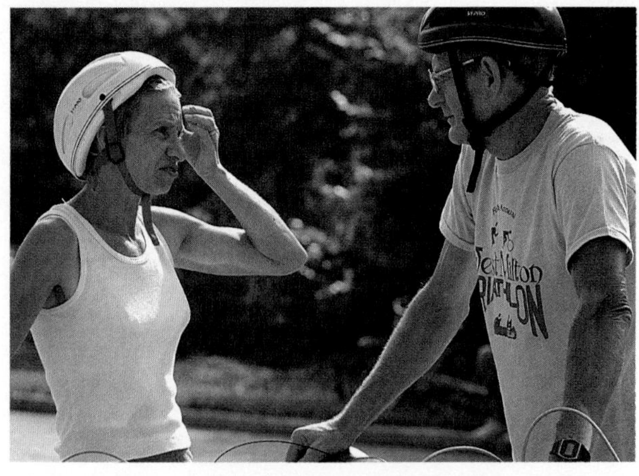

Exercise can prevent or delay many of the physical changes associated with aging.

### Intellectual Power

Mental ability does not decline along with physical vigor. In one study, researchers at Pennsylvania State University were able to reverse the supposedly "normal" intellectual declines of 60- to 80-year-olds by giving them tutoring sessions in problem solving.[5]

Reaction time, intellectual speed and efficiency, nonverbal intelligence, and maximum work rate for short periods may diminish by age 75. However, understanding, vocabulary, ability to remember key information, and verbal intelligence remain about the same.

**STRATEGY FOR CHANGE**

**Boosting Your Brain Power**

- Remain mentally active. Just as you have to use your body to keep it at its peak, you have to exercise your brain regularly to prevent its deterioration.
- Keep pushing your limits. Most people have a certain level of stimulation at which they function best.
- Allow yourself more time to learn new material or perform difficult tasks.
- If any sudden, dramatic changes in mental ability occur, get prompt medical attention. Don't assume they're part of normal aging, because they aren't.

### Memory

Although certain aspects of memory falter with time, most people can compensate for them by relying on simple coping strategies. Some people have better

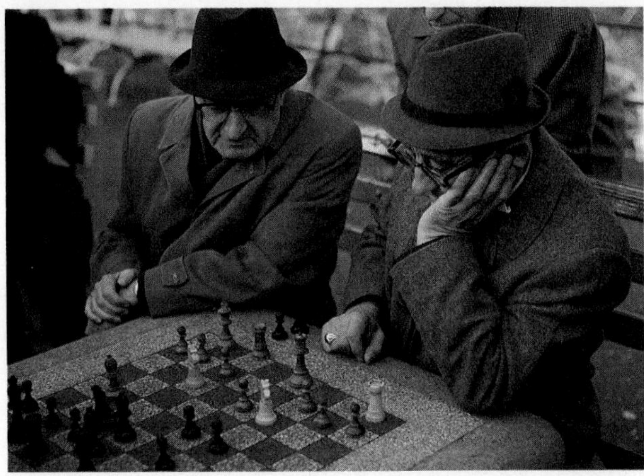

Just as exercise shapes up the aging body, mental challenges can sharpen the aging brain.

memories in their seventies than others do in their thirties. And at any age, people can improve their recall.[6]

The most frequent problem for people over age 60 is remembering names. They recognize a person or know how to use an object, but they can't produce the name. This problem occurs most with words they don't use very often. For example, they may want to think of the word for a game played with a small white ball and paddles. Instead of coming up with *Ping-Pong,* the nearest they can come is *tennis.* The best approach is to relax and try filling in the details of its context so they can visualize it clearly. The harder they try and the more anxious they become, the more difficult remembering will be.

Beginning in their forties, individuals may find it more difficult than younger people to recall newly learned information. The reason may be that they didn't learn the information as well in the first place. Older people often don't spend as much time organizing the material they want to master as young people do.

**STRATEGY FOR CHANGE**

**When Should You Worry About Memory Loss?**

At any age, occasional forgetfulness, memory lapses, and misplacing everyday objects are common. What's *not* normal are any of the following:

- frequent difficulty completing a sentence because of forgetting what you want to say or the words with which to say it
- misplacing important items, such as money or bank records
- frequent confusion
- forgetting how to use common items or perform simple tasks
- getting lost or disoriented in familiar places, especially at home
- difficulty identifying the month or season
- dizzy spells or severe headaches accompanying memory loss

A number of illnesses—including depression, kidney disease, alcoholism and Alzheimer's disease—can cause these symptoms. Only thorough medical and neurological examinations can pinpoint the specific problem.

## Mental Health

The elderly are not more vulnerable to mental illness. No psychiatric disorders occur more frequently in the elderly, and some become less likely with age.[7] Even depression—which is not uncommon among the elderly—strikes less often in old age than at earlier stages of the life cycle. Often, those most likely to become depressed have lost a spouse and have few social supports. The social ties of the elderly are most

**HEALTH HEADLINE**

**Emotional Health at Age 65**

The secret of emotional well-being at retirement age is not professional success or happy marriage, but an ability to cope with life's setbacks without blame or bitterness, according to a study of 173 Harvard College graduates begun in the 1940s. Problems in childhood (such as being poor or orphaned) had almost no effect on psychological health at age 65; being close to brothers and sisters at college age did have a great impact. Traits that were important at college age, such as making friends easily, became unimportant later in life. However, students who had been good at practical organization in college were among the healthiest in mind at 65—they were rated by psychiatrists as "steady, stable, dependable, thorough, sincere, and trustworthy."

SOURCE: Goleman, Daniel. "Men at 65: New Findings on Well-being," *New York Times,* January 16, 1990.

likely to fray as they retire, move, or lose spouses and close friends.

### Sexual Activity

Sexual activity does not end in later life. However, aging does cause some changes in sexual response: Women produce less vaginal lubrication; it may take longer for an older man to achieve an erection and longer for him to attain another after ejaculation. Both sexes experience fewer contractions during orgasm. However, none of these changes reduces sexual pleasure or desire.

**STRATEGY FOR CHANGE**

**Ingredients for a Long and Healthy Life**

By changing your health habits, you may be able to "buy" yourself extra years of life and health. Here's how:

- *Smoking.* If you smoke two or more packs of cigarettes a day, you are essentially trading a minute of life for a minute of smoking. You can expect to lose 8.3 years of life you might have lived as a nonsmoker.
- *Drinking.* Moderate drinkers seem to live longer than either heavy drinkers or nondrinkers. Drinking in excess can lead to cirrhosis of the liver, car accidents, pneumonia, high blood pressure, diabetes, and many other life-threatening conditions.
- *Eating.* Some believe a bad diet can decrease the average life span 6 to 10 years. Certainly, diet may have a lot to do with your risk of heart disease, bowel or breast cancer, and other disorders.
- *Weight.* Your weight can make a difference in your predisposition to heart attacks, strokes, kidney disease, diabetes, and other disorders.
- *Exercise.* Exercise may add 6 to 9 years to your life. The fitter you are, the longer you can expect to live.
- *Stress.* Stress can make intense demands upon the body and may make some people prone to heart attacks. Learning to control stress can lessen the toll it takes on well-being.
- *Interest in life.* Job satisfaction and interest in others and in the future can make a big difference in life span. People who lose their jobs or a spouse or who retire without other interests, may lose years too. Anything that improves the quality of life may well increase its quantity.

## PROBLEMS OF THE ELDERLY

Sadly, life's final decades aren't always golden. Senior citizens may have to deal with physical, economic, social, and psychological challenges.

### Health Problems

The chances of becoming sick or physically disabled increase with age. The National Institute on Aging points out that the symptoms of some diseases may be different for older people—a heart attack may occur without chest pains, and appendicitis without abdominal tenderness—so they may not seek prompt treatment. Sometimes an older adult's illness or disability is temporary, but often it persists for the remainder of that person's life. Many older people have several health problems, requiring several medications, at the same time. The drugs may interact and cause a confusing array of symptoms and reactions.

**Osteoporosis** is a condition in which losses in bone density become so severe that a bone can break after slight trauma or injury. Among those who live to age 90, 32 percent of women and 19 percent of men suffer hip fractures as the result of osteoporosis. Compared to black women, white and Asian women are at greater risk for osteoporosis, probably because they have smaller bone masses.

Three separate factors contribute to osteoporosis:

- a decline in bone mass that begins in the twenties and thirties in both men and women
- in women, a decline in bone loss after menopause, when levels of the female hormone estrogen decline
- preventable risk factors, including cigarette smoking, heavy alcohol intake, and inadequate calcium

The best time to prevent osteoporosis is during young adulthood. By getting sufficient calcium, particularly during the growth spurt of adolescence, you can produce a heavier, denser skeleton and thus face less risk of the complications of bone loss later in life. Adequate dietary calcium throughout one's life—especially in childhood, adolescence, and young adulthood—is necessary to maintain bone density.[8]

Estrogen helps protect women against bone loss, and the Food and Drug Administration has approved its use to prevent osteoporosis in postmenopausal women. However, because of possible risks associated with estrogen supplements (including an in-

**osteoporosis** A condition in which loss of bone density results in easily broken, brittle bones.

creased danger of cancer of the uterus), estrogen is recommended only for women at high risk for osteoporosis, and estrogen use requires careful follow-up. (Estrogen is usually combined with progestin, another hormone, to reduce the danger of cancer.) Researchers are investigating other therapies for osteoporosis.

Exercise may help prevent osteoporosis. The most helpful form seems to be a combination of aerobic training and weight lifting (see Chapter 5). However, too much exercise can increase the danger of bone loss. Young ballet dancers and women athletes who diet or exercise so extensively that their menstrual periods stop or become irregular may weaken their bones and develop curvature of the spine (scoliosis) or stress fractures in their feet. Those who overexercise are at higher risk of bone injuries later in life.

## Medication Abuse

Although the use of street drugs is rare among the elderly, misuse and abuse of prescription and over-the-counter medications are common. In part, the reason is that health practitioners prescribe more drugs to people over age 65 than to any other group in society. Older Americans consume one-quarter of all drugs prescribed in the United States.[9]

The most commonly misused drugs are sleeping pills, tranquilizers, pain medications, and laxatives. Sometimes a person innocently takes more than the prescribed dose or takes several prescriptions simultaneously. Other older people are aware of their overreliance on drugs but don't like the way they feel when they don't take the pills.[10]

One in seven elderly men and women use tran-

### STRATEGY FOR CHANGE

#### Preventing Osteoporosis

- Make sure you get adequate calcium. The minimum recommended amount for adults over 25 is 1,000 mg per day; researchers recommend 1,500 mg per day for postmenopausal women. Two excellent sources of calcium are milk (275 mg in an 8-ounce glass) and sardines (370 mg in 3 ounces with bones). (See Chapter 4 for more information on calcium-rich foods.)
- Exercise regularly, but not excessively.
- Watch your caffeine intake, and put some skim milk in your coffee. In a Washington State University study, caffeine increased the amount of calcium lost in urine by 65 percent, but drinking the equivalent of 1/3 cup of milk with two small cups of coffee canceled out the loss.
- Drink only moderately. More than two or three drinks of alcohol a day impairs intestinal calcium absorption.
- Don't smoke. Smokers tend to be thin (a risk factor for osteoporosis) and to enter menopause earlier, thus extending the period of jeopardy resulting from estrogen loss.
- Let the sunshine in. Vitamin D, a vitamin produced in the skin in reaction with sunlight, boosts calcium absorption. Get a few minutes of midday sun in summer; stay out longer in winter. (Note: You never need to stay out so long that you burn.)
- If you're at high risk (that is, white or Asian, small-boned, with a family history of osteoporosis), seek a doctor's advice about estrogen supplements after menopause.

### HEALTH HEADLINE

#### Eat Less, Live Longer?

How would you like to extend your life span by 50 percent or more; prevent heart disease, diabetes, and kidney problems; decrease your risk of cancer; and delay the usual signs of aging, including gray hair? The only catch: You have to cut back to 60 to 65 percent of the calories you usually eat.

Numerous studies of rats, mice, and simpler animals have found that a significant reduction in food intake can lengthen life, prevent disease, and slow down the aging process. Though most laboratory mice live about 36 months, for example, those on a restricted diet have lived to 55 months. Studies are underway to determine what effect calorie restriction might have on monkeys. There is no evidence that less food might mean longer life for humans, but some researchers speculate that a restricted diet might boost the maximum human life span from 110 to 170 years.

SOURCE: Angier, Natalie. "Diet Offers Tantalizing Clues to Long Life," *New York Times*, April 17, 1990.

SELF-SURVEY

## What Is Your Aging IQ?

***True or False***

1. Everyone becomes "senile" sooner or later, if he or she lives long enough.
2. American families have by and large abandoned their older members.
3. Depression is a serious problem for older people.
4. The number of older people is growing.
5. The vast majority of older people are self-sufficient.
6. Mental confusion is an inevitable, incurable consequence of old age.
7. Intelligence declines with age.
8. Sexual urges and activity normally cease between the ages of 55 and 60.
9. If a person has been smoking for 30 to 40 years, it does no good to quit.
10. Older people should stop exercising, and rest.
11. As you grow older, you need more vitamins and minerals to stay healthy.
12. Only children need to be concerned about calcium for strong bones and teeth.
13. Extremes of heat and cold can be particularly dangerous to older people.
14. Many older people are hurt in accidents that could have been prevented.
15. More men than women survive to old age.
16. Deaths from stroke and heart disease are declining.
17. Older people on the average take more medications than younger people.
18. Snake-oil salesmen are as common today as they were on the frontier.
19. Personality changes with age, as does hair color and skin texture.
20. Sight declines with age.

***Answers***

1. *False.* Even among those who live to be 80 years or older, only 20 to 25 percent develop Alzheimer's disease or some other incurable form of brain disease. *Senility* is a meaningless term that should be discarded.
2. *False.* The American family is still the number one caretaker of older Americans. Most older people live close to their children and see them often; many live with their spouses. In all, 8 out of 10 men and 6 out of 10 women live in family settings.
3. *True.* Depression, loss of self-esteem, loneliness, and anxiety can become more common as older people face retirement, the deaths of relatives and friends, and other such crises—often at the same time. Fortunately, depression is treatable.
4. *True.* Today, 12 percent of the U.S. population is 65 years or older. By the year 2030, one in five people will be over 65 years of age.
5. *True.* Only 5 percent of the older population live in nursing homes; the rest are basically healthy and self-sufficient.

quilizers; half of them are psychologically dependent on the drugs and feel they could not get along without them. Others take sleeping pills every night and believe they couldn't rest without drugs. A physician's supervision is necessary to ensure safe withdrawal from these medications.

### Financial Limitations

About 13 percent of the nearly 30 million Americans over age 65 live below the poverty line (about $10,000 for an individual, $13,000 for a couple) (see Figure 17-2). The poverty rate is highest among women, minorities, those who live alone, the unmarried, and the rural elderly.[11]

As many as 8 million older Americans are economically vulnerable. Their incomes are less than twice

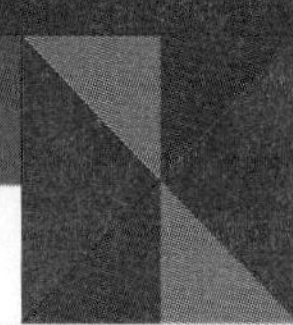

6. *False.* Mental confusion and serious forgetfulness in old age can be caused by Alzheimer's disease or other conditions that cause incurable damage to the brain, but some 100 other problems can cause the same symptoms. A minor head injury, a high fever, poor nutrition, adverse drug reactions, and depression can all be treated and the confusion cured.
7. *False.* Intelligence per se does not decline without reason. Most people maintain their intellect or improve as they grow older.
8. *False.* Most older people can lead an active, satisfying sex life.
9. *False.* Stopping smoking at any age not only reduces the risk of cancer and heart disease, but also leads to healthier lungs.
10. *False.* Many older people enjoy and benefit from exercises such as walking, swimming, and bicycle riding. Exercise at any age can help strengthen the heart and lungs and lower blood pressure. See your physician before beginning a new exercise program.
11. *False.* Although certain requirements, such as that for "sunshine" vitamin D, may increase slightly with age, older people need the same amounts of most vitamins and minerals as do younger people. Older people, in particular, should eat nutritious food and cut down on sweets, salty snack foods, high-calorie drinks, and alcohol.
12. *False.* Older people require fewer calories, but adequate intake of calcium for strong bones can become more important as you grow older. This is particularly true for women, whose risk of osteoporosis increases after menopause. Milk and cheese are rich in calcium, as are cooked dried beans, collards, and broccoli. Some people need calcium supplements as well.
13. *True.* The body's thermostat tends to function less efficiently with age, and the older person's body may be less able to adapt to heat or cold.
14. *True.* Falls are the most common cause of injuries among the elderly. Good safety practices, including proper lighting and nonskid carpets, can help prevent serious accidents.
15. *False.* Women tend to outlive men by an average of eight years. There are 150 women for every 100 men over age 65, and nearly 250 women for every 100 men over age 85.
16. *True.* Fewer men and women are dying of stroke or heart disease. This has been a major factor in the increase in life expectancy.
17. *True.* The elderly consume 25 percent of all medications and, as a result, have many more problems with adverse drug reactions.
18. *True.* Medical quackery is a $10 billion business in the United States. People of all ages are commonly duped into "quick cures" for aging, arthritis, and cancer.
19. *False.* Personality doesn't change with age. Therefore, all old people can't be described as rigid and cantankerous. You are what you are for as long as you live. But you can change what you do to help yourself enjoy good health.
20. *False.* Although changes in vision become more common with age, any change in vision, regardless of age, is related to a specific disease. If you are having problems with your vision, see your doctor.

SOURCE: U.S. Department of Health and Human Services, Bethesda, Md.: U.S. Government Printing Office, 1986.

the poverty level, and a serious illness, the loss of their home in a fire or flood, or other unexpected catastrophes could easily plunge them into poverty.

A lack of money limits the options of the elderly and can impair their health. They may not be able to afford nutritious food, regular health checkups, new eyeglasses or hearing aids, or the small pleasures that make life enjoyable.

## Housing

Nearly half of all Americans over age 65 own their own homes. Fewer than 5 percent live in nursing homes. The percentage of those in nursing homes rises with age, from barely 1 percent of men and women under age 74, to 22 percent of those age 85 or older.[12]

Housing can become a major problem for the elderly poor. They may have to live in low-rent apart-

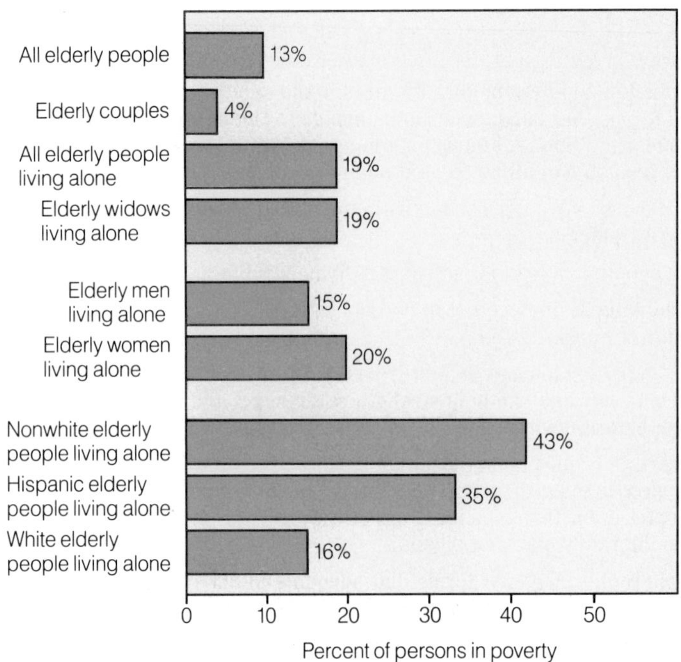


SOURCE: The Commonwealth Fund Commission on Elderly People Living Alone.

**FIGURE 17-2** Poverty rates among those age 65 and older, 1987.

ments in dangerous neighborhoods, where they are vulnerable to street criminals. Some end up isolated in tiny rooms, fearful of muggers, burglars, or simple safety hazards, such as dark and slippery staircases.

## Need for Help in Daily Living

As Figure 17-3 shows, many noninstitutionalized older adults need the help of another person to perform some activity of daily living. Some researchers estimate that one in five of these people need help with tasks such as dressing, walking, bathing, or shopping.[13] In the past, aging parents tended to live with their children's families. That's changed dramatically, however—not just because children live farther away or may be separated or divorced, but also because the older parents seem to prefer their independence. Problems can develop, though, when declining health or increasing disability makes it more difficult for the elderly to manage on their own.

Increasingly, older Americans are turning to their own peers for assistance. The percentage of individuals age 85 and older providing such care is almost as high as the percentage of 25- to 34-year-olds caring for the elderly.

Adult day centers and group retirement homes are another alternative for dealing with the problems of infirmity and old age. They help fill the gap between living at home and entering a nursing home. There are two types of these facilities: health centers, which focus on providing medical services, such as physical therapy, and social centers, which emphasize recreational and social activities.

## Loneliness

More than half of Americans over age 65 are married or live together in two-person households. However, for women, who generally outlive their husbands, the likelihood of living alone rises with time. Whereas 7 out of 10 men age 75 or older are still married and living with their spouses, 7 out of 10 women in that age group are widowed.[14] "We have our children and grandchildren and friends," says one woman in her eighties who lives in an apartment complex for elderly widows. "But we do miss our men."

## Senility

Typically, victims of senility show symptoms such as failing memory, errors in judgment, declining ability to work with numbers, and irritability. However, none of these symptoms by itself is an indication of senility. Only 5 to 10 percent of people over age 65 show serious mental deterioration. About 25 percent of the actual cases of senility—or senile dementia, as doctors call it—are caused by brain tumors, abnormal thyroid activity, some drug effects, and depression;

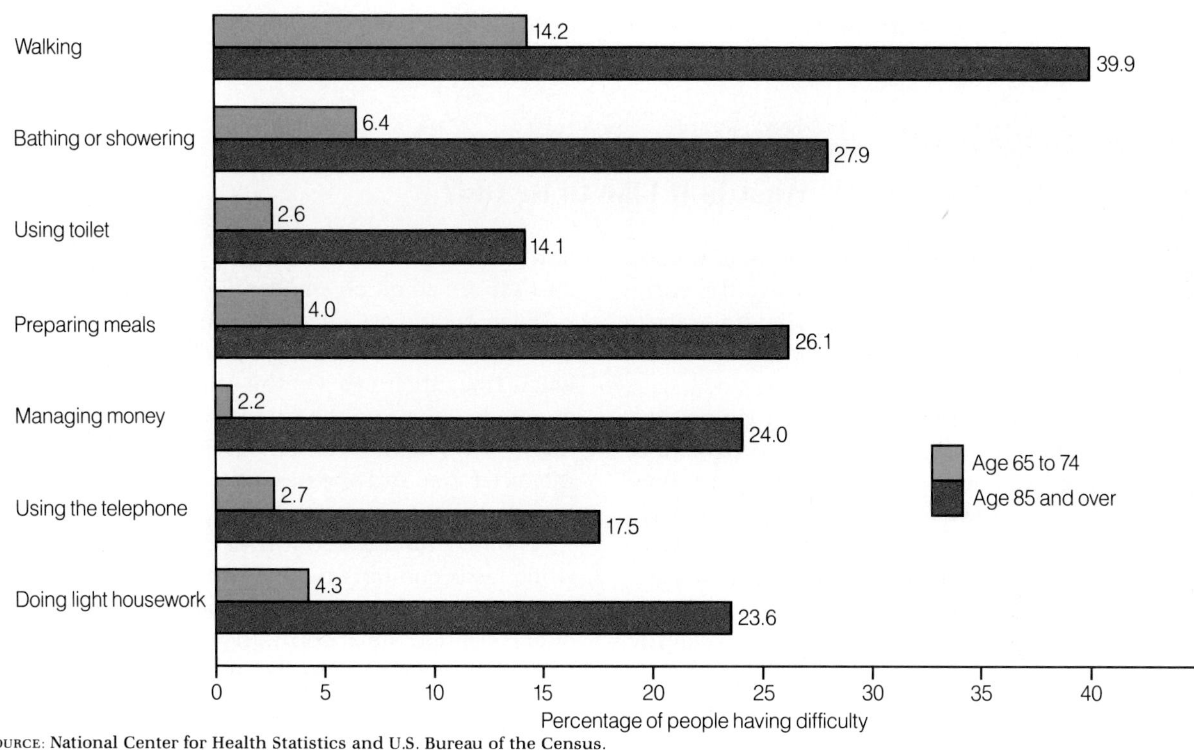


SOURCE: National Center for Health Statistics and U.S. Bureau of the Census.

**FIGURE 17-3** Problems of daily living for older adults.

in these cases, senility can be reversed. Many of the remaining cases are caused by Alzheimer's disease.[15]

## Alzheimer's Disease

The victims of **Alzheimer's disease,** described as the slow death of the mind, gradually lose their memories, their intellects, their personalities, and eventually their lives. Alzheimer's may afflict twice as many Americans as doctors once thought: a total of 4 million men and women over age 65. In a Harvard Medical School study reported in the *Journal of the American Medical Association,* researchers used a variety of neurological and cognitive tests to examine 3,623 elderly residents in Boston. They diagnosed "probable" Alzheimer's for 3 percent of those 65 to 74, 19 percent of the 75- to 84-year-olds, and 47 percent of those 85 or older.[16,17]

Alzheimer's remains a puzzling medical mystery. Until a decade or so ago, physicians assumed that mental impairment was an inevitable consequence of aging. They blamed symptoms such as a poor memory or confusion on hardening of the arteries of the brain. However, autopsies performed on the brains of Alzheimer's victims showed something quite different: missing brain cells and knots of tangled nerve fibers.[18]

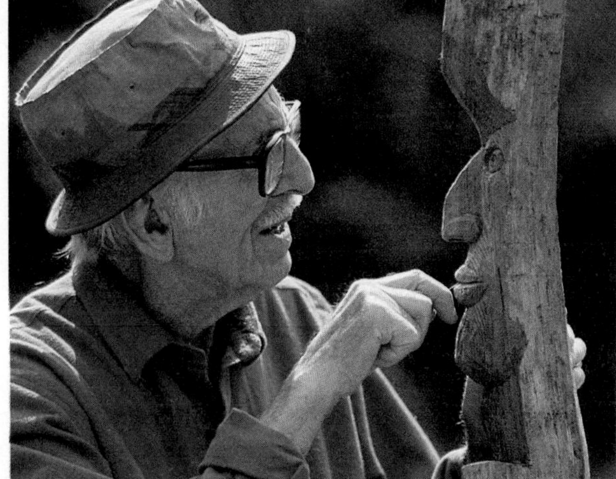

Hobbies remain a source of enjoyment and gratification throughout life.

**Alzheimer's disease** A progressive deterioration of intellectual powers due to physiological changes within the brain; symptoms include diminishing ability to concentrate and reason, disorientation, depression, apathy, and paranoia.

HEALTH SPOTLIGHT

## What Is It Like to Be Old?

"Everything is farther away than it used to be. It is even twice as far to the corner, and they have added a hill. I have given up running for the bus; it leaves earlier than it used to.

"It seems to me they are making the stairs steeper than in the old days. And have you noticed the smaller print they use in newspapers? There is no sense asking anyone to read aloud anymore, as everybody speaks in such a low voice I can hardly hear them.

"The material in dresses is so skimpy now, especially around the hips and waist, that it is almost impossible to reach one's shoelaces. And the sizes don't run the way they used to. The 12s and 14s are so much smaller.

"Even people are changing. They are so much younger than they used to be when I was their age. On the other hand, people my own age are so much older than I am. I ran into an old classmate the other day, and she has aged so much that she didn't recognize me.

"I got to thinking about the poor dear while I was combing my hair this morning; and in so doing, I glanced at my own reflection. Really now, they don't even make good mirrors like they used to."

SOURCE: A letter from an anonymous correspondent, reprinted by Ann Landers.

Alzheimer's is diagnosed through a combination of physical, psychiatric, and neurological examinations. Precise testing is crucial because many conditions—including brain tumors, infections, abnormal thyroid function, vitamin and nutrition deficiencies, alcoholism, and a series of small strokes—can mimic Alzheimer's.

As Alzheimer's progresses, patients have more trouble concentrating and reasoning. They may feel disoriented and lose their ability to recall words or form sentences. Later, they may show signs of paranoia, extreme depression, or apathy. Because they may wander away from home and get lost, some require close supervision either at home or in a nursing facility.

Many hospitals provide outpatient day therapy that seems to help Alzheimer's patients orient themselves. Staff members use large clocks and calendars to remind the patients of the time and day, provide photographs of themselves and the group to help the patients recall faces, label cupboards so items can more easily be found, and so on.

Some experimental drugs have helped patients temporarily, and early behavioral treatment may delay mental deterioration. Even those with severe cases benefit from adequate rest, exercise, intellectual stimulation, social contacts, balanced and regular meals, and elimination of nonessential drugs.

Researchers feel that they are close to a breakthrough in understanding the complex causes of Alzheimer's disease. Among the possible culprits are a virus, a genetic defect, and a combination of the two. Scientists already know that Alzheimer's victims lack certain crucial brain chemicals, so they are experimenting with drugs that may restore the natural chemical balance.[19]

Alzheimer's can take an enormous toll on the relatives of victims of the disease. Often they must watch helplessly as a loved one slowly becomes a stranger to them. Many hospitals and community mental health centers provide counseling and support groups for spouses and children of Alzheimer's patients.

### Mental Illness

The American Psychiatric Association estimates that 15 to 25 percent of the aged have significant symptoms of mental illness. Although more than 75 percent of the depressed elderly improve with treatment, the elderly are among the least likely to get the help they need. Services to senior citizens account for only 3 percent of those provided by therapists and clinics.[20]

In some communities, support groups for the aged—some focusing on specific issues, such as recent retirement, and some dedicated to sharing perspectives on a wide range of mutual problems—help older Americans deal with psychological problems.

### Elder Abuse

According to estimates from congressional committees on the aging, the number of cases of abused, neglected, or exploited elderly in the United States ranges from 600,000 to 1 million, or 4 percent of the elderly population. Abuse can take the form of deprivation, assault, or even rape. The average victim is age 75 or older and, more often, a woman. Usually the victim must rely on the abuser for food and shelter. Often, the abuser has drinking, drug, marital, or financial problems. Frightened that they have nowhere else to go, the elderly rarely report incidents of family abuse to police. In several communities, family service organizations are encouraging elderly victims to seek help and are also offering counseling to victims' children.

## HOW LONG CAN YOU LIVE?

As life expectancy has pushed higher, scientists have speculated that it may be possible to extend life not just by years, but by decades. According to one theory, gradually restricting caloric intake to about 40 percent less than needed to maintain normal body weight might allow people to live to the extremely ripe old age of 140 (see "Health Headlines" in this chapter). Other researchers believe that antioxidants—protective substances, including vitamins A, C, and E, and the mineral selenium (see Chapter 4)—might slow the aging process. However, all these theories remain long on promises and short on proof.[21]

### Wearing Out or Rusting Out?

Many scientists believe that the issue isn't the quantity, but the quality, of life and that the ideal life span, from a health perspective, is less than 100 years. In their book *Vitality and Aging*, Dr. James Fries and Dr. Lawrence Crapo of Stanford University School of Medicine make the case that the ideal life span is approximately eighty-five years.[22] Between 1900 and 1980, the average length of life rose from 47 to 73 years, they point out, but the same percentage of the population still lives to 85 years. The statistics on human longevity, they say, have remained unchanged in the past 100,000 years. The authors believe two reasons, limited cell doubling and declining organ reserve, may account for this.

*Cell doubling* refers to the number of cell doublings needed to replace dead cells. The capacity for cell doubling may be finite in the average life span of each species. Human cells double about fifty times; after that, new cells fail to grow, even though nutrients and other conditions remain the same.

*Organ reserve* refers to the functional capacity of human organs—including the heart, lungs, kidneys, and liver—to sustain life. This organ reserve allows a person's body to restore homeostasis—the body's internal balance—when it is disturbed by some sort of outside influence. In a young adult this capacity is 4 to 6 times greater than that needed for survival. However, organ reserve begins to decline at about age 30, and the eventual result is natural death, even without disease.

### The Toll of Stress

Over the years the wear and tear of daily living may leave us less able to cope with stress. When scientists study older people's response to experimental stressors (such as lowering blood pressure or temperature), their levels of norepinephrine (adrenalin), the hormone involved in the fight-or-flight response, go up higher and stay up longer than in young people. In other words, the aging person seems to overrespond to stress. Chronically high levels of norepinephrine can cause a variety of problems, including high blood pressure, anxiety, and poor sleep.

**STRATEGY FOR CHANGE**

**How to Live to Be 100 Years Old**

The Committee for an Extended Lifespan, in San Marcos, California, collected information on 1,000 centenarians, men and women who have lived 100 years or more. Here's what they can teach us about how to survive for a century:[23]

- Do nothing in excess. The centenarians who drink do so in moderation. Those who use tobacco indulge in cigars, pipes, or chewing.

The few that smoke cigarettes do not inhale. Few are fat. They are not given to binges of any kind.

- Get up early. The centenarians are early risers. Usually, this means they go to bed early, too.
- Have faith in some higher power. A high proportion have led what they consider a spiritual life, accepting all experiences as "God's will."
- Keep busy. Few are dreamers or loungers. The majority attribute their long survival to hard work.
- Take care of yourself. Centenarians are as self-sufficient as possible.

## LIVING IN AN AGING SOCIETY

The population of America is growing older (see Figure 17-4), and the "graying" of America will affect nearly every aspect of life in this country, including the following:

- *Retirement Costs*—Social Security taxes on workers will have to be increased unless the retirement age is raised or other changes are made to lessen the demand on the Social Security system.
- *Health Costs*—Medical costs for people over age 65 are twice those for people under age 65, who might be required to carry some of the burden for an aging population.
- *Aging and Education*—By the year 2000 there will be more Americans over age 55 than of elementary- and secondary-school age.
- *"Gray Power" Politics*—Senior citizens go to the polls in larger numbers than younger voters. With such voting power, programs for the elderly may make up a larger share of future federal budgets.

## MAKING THIS CHAPTER WORK FOR YOU

### Getting Older and Better

**The key to being healthy in your later years is having good health habits throughout life. Many of the physical changes that accompany aging—such as the decline in heart and lung functioning, slowing of circulation and metabolism, loss of muscular strength, and slowing of reaction time—can be delayed by regular exercise and a nutritious diet.**

**FIGURE 17-4** Because of better health and medical care, more people are living longer. By the year 2000—less than 10 years from now—almost 30 million Americans will be over 55.

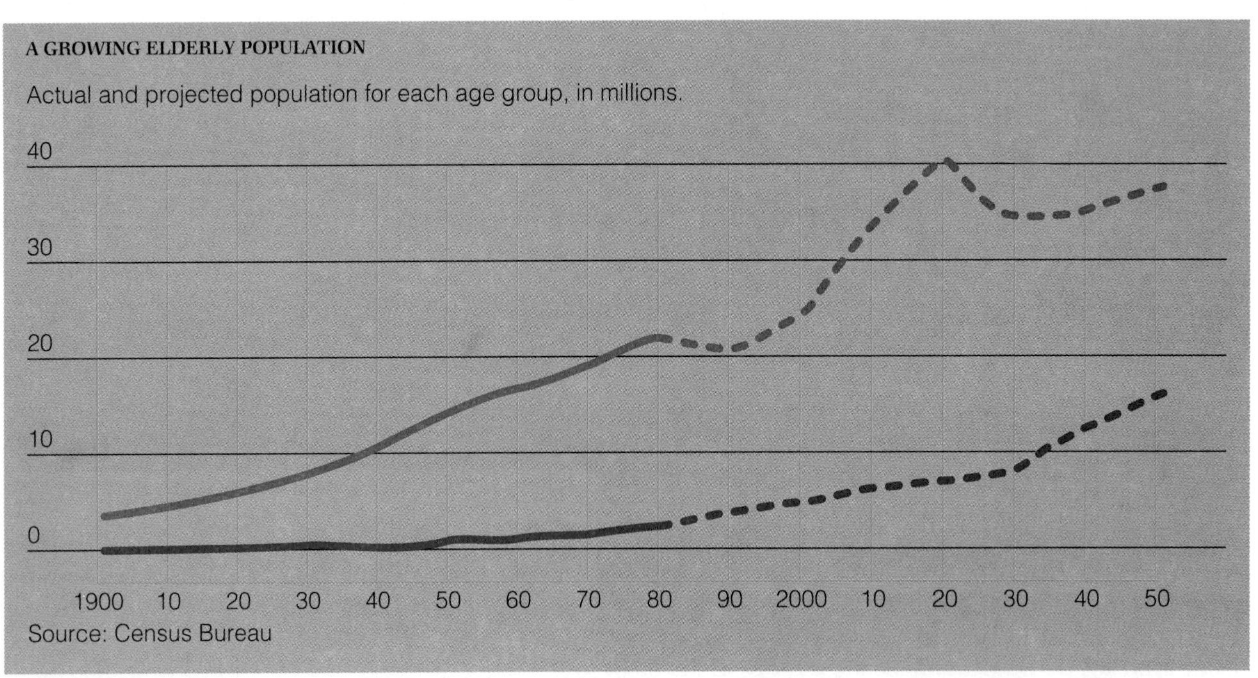

## WHAT DO YOU THINK?

Who's happier: older people or young adults? According to social psychologist Dr. Carin Rubinstein, "Old people in general feel psychologically better than young people. They have fewer worries about themselves and how they look to other people; they have higher self-esteem; they aren't as lonely as people think they are." Are you surprised? Why? What do you think most affects happiness in a young person? In an older person?

Imagine a time in the future when your aged mother suffers a stroke. The doctors tell you that she will require constant care for the rest of her life. Neither your mother's insurance nor the government pays for such help. Medicaid will pay for a nursing home only after your mother has used up all the money she has. What would you do? What options would you have? Can you do anything now to plan for such a situation?

Steve just found out that his widowed grandmother is moving to a one-bedroom apartment with a male friend. Steve is upset by the news and tells his grandmother that she "is too old for such foolishness." Can you understand his attitude? How would you feel if it were your grandmother? If you were Steve's grandmother, what would you say to help him accept your decision?

Most intellectual abilities do not diminish with age, although some, such as the ability to remember newly learned information, do decline. Sexual interest does not diminish with age, although sexual activity may decrease because of a lack of partners.

In older people drugs may cause different reactions than in younger people, and diseases may have different symptoms. Osteoporosis, a major health problem for elderly people, can be prevented by exercise; increased calcium intake; and, in women, estrogen supplements. Abuse of prescription and over-the-counter drugs is a common problem among the elderly.

Many older Americans lack the financial resources for basic necessities such as regular health care and a nutritious diet. Almost half of all elderly Americans own their homes; however, for older adults who are poor, finding safe and affordable housing is a major problem. Because of illness or disability, about one in five older adults needs assistance in performing the activities of daily living. Because women tend to outlive their spouses, there is great likelihood that they will live out their elderly years alone.

Senility can be the result of a brain tumor; abnormal thyroid activity; drug side effects; depression; or Alzheimer's disease, a condition in which the mind slowly deteriorates. Its possible causes include a virus, a genetic defect, and a combination of the two. Elderly people may also become victims of abuse, sometimes at the hands of their own children.

You may think that aging is something that concerns only your parents or teachers. But stop and ask yourself: What will you be like in twenty, thirty, or forty years? To some degree, you may find the answer today. Just as you were a different person ten years ago, you will undoubtedly be a different person decades from now. Here are some rules to remember for growing better as you grow older:

- Read something informative and interesting every day, if only for a few minutes.
- Stay flexible and curious. Avoid emotional and mental ruts.
- Stay in contact with other people of all ages and experiences. Make the effort to invite them to your home, or arrange to go out with them.
- Practice the art of good listening.
- On a regular basis, perhaps once a week, do something to help another person.
- Greet each day with a specific goal—to play a game of golf, write letters, clean the workroom, or visit a friend.

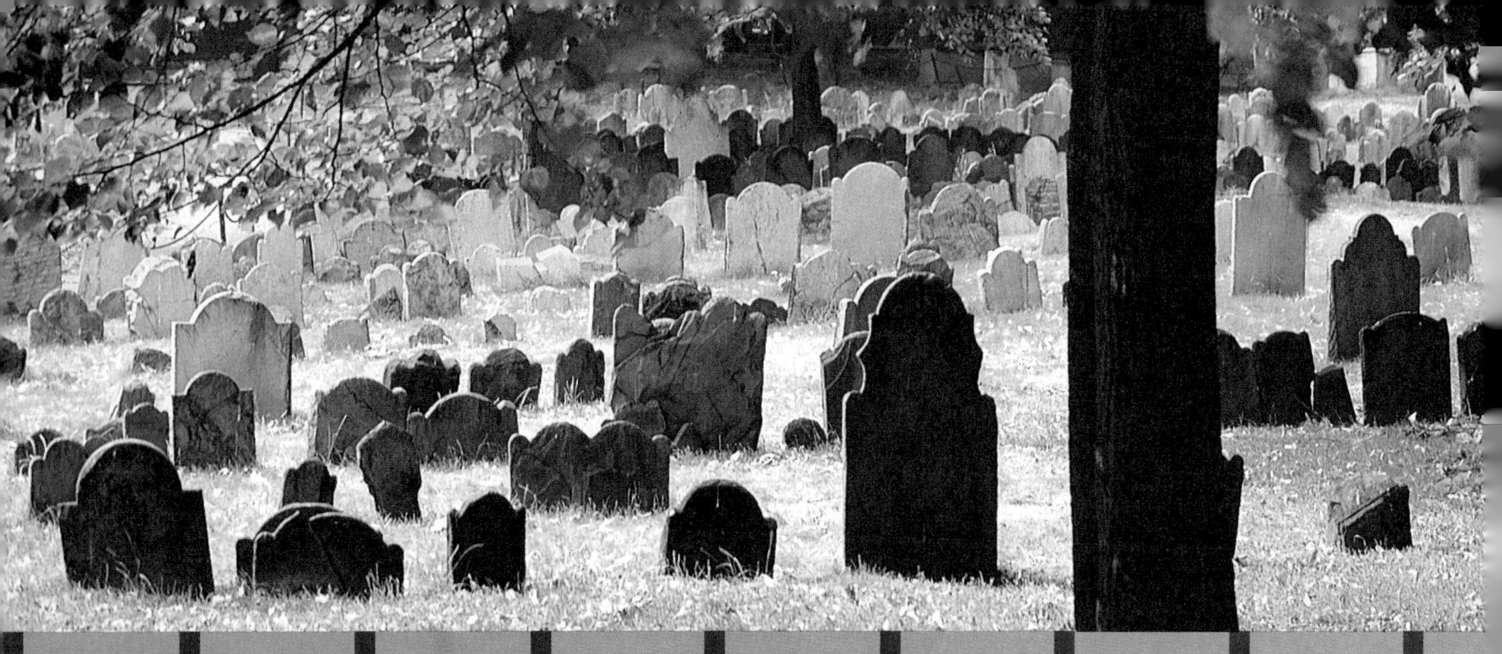

# 18 THE FINAL CHAPTER: COMING TO TERMS WITH DEATH

In this chapter

What is death?

Denying death

Facing life's end

Grief

Practical arrangements

Preparing for your death

Making this chapter work for you: Understanding the meaning of death

*No one gets out of this life alive.* Death is the natural completion of things, as much a part of the real world as life itself. If you are in your late teens or twenties, death may seem unimaginable. That's normal: At all ages, we struggle to deny the reality of death.

Yet we never escape. We lose grandparents, uncles and aunts, parents, friends, coworkers, teachers, and neighbors. As parents, we may lose our children; as partners, we may lose the persons we love most. With every loss, part of us dies; yet each loss also reaffirms how precious life is.

The death that most frightens and fascinates us is our own. We hope that it will not come for a long, long time. We also hope that when it does come, we will be able to face it with dignity and courage; and we wonder—as have all who've come before us—what, if anything, waits beyond death.

This chapter explores the meaning of death, describes the process of dying, provides practical information on medical and legal arrangements, and offers advice on comforting the dying and helping their survivors.

## WHAT IS DEATH?

Because machines can now keep alive people who, in the past, would have died, the definition of death has become more complex. Among the possible ways of defining death are the following:

- *Functional Death*—The end of all vital functions, such as heartbeat and respiration.
- *Cellular Death*—Many cells die gradually, at different rates, some time after the heart stops. If placed in a tissue culture or, as is the case with various organs, transplanted to another body, some cells can remain alive indefinitely.
- *Cardiac Death*—The moment when the heart stops beating.
- *Brain Death*—The end of all brain activity, indicated by an absence of electrical activity (confirmed by a test called an electroencephalogram); a lack of reflexes, response to stimuli, and movement; and an absence of breathing.
- *Spiritual Death*—Many religions define this as the moment when the soul leaves the body.

The traditional legal definition of death is failure of the lungs or heart to function. However, because modern medicine is often able to maintain respiration and circulation by artificial means, most states have declared that an individual is considered dead only when the brain, including the brain stem, completely stops functioning. Brain-death laws do not allow medical staff to "pull the plug" if there is any hope of sustaining life.

## DENYING DEATH

Most of us don't quite believe that we're going to die. Whereas a reasonable amount of denial helps us focus on the day-to-day realities of living, excessive denial can be life-threatening. Many drivers, for instance, refuse to buckle up their seat belts, because they deny that a drunk driver might collide with them. Cigarette smokers deny that lung cancer will ever strike them. People who eat high-fat meals deny that they'll ever suffer a heart attack.

One important factor in denial is the nature of the threat. It's easy to believe death is at hand when someone points a gun at you. It is harder to believe cigarette smoking might cause your death 20 or 30 years down the line.

## FACING LIFE'S END

Most people who have a fatal, or **terminal,** illness, prefer to know the truth about their health and chances for recovery. Even when they are not officially informed by a doctor or relative, most fatally ill people know or strongly suspect they are dying.

Dying people usually make it clear whether they want to talk about death and to what extent. The most frequent concern is how much time is left. Usually physicians can give only a rough estimate, such as "several weeks or months."

One way of reducing the mystery and fear of death is to learn more about it. The more we all learn about the process of dying and about what can be done to help more people die in peace, the better we can understand and offer support to the terminally ill.

**terminal illness** The final stages of a fatal illness.

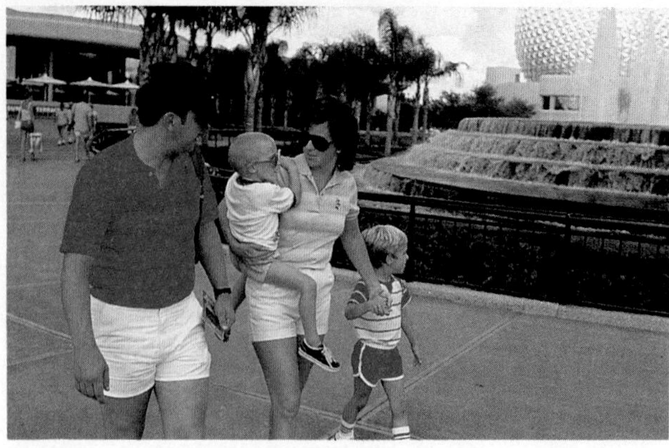

These parents of a terminally ill child are trying to make the most of every remaining day of his life.

## The Emotional Experience of Dying

Psychiatrist Elisabeth Kubler-Ross, who has studied the process of dying, has identified five typical stages of reaction:[1]

1. *Denial ("No, not me.")*—On learning that death is coming, a terminally ill patient rejects the news. The denial overcomes the initial shock and allows the person to begin to gather together his or her defenses. Denial, at this point, is a healthy defense mechanism. It can become distressful, however, if it is reinforced by the relatives and friends of the dying patient.
2. *Anger* ("Why me?")—In the second stage, the dying person begins to feel resentment and rage toward his or her impending death. The anger may be directed at the patient's family and caregivers, who can do little but try to endure such encounters, comfort the patient, and help him or her on to the next stage.
3. *Bargaining ("Yes, me, but . . .")*—In this stage, a patient may try to bargain, usually with God, for a way to reverse, or at least postpone, dying. The patient may promise, in exchange for recovery, to do good works or to see his or her family more. Alternatively, he or she may say "Let me live long enough to see my grandchild born," or ". . . to see the spring again."
4. *Depression ("Yes, it's me.")*—In the fourth stage, the patient gradually realizes the full consequences of his or her condition. This may begin as grieving for health that has been lost and then become anticipatory grieving for the loss that is to come of friends, loved ones, and life itself. This is perhaps the most difficult time, and the dying person should not be left alone. Neither should one try to cheer the patient, for he or she must be allowed to grieve.
5. *Acceptance ("Yes, me; and I'm ready.")*—In this last stage, the person has accepted the reality of his or her death: The moment looms as neither frightening nor painful, neither sad nor happy—only inevitable. As the person waits for the end of life, he or she may ask to see fewer visitors, to separate from other people, and perhaps to turn to just one person for support.

Several stages may exist at the same time. Some may occur out of sequence. Each stage may take days, or only hours or minutes. Throughout, denial may come back to assert itself unexpectedly—and hope for a medical breakthrough or a miraculous recovery is forever present.

Not all people go through such well-defined stages in the dying process. Some specialists have commented that the way a person faces death is a mirror of the way he or she has faced other major stresses in life: Those who have had the most trouble adjusting to other crises will have the most trouble adjusting to the news of their impending death.

The family of a dying person also experiences a spectrum of often wrenching emotions. Family members too may deny the verdict of death, rage at the doctors and nurses who can't do more to save their loved one, bargain with God to give up their own health if necessary, sink into helplessness and depression, and finally accept the reality of their anticipated loss.

**STRATEGY FOR CHANGE**

### How to Help a Dying Person

Although you may be reluctant to visit, your presence can convey the message that the dying person has not been abandoned.

- Don't worry about what to say. Your words matter less than your presence. Just being there, holding hands, is a comfort.
- Listen. Dying people often need someone to listen as they talk through their feelings. Such discussions don't make them more upset but help them come to terms with what is happening.
- Be genuine. Don't try to look or act cheerful. Your loved one will see through you and feel more isolated than before. It's better to let your sadness and concern show.
- Don't try to explain or rationalize what has happened. Offer consolation and reassurance.

## HALES INDEX

Number of comatose patients being kept alive artificially: 10,000

Percentage of physicians who favor withdrawal of life support systems from hopelessly ill or comatose patients if family requests: 78
Percentage of Americans who believe doctors should be allowed to withdraw life-sustaining equipment if patient has left a living will: 81

Percentage who believe doctors should administer lethal injections or drugs in such cases: 57

Percentage who believe families and doctors, not lawmakers, should decide about ending the lives of comatose patients: 81

Number of states that heed living wills: 40

Number of members of the pro-euthanasia Hemlock Society: 32,000

Number of individuals still depressed four years after losing a spouse: 2 in 5

Estimated number of AIDS patients who've committed suicide: 1,000

SOURCES: **1** Gibbs, Nancy. "Love and Let Die," *Time,* March 19, 1990. **2, 3, 4, 5** Gianelli, Diane. "Would Aiding in Dying Make MDs Hired Killers?" *American Medical News,* February 16, 1990. **6** Rymer, Russ. "The Judge," *Hippocrates,* May/June 1988. **7** Cooke, Patricia. "The Gentle Death," *Hippocrates,* September/October 1989. **8** Goleman, Daniel. "New Studies Find Many Myths about Mourning," *New York Times,* August 8, 1989. **9** Mydans, Seth. "AIDS Patients' Silent Companion Is Often Suicide, Experts Discover," *New York Times,* February 25, 1990.

## Life Before Death

Even when patients cannot be cured, medical care can help them feel more comfortable by relieving discomfort and pain. Some patients require sophisticated treatments available only in hospitals. Others prefer to go home, where they feel more like individuals, remain part of their families, and avoid some of the feelings of isolation.

The National Institute on Aging has compiled the findings and observations of researchers who've studied the experience of dying. Here's what they found:[2]

- Dying patients under the age of 50 have greater mental and physical distress than those age 50 and older.
- Levels of depression and anxiety vary with the length and discomfort of the terminal illness.
- People dying at home are more likely to be fully alert before death; less likely to be suffering from vomiting, incontinence, or bedsores; and less likely to experience unrelieved physical distress than are hospitalized patients. (However, patients in hospitals may have been sicker initially and thus more likely to suffer distress.)
- Terminal patients develop similar physical symptoms, such as pain, difficulty breathing and swallowing, nausea, vomiting, persistent cough, weakness, hiccups, and loss of appetite. More than half also exhibit mental symptoms, including fear, depression, uncoordinated thinking, lack of interest, hallucinations, irritability, forgetfulness, lack of concentration and judgment, delusions, auditory and visual illusions, and unconsciousness. Patients with strong religious beliefs—or a total absence of them—show less fear than do those with weaker religious convictions.

Patients seem to be more afraid of pain, physical distress, or chronic disability than they are of death itself. Immediately before death, patients need less pain-relieving medication and often seem more vital, appreciate food again, and appear generally improved.

### Pain Relief

In the past, medical professionals often gave drugs to a terminal patient on an "as-needed" basis—that is, when the pain got so bad that the person asked for relief. Because this can result in the person's last hours being a cycle of anxiety, anger, and pain, drugs are now often given on a regular, timed basis, beginning with a small dose and gradually increasing until the patient is pain-free, with each subsequent dose given before the previous one has worn off.

In addition to standard painkillers, researchers have also experimented with restricted drugs such as marijuana (for the relief of nausea in cancer patients undergoing chemotherapy), heroin (as a painkiller for people who do not respond well to other narcotics), and LSD (to reduce pain and alleviate fears).

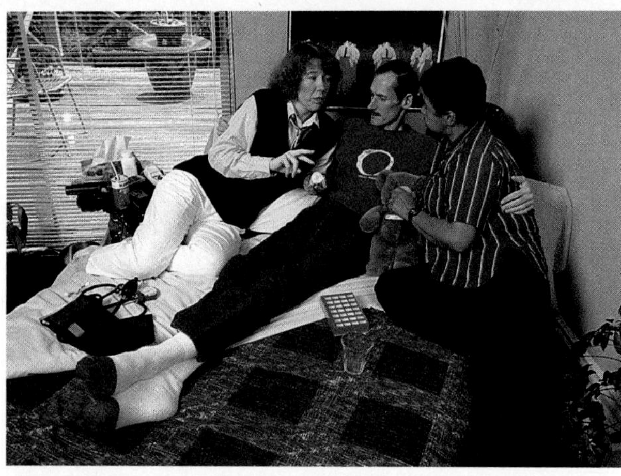

Hospices create a caring, comforting environment that allows dying patients to spend their final days surrounded by those they love.

## Hospice: Caring When Curing Isn't Possible

In **hospice** programs caregivers help dying men and women live their final days to the fullest, as free as possible from disabling pain and mental anguish, often in their own homes or in a special setting for the terminally ill. Hospice workers generally work in teams, usually consisting of a nurse, physician, social worker, and chaplain, and trained volunteers. Others, such as physical therapists, may join the team when needed. These workers provide the comfort, support, and care dying patients need until they do die.

Hospices offer a combination of medical and emotional care that involves not only the patient, but also the family or others concerned with caring for the patient. Most hospice patients have life expectancies of six months or less and no longer are receiving treatments aimed at curing their diseases. When someone is available to provide care, patients remain in their own homes. Hospice nurses regularly visit all home patients and are available around the clock.

For patients requiring care that the family cannot provide, 24-hour care is available at many hospice facilities. Unlike a traditional hospital, where the focus is on diagnosis, cure, and treatment, a hospice works to make what is left of life pain-free and comfortable. Visiting hours for relatives and friends are flexible, with no restrictions on visits by children and grandchildren. Hospice services are covered, in full or part, by most major insurance companies.

## Sustaining Life: Who Decides When to Pull the Plug

Increasingly, doctors and lawyers are recognizing a patient's right to die. The courts have upheld that "the right of a competent adult patient to refuse medical treatment is a constitutionally guaranteed right which must not be abridged." Medical ethicists have developed guidelines for health-care professionals. Such guidelines state that dying patients or their families should be able to refuse life-sustaining treatments, including transfusions and feeding tubes.[3]

Families have gone to court for permission to disconnect respirators or feeding tubes for patients who have spent years in a vegetable-like state. One 82-year-old patient sued the doctors who resuscitated him after a heart attack for "wrongful life."[4]

## Euthanasia: "Mercy Death"

Passive **euthanasia,** sometimes called **dyathanasia,** is the ending of extraordinary methods of sustaining life and may take the form of withholding oxygen, intravenous feeding, or other life-sustaining medical techniques from a terminally ill patient. Euthanasia, which is illegal, is the active form of so-called mercy death for terminally ill patients in extreme pain.

## Suicide

One of the main causes of suicide is illness, especially terminal illness. Approximately three-quarters of those who commit suicide consult a physician, most with medical complaints, within the six-month period prior to their deaths (see Chapter 2).

Disease, medication, and the fear of pain or of being a burden to the family can breed depression, a primary factor among those who attempt suicide. Fatally ill individuals who talk about suicide should be taken seriously; family physicians can arrange for them to talk with psychotherapists.

## Out-of-Body Experiences

Some individuals who have survived a close brush with death have reported watching, from several feet in the air, resuscitation attempts on their own bodies or a sense of passing into a foreign region or dimension. These experiences were not perceived as unpleasant or terrifying, but rather as going through darkness and then entering a brightly lit space of beauty and calm. Whereas some see such reports as proof of an afterlife, others have suggested that they are invented experiences caused by the mind's attempt to fill a psychological vacuum.

**hospice** A program of care, based either at home or in a home-like facility, that provides supportive care for terminally ill persons and their families.
**euthanasia** A passive or active method of painlessly causing death for terminally ill patients.
**dyathanasia** Ending extraordinary methods of sustaining life.

SELF-SURVEY

## How Do You Feel About Death?

***Purpose***
This questionnaire is not designed to test your knowledge. Instead it should encourage you to think about your present attitudes toward death and how these attitudes may have developed.

***Directions***
Answer the questions to the best of your knowledge, by circling the appropriate letter.

1. Who died in your first personal involvement with death?
   a. grandparent or great-grandparent
   b. parent
   c. brother or sister
   d. friend or acquaintance
   e. stranger
   f. public figure
   g. animal
2. To the best of your memory, at what age were you first aware of death?
   a. under 3 years
   b. 3 to 5 years
   c. 5 to 10 years
   d. 10 years or older
3. When you were a child, how was death talked about in your family?
   a. openly
   b. with some sense of discomfort
   c. only when necessary and then with an attempt to exclude children
   d. as though it were a taboo subject
   e. never recall any discussion
4. Which of the following best describes your childhood conceptions of death?
   a. heaven-and-hell concept
   b. afterlife
   c. death as sleep
   d. cessation of all physical and mental activity
   e. mysterious and unknowable
   f. something other than the above
   g. no conception
   h. can't remember
5. To what extent do you believe in a life after death?
   a. strongly believe in it
   b. tend to believe it
   c. uncertain
   d. tend to doubt it
   e. convinced it does not exist
6. Regardless of your belief about life after death, what is your wish about it?
   a. I strongly wish there were a life after death.
   b. I am indifferent about life after death.
   c. I definitely prefer that there not be a life after death.
7. Has there been a time in your life when you wanted to die?
   a. yes, mainly because of great physical pain
   b. yes, mainly because of great emotional upset

## SELF-SURVEY

c. yes, mainly to escape an intolerable social or interpersonal situation
d. yes, mainly because of great embarrassment
e. yes, for a reason other than above
f. no

8. What does death mean to you?
   a. the end, the final process of life
   b. the beginning of a life after death, a transition, a new beginning
   c. a joining of the spirit with a universal cosmic consciousness
   d. a kind of endless sleep, rest and peace
   e. termination of this life but survival of the spirit
   f. don't know
   g. other (specify) ______________
9. What aspect of your own death is the most distasteful to you?
   a. I could no longer have any experiences.
   b. I am afraid of what might happen to my body after death.
   c. I am uncertain about what might happen to me if there is a life after death.
   d. I could no longer provide for my dependents.
   e. It would cause grief to my relatives and friends.
   f. All my plans and projects would come to an end.
   g. The process of dying might be painful.
   h. Other (specify) ______________
10. How do you rate your present physical health?
    a. excellent
    b. very good
    c. moderately good
    d. moderately poor
    e. extremely bad
11. How do you rate your present mental health?
    a. excellent
    b. very good
    c. moderately good
    d. moderately poor
    e. extremely poor
12. Based on your present feelings, what is the probability of your taking your own life in the near future?
    a. extremely high (feel very much like killing myself)
    b. moderately high
    c. between high and low
    d. moderately low
    e. extremely low (very improbable that I would kill myself)
13. In your opinion, at what age are people most afraid of death?
    a. up to 12 years
    b. 13 to 19 years
    c. 20 to 29 years
    d. 30 to 39 years
    e. 40 to 49 years
    f. 50 to 59 years

g. 60 to 69 years
h. 70 years and over

14. When you think of your own death (or when circumstances make you realize your own mortality), how do you feel?
a. fearful
b. discouraged
c. depressed
d. purposeless
e. resolved, in relation to life
f. pleasure, in being alive
g. other (specify) ______________

15. What is your present orientation to your own death?
a. death-seeker
b. death-hastener
c. death-accepter
d. death-welcomer
e. death-postponer
f. death-fearer

16. If you were told that you had a terminal disease and a limited time to live, how would you want to spend your time until you died?
a. I would make a marked change in my life-style to satisfy hedonistic needs (travel, sex, drugs, or other experiences).
b. I would become more withdrawn—reading, contemplating, or praying.
c. I would shift from my own needs to a concern for others (family and friends).
d. I would attempt to complete projects, to tie up loose ends.
e. I would make little or no change in my life-style.
f. I would try to do one very important thing.
g. I might consider committing suicide.
h. I would do none of these.

17. How do you feel about having an autopsy done on your body?
a. approve
b. don't care one way or the other
c. disapprove
d. strongly disapprove

Now examine your attitudes toward death and discuss your feelings with classmates, friends, and family. Although we read about death in the newspapers every day, we rarely come in close contact with it. Our society tends to reinforce the denial of death. By completing this questionnaire, you are taking a step toward facing the reality of death.

SOURCE: Shneidman, Edwin. "You and Death Questionnaire," *Psychology Today*, August 1970.

## GRIEF

An estimated 8 million Americans lose a member of their immediate family each year. The death of a loved one may be the single most upsetting and feared event in a person's life. According to one survey, college students listed death of a relative as their greatest fear, even outweighing fear of their own deaths.[5]

The death of a family member produces a wide range of reactions, including anxiety, guilt, anger, and money worries. Many see the death of an old person as less tragic (usually) than the death of a child or young person. A sudden death is more of a shock than one following long illness. A suicide can be particularly devastating because family members may wonder if they could have prevented it.

The cause of death can also affect the reactions of friends and acquaintances. Some people express less sympathy and support when death is by suicide or homicide.

### HEALTH HEADLINE

#### Willpower Can Delay Death

**The desire to live long enough to celebrate a big event can keep people alive, according to a study of elderly Chinese women in California. During the week before a major family festival, the death rate was abnormally low. The week after the celebration, the death rate was abnormally high. During this particular festival, the oldest woman in the family directs younger women and serves as the focal point of the holiday feast. The researchers also found a dip and peak in death rates around the observance of an individual's birthday or other "personally meaningful" occasions.**

SOURCE: Phillips, D. P. and D. G. Smith. "Postponement of Death until Symbolically Meaningful Occasions," *Journal of the American Medical Association*, vol. 263, no. 14, April 11, 1990.

### STRATEGY FOR CHANGE

#### Knowing What Not to Say

Sometimes poorly chosen words, meant to comfort, only make a grieving person feel worse. Here are some to avoid:

- "It's God's will."
- "You're so strong. It's fortunate this happened to someone like you."
- "Tell me what I can do."
- "I understand."
- "It was a blessing."

Such statements minimize the grieving person's anguish, make the mourner feel guilty about being sad or angry, or seem insensitive.

### The Biology of Grief

Men and women who lose partners, parents, or children endure so much stress that they're at increased risk of serious physical and mental illness, and even of premature death. A two-year study by the National Academy of Sciences of the biology of grief—the most comprehensive scientific review ever of the impact that death has on survivors—found the following:[6,7]

- For widowers under age 75, there is a significant increase in death from accidents, heart disease, and some infectious illnesses. The risk is greatest in the first year but continues for as long as six years among men who don't remarry. There is also an increased likelihood of suicide in the first year, particularly among older widowers.
- For women, mortality may increase in later years after bereavement, but not in the first year. Women seem to stand up better, in part because they "are more likely to cry on a friend's shoulder" and tend to seek greater social support than men.
- Some widows may have increased rates of suicide and death from cirrhosis of the liver. Grief intensifies self-destructive behaviors such as smoking, drinking, and drug use. The greatest risk factors are poor previous mental and physical health and a lack of social support.
- Friends and remarriage offer the greatest protection against health problems.
- Grieving adults may experience mood swings between sadness and anger, guilt and anxiety. They may feel physically sick, lose their appetites, sleep poorly, or fear they're going crazy because they "see" the deceased person on the street, in a restaurant, or wherever they go.

HEALTH SPOTLIGHT

## One Man's Grief

In the following essay, a college student describes what it's like to lose a close friend:

On a December night, Gary was shot and killed on the street. It happened during our junior year of college. For nearly 16 years we had been companions and confidantes, passing through childhood, adolescence, and early adulthood together. Each of us had always provided the other a word of encouragement, an available ear, a shoulder to lean on. In school, sports, and play, we competed as equals; and as our lives unfolded, our friendship developed with the same equality.

Staring at his body in the funeral home left me bewildered: Where had Gary gone? This had happened just as he and I thought we had begun to untangle some of life's intricacies. I was 20 years old, and the confrontation with mortality left me breathless, robbed of my desire to fight.

I went through the motions of being back in school. Each day I attended classes and meals; but every morning I faced the same sadness and anger: *Why* had I awakened? Couldn't I just die in my sleep? One night I had a dream in which Gary was comforting me. His words were assuaging the pain: "Death is friendly. It doesn't hurt. I promise you, I never felt the bullets. I'll see you again someday." I wrapped that dream around my shivering soul.

Then one morning in April, I awoke to the sun pouring into my room and the sound of birds singing outside. Something about awakening that morning was different. A realization drifted up slowly from within: I was *glad* to be alive.

That was the most painful, wonderful discovery. I knew it meant that I would go on with my life, that I was ready and wanted to continue living; but it also confirmed the knowledge that Gary was dead. I finally understood the contradiction: Gary would always be with me; yet I would have to go on living without him.

SOURCE: Journal of the American Medical Association, March 23–30, 1984.

- Grief produces changes in the respiratory, hormonal, and central nervous systems, and may affect functions of the heart, blood, and immune systems.

Men and women's response to the loss of a mate—and subsequent health risks—may depend on how their spouses died. Men whose wives die suddenly face a much greater risk of dying themselves than those whose wives die after a long illness; women whose husbands die after a long illness face greater risk than other widows, according to a University of Utah study reported in *Psychology Today.* The reason may be that, unlike men whose wives die suddenly, those whose wives were chronically ill may have learned how to cope with the loss of their nurturers. On the other hand, women who have spent a long time caring for an ill husband may be at greater risk because of the combined burdens of caregiving and the loss of financial support.[8]

## Methods of Mourning

Psychotherapists refer to grief as work, and it is that—slow, tedious, and painful. Yet only by working through grief can bereaved individuals make their way back to the living world of hope and love.

Psychotherapists define normal grief as a predictable succession of stages of resolution. In pathologic grief, the bereaved person stops somewhere in the midst of the process of normal grieving and may become clinging and overreliant; pine for the deceased; or show signs of denial, avoidance, or anxiety.[9]

Grief is, as one researcher put it, "an individual journey." Some people resolve their grief and accept death as "God's will" or as "something that happens." Others deal with their grief by keeping busy to take their minds off their losses. For many, grief can long remain an everyday presence in life.

New studies on grief, reviewed in the *Journal of Clinical and Consulting Psychology,* indicate that mourning can take many forms. About a quarter to two-thirds of widows and widowers are not greatly distressed by their losses. Those who lose children or spouses in car accidents are most likely to remain depressed and anxious years later. One of the most devastating losses is the death of a child killed by a drunk driver. Many years afterward parents cannot find any "meaning" in what happened.[10]

**STRATEGY FOR CHANGE**

**Grieving for Someone You Love**

- Accept your feelings as normal. Don't try to deny emotions such as anger, guilt, despair, emptiness, confusion, anxiety, relief, or fear.
- Let others help you. (It will make them feel better too.)
- Express your feelings—through tears, recollections, and talking about them with others—so that you can accept the loss.
- Don't feel that you must be strong and brave and silent, though you have every right to keep your grief private.
- Face each day as it comes. Give yourself time—more than you ever imagined—for the pain to ebb, the scars to heal, and the rest of your life to begin.

**HEALTH HEADLINE**

**When Parents Die**

**Even in adulthood, individuals who lose their parents may feel like orphaned children, according to researchers at the University of Southern California School of Social Work. One to five years after a parent's death, at least 25 percent of those studied cried or became upset when they thought of the dead parent. More than 20 percent continued to be preoccupied with thoughts of the parent. An especially common response was a feeling of being orphaned and no longer fitting into the role of being anyone's child.**

SOURCE: Larsen, David. "The 'Orphaned' Adult," *San Francisco Chronicle*, February 2, 1990.

### Helping the Survivors

Though we grieve for the dead, the living are the ones who need our help. Bereavement is such an intense loss that survivors may be too numb or too stunned to ask for help. Family and friends must take the initiative and spend time with them, even if that means sitting together silently. Offer empathy and support and let the grieving person know with verbal and nonverbal expressions that you care and wish to help.

Most bereaved people do not need professional psychological counseling. However, you should urge a friend or relative to seek help if he or she shows no sign of grieving or exhibits as much distress a year after the loss as during the first months. The family members of a suicide victim are most likely to need and benefit from professional help in sorting out their feelings of failure, anger, and sorrow.

**STRATEGY FOR CHANGE**

**How to Comfort Grieving Friends**

- Be there. Your presence will let your friend know you care. A hug can communicate more than a thousand words.
- Listen. Bereaved individuals need to talk out their feelings—often again and again.
- Write a simple note. A few phrases, such as "I want to let you know I'm thinking of you and praying for you," mean a great deal. A small gift, such as a book or a plant, is also thoughtful.
- Invite your friend to do something with you. Choose something you know your friend might enjoy—a walk in the country or a concert.
- Don't give your help over the first few days or weeks only, and then withdraw. Grieving people continue to need support for many months. The first anniversary of a death or the first holiday spent alone can be particularly miserable.

## PRACTICAL ARRANGEMENTS

At a time of great emotional pain, grieving family members must cope with medical, legal, and practical arrangements, including obtaining a medical certificate of the cause of death, registering the death, and making funeral arrangements. They may also want to arrange for organ donations and, in some circumstances, an autopsy.

## Funeral Arrangements

Memorial societies are voluntary groups that help people plan in advance for death. They obtain services at moderate cost; keep the arrangements simple and dignified; and—most important, perhaps—ease the emotional and financial burden on the rest of the family when death finally does come.

A body can be either buried or cremated. Burial requires the purchase of a cemetery plot, which many families do decades before death. For cremation (incineration of the remains), you must complete some additional formalities, with which the funeral director can help you. After a cremation, you can either collect the ashes to keep, bury, or scatter for yourself or ask the crematorium to dispose of them.

The tradition of a funeral may help survivors come to terms with the death, enabling them both to mourn their loss and to celebrate the dead person's life. Alternatively, the body may be disposed of immediately, through burial, cremation, or bequeathal to a medical school; a memorial service can be held at some time thereafter.

Funerals are usually held 2 to 4 days after death. Many have two parts: a religious ceremony at a church or funeral home and a burial ceremony at the grave site. A memorial service is also a possibility; the body is not present, which may change the focus of the service from the person's death to his or her life.

## Autopsies

An **autopsy** is a detailed examination and dissection of a body after death, also called a postmortem exam. The two types of autopsies are medicolegal autopsies and medical/educational autopsies.

A *medicolegal* autopsy is performed to establish the cause of death and to gather information about the death for use as evidence in any legal proceedings. It is done to detect any crimes and to help identify the proper person for prosecution, to investigate possible industrial hazards or contagious diseases that may endanger the public health, or to establish the cause of death for insurance purposes.

A *medical/educational* autopsy is performed, usually in the hospital where the person died, to increase medical knowledge and to determine a more exact cause of death. It may be requested by either the attending physician or the family, but it cannot be performed without the family's permission.

**autopsy** The detailed examination and dissection of a dead body.

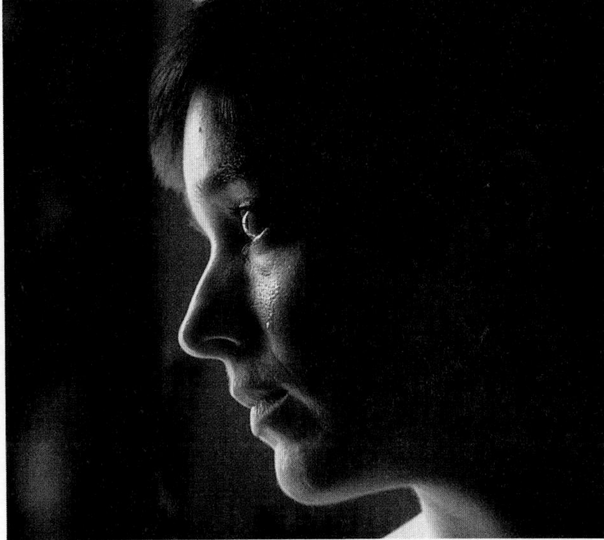

Friends and family members who lose loved ones must work through the pain of grief in order to make their way back to the living world of hope and love.

# PREPARING FOR YOUR DEATH

Throughout this book we have stressed the ways in which you decide how well and how long you live. You can also make decisions about the end of your life, particularly its impact on other people. Ask yourself the following three questions:

- Would I like my bodily systems to be kept functioning by extraordinary life-sustaining measures, even though my natural systems have failed?
- Would I like the state to decide how to distribute my property or provide for my children (if any), or my family to decide how to handle my funeral arrangements?
- Would I care to give someone the same possibilities for life that I have had?

Various forms of wills can ensure that your wishes are heeded.

## The "Living Will"

If you were severely injured in an accident, would you want to be kept alive in a nearly vegetative state? As Figure 18-1 shows, you may be able to prevent this possibility with a "living will" card that you should carry in your wallet. Most states recognize living wills as legally binding, and recent court decisions have upheld the individual's right to refuse medical treatment or resuscitation attempts.[11]

## The Holographic Will

Perhaps you think that only rich or older people need to write wills. However, if you are married, have chil-

TO MY FAMILY, MY PHYSICIAN, MY LAWYER, MY CLERGYMAN
TO ANY MEDICAL FACILITY IN WHOSE CARE I HAPPEN TO BE
TO ANY INDIVIDUAL WHO MAY BECOME RESPONSIBLE FOR MY HEALTH, WELFARE OR AFFAIRS

Death is as much a reality as birth, growth, maturity and old age—it is the one certainty of life. If the time comes when I, ______________________ can no longer take part in decisions for my own future, let this statement stand as an expression of my wishes, while I am still of sound mind.

If the situation should arise in which there is no reasonable expectation of my recovery from physical or mental disability, I request that I be allowed to die and not be kept alive by artificial means or "heroic measures". I do not fear death itself as much as the indignities of deterioration, dependence and hopeless pain. I, therefore, ask that medication be mercifully administered to me to alleviate suffering even though this may hasten the moment of death.

This request is made after careful consideration. I hope you who care for me will feel morally bound to follow its mandate. I recognize that this appears to place a heavy reponsibility upon you, but it is with the intention of relieving you of such responsibility and of placing it upon myself in accordance with my strong convictions, that this statement is made.

Signed ______________________

Date ______________________

Witness ______________________

Witness ______________________

Copies of this request have been given to ______________________

______________________

______________________

______________________

______________________

**FIGURE 18-1** Example of the "living will." Copies may be obtained from the Euthanasia Educational Council (250 W. 57th St., New York, NY 10019).

dren, or own property, you should hire a lawyer to draw up a will or you can write a **holographic will** yourself by specifying who you wish to raise your children or who should have your property. If you don't (if you die intestate, without a will), the state will make these decisions for you. Even a modest estate can be tied up in court for a long period of time, depriving family members of money when they need it most.

UNIFORM DONOR CARD

OF ______________________
Print or type name of donor

In the hope that I may help others, I hereby make this anatomical gift, if medically acceptable, to take effect upon my death. The words and marks below indicate my desires.

I give: (a) _____ any needed organs or parts
(b) _____ only the following organs or parts

______________________
Specify the organ(s) or part(s)

for the purposes of transplantation, therapy, medical research or education;

(c) _____ my body for anatomical study if needed.

Limitations or special wishes, if any: ______________________

**FIGURE 18-2** Example of a uniform donor card.

STRATEGY FOR CHANGE

### Drawing Up a Will

Many states will recognize a handwritten (not typed) statement by you, through which you can accomplish the following:

- Name a family member or friend as the executor, the person who sees that your wishes are carried out.
- List the things you own and to whom you want them to go; include addresses and telephone numbers, if possible.
- Select a guardian for your children, if any, presumably someone whose ideas about raising children are similar to your own. Be sure they want the responsibility.
- Specify any funeral arrangements.
- Be sure to keep the will in a safe place, where your executor, family members, or closest beneficiary can get to it quickly and easily; tell them where it is.

**holographic will** A will wholly in the handwriting of its author.

## W H A T D O Y O U T H I N K ?

In 20 cases over the last fifty years, family members accused of "mercy killings" of fatally ill relatives have gone to trial. One was a father who held off hospital workers with a pistol while he unplugged his baby's respirator. Another was a man who suffocated his wife with a pillow. Only three of the defendants were sentenced to jail. Do you think these individuals should have been put on trial? Should all have been punished? Are there circumstances that would make mercy killing a crime in some cases but not in others?

Some gravely ill AIDS patients have killed themselves, and many individuals who are infected with the virus that causes AIDS say they plan to do the same if they develop disabling and painful complications of the disease. Do you think they have the right to end their own lives? What would you do if someone with a terminal disease asked your help in preparing for his or her suicide?

What if you were hooked up to artificial respirators and feeding tubes? Would you want doctors to do everything possible to fight for your life? Or would you want to spend months or even years totally unaware of your surroundings? Would you prepare a legal document, before you even became ill, instructing doctors not to resort to extraordinary means to keep you alive? Why or why not?

### The Gift of Life

If you are at least 18 years old, you can fill out a donor card, agreeing to designate, in the event of your death, any needed organs or tissues for transplantation (see Figure 18-2). The card should be filled out and signed in the presence of two witnesses, who also sign it. Attach it to the back of your driver's license or ID card. (Whole body donations require other arrangements.)

## MAKING THIS CHAPTER WORK FOR YOU

### Understanding the Meaning of Death

Many states define death as the end of all functioning of the brain, including those parts of the brain that control breathing and circulation. But while death itself is an end, dying can be a long, complex process.

Individuals with fatal illnesses may go through various emotional stages: denial, anger, bargaining, depression, and acceptance. Often, dying patients share common physical and mental symptoms.

Pain medications on a regular, timed basis relieve the discomfort of the fatally ill. The hospice program provides care to fatally ill patients and their families. "Mercy death" includes both euthanasia and dyathanasia. Dyathanasia refers to withholding or stopping any extraordinary measures to sustain life. Euthanasia, which is illegal, may involve active participation in ending a dying person's life.

Grief encompasses many feelings—including sadness, anger, guilt, despair, confusion, relief, and fear—and has profound effects on the body. Survivors continue to need the understanding and help of friends and relatives.

With the help of memorial societies, people can make advance arrangements for their funerals. An autopsy may be performed to determine the cause of death to increase medical knowledge.

With a living will, a person can indicate his or her wishes about the use of extraordinary measures to keep bodily systems functioning. In many states, a handwritten holographic will is considered a legal document. People over 18 years of age can designate that, in the event of their death, their organs are to be donated to others.

Thinking about death can be difficult. Yet realizing that life will not go on forever is what makes every day, every minute, of living so precious. As Elisabeth Kubler-Ross observed in *Death: The Final Stage of Growth:*

> When you live as if you'll live forever, it becomes too easy to postpone the things you know that you must do. You live your life in preparation for tomorrow or in remembrance of yesterday; and meanwhile, each today is lost. In contrast, when you fully understand that each day you awaken could be the last you have, you take the time that day to grow, to become more of who you really are, to reach out to other human beings.

# YOUR HEALTH CARE AND SURVIVAL GUIDE

## STRATEGIES FOR SAFETY

Accidents don't always have to happen. Sometimes we do not place enough importance on safety guidelines. This section includes recommendations for common-sense safety, including safety at home, with children, on the road, in the water, and on the job. Turn to page A-2 for specifics.

## EMERGENCY!

An emergency is a situation in which you must think and act quickly. Have your basic emergency system in place: Keep emergency telephone numbers handy; know the fastest route to your local emergency room; and keep a supply of basic first-aid items in a convenient place. Use this section either to brush up on your knowledge or to refer to in the event of an emergency. Turn to page A-4.

## MINOR HEALTH PROBLEMS

Minor health problems may occur to any of us at any time. This section will help you identify when you may treat those problems at home, and how you should treat them. It will also tell you when you should consult a doctor. Use it for handy reference. Turn to page A-13.

## YOUR BODY'S WARNING SIGNALS

It is often hard to know how serious a symptom is. We might mistakenly assume that a minor problem is the sign of a dread disease—or we may dismiss a warning signal as trivial. In either case, we may not take proper steps for treatment. This section can help you identify health warnings that may or may not be serious, but that should never be ignored. Turn to page A-14.

# STRATEGIES FOR SAFETY

Accidents don't always have to happen. Sometimes we let them happen—by not placing enough importance on safety guidelines. Chapter 14 presents basic information on accidents; this section presents some additional recommendations for avoiding them.

## At Home

Every year home accidents claim more than 24,000 lives and cause nearly 25 million injuries. To ensure your own and your family's safety:

- Wash knives, cutting boards, and other utensils in hot soapy water after use, especially after using them to cut or mix raw meat, fish, or poultry, to prevent the spread of disease-causing organisms.
- Do not serve raw fish, meat, or poultry, which may contain dangerous organisms.
- When serving, keep hot foods hot (at a temperature of 140°F) and cold foods cold (38°F). Heat kills the bacteria that can cause food poisoning; refrigeration slows their spread.
- Do not allow frozen foods to stand at room temperature before cooking.
- Wash all produce thoroughly to remove surface pesticides.
- Wear gloves whenever using household cleaning products. Read labels carefully and use only in well-ventilated rooms.
- Never combine cleaning products. This could produce a dangerous chemical reaction.
- Maintain oil and natural gas-fired furnaces in good working order to avoid emission of carbon monoxide and fire hazards.
- Use kerosene heaters only if people are at home and awake. If they malfunction, such heaters can suffocate sleepers.
- To prevent home fires, follow electrical safety rules, store flammable materials in fireproof containers, and keep matches and cigarette lighters out of children's reach.
- Install at least one fire detector on each floor.
- In case of a fire, get out of the house as quickly as possible. Crawl along the floor, away from the heat and smoke. Cover your mouth with a wet cloth to prevent smoke inhalation.
- Post the number of the local emergency service and Poison Control Center near each phone in the house.
- To prevent falls, be careful getting in and out of the tub, using ladders, or going up and down stairs.

## Protecting Children

Here are some preventive measures to take for those in the curiosity years:

- *For babies, 6 to 12 months.* Make sure low shelves, cupboards, and storage areas, particularly in the kitchen and bathrooms, have nothing remotely poisonous—that means anything you can think of that doesn't belong in a baby's mouth.
- *For small children, ages 1 to 2.* Toddlers have the highest accident rate of any age group, since they can stand and reach above eye level. Make sure things on countertops, such as cleansers, bleaches, and polishes, are secured.
- *For children ages 2 to 5.* Check high shelves and medicine cabinets. Put all drugs in childproof containers.
- *For all.* Plants are the number-one poisoning agent; keep out of children's reach. Most poisonous bulbs: daffodil, hyacinth, narcissus. Most poisonous leaves: crocus, elephant ears, English ivy, foxglove, iris, lily of the valley, oleander, philodendron, rhubarb (leaves), wisteria, yew.

## On the Road

Car accidents claim 50,000 lives and cause 2 million serious injuries each year. Careless or reckless driving is responsible for more than 95 percent of car accidents; alcohol contributes to about half of those. Here is what you can do to drive and ride safely:

- Always wear your safety belt.
- Never drink and drive nor get into a car if you suspect the driver may be intoxicated.

- Make sure small children are in child-safety seats.
- Don't exceed the speed limit. Drive slower if weather conditions are bad.
- Maintain your car properly, checking windshield wipers and tires when necessary.
- If you become exhausted, pull over and rest as long as necessary. Fatigue is second only to alcohol as a cause of serious accidents.
- If you're a bicyclist, know the traffic rules, yield right-of-way appropriately, signal turns properly, obey stop signs, don't weave in and out of traffic, don't ride in the center of the street or against traffic flow.
- Wear a helmet. Be sure your bike has reflectors on the front, back, and both wheels, as well as taillights and headlights for night use.

## In the Water

Drownings claim more than 6,000 lives a year. Many of these deaths could be prevented. Here is what you need to know to enjoy the water safely:

- Learn "drownproofing," or ways of treading water or moving with minimal output of energy.
- If thrown from a boat or canoe, stay with the craft and use it for support.
- Wear a personal flotation device whenever you're boating, rafting, or canoeing.
- Don't drink. Alcohol contributes to the recklessness that leads to many water accidents.
- Find out about currents, undertows, or sharp underwater rocks before swimming in a strange place.

## On the Job

Many different types of workers, from laboratory technicians to professional artists, must use dangerous chemicals. Here are some safety guidelines to follow if you work with potentially dangerous substances:

- Make sure your workspace is adequately ventilated. This doesn't mean a fan, which just blows dust and fumes around, but the equivalent of a filtered vacuum cleaner at the source of the toxic material.
- Be careful with storage and handling of flammable solvents.
- Label all toxic materials clearly and carefully. Store them in nonbreakable containers. Discard according to instructions.
- Wash thoroughly with soap and water before taking a break.
- Do not eat or smoke when using toxic materials.
- Don't sweep up; vacuum or wet mop.
- Wear appropriate protective gear: air respirators, goggles, gloves, etc.

# EMERGENCY!

By definition, an emergency is a situation in which you have to think and act fast. Start by assessing the circumstances. Shout for help if you're in a public place. Look for any possible dangers to you or the victim, such as a live electrical wire or a fire. Seek medical assistance as quickly as possible. Dial 911, the operator, or a local emergency phone number, and keep it near every phone in your house. Don't attempt rescue techniques, such as cardiopulmonary resuscitation (CPR), unless you are trained. If you have a car, be sure you know the shortest route from your home to the nearest 24-hour hospital emergency department.

### SUPPLIES

Every home should have a kit of basic first-aid supplies kept in a convenient location out of the reach of children. Stock it with the following:

- → Bandages
- → Sterile gauze pads and bandages
- → Adhesive tape
- → Scissors
- → Cotton balls or absorbent cotton
- → Cotton swabs
- → Thermometer
- → Syrup of Ipecac to induce vomiting
- → Antibiotic ointments
- → Sharp needle
- → Safety pins
- → Calamine lotion

Keep a similar kit in your car or boat. You might want to add some extra items from your home, such as a flashlight, soap, blanket, paper cups, and any special equipment that a family member with a chronic illness may need.

## BLEEDING

Blood loss is frightening and dangerous. Direct pressure stops external bleeding. Since internal bleeding can also be life-threatening, you must be aware of the warning signs.

### FOR AN OPEN WOUND

1. Apply direct pressure over the site of the wound. Cover the entire wound.
2. Use sterile gauze, a sanitary napkin, a clean towel, sheet, or handkerchief or, if necessary, your washed bare hand. Ice or cold water in a pad will help stop bleeding and decrease swelling.
3. Apply firm, steady pressure for 5 to 15 minutes. Most wounds stop bleeding within a few minutes.
4. If the wound is on a foot, hand, leg, or arm, use gravity to help slow the flow of blood. Elevate the limb so it is higher than the victim's heart.
5. If the bleeding doesn't stop, press harder.
6. Seek medical attention if the bleeding was caused by a serious injury, if stitches will be needed to keep the wound closed, or if the victim has not had a tetanus booster within the last 10 years.

### FOR INTERNAL BLEEDING

1. Suspect internal bleeding if a person coughs up blood, vomits red or brown material that looks like coffee grounds, passes blood in urine or stool, or has black, tar-like bowel movements.
2. Do not let the victim take any medication or fluids by mouth until seen by a doctor because surgery may be necessary.
3. Have the victim lie flat. Cover him or her lightly.
4. Seek immediate medical attention.

### FOR A BLOODY NOSE

1. Have the victim sit down, leaning slightly forward so the blood does not run down his or her throat. The person should spit out any blood in his or her mouth.
2. Use thumb and forefingers to pinch the nose. If the victim can do the pinching, apply a cold compress to the nose and surrounding area.
3. Apply pressure for 10 minutes without interruption.
4. If pinching does not work, gently pack the nostril with gauze or a clean strip of cloth. Do not use absorbent cotton, which will stick. Let the ends hang out so you

can remove the packing easily later. Pinch the nose, with the packing in place, for 5 minutes.

5 If a foreign object is in the nose, do not attempt to remove it. Ask the person to blow gently. If that does not work, seek medical attention.

6 The nose should not be blown or irritated for several hours after a nosebleed stops.

## BREATHING PROBLEMS

If a person appears to be unconscious, approach carefully. The victim may be in contact with electrical current. If so, make sure the electricity is shut off before touching the victim. The first function you should check is respiration. Tap or shake the victim's shoulder gently, shouting, "Are you all right?" Look for any signs of breathing: Can you hear breath sounds? Can you feel breath on your cheek? If the person is breathing, do not perform mouth-to-mouth resuscitation.

If you aren't certain if the victim is breathing, or if there are no signs of breath, follow these steps:

1 Lay the person on his or her back on the floor or ground. Roll the victim over if necessary, being careful to turn the head with the remainder of the body as a unit to avoid possible neck injury. Loosen any tight clothing around the neck or chest.

2 Check for any foreign material in the mouth or throat and remove it quickly.

3 Open the airway by tilting the head back and lifting the chin up.

4 Pinch the nostrils shut with your thumb and index finger.

5 Take a deep breath, open your mouth wide and place it securely over the victim's and give two slow breaths, each lasting 1 to $1\frac{1}{2}$ seconds. Remove your mouth, turn your head and check to see if the victim's chest rises and falls. If you hear air escaping from the victim's mouth and see the chest fall, you know that you are getting air into the lungs.

6 Repeat once every 5 seconds (12 breaths per minute) until professional help takes over, or the victim begins breathing on his or her own. It may take several hours to revive someone. If you stop, the victim may not be able to breathe on his or her own. Once the person does begin to breathe independently, always get professional help.

7 If air doesn't seem to be entering the chest, or the chest doesn't fall between breaths, tilt the head further back. If that doesn't work, follow the directions for choking emergencies later in this section.

8 If the victim is a child, do not pinch the nose shut. Cover both the mouth and nose with your mouth, and place your free hand very lightly on the child's chest. Use small puffs of air rather than big breaths. Feel the chest inflate as you blow, and listen for exhaled air. Repeat once every 3 seconds (20 breaths per minute).

## BROKEN BONES

If you suspect that a person has broken a leg, do not move him or her unless there is immediate danger.

1 Check for signs of breathing. If there is none or breathing is very weak, administer mouth-to-mouth resuscitation.

2 If the person is bleeding, apply direct pressure on the site of the wound.

3 Try to keep the victim warm and calm.

4 Do not try to push a broken bone back into place if it is sticking out of the skin. You can apply a moist dressing to prevent it from drying out.

5 Do not try to straighten out a fracture.

6 Do not allow the victim to walk.

7 Splint unstable fractures to prevent painful motion.

## BURNS

1 If fire caused the burn, cool with water to stop the burning process.

2 Remove the victim's garments and jewelry and cover him or her with clean sheets or towels.

3 Call for help immediately.

4 If chemicals caused the burn, wash with cool water for at least 20 minutes. Chemical burns of the eye require immediate medical attention after flushing with water for 20 minutes.

## CHOKING

A person with anything stuck in the throat and blocking the airway can stop breathing, lose consciousness, and die within 4 to 6 minutes. A universal signal of distress because of choking is clasping the throat with one or both hands. Other signs are an inability to talk and noisy, difficult breathing. You need to take immediate action, but NEVER slap the victim's back. This could make the obstruction worse.

If the victim can speak, cough, or breathe, do not interfere. Coughing alone may dislodge the foreign object. If the choking continues without lessening, call for medical help.

If the victim cannot speak, cough, or breathe but is conscious, use the Heimlich maneuver as described below:

1 Stand behind the victim (who may be seated or standing) and wrap your arms around his or her waist.

2 Make a fist with one hand and place the thumbside of your fist against the victim's abdomen, just above the navel. Grasp your fist with your other hand and press into his or her abdomen with a quick, upward thrust. Do not exert any pressure against the rib cage with your forearms.

3 Repeat this procedure until the victim is no longer choking or loses consciousness.

4 If the person is lying facedown, roll the victim over. Facing the person, kneel with your legs astride his or her hips. Put the heel of one hand below the rib cage and place your other hand on top. Press into the abdomen with a quick, upward thrust. Repeat thrusts as needed.

5 If you start choking when you're by yourself, place your fist below your rib cage and above your navel. Grasp this fist with your other hand and press into your abdomen with a quick, upward thrust. You also can lean over a fixed, horizontal object, such as a table edge or chair back, and press your upper abdomen against it with a quick, upward thrust. Repeat as needed until you dislodge the object.

### IF THE VICTIM IS UNCONSCIOUS

1 Place him or her on the ground and give mouth-to-mouth resuscitation as described earlier.

2 If the victim does not start breathing and air does not seem to be going into his or her lungs, roll the victim onto his or her back and give one or more manual thrusts: Place one of your hands on top of the other with the heel of the bottom hand in the middle of the abdomen, slightly above the navel and below the rib cage. Press into the abdomen with a quick, upward thrust. Do not push to either side. Repeat 6 to 10 times as needed.

3 Clear the airway. Hold the victim's mouth open with one hand and use your thumb to depress the tongue. Make a hook with the pointer finger of your other hand and, using a gentle, sweeping motion, reach into the victim's throat and feel for a swallowed foreign object in the airway.

4 Repeat the following steps in this sequence:
→ 6 to 10 abdominal thrusts
→ Probe in mouth
→ Try to inflate lungs
→ Repeat

5 If the victim suddenly seems okay, but no foreign material has been removed, take him or her directly to the hospital. A foreign object, such as a fish or chicken bone or other jagged object, could do internal damage as it passes through the victim's system.

### IF THE VICTIM IS A CHILD

1 If the child is coughing, do nothing. The coughing alone may dislodge the object.

2 If the airway is blocked and the child is panicky and fighting for breath, do NOT probe the airway with your fingers to clear an unseen foreign object. You might push the material back into the airway, worsening the obstruction.

3 For an infant younger than a year, hang the child over your arm so that the head is lower than the trunk. Using the heel of your hand, administer 4 firm blows high on the back between the shoulder blades. For a bigger child, follow the same procedure, but invert the child over your knee rather than your arm.

4 After 4 back blows, perform 4 chest thrusts (the Heimlich maneuver as described above).

## DROWNING

A person can die of drowning 4 to 6 minutes after breathing stops. While prevention is the wisest course, follow these steps in case of a drowning emergency:

1 Get the victim out of the water fast. Be extremely cautious, because a drowning person may panic and grasp at a rescuer, endangering that individual as well. If possible, push a branch or pole within the victim's reach.

2 If the victim is unconscious, use a flotation device if at all possible. Carefully place the person on the device. Once out of the water, place the victim on his or her back.

3 If the victim is not breathing, start mouth-to-mouth resuscitation. Continue until the person can breathe unassisted or help arrives. (Note that it may take an hour or two for a drowning victim to resume independent breathing.) Do not leave the victim alone for any reason.

4 Once the person is breathing without assistance, even if he or she is still coughing, you need only stay nearby until professional help arrives.

## ELECTRICAL SHOCK

1 If you suspect that an electrical shock has knocked a person unconscious, approach very carefully. Do not touch the victim unless the electricity has been turned off.

2 Shut off the power at the plug, circuit breaker, or fuse box. Simply shutting off an appliance does not remove the shock hazard. Use a dry stick to move a wire or

downed power line from the victim. Keep in mind that you also are in danger until the power is off.

3 If the person's breathing is weak or has stopped, follow the steps for mouth-to-mouth resuscitation.

4 Even if the victim returns to consciousness, call for medical help. While waiting, cover the victim with a blanket or coat to keep him or her warm. Place a blanket underneath the body if the surface is cold. Be sure the person lies flat if conscious, with legs raised. If the victim is unconscious, place him or her on one side, with a pillow supporting the head. Do not give the victim anything to eat or drink.

5 Electrical burns can extend deep into the tissue, even when they appear minor. Do not put butter, household remedies, or sprays on burns without a doctor's instruction. Do not use ice or cold water on an electrical burn that is more than two inches across.

## HEART ATTACK

Chest pain can be caused by indigestion, strained muscles, or lung infections. The warning signs of a heart attack are:

→ Intense pain that lasts for more than 2 minutes, produces a tight or crushing feeling, is centered in the chest, or spreads to the neck, jaw, shoulder, or arm
→ Shortness of breath that is worse when the person lies flat and improves when the person sits
→ Heavy sweating
→ Nausea or vomiting
→ Irregular pulse
→ Pale or bluish skin or lips
→ Weakness
→ Severe anxiety, feelings of doom

If an individual develops these symptoms:

1 Call for emergency medical help immediately.

2 Have the person sit up or lie in a semi-reclining position. Loosen tight clothing. Keep him or her comfortably warm.

3 If the person loses consciousness, turn on his or her back and check for breathing and pulse. If vomiting occurs, turn the victim's head to one side and clean the mouth.

4 If the person has medicine for angina pectoris (chest pain) and is conscious, help him or her take it.

5 If the person is unconscious, and you are trained to perform cardiopulmonary resuscitation (CPR), check for a pulse at the wrist or neck. If there is none, begin CPR in conjunction with mouth-to-mouth resuscitation. Do not attempt CPR unless you are trained. It is not a technique you can learn from a book.

## POISONING

Many common household substances, including glue, aspirin, bleaches, and paint, can be poisonous. Make sure you know the emergency numbers for the Poison Control Center and Fire Department Rescue Squad. Keep them near your telephone. Be prepared to provide the following information:

→ Kind of substance swallowed
→ How much was swallowed
→ If a child or adult swallowed the substance
→ Symptoms
→ Whether or not vomiting has occurred
→ Whether you gave the person anything to drink
→ How much time it will take to get to an emergency room

The Poison Control Center or rescue team will tell you whether or not to induce vomiting or neutralize a swallowed poison. Here are some additional guidelines:

1 Always assume the worst if a small child has swallowed or might have swallowed something poisonous. Call the local Poison Control Center or emergency number (911 in many areas). Keep the suspected item or container with you to answer questions.

2 Do not give any medications unless a physician or the Poison Control Center instructs you to do so.

3 Do *not* follow the directions for neutralizing poisons on the container unless a doctor or the Poison Control Center confirms that they are appropriate measures to take.

4 If the child is conscious, give moderate doses of water to dilute the poison.

5 If a poisoning victim is unconscious, make sure he or she is breathing. If not, give mouth-to-mouth resuscitation. Do not give anything by mouth or attempt to stimulate the person. Call for emergency help immediately.

6 If the person is vomiting, make sure he or she is in a position in which they cannot choke on what is brought up.

7 While vomiting is the fastest way to expel swallowed poisons from the body, you should never try to induce vomiting if the person has swallowed any acid or alkaline substance, which can cause burns of the face, mouth, and throat (examples include ammonia, bleach, dishwasher detergent, drain and toilet cleaners, lye, oven cleaners, or rust removers), or petroleumlike products, which produce dangerous fumes that can be inhaled during vomiting (examples include floor polish, furniture wax, gasoline, kerosene, lighter fluid, turpentine, and paint thinner).

## MINOR HEALTH PROBLEMS

| Problem | What It Is | How It Develops | How to Prevent It |
|---|---|---|---|
| **Acne** | Eruption of pimples and blackheads caused by increased skin oils (typical in adolescence). | Skin oils accumulate in openings of oil glands and hair follicles. Bacteria grow and cause changes in the secretions that are irritating to the surrounding skin. | Scrub the face several times a day with a washcloth and soap to remove skin oils; avoid skin creams and greases. |
| **Athlete's Foot** | A common infection that most people develop at some time, even if they aren't athletes. | A fungus found on the skin spreads to the environment (such as a floor), where it can infect others. | Keep feet clean and dry. Change socks often. Use medicated food powder during warm weather. |
| **Common Cold** | A viral infection affecting nasal passages, mucous membranes of the eyes, and frequently the throat and ears. | The virus spreads from person to person. | Stay away from infected people as much as possible. Wash your hands carefully after being with someone with a cold. |
| **Discharge from the Penis** | Thick mucous secretions from the penis. | After contact with someone with a sexually transmitted disease (usually gonorrhea or syphilis). | Use of condoms; urination after sexual intercourse. |
| **Ear Pain or Discharge** | Pressure caused by a build-up of fluid in the middle ear (the portion behind the ear drum). | Typical causes are cold, flu, allergies, or air pressure changes during plane trips, as well as infection. Ear discharges may be the result of "swimmers' ear," an irritation, or mild bacterial infection. | Avoid obvious carriers of cold/ flu viruses and any substances to which you know you are allergic. |
| **Eye Pain or Discomfort** | Discomfort or feeling of tiredness in the eyes. | Pain behind, over, or under eye may be the result of a sinus problem. Various infections, including flu, can make eyes temporarily sensitive to light. Burning and itching are usually caused by conjunctivitis, an inflammation of eye membrane triggered by pollution, chemicals, or allergies. | Staying inside during peak pollution periods may help. |
| **Flu** | Viral infection of the breathing passages. | Inhalation of the virus, which is most prevalent from January to April. | Avoid known carriers. |

## MINOR HEALTH PROBLEMS

| How to Recognize It | What You Can Do | When to Call the Doctor |
|---|---|---|
| Increase in pimples or blackheads (which are formed when air causes a chemical change in the keratin plugs in hair follicles). | Use abrasive soap to reduce oiliness of the skin or over-the-counter medications containing benzoyl peroxide. Hot drying compresses or agents may help. | If you cannot control the problem on your own. He or she may prescribe medications containing retinoic acid (retin A), which have proven highly effective. |
| Itching, peeling, formation of cracks in skin; sometimes pain and bleeding. Usually affects both feet. | Use over-the-counter antifungal ointments or powders on the infected area. | If symptoms don't improve in a week; if you develop a fever or the foot becomes red, swollen, or tender; or if you develop red streaks up the leg (indicating a secondary bacterial infection). |
| Stuffy or runny nose, aches and pains, sore throat, cough, watery eyes, clogged ears, low-grade fever. | Rest, aspirin or acetaminophen for pain, medications for specific symptoms. | If you develop a high fever, persistent cough, earache, or other severe symptoms. |
| Difficulty in urinating, pain, tenderness and swelling of the testicles; other symptoms possible, such as sore throat. | No home treatment. | As soon as symptoms develop—to begin antibiotic treatment. |
| Feelings of stuffiness that persist for several days. | Moisture and humidity help, so stand in a steamy shower or use a vaporizer. Aspirin or acetaminophen relieve pain. | If the stuffiness doesn't clear up or if you develop problems hearing. Medications, including antibiotics if necessary, provide quick relief. |
| Burning, itchiness, sensitivity to light. Serious bacterial infections (which always require treatment) produce thick pus. | No real home treatment other than avoiding light and resting the eyes if fatigue or flu is the cause of pain. | If eye pain persists or worsens over a period of weeks, which could indicate glaucoma, a build-up of pressure within the eye that can impair vision if untreated. |
| Fever and dry cough. May develop headaches and muscle aches. Minor sore throat. | Aspirin for adults; acetaminophen for children and teenagers; liquids, bed rest. | If you don't improve after 2 or 3 days, if you cough up sputum, or if you seem to improve then take a turn for the worse (a possible indicator of bacterial pneumonia). |

## MINOR HEALTH PROBLEMS

| Problem | What It Is | How It Develops | How to Prevent It |
|---|---|---|---|
| **Heartburn** | Irritation of the stomach or esophagus (tube leading from mouth to stomach). | Stomach acids irritate the lining or push up into the esophagus. | Avoid substances that aggravate the problem, including spicy foods, coffee, tea, and alcohol. Don't lie down after eating. Don't wear tight-fitting clothes. Don't eat or drink for 2 hours before bedtime. |
| **Infected Wound (Blood Poisoning)** | Bacterial infection of a wound that may spread to the bloodstream. | An infected wound festers for 2 or 3 days and bacteria grow, increasing redness, pain, and swelling. | Keep a wound clean, leaving it open to the air if possible. If you use a bandage, change it often. Soak and wash a wound gently several times a day to remove dirt and keep the scab soft. |
| **Mononucleosis** | A common viral infection that only rarely causes serious complications, such as a ruptured spleen. | Oral contact with an infected individual, including kissing. | Avoid oral contact with infected persons. |
| **Mouth Sore** | A cold sore, fever blister, canker sore, or other lesion or break in the mucous membranes of the mouth. | A virus, such as herpes, causes fever blisters and cold sores. An injury, such as accidentally biting the lip or tongue, can cause a canker sore. Allergic reactions to drugs also can cause mouth sores. | Avoid oral contact with anyone with an open mouth sore. |
| **Nosebleed** | Recurrent or frequent bleeding from the nose. | Picking of the nose, irritation by a virus, or vigorous nose blowing. | Because nosebleeds are more common in winter when viruses are common and heated indoor air becomes dry, a humidifier can help. |
| **Sore Throat** | Usually a viral infection. Streptococcus bacteria can cause a severe sore throat. | Exposure to infected individuals. | Avoid infected people; wash hands carefully. |
| **Sunburn** | A serious burn caused by overexposure to ultraviolet light. | Ultraviolet light—either from the sun or artificial lights—causes a chemical reaction in the skin. | Limit time in sun or tanning booths. Always use sunscreens, and make sure your eyes are shielded. |

# MINOR HEALTH PROBLEMS

| How to Recognize It | What You Can Do | When to Call the Doctor |
|---|---|---|
| Burning, painful sensation just below breastbone or ribs. | Nonabsorbable antacids taken every 1 to 2 hours; or milk may provide some relief. | If pain is intense or lasts for more than 3 days. |
| Fever of more than 99.6°F; increase in pain; redness or swelling; thick smelly pus draining from the wound. | Frequent cleaning of the wound and changes of bandages. | If a wound is not healing and you develop a fever. If you see red streaks around the wound. |
| Fever; sore throat; swollen glands in neck, armpit, and groin; general aches; fatigue. | Bed rest, no strenuous activity or contact sports (because of danger to the spleen). | If a high fever, severe sore throat, or other symptoms persist for more than a week, primarily to rule out other more serious conditions. |
| Cold sores or canker sores start as blisters and then change to small spots with white centers. | Cold liquids and popsicles are soothing. Nonprescription medications also provide relief. | If the lesion developed shortly after you began taking a medication or if a sore persists for more than 3 weeks. |
| Noticeable blood loss. | Squeeze the nose between thumb and forefinger just below the hard portion of the nose for about 5 minutes. See emergency guidelines for bleeding earlier in this section. | If nosebleeds recur, become more frequent, and are not associated with a cold or other infection. |
| Discomfort or dry, burning sensation in throat; difficulty in swallowing. | Throat lozenges; warm liquids. | If you develop a high fever, markedly swollen neck glands, or severe pain on swallowing, or if the sore throat lasts for more than a week. Doctor will test for strep throat, which can lead to abscesses around the tonsils, middle-ear infections, inflammation of kidneys, or rheumatic fever. |
| The pain of sunburn becomes worse 6 to 48 hours after exposure. Blistering indicates a serious, second-degree burn. | For relief, try cool compresses or baths (add baking powder or Aveeno to the tub). Aspirin eases pain. | If you experience vision problems or if burn is very severe. |

## MINOR HEALTH PROBLEMS

| Problem | What It Is | How It Develops | How to Prevent It |
|---|---|---|---|
| **Urinary Difficulty (Women)** | Frequent, painful, or bloody urination in women usually is a sign of bladder infection or cystitis. | Bacteria from rectum and vagina are transferred to the bladder, causing infection. Women are more susceptible because their urethras (the tube leading from the bladder to outside the body) are shorter than men's. | Women who experience frequent attacks should urinate after intercourse to wash bacteria out of the urethra and bladder. |
| **Urinary Difficulty (Men)** | Frequent, painful, or bloody urination. | The most common causes are bladder infections, viral infections, excessive use of caffeine-containing beverages, infection of the prostate gland, and venereal disease. | Cutting back on caffeinated beverages may help if they are the true culprit. |
| **Vaginal Infection** | Infection most often caused by bacteria, candida (a fungus), or trichomonas (a protozoa). | Use of oral contraceptives or a course of antibiotics for another infection may increase susceptibility to bacterial and yeast infections, which also can be transmitted sexually; trichomonas is usually transmitted sexually. | The use of condoms and spermicides helps reduce the risk of sexually transmitted infections. |

## MINOR HEALTH PROBLEMS

| How to Recognize It | What You Can Do | When to Call the Doctor |
|---|---|---|
| Frequent urge to urinate, often accompanied by pain or burning. | Drink a lot of fluids, particularly fruit juices. Cranberry juice is especially good because it has a natural antibiotic. | If you develop fever or pain along the sides of your middle back (an indication of kidney infection), or if symptoms persist or intensify. The usual treatments are antibacterial agents. |
| Absence of other telltale symptoms, such as vomiting, back pain, and chills (signs of kidney infection). | Drink plenty of fluids, up to several gallons in the first 24 hours, especially fruit juices. | If symptoms persist for 24 hours or recur. |
| Vaginal discharge, itching, burning. | Creams or douches containing antibiotic, antiyeast, or antiprotozoa medications. | When symptoms persist. |

# YOUR BODY'S WARNING SIGNALS

Often it's hard to know how serious a symptom is. We might assume that a minor problem is a sign of a dread disease and feel panic-stricken. Or we may dismiss a warning signal of a potentially serious illness as trivial. In either circumstance, we may put off getting treatment that could help us feel better faster. The following guide can help you identify health warnings that may or may not be serious, but that should never be ignored.

## Abdominal Pain

Minor problems, such as gas or a viral infection, trigger most abdominal pain. Many women occasionally feel pain in the lower abdomen at mid-cycle; this usually accompanies the release of an egg at ovulation. Premenstrual pain can indicate endometriosis, the growth of uterine lining cells in the abdominal cavity. Severe and persistent pain, especially in a woman who believes she may be pregnant, can indicate an ectopic pregnancy, in which the fertilized egg implants itself outside the uterus. Pain can signal that the developing amniotic sac has ruptured, requiring immediate attention. Appendicitis, another potential emergency, usually causes pain first around the navel or just below the breast bone and later in the right lower quarter of the abdomen.

## Back Pain

This common woe knocks millions of Americans off their feet every year. Most low-back pain involves a spasm of the large supportive muscles alongside the spine, usually triggered by exertion, lifting, or injury. Women are particularly vulnerable during pregnancy when hormones loosen ligaments and joints. Muscular strains require rest and time for natural healing.

If the pain is the result of a blow or fall, or if you don't feel any better after a week, see a physician. You should also seek medical care if the pain extends beyond the lower back to the legs, a signal of pressure on the sciatic nerve that could be the result of a slipped disc, a rupture of one of the spine's built-in "shock absorbers."

## Bad Breath

A thick bowl of onion soup could make anyone's breath less than kissably sweet. But persistent bad breath is more than an embarassment and can indicate either a dental or a medical problem. A prime suspect is peridontal or gum disease. Odor can come from bacteria, by-products of their activity, food and debris on the teeth and gums, and eventually from rotting bone. Decayed or abcessed teeth also can sour breath. Possible medical culprits include post-nasal drip, indigestion, and hiatal hernia (back-up of stomach acids into the esophagus).

## Bowel Changes

By medical definition, diarrhea refers to a minimum of six unformed stools in 24 hours. Possible reasons are medications, food allergies, food poisoning or, especially if you've been traveling, an intestinal infection, such as dysentery. Whatever the cause of diarrhea, the greatest risk is dehydration. Seek medical care if you're in severe pain, if stools are black or bloody, or if diarrhea recurs frequently.

## Breast Changes in Women

Any woman who feels tenderness, pain, or a lump in one or both breasts should see her doctor to determine whether she has a benign cyst or a cancerous tumor. Other changes to check for during regular breast self-examinations are thickening, swelling, puckering, dimpling, skin irritation, distortion or scaliness of nipples, and nipple discharge.

## Breathing Problems

If you huff and puff after climbing a flight of stairs, you may simply be out of shape. Among young adults, difficulty breathing is likely to be hyperventilation syndrome, a feeling of being unable to get sufficient air into the lungs; anxiety is the true culprit. Breathlessness without exertion can be an allergic reaction or an asthma attack (especially the first such episode). If you're suffering genuine air hunger, you could have a serious infection or an accumulation of fluid or a blood clot (a pulmonary embolism) in your lungs. The diagnosis will depend on your other symptoms.

## Changes in Vision

Some drugs, such as antidepressants and antihistamines (found in many cold and allergy medications), can cause blurred vision. Ask your doctor about any prescription or over-the-counter drugs you're taking. If one eye is blurred and you are seeing flashing lights or floating spots, but the eye is not painful, you may have retinal detachment, a separation of the light-sensitive cells that line the back of the eyeball.

## Coughing

A cough is one of the body's basic defense mechanisms, an effective way of expelling abnormal material. Most doctors agree that it's best not to stifle a "productive" cough, one that brings up mucus and phlegm from the lungs. If you spike a fever, and you're coughing up rusty or foul material, you may have a bacterial infection and need treatment. A good rule of thumb is to seek help if you develop a cough unlike any you've had before.

A persistent dry cough is usually the result of smoking, allergies, chemical irritants, or a viral infection. The nagging, tickling cough of bronchitis may linger for 2 or 3 weeks; self-care measures, such as sucking on lozenges, provide some relief. Even in smokers, coughing rarely is a sign of cancer.

## Fainting or Dizziness

If you've also noticed a hearing loss or noises in your ear, the problem may be Meniere's disease, which causes an increase in fluid in the part of the inner ear that controls balance. If you have any form of heart disease and your heartbeat slows or speeds up before you feel faint, you may have developed a heart rate or rhythm problem requiring medical attention.

## Fatigue

The causes of this common complaint can be as obvious as too many late nights or as hard to pinpoint as subtle shifts in hormones at different stages of a woman's menstrual cycle. Fatigue that waxes and wanes or worsens late in the day usually is the result of too little sleep or exercise, crash dieting, heavy smoking, or drinking. Some common medications, including antihistamines, tranquilizers, and certain antihypertension treatments, often induce weariness.

Bone-deep tiredness can be part of premenstrual syndrome or an early symptom of pregnancy. Fatigue that drags at you from dawn to dusk, day after day, usually has a medical cause, such as iron-deficiency anemia, hypothyroidism (too little thyroid hormone), or infectious diseases, including mononucleosis and chronic Epstein-Barr virus, a mysterious ailment that produces debilitating fatigue (see Chapter 15).

## Fever

Fever (which refers to any elevation of temperature above 100°F) is your body's way of fighting back against a bacterial or viral invasion. Fever up to 102°F activates protective white cells and kills some pathogens, but the height of a temperature doesn't necessarily indicate how serious the problem is. That depends on other symptoms, such as ear ache, sore throat, or abdominal pain.

The greatest danger of an extremely high temperature, particularly in children, is a seizure or convulsion. If fever doesn't respond to standard treatment (such as aspirin or acetaminophen) or persists for more than 5 days, you should see a physician.

## Headache

Stress or tension in the muscles of the neck, scalp, and jaw produce most pains in the head. A migraine—a headache accompanied by nausea, visual hallucinations such as flashing lights, and one-sided pain—is caused by constriction of blood vessels and can be a response to stress. A cluster headache—characterized by stabbing pain around the eye or temple—may be triggered by alcohol or nicotine.

Many headache sufferers are sensitive to chemicals in foods, including MSG (often used in Chinese cooking) and tyramine (found in red wine, chocolate, citrus fruits, some cheeses, and yogurt). If you wake up with headaches several times a week, you could have high blood pressure. While headache sufferers often worry about brain tumors, that possibility is exceedingly remote.

## Heart Palpitations

Normally your heart beats between 72 and 80 times per minute. People who complain of palpitations *perceive* their hearts as beating harder or irregularly, whether or not they are. The sense that your heart is pounding fiercely within your chest is almost always related to anxiety. Extra heart beats—even as many as 3 per minute—are common and present no risk. However, continued irregular heart beats, chest pain, and shortness of breath are classic signs of a heart attack.

## Muscle and Joint Pains

After spring gardening or a long hike, you expect sore muscles, and such aches and pains do not require medical attention. But you should see a doctor for muscle or joint pain, if any of the following conditions occur: Only one joint is hot or painful (this could be an infection); you have a fever (a sign of more widespread disease); you feel tingling or a pins-and-needles sensation (which could indicate nerve inflammation); or the pain or stiffness lasts for 6 weeks (an indication of a chronic problem, such as arthritis).

## Hoarseness or Sore Throat

Most hoarseness—with or without a sore throat—is a sign of a cold or inflammation of the vocal cords. But if it persists for more than a week, you could have a polyp on your larynx. Garden-variety sore throats are more of a nuisance than a threat, yet doctors generally want to rule out streptoccocal bacteria as a cause. Physicians don't give antibiotics for strep to decrease discomfort, but to prevent the real and serious complications of strep infection (including damage to the heart and kidneys).

## Insomnia

An estimated 100 million Americans suffer from occasional or chronic sleep disturbances. Some sleep problems are simply bed problems, caused by old, saggy, or too-small mattresses. Caffeine, nicotine, and alcohol also can sabotage a good night's sleep. Stress may be the most sinister—and common—sleep disrupter; regular exercise and relaxation exercises help many people unwind. If your sleep problems persist for more than 3 weeks or become so severe that they interfere with daytime functioning, see your physician. You could have an underlying psychological problem, such as depression, or a sleep disorder, such as apnea.

## Itching

Complaints of raw, irritated skin go up when the temperature goes down because the combination of outdoor cold and indoor heating dries the skin. Itching that persists for more than 6 weeks in any season may have a medical cause. Often it's a chemical reaction, called contact dermatitis. Only a certain part of the body may be affected, such as the neck or wrist under a piece of jewelry.

In addition to checking for irritants, a physician will ask about other symptoms, since itchiness can be a sign of many diseases, including thyroid disorders and diabetes. Declining levels of estrogen, beginning after age 35, can make skin exquisitely sensitive. Some women feel perpetually itchy, as if—as one sufferer put it—"bugs are crawling under the skin."

## Moles, Lumps, and Bumps

The vast majority of skin changes are harmless. Hard, solid lumps are likely to be boils, infections underneath the skin. However, you should watch for any new bumps that are shiny or pearly with blood vessels over their surface or any that look like large warts. They could be basal or squamous cell skin cancers, which are not life-threatening, but must be removed. Warning signs for a more threatening form of skin cancer, melanoma, are moles that grow, become itchy, change color (turning red, gray, blue, black, or brown), have notched borders, are asymmetrical, or have odd configurations. (See Chapter 14 for more on skin cancers.) If you notice any of these changes, see a doctor as soon as possible.

## Nausea and Vomiting

Few symptoms make us feel so wretched so quickly. While you may feel nauseous or vomit simply because you've drunk too much alcohol or eaten something that didn't agree with you, severe bouts of nausea and vomiting indicate food poisoning. Vomiting is the body's way of getting rid of toxic material. The greatest danger is of dehydration.

Recurrent nausea—especially first thing in the morning—is one of the classic signs of pregnancy. Diabetes and medications also can cause vomiting, so you should check with your physician. Seek prompt medical care if the vomited material is black or bloody or if you develop severe pain. These can be signs of gastritis (inflammation of the stomach) or ulcers.

## Rectal Bleeding

This problem is rarely as serious as it seems, although it can be very frightening. Hemorrhoids and tears in the rectum are the primary causes of bright red bleeding. Blood in the stool is rarely a sign of colon cancer, which does not bleed rapidly.

## Skin Rashes

Most people seek help for an itching, spreading, or oozing skin rash quickly for one simple reason: it's making them too miserable to wait. Many rashes are allergic or chemical reactions, but some can be infectious. Impetigo, for instance, is a bacterial infection that causes crusty, scaly patches. If you have several lesions, see a doctor because the infection can continue to spread.

## Urinary Changes

Discomfort while urinating is a classic sign of urinary tract infections, which occur in one of every five women every year. Sometimes drinking large amounts of fluids helps to flush out bacteria, but you should seek medical treatment if the problem persists or worsens.

If your urine has an unusual smell or look, the cause may be medications, such as drugs that thin the blood to prevent blood clots. If your urine is pink, red, or smoky brown, you may have a urinary tract disorder, such as cystitis, or a serious kidney infection (other symptoms include high fever, nausea, vomiting).

## Weakness, Numbness, or Tingling in the Face, Arms, or Legs

Loss of sensation or a prickling sensation could be a sign of a transient ischemic attack (TIA) or a stroke, especially if you also experience difficulty speaking, blurred vision, confusion, and dizziness. While the effects of stroke can be extremely disabling and last for more than 24 hours, the symptoms of a TIA last for only a few minutes or hours. Nearly half of those who have TIAs are apt to have a stroke within 5 years. Some physicians suggest preventive treatments, such as daily aspirin, to reduce the risk of blood clots.

## Weight Loss Without Dieting

While most people worry far more about putting on pounds than shedding them, unplanned weight loss can be troubling. The most common reasons are changes in diet, exercise, or anxiety.

Any chronic illness seems to put stress on the body in ways that aren't entirely clear but that can promote weight loss. Examples include arthritis and diabetes. Loss of both weight and appetite is a classic symptom of depression. Another possibility is an overactive thyroid, which can speed up metabolic rate so a person drops several pounds without trying.

# YOUR HEALTH DIRECTORY

In *Your Health,* we emphasize that you shoulder a great deal of responsibility for your health and the quality of your life. Given the complexity of our minds and bodies and the many social and environmental factors that affect us, this responsibility can be a very heavy burden. But your load can be made lighter if you know where to turn for health information, services, and support.

In this directory, you will find over 100 health-related topics and about 250 resources, including hot lines, government agencies, computerized data services, national organizations and foundations, professional groups, self-help groups, and support groups. Many of the organizations and groups listed here have toll-free numbers, and much of the literature available from these organizations is free.

We have included clearinghouses and information centers because they are rich sources of health information. Their main purpose is to collect, help manage, and disseminate information. Clearinghouses often perform other services as well, such as creating original publications and providing tailored responses to individual requests. These organizations also may provide referrals to other groups that can help you.

Many of the groups listed here have local offices or chapters. You can call or write these organizations to find out if there is a branch in your vicinity or you can check the white or yellow pages of your telephone directory.

The purpose of this directory is to help you be in control of your health. If you know where to turn for answers to your questions and if you know what choices you have, you may find that you have more control over your life.

## GENERAL INFORMATION RESOURCES

**National Center for Health Services Research**
Publications Branch
5600 Fishers Lane
Room 18-12
Rockville, MD 20857
(301) 443-2403

**National Center for Health Statistics (NCHS)**
(produces vital statistics and health statistics for the United States)
Scientific and Technical Information Branch
Department of Health and Human Services
6525 Belcrest Road
Room 1064
Hyattsville, MD 20782
(301) 436-8500

**ODPHP National Health Information Clearinghouse**
P.O. Box 1133
Washington, DC 20013-1133
(301) 565-4167
Toll-free: (800) 336-4797

**National Institutes of Health (NIH)**
9000 Rockville Pike
Bethesda, MD 20892
(301) 496-4000

**Public Health Service**
200 Independence Avenue, S.W.
Washington, DC 20201
(202) 245-6867

**Tel-Med Health Information Service**
(provides taped messages on health concerns)
*See white pages of telephone directory for listing*

## DATA CENTERS (ONLINE COMPUTER SERVICES)

**BRS Information Technologies**
1200 Route 7
Latham, NY 12110
(800) 235-1209
in New York (518) 783-1161

**DIALOG Information Services, Inc.**
3460 Hillview Avenue
Palo Alto, CA 94304
(800) 334-2564
(415) 858-2700

**National Library of Medicine MEDLARS Management Section**
Building 38A, Room 4N-421
8600 Rockville Pike
Bethesda, MD 20209
(800) 638-8480;
(301) 496-6193

## RESOURCES BY TOPIC

### Abortion

**National Abortion Federation**
(provides information about abortion and referral for abortion services)
1436 U Street, N.W.
Washington, DC 20009
(202) 667-5881
Consumer Information Hotline:
(800) 772-9100

*See also Family Planning*

### Accident Prevention

**Centers for Disease Control**
1600 Clifton Road, N.E.
Atlanta, GA 30333
(404) 639-3534

**National Safety Council**
425 North Michigan Avenue
Chicago, IL 60611
(312) 527-4800

*See also Automobile Safety; Injury Prevention; Poisoning; Product Safety*

### Adoption

**Adoptees' Liberty Movement Association (ALMA) Society**
(provides assistance for adopted children to locate natural parents and for natural parents to locate relinquished children)
P.O. Box 154
Washington Bridge Station
New York, NY 10033
(212) 581-1568

**AASK (Aid to the Adoption of Special Kids)**
(provides assistance to families who adopt older and handicapped children)
3530 Grand Avenue
Oakland, CA 94610
(415) 451-1748

### Aging

**American Association of Retired Persons**
(provides informational material related to retirement and aging)
1909 K Street, N.W.
Washington, DC 20049
(202) 872-4700

**Gray Panthers**
311 S. Juniper Street
Suite 601
Philadelphia, PA 19107
(215) 545-6555

*See also white or yellow pages of telephone directory for listing of local chapter*

**National Council on the Aging, Inc.**
(provides information on aging to the public and to health professionals)
646 Washington Street
Washington, DC 21502
(301) 724-5626

### AIDS (Acquired Immune Deficiency Syndrome)

**National STD Hotline**
(800) 227-8922

**National AIDS Hotline**
(800) 342-AIDS

**San Francisco AIDS Foundation**
25 Van Ness Street
San Francisco, CA 94102
(415) 864-4376

**Shanti**
(provides counseling and assistance to persons with AIDS)
525 Howard Street
San Francisco, CA 94105
(415) 777-2273

**Surgeon General's Report on Acquired Immune Deficiency**
Single copies available free by contacting:
Public Health Service
Office of Communications
200 Independence Avenue, S.W.
Washington, DC 20201
(202) 245-6867

*See also Sexually Transmitted Diseases; Terminal Illness*

### Alcohol Abuse and Alcoholism

**Al-Anon and Alateen**
(support groups for friends and relatives of alcoholics)
P.O. Box 862
Midtown Station
New York, NY 10018
(212) 302-7240
(800) 356-9996

*See also white pages of telephone directory for listing of local chapter*

**Alcohol Hotline**
Toll-free: (800) ALCOHOL

**Alcoholics Anonymous** 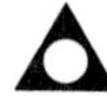
P.O. Box 459
Grand Central Station
New York, NY 10017
(212) 686-1100

*See also white pages of telephone directory for listing of local chapter*

**Children of Alcoholics Foundation**
200 Park Avenue
31st Floor
New York, NY 10166
(212) 351-2680

**National Clearinghouse for Alcohol Information**
P.O. Box 2345
Rockville, MD 20852
(301) 468-2600

**National Institute on Alcohol Abuse and Alcoholism**
5600 Fishers Lane
Rockville, MD 20857
(301) 443-3860

**Women For Sobriety, Inc.**
(support group for women with drinking problems)
P.O. Box 618
Quakertown, PA 18951
(215) 536-8026

*See also Drug Abuse; Drunk Driving Groups*

### Allergy

*See Asthma; Lung Disease*

## Alzheimer's Disease

**Alzheimer's Disease and Related Disorders Association**
70 E. Lake Street
Chicago, IL 60601
(312) 853-3060
(800) 621-0379
in Illinois (800) 572-6037

*See also Aging*

## Anorexia

*See Eating Disorders*

## Arthritis

**Arthritis Foundation**
1314 Spring Street, N.W.
Atlanta, GA 30309
(404) 872-7100

## Asthma

**Asthma and Allergy Foundation of America**
1717 Massachusetts Avenue, N.W.
Suite 305
Washington, DC 20036
(202) 265-0265

**National Jewish Lung Line**
(information + referral service)
(800) 222-LUNG

*See also Lung Disease*

## Automobile Safety

**American Automobile Association**
8111 Gatehouse Road
Falls Church, VA 22047
(703) 222-6000

*See also white or yellow pages of telephone directory for listing of local chapter*

**Insurance Institute for Highway Safety**
1005 North Glebe Road
Arlington, VA 22201
(703) 247-1500

**National Highway Traffic Safety Administration**
Office of Publications
400 7th Street, S.W.
Room 6170
Washington, DC 20590
(202) 366-2587

**Auto Safety Hotline**
(for consumer complaints about auto safety and child safety seats and requests for information on recalls)
(800) 424-9393

*See also Drunk Driving Groups*

## Birth Control

**American College of Obstetricians and Gynecologists**
(provides literature and contraceptive information)
409 12th Street, S.W.
Washington, DC 20024
(202) 638-5577

**Association for Voluntary Surgical Contraception**
(provides information and referrals to individuals considering tubal ligation or vasectomy)
122 East 42d Street
New York, NY 10168
(212) 351-2555

*See also Family Planning*

## Birth Defects

**Cystic Fibrosis Foundation**
2250 North Druid Hills Road
Suite 275
Atlanta, GA 30329
(404) 325-6973

**March of Dimes Birth Defects Foundation**
**Public Health Education Foundation**
1275 Mamaroneck Avenue
White Plains, NY 10605
(914) 428-7100

*See also white pages of telephone directory for listing of local chapter*
*See also Down's Syndrome; Inherited Diseases; Sickle-Cell Anemia*

## Blindness

**American Foundation for the Blind**
15 W. 16th Street
New York, NY 10011
(212) 620-2000
(800) 232-5463

**National Federation of the Blind**
1800 Johnson Street
Baltimore, MD 21230
(301) 659-9314

**National Library Service for the Blind and Physically Handicapped**
Library of Congress
1291 Taylor Street, N.W.
Washington, DC 20542
(202) 707-5100
(800) 424-8567

## Blood Banks

**American Red Cross**
17th and D Streets, N.W.
Washington, DC 20006
(202) 737-8300

*See also white or yellow pages of telephone directory for listing of local chapter*

## Brain

**Brain Research Foundation**
208 S. La Salle Street
Suite 1426
Chicago, IL 60604
(312) 782-4311

*See also Neurological Disorders; Stroke*

## Breast Cancer

**Reach to Recovery**
(support program for women who have undergone mastectomies as a result of breast cancer)
American Cancer Society
1599 Clifton Road
Atlanta, GA 30329
(404) 320-3333

*See also Cancer*

## Bulimia

*See Eating Disorders*

## Burn Injuries

**National Burn Victim Foundation**
308 Main Street
Orange, NJ 07050
(201) 731-3112

**Phoenix Society**
(self-help organization for burn victims and their families)
National Organization for Burn Victims
11 Rust Hill Road
Levittown, PA 19056
(215) 946-4788

## Cancer

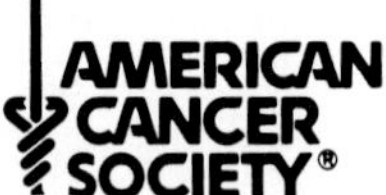


1599 Clifton Road
Atlanta, GA 30329
(404) 320-3333

*See also white pages of telephone directory for listing of local chapter*

**Cancer Connection**
(support group that matches cancer patients with volunteers who are cured, in remission, or being treated for same type of cancer)
H&R Block Building
4410 Main
Kansas City, MO 64111
(816) 932-8453

**Cancer Information Service**
(supplies cancer information to general public)
National Cancer Institute
9000 Rockville Pike
Bethesda, MD 20205
(301) 496-4000
(800) 4-CANCER

**Leukemia Society of America, Inc.**
733 Third Avenue
New York, NY 10017
(212) 573-8484

*See also Breast Cancer; DES Exposure; Lung Disease; Smoking and Tobacco; Terminal Illness*

## Child Abuse

**Child Assault Prevention (CAP) Project**
**National Assault Prevention Center**
(provides services to children, adolescents, mentally retarded adults and elderly)
P.O. Box 02015
Columbus, OH 43202
(614) 291-2540

**Clearinghouse on Child Abuse and Neglect Information**
P.O. Box 1182
Washington, DC 20013
(703) 821-2086

**National Child Abuse Hotline**
(800) 422-4453

**National Committee for the Prevention of Child Abuse (NCPCA)**
(provides literature on child abuse prevention programs)
332 S. Michigan Avenue
Suite 950
Chicago, IL 60604
(312) 663-3520

**Parents Anonymous**
(self-help group for abusive parents)
6733 South Sepulveda
Suite 270
Los Angeles, CA 90045
(800) 352-0386 in California
(800) 421-0353 (outside California)

*See also Missing and Runaway Children; Sexual Abuse and Assault*

## Child Health and Development

**National Center for Education in Maternal and Child Health**
38th and R Streets, N.W.
Washington, DC 20007
(202) 625-8400

**National Institute of Child Health and Human Development**
9000 Rockville Pike
Bethesda, MD 20892
(301) 496-4000

*See also Infant Care; Marriage and Family; Parent Support Groups*

## Childbirth

**American College of Nurse-Midwives**
(RNs who provide services through the maternity cycle)
1522 K Street, N.W.
Suite 1120
Washington, DC 20005
(202) 347-5445

**American College of Obstetricians and Gynecologists**
409 12th Street, S.W.
Washington, DC 20024
(202) 638-5577

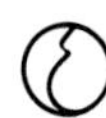

**American Society for Psychoprophylaxis in Obstetrics**
(provides information about the Lamaze method)
1840 Wilson Boulevard
Suite 204
Arlington, VA 22201
(703) 524-7802

**International Childbirth Education Association**
P.O. Box 20048
Minneapolis, MN 55420
(612) 854-8660

**National Association of Parents and Professionals for Safe Alternatives in Childbirth**
(provides information and support for alternatives in birth experiences)
Route 1, Box 646
Marble Hill, MO 63764
(314) 238-2010

**Parent Care**
(resource for parents of premature and high-risk infants)
101 1/2 South Union Street
Alexandria, VA 22314
(703) 836-4678

*See also Infant Care; Pregnancy; Women's Health*

## Chiropractic

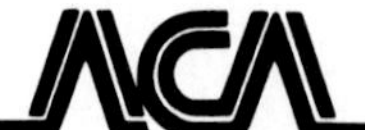


**American Chiropractic Association**
1701 Clarendon Blvd.
Arlington, VA 22209
(800) 368-3083

## Cocaine Abuse

**Cocaine Anonymous World Services**
3740 Overland Avenue

Suite G
Los Angeles, CA 90034
(213) 559-5833

*See white pages of telephone directory for listing of local chapter*

**CokEnders**
1240 Powell
Emeryville, CA 94608
(415) 652-1772

**National Cocaine Hotline**
Toll-free: (800) COCAINE

*See also white pages of telephone directory for listing of local chapter*
*See also Drug Abuse*

## Consumer Information

**Consumer Information Catalog**
(catalog of publications developed by federal agencies for consumers)
Pueblo, CO 81009

**Consumer Information Center (CIC)**
(distributes publications developed by federal agencies for consumers)
General Services Administration
Washington, DC 20405
(202) 566-1794

**Consumer Product Safety Commission Information Service**
Washington, DC 20207
(800) 638-CPSC

**Consumers Union**
(tests quality and safety of consumer products; publishes magazine *Consumer Reports*)
256 Washington Street
Mount Vernon, NY 10550
(914) 667-9400

**Council of Better Business Bureaus**
4200 Wilson Boulevard
Suite 800
Arlington, VA 22209
(703) 276-0100

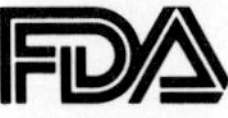

**Food and Drug Administration (FDA)**
Office of Consumer Affairs
Public Inquiries
5600 Fishers Lane (HFE-88)
Rockville, MD 20857
(301) 443-3170

*See also Product Safety*

## Crime Victims

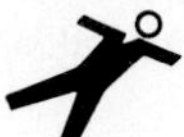

*See white or yellow pages of telephone directory for listings of local Crisis Centers, Rape Centers, Victim's Assistance Programs*

**National Association for Crime Victims Rights**
P.O. Box 16161
Portland, OR 97216
(503) 252-9012

**Victims Anonymous**
(support group for victims of sexual or physical abuse)
9514-9 Reseda Boulevard, No. 607
Northridge, CA 91324
(818) 993-1139

*See also Domestic Violence; Rape; Sexual Abuse and Assault*

## Crisis Intervention Services

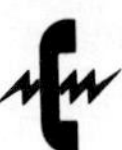

*See white or yellow pages of telephone directory for listings of local Crisis Centers and hotlines*

**National Crises Prevention Institute**
(offers programs on nonviolent physical crisis intervention)
3315K N. 124th Street
Brookfield, WI 53005
(414) 783-5787
(800) 558-8976

*See also Crime Victims; Mental Health; Rape; Sexual Abuse and Assault; Suicide Prevention*

## Deafness

*See Hearing Impairment*

## Death and Grieving

Call local Crisis Intervention Service for referral to agencies providing counseling and care to terminally ill individuals and their families

**SHARE**
(support group for parents who have suffered loss of newborn baby)
c/o St. John's Hospital
800 E. Carpenter Street
Springfield, IL 62769
(217) 544-6464

*See also AIDS; Hospices; Terminal Illness*

## Dental Health

**American Dental Association**
211 E. Chicago Avenue
Chicago, IL 60611
(312) 440-2500

**National Institute of Dental Research Office of Communications**
9000 Rockville Pike
Building 31, Room 2C35
Bethesda, MD 20892
(301) 496-4261

## Depressive Disorders

**Depressives Anonymous**
329 East 62nd Street
New York, NY 10021
(212) 689-2600

**National Depressive and Manic Depressive Association**
Merchandise Mart
P.O. Box 3395
Chicago, IL 60654
(312) 939-2442

*See also Crisis Intervention Services; Mental Health; Suicide Prevention*

## DES (Diethylstilbestrol) Exposure

**DES Action, National**
(support group for persons exposed to DES)
Long Island Jewish-Hillside
Medical Center

New Hyde Park, NY 11040
(516) 775-3450

*See also Cancer; Women's Health*

## Diabetes

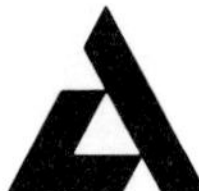


1660 Duke Street
Alexandria, VA 22314
(703) 549-1500

**Juvenile Diabetes Foundation International Hotline**
(800) 223-1138
in New York (212) 889-7575

**National Diabetes Information Clearinghouse**
Box NDIC
Bethesda, MD 20892
(301) 468-2162

## Digestive Diseases

**National Digestive Diseases and Education and Information Clearinghouse**
Box NDDIC
Bethesda, MD 20892
(301) 468-6344

## Disabled

*See Handicapped and Disabled*

## Divorce

*See Marriage and Family; Parent Support Groups*

## Domestic Violence

**Batterers Anonymous**
(self-help group designed to rehabilitate men who abuse women)
1269 N.E. Street
San Bernardino, CA 92405
(714) 355-1100

**National Coalition Against Domestic Violence**
Toll-free: (800) 333-SAFE

*See also Child Abuse; Sexual Abuse and Assault*

## Down Syndrome

**National Association for Down Syndrome (NADS)**
(provides information about Down Syndrome)
1800 Dempster
Park Ridge, IL 60068-1146
(708) 823-7550

**National Down Syndrome Society Hotline**
666 Broadway
New York, NY 10012
(212) 460-9330
(800) 221-4602

## Drug Abuse

**Alcohol, Drug Abuse, and Mental Health Administration**
5600 Fishers Lane
Rockville, MD 20857
(301) 443-2403

**Substance Abuse Prevention**
ADAMHA
Office for Substance Abuse Prevention
5600 Fishers Lane
Rockwall II Building
Rockville, MD 20857
(301) 443-0365

**Narcotics Anonymous**
(support group for recovering narcotics addicts)
P.O. Box 9999
Van Nuys, CA 91409
(818) 780-3951

**National Clearinghouse for Alcohol and Drug Information**
P.O. Box 2345
Rockville, MD 20852
(301) 468-2600
Toll-free: (800) 729-6686

**National Institute on Drug Abuse Helpline**
(800) 662-4357

**PRIDE (Parents' Resource Institute for Drug Education**
50 Hurt Plaza
Suite 210
Atlanta, GA 30303
(404) 577-4500
Toll-free: (800) 67-PRIDE
(taped message)
(800) 241-7946 (pamphlets and information)

*See also Alcohol Abuse and Alcoholism; Cocaine Abuse*

## Drunk Driving Groups

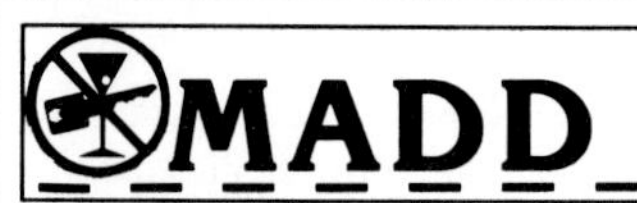


**Mothers Against Drunk Driving (MADD)**
669 Airport Freeway
Suite 310
Hurst, TX 76053
(817) 268-6233
(800) 438-6233

**Remove Intoxicated Drivers (RID)**
P.O. Box 520
Schenectady, NY 12301
(518) 372-0034

**Students Against Drunk Driving (SADD)**
P.O. Box 800
Marlboro, MA 01752
(508) 481-3568

## Eating Disorders

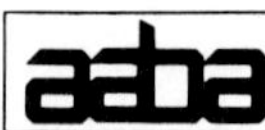


**American Anorexia/Bulimia Association, Inc.**
(self-help group that provides information and referrals to physicians and therapists)
418 E. 76th Street
New York, NY 10021
(212) 734-1114

**Anorexia Nervosa and Related Eating Disorders, Inc.**
(provides information and referrals for people with eating disorders)
P.O. Box 5102
Eugene, OR 97401
(503) 344-1144

**Bulimia and Anorexia Self-Help Hotline**
Toll-free: (800) 762-3334

## Environment

**Environmental Protection Agency (EPA)**
Public Information Center
PM 211-B
401 M Street, S.W.
Washington, DC 20460
(202) 382-2080

**Greenpeace, USA**
1436 U Street, N.W.
Washington, DC 20009
(202) 462-1177

**Sierra Club**
730 Polk Street
San Francisco, CA 94109
(415) 776-2211

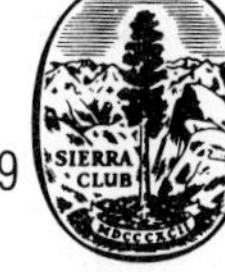


*See also Hazardous Wastes; Nuclear Energy Control and Safety; Pesticides; Radiation Control and Safety*

## Epilepsy

**Epilepsy Foundation of America**
4351 Garden City Dr.
Landover, MD 20785
(301) 459-3700
(800) 332-1000

## Exercise

*See Physical Fitness*

## Family Planning

**Center for Population Options**
(offers programs aimed at reducing teenage pregnancy)
1025 Vermont Avenue
Suite 210
Washington, DC 20005
(202) 347-5700

**Family Life Information Exchange**
P.O. Box 30436
Bethesda, MD 20814
(301) 770-3662

**Planned Parenthood Federation of America**

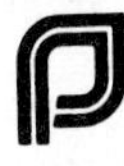

810 Seventh Avenue
New York, NY 10019
(212) 541-7800

*See also white pages of telephone directory for listing of local chapter*
*See also Birth Control; Women's Health*

## Food and Nutrition

*See Nutrition*

## Gay Groups and Services

**National Gay and Lesbian Task Force**
1517 U Street, N.W.
Washington, DC 20009
(202) 332-6483
Crisis Hotline
(800) 221-7044

NGTF

**Federation of Parents and Friends of Lesbians and Gays (Parents FLAG)**
(support group for parents of homosexuals; provides education on gay rights)
P.O. Box 24565
Los Angeles, CA 90024
(213) 472-8952

*See also AIDS*

## Handicapped and Disabled

**American Alliance for Health, Physical Education, Recreation, and Dance**
(provides information about recreation and fitness opportunities for the handicapped)
1900 Association Drive
Reston, VA 22091
(703) 476-3400

**National Library Service for the Blind and Physically Handicapped**
Library of Congress
1291 Taylor Street, N.W.
Washington, DC 20542
(202) 707-5100
(800) 424-8567

**National Rehabilitation Information Center**
8455 Colesville Road
Suite 935
Silver Springs, MD 20910
(301) 588-9284
Toll-free: (800) 34-NARIC

**Special Olympics**
1359 New York Ave., N.W.
Suite 500
Washington, D.C. 20005
(202) 628-3630

## Hazardous Wastes

**Environmental Protection Agency**
Public Information Center
PM 211-B
401 M Street, S.W.
Washington, DC 20460
(202) 382-2080

**Hazardous Waste Hotline**
(800) 424-9346

*See also Environment; Pesticides*

## Health Care

**American Medical Association**
535 North Dearborn Street
Chicago, IL 60610
(312) 645-5000

**American Nurses Association**
2420 Pershing Road
Kansas City, MO 64108
(816) 474-5720

**Medical Self-Care Magazine**
P.O. Box 717
Inverness, CA 94937

*See also Chiropractic; Consumer Information; Dental Health; Holistic Medicine; Homeopathy; Mental Health; Osteopathic Medicine; Surgery*

## Health Education

**Center for Health Promotion and Education**
Centers for Disease Control
Mail Stop A34
1600 Clifton Road, N.E.
Atlanta, GA 30333
(404) 639-3492 or 639-3698

## Hearing Impairment

**American Society for Children**
(Resource group for parents of hard of hearing and deaf children)
814 Thayer Avenue
Silver Springs, MD 20910
(301) 585-5400

**Better Hearing Institute**
(provides educational and resource materials on deafness)
Box 1840
Washington, DC 20013
(703) 642-0580
Toll-free: (800) EAR-WELL

## Heart Disease

**American Heart Association**
7320 Greenville Avenue
Dallas, TX 75231
(214) 373-6300
*See also white pages of telephone directory for listing of local chapter*

**NHLBI Educational Program Information Center**
(provides information on cardiovascular risk factors)
4733 Bethesda Avenue
Suite 530
Bethesda, MD 20814
(301) 951-3260

**Mended Hearts**
(support group for persons who have undergone heart surgery and their families)
c/o American Heart Association
7320 Greenville Avenue
Dallas, TX 75231
(214) 706-1442

**National Heart, Lung, and Blood Institute**
(provides information on cardiovascular disease)
9000 Rockville Pike
Building 31, Room 4A21
Bethesda, MD 20892
(301) 496-4236
*See also Hypertension; Stroke*

## High Blood Pressure

*See Hypertension*

## Holistic Medicine

**American Holistic Medical Association**
2002 Eastlake Avenue
Seattle, WA 98102
(206) 322-6842

## Homeopathy

**National Center for Homeopathy**
1500 Massachusetts Avenue, N.W.
Suite 42
Washington, DC 20005
(202) 223-6182

## Homosexuality

*See Gay Groups and Services*

## Hospices

**National Hospice Organization**
1901 N. Fort Moore Street
Suite 901
Arlington, VA 22209
(703) 243-5900

## Hypertension

**NHLBI Educational Program Information Center**
(provides information on cardiovascular risk factors)
4733 Bethesda Avenue
Suite 530
Bethesda, MD 20814
(301) 951-3260

**National Heart, Lung, and Blood Institute**
(provides information on cardiovascular diseases)
9000 Rockville Pike
Building 31, Room 4A21
Bethesda, MD 20892
(301) 496-4236
*See also Heart Disease*

## Hypnosis

**American Society of Clinical Hypnosis**
2200 E. Devon Avenue
Suite 291
Des Plaines, IL 60018
(708) 297-3317

## Immunization

**Center for Prevention Services**
Centers for Disease Control
1600 Clifton Road, N.E.
Atlanta, GA 30333
(404) 639-3534

## Incest

*See Child Abuse; Sexual Abuse and Assault*

## Infant Care

**American Red Cross**
(offers classes to expectant parents to prepare them for care and nurturing of infant)
17th and D Streets, N.W.
Washington, DC 20006
(202) 737-8300
*See also white pages of telephone directory for listing of local chapter*

**Beechnut Nutrition Hotline**
(800) 523-6633

**La Leche League International**
(provides information and support to women interested in breast feeding)
9616 Minneapolis
Franklin, IL 60131
(708) 455-7730
*See also Child Health and Development; Childbirth; Pregnancy*

## Infectious Diseases

**Centers for Disease Control**
1600 Clifton Road, N.E.
Atlanta, GA 30333
(404) 639-3534
*See also Sexually Transmitted Diseases*

## Infertility

**Resolve, Inc.**
(offers counseling, information, and support to people with problems of infertility)
5 Water Street
Arlington, MA 02174
(617) 643-2424

*See also white pages of telephone directory for listing of local chapter*

**In-Vitro Fertilization**
Eastern Virginia Medical School
The Howard and Georgeanna Jones Institute for Reproductive Medicine
825 Fairfax Avenue
Norfolk, VA 23507
(804) 446-8948

## Inherited Diseases

**National Clearinghouse for Human Genetic Disease**
(provides information about inherited diseases; publishes directory of genetic counseling services)
National Center for Education in Maternal and Child Health
38th and R Streets, N.W.
Washington, DC 20057
(202) 625-8400

*See also Birth Defects; Sickle-Cell Anemia*

## Injury Prevention

**Center for Environmental Health**
Centers for Disease Control
1600 Clifton Road, N.E.
Atlanta, GA 30333
(404) 639-3534

**National Injury Information Clearinghouse**
5401 Westbard Avenue
Room 625
Washington, DC 20207
(301) 492-6424

*See Accident Prevention; Automobile Safety; Poisoning; Product Safety*

## Kidney Disease

**American Kidney Fund**
(provides information on financial aid to patients, organ transplants, and kidney-related diseases)
6110 Executive Boulevard
Suite 1010
Bethesda, MD 20852
(301) 986-1444
(800) 638-8299

**American Association of Kidney Patients**
One Davis Boulevard
Suite LL1
Tampa, FL 33606
(813) 251-0725

**National Kidney Foundation**

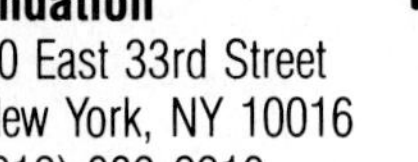

30 East 33rd Street
New York, NY 10016
(212) 889-2210

## Learning Disorders

**Association for Children and Adults with Learning Disabilities**
4156 Library Road
Pittsburgh, PA 15234
(412) 341-1515

## Liver Disease

**American Liver Foundation**
1425 Pompton Avenue
Cedar Grove, NJ 07009
(201) 857-2626
(800) 223-0179

## Lung Disease

AMERICAN LUNG ASSOCIATION

1740 Broadway
New York, NY 10019
(212) 315-8700

**NHLBI Educational Program Information Center**
(provides information on cardiovascular risk factors)
4733 Bethesda Avenue
Suite 530
Bethesda, MD 20814
(301) 951-3260

**National Jewish Hospital/National Asthma Center**
(800) 222-LUNG

*See also Asthma; Cancer; Smoking and Tobacco*

## Lupus Erythematosus

**Lupus Foundation of America**
1717 Massachusetts Avenue, N.W.
Suite 203
Washington, DC 20036
(202) 328-4550
Toll-free: (800) 558-0121

## Marriage and Family

**Displaced Homemakers Network**
(national advocacy group for women over 35 who have lost their primary means of support through death, divorce, or disabling of spouse)
1411 K Street, N.W.
Suite 930
Washington, DC 20005
(202) 628-6767

**Equal Rights for Fathers**
P.O. Box 90042
San Jose, CA 95109-3042
(415) 454-3237

**Family Service America**
11700 West Lake Park Drive
Milwaukee, WI 53224
(414) 359-2111

*See also white or yellow pages of telephone directory for listing of local chapter*

**Single Parent Resource Center**
1165 Broadway
Room 504
New York, NY 10001
(212) 213-0047

**Stepfamily Association of America**
(provides information and publishes quarterly newsletter)
215 Centennial Mall South
Suite 212
Lincoln, NB 68508
(402) 477-7837

*See also Family Planning; Parent Support Groups*

## Medical Care

*See Health Care*

## Medical Identification

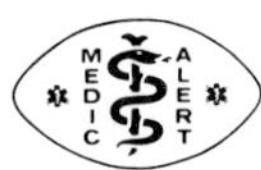


**Medic-Alert Foundation International**
(provides those with medical problems bracelets or neck chains with special emblems to alert medical or law enforcement personnel)
2323 Colorado
Turlock, CA 95381
(209) 668-3333
(800) ID-ALERT

## Medications (Prescription and Over-the-Counter)

**Food and Drug Administration (FDA)**
Office of Consumer Affairs
Public Inquiries
5600 Fishers Lane (HFE-88)
Rockville, MD 20857
(301) 443-3170

*See also Consumer Information*

## Mental Health

**American Psychiatric Association**
1400 K Street, N.W.
Washington, DC 20005
(202) 682-6000

**American Psychological Association**
1200 17th Street, N.W.
Washington, DC 20036
(202) 955-7600

**National Alliance for the Mentally Ill**
(self-help advocacy organization for persons with schizophrenia and depressive disorders and their families)
2101 Wilson Boulevard
Suite 302
Arlington, VA 22201
(703) 524-7600

**National Institute of Mental Health**
Information Resources and Inquiries Branch
5600 Fishers Lane
Room 15C05
Rockville, MD 20857
(301) 443-4515

**National Mental Health Association**
1021 Prince Street
Alexandria, VA 22314-2971
(703) 684-7722

**Recovery, Inc.**
(self-help group for former mental patients)
Association of Nervous and Former Mental Patients
802 North Dearborn Street
Chicago, IL 60610
(312) 337-5661

*See also Crisis Intervention Services; Depressive Disorders; Suicide Prevention*

## Mental Retardation

**National Association for Retarded Citizens**
P.O. Box 6109
Arlington, TX 76005
(817) 640-0204

*See also Down's Syndrome*

## Missing and Runaway Children

**Adam Walsh Child Resource Center**
311 South Dixie Highway
Suite 244
W. Palm Beach, FL 33405
(407) 833-9080

**Childfind**
P.O. Box 277
New Paltz, NY 12561
(800) 426-5678; (914) 255-1848

**National Center for Missing and Exploited Children**
2101 Wilson Boulevard
Suite 550
Arlington, VA 22201
(800) 843-5678

**Runaway Hotline**
(800) 231-6946
in Texas (800) 392-3352

## Neurological Disorders

**National Institute of Neurological and Communicative Disorders and Stroke**
National Institutes of Health
9000 Rockville Pike
Bethesda, MD 20205
(301) 496-4000

*See also Alzheimer's Disease; Brain; Mental Health; Stroke*

## Nuclear Energy Control and Safety

**Council for a Livable World**
(promotes nuclear arms control)
100 Maryland Avenue, N.E.
Washington, DC 20002
(202) 543-4100

**SANE/Freeze: Committee for a Sane Nuclear Policy**
(promotes nuclear freeze policy)
1819 H Street, N.W.
Suite 1000
Washington, DC 20006
(202) 862-9740

## Nutrition

**American Institute of Nutrition**
9650 Rockville Pike
Bethesda, MD 20814
(301) 530-7050

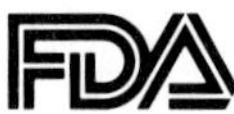


**Food and Drug Administration**
Office of Consumer Affairs
Public Inquiries
5600 Fishers Lane (HFE-88)
Rockville, MD 20857
(301) 443-3170

**Food and Nutrition Board**
Institute of Medicine
2101 Constitution Avenue, N.W.
Washington, DC 20418
(202) 334-2238

**National Nutrition Education Clearinghouse**
Society for Nutrition Education
1700 Broadway

Suite 300
Oakland, CA 94612
(415) 444-7133

## Obesity

*See Nutrition; Weight Control*

## Occupational Safety and Health

**Clearinghouse for Occupational Safety and Health Information**
Centers for Disease Control
National Institute for Occupational Safety and Health
5600 Fishers Lane
Rockville, MD 20857
(202) 472-7134

## Organ Donations

**Living Bank**
(provides information and acts as registry and referral service for people wanting to donate organs for research or transplantation)
(800) 528-2971
in Texas (713) 528-2971

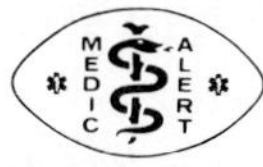


**Medic-Alert Organ Donor Program**
2323 Colorado
Turlock, CA 95381-1009
(209) 668-3333
(800) ID-ALERT

## Osteopathic Medicine

**American Osteopathic Association**
142 East Ontario
Chicago, IL 60611
(312) 280-5800

## Parent Support Groups

**National Organization of Mothers of Twins Clubs, Inc.**
P.O. Box 23188
Albuquerque, NM 87192-1188
(505) 275-0955

**Parents Anonymous**
(self-help group for abusive parents)
6733 S. Sepulveda
Suite 270
Los Angeles, CA 90045
(213) 410-9732
(800) 421-0353
in California (800) 352-0386

**Parents Without Partners**
8807 Colesville Road
Silver Spring, MD 20910
(301) 588-9354
*See also white pages of telephone directory for listing of local chapter*

**Toughlove**
(support group for parents of problem teenagers)
P.O. Box 1069
Doylestown, PA 18901
(215) 348-7090
(800) 333-1069
*See also Marriage and Family*

## Pesticides

**National Pesticide Telecommunications Network**
Texas Tech University
School of Medicine
Dept. of Preventive Medicine, Health Science Center
4th and Indiana
Lubbock, TX 79430
(806) 743-3091
Toll-free: (800) 858-7378
*See also Environment; Hazardous Wastes*

## Phobias

**PASS Group**
(support group to help treat agoraphobics)
P.O. Box 1614
Williamsville, NY 14221
(716) 689-4399

**Anxiety Disorders Association of America**
(provides information about phobias and referrals to therapists and support groups)
6000 Executive Boulevard
Suite 200
Rockville, MD 20852
(301) 231-9350

**TERRAP (TERRitorial APprehensiveness)**
(headquarters for national network of treatment clinics for agoraphobia)
648 Menlo Avenue
Suite 5
Menlo Park, CA 94025
(415) 327-1312
*See also Mental Health*

## Physical Fitness

*See yellow and white pages of telephone directory for listings of local health clubs and YMCAs, YWCAs, and Jewish Community Centers*

**Aerobics International Research Society**
12330 Preston Road
Dallas, TX 75230
(800) 635-7050

**American Running and Fitness Association**
2001 S Street, N.W.
Suite 540
Washington, DC 20001
(202) 667-4150

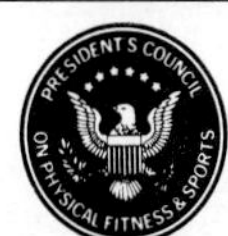


**President's Council on Physical Fitness and Sports**
450 5th Street, N.W.
Suite 7103
Washington, DC 20001
(202) 272-3430

**Women's Sports Foundation**
342 Madison Avenue
Suite 728
New York, NY 10017
Toll-free: (800) 227-3988

## Physicians

*See Health Care*

## Poisoning

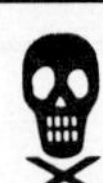

*See emergency numbers listed at the front of the telephone directory for telephone number of local Poison Control Center or call directory assistance for toll-free hotline number for your area*

*See also Accident Prevention; Injury Prevention*

## Pregnancy

**National Center for Education in Maternal and Child Health**
38th and R Streets, N.W.
Washington, DC 20057
(202) 625-8400

*See also Childbirth; Family Planning; Infant Care; Women's Health*

## Product Safety

**Consumer Product Safety Commission**
Washington, DC 20207
(800) 638-CPSC

*See also Accident Prevention; Consumer Information; Injury Prevention*

## Radiation Control and Safety

**Center for Devices and Radiological Health**
Office of Consumer Affairs
5600 Fishers Lane
HFC-210
Rockville, MD 20857
(301) 443-4190

**National Institute of Environmental Sciences**
P.O. Box 12233
Research Triangle Park, NC 27709
(919) 541-3345

*See also Environment*

## Rape

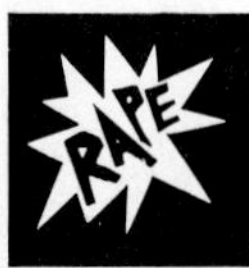


*See white pages of telephone directory for listing of local Rape Centers*

**National Clearinghouse on Marital and Date Rape**
(for profit referral service)
2325 Oak Street
Berkeley, CA 94708
(415) 548-1770

**National Coalition Against Sexual Assault (NCASA)**
2428 Ontario Road, N.W.
Washington, DC 20009
(202) 483-7165

## Reye's Syndrome

**National Reye's Syndrome Foundation**
426 North Lewis
Bryan, OH 43506
Toll-free: (800) 233-7393

## Self-Care/Self-Help

**National Self-Help Clearinghouse**
(provides information about self-help groups)
25 W. 43rd Street
Room 620
New York, NY 10036
(212) 642-2944

**Self-Help Institute**
(provides information about self-help groups)
1600 Dodge Avenue
Suite S-122
Evanston, IL 60201
(708) 328-0470

## Sex Education

**American Association of Sex Educators, Counselors, and Therapists**
435 North Michigan
Suite 1717
Chicago, IL 60611
(312) 644-0828

**Center for Population Options**
(develops programs and material to educate teenagers on sex and sexual responsibility)
1025 Vermont, N.W.
Suite 210
Washington, DC 20005
(202) 347-5700

**Planned Parenthood Federation of America**
810 Seventh Avenue
New York, NY 10019
(212) 541-7800

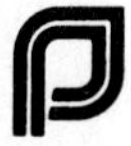

*See also white pages of telephone directory for listing of local chapter*

**Sex Information and Education Council of the United States (SIECUS)**
(maintains an information clearinghouse on all aspects of human sexuality)
130 West 42nd Street
Suite 2500
New York, NY 10036
(212) 819-9770

*See also Family Planning*

## Sex Therapy

**American Association of Sex Educators, Counselors, and Therapists**
435 N. Michigan
Suite 1717
Chicago, IL 60611
(312) 644-0828

## Sexual Abuse and Assault

**National Assault Prevention Center**
(provides services to children, adolescents, mentally retarded adults and elderly)
P.O. Box 02015
Columbus, OH 43202
(614) 291-2540

**National Committee for Prevention of Child Abuse**
332 S. Michigan Avenue
Suite 1600
Chicago, IL 60604
(312) 663-3520

**Parents United**
(support group for individuals and families who have experienced sexual molestation as children)
P.O. Box 952
San Jose, CA 95108
(408) 453-7616

**Victims Anonymous**
(support group for victims of sexual or physical abuse)
9514-9 Reseda Boulevard, No. 607
Northridge, CA 91324
(818) 993-1139

*See also Child Abuse; Rape*

## Sexual Difficulties

**Impotence Information Center**
(provides information on causes and treatment of impotence)

P.O. Box 9
Minneapolis, MN 55440
(800) 843-4315
in Minnesota (612) 933-4666

**Sexaholics Anonymous**
(self-help group for sexual addicts)
P.O. Box 300
Simi Valley, CA 93062
(818) 704-9854

*See also Sex Therapy*

## Sexually Transmitted Diseases

**Center for Prevention Services**
Centers for Disease Control
1600 Clifton Road, N.E.
Atlanta, GA 30333
(404) 329-1819

**Herpes Resource Center**
Box 13827
Research Triangle Park, NC 27709
(919) 361-2742

**National STD Hotline**
(800) 227-8922

*See also AIDS; Sex Education*

## Sickle-Cell Anemia

**Center for Sickle Cell Disease**
2121 Georgia Avenue, N.W.
Washington, DC 20059
(202) 806-7930

## Skin Disease

**National Psoriasis Foundation**
6443 S.W. Beaverton Highway
Suite 210
Portland, OR 97221
(503) 297-1545

## Sleep and Sleep Disorders

**American Narcolepsy Association**
P.O. Box 1187
San Carlos, CA 94070
(415) 591-7979

**Better Sleep Council (of the international Sleep Products Association)**
333 Commerce Street
Alexandria, VA 22314
(703) 683-8371

**American Sleep Disorders Association**
604 Second Street, S.W.
Rochester, MN 55902
(507) 287-6006

## Smoking and Tobacco

**Action on Smoking and Health (ASH)**
(provides information on nonsmokers' rights and related subjects)
2013 H Street, N.W.
Washington, DC 20006
(202) 659-4310

(provides information about quitting smoking and smoking cessation programs)
1599 Clifton Road
Atlanta, GA 30329
(404) 320-3333

*See also white pages of telephone directory for listing of local chapter*

**American Heart Association**
(provides information about quitting smoking and smoking cessation programs)
7320 Greenville Avenue
Dallas, TX 75231
(214) 373-6300

*See also white pages of telephone directory for listing of local chapter*

**American Lung Association**
(provides information about quitting smoking and smoking cessation programs)
1740 Broadway
New York, NY 10019
(212) 315-8700

*See also white pages of telephone directory for listing of local chapter*

**Breathe-Free Plan To Stop Smoking**
6830 Laurel Street, N.W.
Washington, DC 20012
(202) 722-6724

**Group Against Smokers' Pollution (GASP)**
(provides information on nonsmokers' rights and related subjects)
P.O. Box 632
College Park, MD 20740
(301) 577-6427

**SmokEnders**
(for profit organization teaching smokers to quit using Rogers method)
18551 Von Karman Avenue
Irvine, CA 92715
(714) 854-2273

*See also Cancer; Heart Disease; Lung Disease*

## Stress Reduction

*See white or yellow pages of telephone directory for listings on Biofeedback Therapy and Training, Crisis Centers, Meditation*

**Biofeedback Society of America**
10200 W. 44th Avenue
Suite 304
Wheat Ridge, CO 80033
(303) 422-8436

*See also Mental Health; Physical Fitness*

## Stroke

**Council on Stroke**
American Heart Association
7320 Greenville Avenue
Dallas, TX 75231
(214) 373-6300

**National Institute of Neurological and Communicative Disorders and Stroke**
National Institutes of Health
9000 Rockville Pike
Bethesda, MD 20205
(301) 496-4000

**Stroke Club International**
(group for stroke victims)
805 12th Street
Galveston, TX 77550
(409) 762-1022

*See also Heart Disease*

## Stuttering

**National Center for Stuttering**
200 East 33rd Street
New York, NY 10016
Toll-free: (800) 221-2483

## Sudden Infant Death Syndrome (SIDS)

**National Sudden Infant Death Syndrome Foundation**
(provides information and referrals for families who have lost an infant because of SIDS)
2320 Glenview Road
Glenview, IL 60025
(708) 657-8080
(800) 221-7437

## Suicide Prevention

*See white pages of telephone directory for listing of Suicide Prevention Centers; also see listings for Crisis Centers*

**American Association of Suicidology**
2459 S. Ash
Denver, CO 80222
(303) 692-0985

**National Adolescent Suicide Hotline**
(800) 621-4000

**Youth Suicide National Center**
445 Virginia Avenue
San Mateo, CA 94402
(415) 347-3961

*See also Crisis Intervention Services; Depressive Disorders; Mental Health*

## Surgery

**National Second Surgical Opinion Program**
(800) 638-6833
in Maryland (800) 492-6603

*See also Health Care*

## Terminal Illness

**Concern for Dying**
(promotes research on death and dying and works for the right of terminally ill persons to refuse extraordinary life-prolonging measures)
250 W. 57th Street, Room 831
New York, NY 10107
(212) 246-6942
(800) 248-2122

**The Hemlock Society**
(promotes tolerance of the right of terminally ill persons to end their lives in a planned manner)
P.O. Box 11830
Eugene, OR 97440
(503) 342-5748

**Make-A-Wish Foundation of America**
(dedicated to granting the special wishes of terminally ill children)
2600 North Central Avenue
Suite 936
Phoenix, AZ 85004
(602) 240-6600

**Make Today Count**
(self-help group for persons with terminal illness)
101 1/2 South Union Street
Alexandria, VA 22314
(703) 548-9674

*See also AIDS; Cancer; Death and Grieving; Hospices*

## Toxic Substances

*See Hazardous Wastes; Pesticides; Poisoning*

## Victims of Violent Crimes

*See Crime Victims; Domestic Violence; Rape; Sexual Abuse and Assault*

## Weight Control

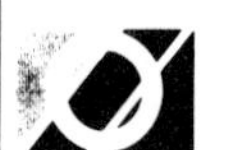

OVEREATERS ANONYMOUS

P.O. Box 92870
Los Angeles, CA 90009
(213) 542-8363

*See also white pages of telephone directory for listing of local chapter*

**Thin Within**
*See white pages of telephone directory for listing of local chapter*

**TOPS (Take Off Pounds Sensibly)**
P.O. Box 07360
4575 S. Fifth Street
Milwaukee, WI 53207
(414) 482-4620

*See also white pages of telephone directory for listing of local chapter*

**Weight Watchers International, Inc.**

Jericho Atrium
500 North Broadway
Jericho, NY 11753-2196
(516) 939-0400

*See also white pages of telephone directory for listing of local chapter*
*See also Nutrition; Physical Fitness*

## Wellness

**Wellness Associates**
(publishes the Wellness Inventory, a questionnaire that individuals can use to determine their level of wellness)
12347 DuPont Road
Sebastapol, CA 95472
(707) 874-1456, x1466

## Women's Health

**Boston Women's Health Book Collective**
(publishes *Our Bodies, Ourselves*, a well-known book on women's health)
240A Elm Street
Sommerville, MA 02144
(617) 625-0271

**National Women's Health Network**
1325 G Street, N.W.
Washington, DC 20005
(202) 347-1140

**Premenstrual Syndrome Action**
(provides information to public and health professionals about PMS)
P.O. Box 16292
Irvine, CA 92713
(714) 854-4407
(800) 272-4PMS (U.S.)
(800) 332-4PMS (in CA)

*See also Childbirth; Family Planning; Pregnancy*

# GLOSSARY

**abortion** A procedure to remove uterine contents after pregnancy has occurred.

**abscess** A localized accumulation of pus and disintegrating tissue.

**absorption** The passage of substances into or across membranes or tissues.

**acid rain** Rain with a high concentration of acids produced by air pollutants emitted during the combustion of fossil fuels; damages plant and animal life and buildings.

**acquaintance rape** Rape by a person known by the victim.

**acquired immune deficiency syndrome (AIDS)** A fatal disease caused by a virus that destroys the ability of the immune system to fight disease; transmitted primarily by sexual contact and the contaminated needles of drug users and, less commonly, through contaminated blood products.

**act-alike** A drug manufactured to get around state laws prohibiting look-alikes.

**active immunity** Immunity resulting from the body's production of antibodies in response to a pathogen or a vaccine.

**adaptation** Any change in structure, form, or behavior to suit a new situation.

**adaptive response** The body's attempt to reestablish homeostasis.

**addiction** A state of compulsive physiological need for a habit-forming substance.

**additive** Characterized by a combined effect that is equal to the sum of the individual effects.

**additives** A substance added to food to enhance certain qualities, such as appearance, taste, or freshness.

**aerobic exercise** Exercise requiring oxygen; exercise in which sufficient or excess oxygen is continually supplied to the body.

**aggression** Forceful behavior with intent to dominate.

**AIDS-related complex (ARC)** See *pre-AIDS*.

**alarm** The first stage of the General Adaptation Syndrome, or stress response, in which the body prepared for fight or flight.

**alcoholic** A person whose drinking interferes on a continuing basis with a major aspect of his or her life.

**allergy** A hypersensitivity to a particular substance or to an environmental condition.

**altruism** An unselfish concern for the welfare of others.

**altruistic egotism** A way of adapting in which a person cooperates with others by giving help and, in return, receives help as well as a sense of self-worth.

**Alzheimer's disease** A progressive deterioration of intellectual powers due to physiological changes within the brain; symptoms include diminishing ability to concentrate and reason, disorientation, depression, apathy, and paranoia.

**amenorrhea** The absence or suppression of menstruation.

**amnion** The innermost membrane of the sac enclosing the embryo or fetus.

**anabolic steroid** A drug derived from testosterone and approved for medical use but often used by athletes to increase their musculature and weight.

**anaerobic exercise** Exercise not using oxygen for energy production; exercise in which the body develops an oxygen deficit.

**analgesic** A medication that relieves pain without inducing a loss of consciousness.

**androgyny** The expression of both masculine and feminine traits.

**aneurysm** A localized, blood-filled sac in an artery wall; caused by dilation or weakening of the artery wall.

**angina pectoris** A severe, suffocating chest pain caused by a brief lack of oxygen to the heart.

**anorexia nervosa** A psychological disorder in which refusal to eat and/or an extreme loss of appetite leads to malnutrition, severe weight loss, and possibly death.

**antagonistic** Opposing or counteracting.

**antibiotic** A substance produced by one type of microorganism that is toxic to other types of microorganisms; in dilute solutions, used to treat infectious diseases.

**antibody** A specialized protein produced by the body; combines with a specific antigen to play the central role in immunity to specific pathogens.

**antigen** Any of a number of substances—including toxins, foreign proteins, and microorganisms—which, when introduced to the body, cause antibody formation.

**antihistamine** A medication used to treat allergic reactions and cold symptoms; inactivates histamine, a substance found in body tissues that plays a role in allergic reactions.

**anxiety** A feeling of apprehension and dread, with or without a known cause; may range from mild to severe and may be accompanied by physical symptoms.

**aortic aneurysm** A blood-filled sac in the aorta; caused by dilation or weakening of the blood vessel wall.

**arrhythmia** Any irregularity in the rhythm of the heartbeat.

**arteriosclerosis** Any of a number of chronic diseases characterized by degeneration of the arteries and hardening and thickening of arterial walls.

**arthritis** An inflammation of the joints.

**asbestos** A mineral widely used for building insulation; has been linked to lung and gastrointestinal cancer.

**assertiveness** The ability to be open and frank, especially in declaring one's rights.

**asthma** A disease or allergic response characterized by bronchial spasms and difficult breathing.

**atherosclerosis** A form of arteriosclerosis in which fatty substances are deposited on the inner walls of blood vessels.

**atrial fibrillation** A condition characterized by an irregular, abnormally rapid heartbeat.

**atrium** (*plural:* **atria**) Either of the two upper chambers of the heart, which receive blood from the veins.

**atrophy** To waste away.

**autoimmune disorder** Any of several disabling conditions in which the immune system attacks body tissues, causing progressively worse degeneration.

**autopsy** The detailed examination and dissection of a dead body.

**aversion therapy** A treatment that attempts to help a person overcome a dependence or a bad habit by making the person feel disgusted or repulsed by the habit.

**ballistic stretching** A potentially hazardous form of stretching that involves bouncing or jerking; can cause the muscles to contract rather than stretch.

**basal body temperature** The body temperature upon waking, before any activity.

**basal metabolic rate** The number of calories required to maintain life-sustaining activities for a specified period of time.

**behavioral modification** An approach to psychological problems that focuses on a symptom and aims to eliminate it by rewarding desired behavior; by punishing unwanted behavior; or by gradual reconditioning, which eliminates the source of the problem.

**behavioral toxicity** Having harmful effects on an individual's actions and attitudes.

**behaviorism** A branch of psychology that views normal and abnormal behavior as the product of conditioned responses to stimuli.

**benign** Harmless; not malignant.

**beryllium** A toxic metallic element that forms hard alloys with other metals and is a good electrical conductor; considered a dangerous pollutant.

**biodegradable** Capable of being broken down into harmless components, especially by the action of bacteria, sunlight, and heat.

**biofeedback** Information about some activity that has just taken place in the body.

**bisexual** The sexual attraction to, and relationships with, people of either sex; a person who is attracted in such a way.

**blood alcohol concentration (BAC)** The amount of alcohol in a person's blood.

**bradycardia** An abnormally slow heart rate, below 60 beats per minute.

**brief psychotherapy** Short-term, structured treatments focusing on a specific emotional problem.

**bulimarexia** A psychological disorder that results in the self-starvation symptoms of anorexia nervosa and the binge-purge behaviors of bulimia.

**bulimia nervosa** Episodic binge eating, often followed by forced vomiting, and accompanied by a persistent overconcern with body shape and weight.

**burnout** A state of physical, emotional, and mental exhaustion resulting from constant or repeated emotional pressure.

**cadmium** A toxic metallic element common in industrial waste and as a component of environmental pollution; used industrially in electroplating and in atomic fusion.

**calorie** The amount of heat required to raise the temperature of 1 gram of water by 1 degree Celsius (the calorie of popular usage is actually 1,000 times larger than the calorie of science).

**cancer** A disease in which a malignant cellular tumor that is capable of spreading to other parts of the body develops.

**capillary** A network of minute blood vessels connecting tiny arteries to tiny veins.

**carbohydrate** An organic compound—such as starch, sugar, or glycogen—composed of carbon, hydrogen, and oxygen; a source of bodily energy.

**carbon monoxide** A colorless, odorless gas that is a by-product of engine exhaust and burning tobacco; displaces oxygen on the hemoglobin molecules of red blood cells.

**carcinogen** A substance that produces cancerous cells or enhances their development and growth.

**cardiopulmonary resuscitation (CPR)** A method of artificial stimulation of the heart and lungs.

**cardiovascular disease** Disorders of the blood and heart.

**cardiovascular fitness** The ability of the heart and blood vessels to work efficiently.

**celibacy** Abstention from sexual activity.

**cerebral embolism** A sudden obstruction of a blood vessel in the brain by an abnormal particle or clot.

**cerebral hemorrhage** The rupturing of a blood vessel in the brain.

**cerebral thrombosis** The formation of a blood clot in a blood vessel of the brain.

**cerebrovascular accident** A condition in which a cerebral blood vessel is blocked.

**cervical cap** A cup-shaped device that is inserted into the vagina to cover the cervix and prevent the passage of sperm into the uterus during sexual intercourse.

**cervix** The opening between the vagina and the uterus.

**cesarean delivery** The surgical procedure in which an infant is delivered through an incision made in the abdominal wall and uterus.

**chanchroid** A soft, painful sore or localized infection usually acquired through sexual contact.

**chancre** A sore or ulcer at the entry point of a pathogen; the first sign of syphilis.

**chlamydia** A sexually transmitted disease caused by *Chlamydia trachomatis,* which is often asymptomatic in women but sometimes characterized by urinary pain; if undetected and untreated, may result in pelvic inflammatory disease.

**chlorofluorocarbons (CFCs)** A group of gases that, when emitted into the atmosphere, may damage the ozone layer.

**cholesterol** A type of fat.

**chromosomes** The structures in the cell nucleus that carry the heredity factors (genes); composed of DNA and protein.

**chronic bronchitis** A persistent inflammation of the bronchi due to irritation by air pollutants and tobacco smoke.

**chronic obstructive lung disease (COLD)** Any one of several lung diseases, characterized by obstruction of breathing; includes emphysema and bronchitis.

**circumcision** The surgical removal of the foreskin of the penis.

**cirrhosis** A chronic disease, especially of the liver, characterized by a degeneration of cells and excessive scarring.

**clitoris** A small erectile structure on the female, corresponding to the penis on the male.

**coitus** See *intercourse.*

**collateral circulation** The development of small blood vessels that detour blood through damaged heart-muscle tissue.

**colpotomy** A surgical sterilization procedure in which the fallopian tubes are ligated or occluded through an incision made in the wall of the vagina.

**combination pill** A type of oral contraceptive containing synthetic estrogen and progestin.

**complementary protein** An incomplete protein that, when combined with another incomplete protein, provides all the amino acids essential for protein synthesis.

**complete protein** A protein that contains all the amino acids needed by the body for growth and maintenance.

**complex carbohydrate** A starch found in cereals, fruits, and vegetables.

**compliance** The act of carefully following treatment instructions.

**conditioning** In sports, to bring one's body to a state of physical fitness.

**condom** A sheath worn over the penis during sexual acts, to prevent conception and/or the transmission of disease.

**conscious** In Freudian theory, the feelings, thoughts, and impressions of which a person is aware.

**contraceptive sponge** A small polyurethane sponge that contains a spermicide and is designed to fit over the cervix to prevent conception.

**Cowper's glands** The small glands that discharge into the male urethra.

**crack** A smokeable form of cocaine that is highly addictive.

**crisis intervention** Immediate response to a dangerous situation.

**cross-addiction** A state of physical dependence in which physiological need for one psychoactive substance leads to dependence on similar substances.

**cross-tolerance** The capacity to endure the effects of psychoactive substances similar to one for which a tolerance has developed.

**cumulative** Characterized by an increase in effects upon successive additions of the same or another substance.

**cyanosis** A blueness of the skin due to an excess of reduced hemoglobin in the blood; caused by insufficient oxygen.

**date rape** An acquaintance rape in which the rapist is someone with whom the victim has gone out on a date.

**decibel (dB)** A unit for measuring noise levels.

**defense mechanism** Any of several irrational processes that work unconsciously to enable a person to cope with a difficult situation or problem.

**delirium tremens (DTs)** The delusions, hallucinations, and agitated behavior following withdrawal from long-term chronic alcohol abuse.

**denial** A refusal to accept reality.

**deoxyribonucleic acid (DNA)** A complex protein found in all living cells; carries the organism's genetic information.

**depressant** A drug that relaxes the central nervous system.

**designer drug** An illegally manufactured psychoactive drug that has dangerous physical and psychological effects.

**detoxification** The removal of a poisonous or harmful substance (such as a drug) from the body; a therapy for alcoholics in which they are denied alcohol in a controlled environment.

**diabetes mellitus** A disease in which the inadequate production of insulin leads to failure of the body tissues to break down carbohydrates at a normal rate.

**diaphragm** A round, flexible rubber disk that is inserted into the vagina to cover the cervix and prevent the passage of sperm into the uterus during sexual intercourse.

**diastole** The period between contractions in the cardiac cycle; when the heart relaxes and dilates as it fills with blood.

**diastolic blood pressure** The force exerted on the walls of a blood vessel by the blood during relaxation and dilation of the heart, during which time the heart fills with blood.

**dilation** The opening up of the cervix before delivery.

**dilation and curettage (D and C)** A procedure in which the cervix is dilated and the contents of the uterus are removed with a scraping instrument (a curette).

**dilation and evacuation (D and E)** The removal of the contents of the uterus through use of medical instruments.

**dioxins** A family of chemicals widely used in industry and as a defoliant; some forms are believed to be extremely toxic.

**displacement** Substituting a person, thing, or image for something that has an emotional meaning.

**distress** A negative stress, which may result in illness.

**dominant trait** A specific trait, determined by a gene on a chromosome, that will prevail over another, recessive trait.

**Down syndrome** A genetic disorder leading to some degree of physical and mental retardation, caused by an extra number 21 chromosome.

**drug** Any substance other than food that, when taken, affects body functions and structures.

**drug abuse** The excessive use of a drug that has dangerous side effects.

**drug misuse** The use of a drug for a purpose other than its original intent.

**dyathanasia** Ending extraordinary methods of sustaining life.

**dysmenorrhea** Painful menstruation.

**dyspareunia** A sexual difficulty in which a woman experiences pain during sexual intercourse.

**edema** An abnormal accumulation of fluid in body parts or tissues; swelling.

**effacement** The thinning of the cervix before delivery.

**ego** In Freudian theory, one of the three divisions of the psyche; a person's consciousness or awareness of self.

**ejaculation** The sudden ejection of semen from the penis at orgasm.

**embryo** An organism in its early stage of development; in humans, the embryonic period lasts from about the second to the eighth week of pregnancy.

**emotional health** The ability to express and acknowledge one's feelings and moods.

**emphysema** A condition caused by overdistention of the pulmonary alveoli or by the abnormal presence of air or gas in the body's tissues.

**endurance** The ability to withstand the stress of physical exertion.

**epididymis** A collection of coiled tubes adjacent to each testis, where sperm are stored.

**epilepsy** A neurological disorder characterized by severe convulsions.

**erogenous** Sexually sensitive.

**estrogen** The female sex hormone that stimulates female secondary sex characteristics.

**ethanol** See *ethyl alcohol.*

**ethyl alcohol** The intoxicating agent in alcoholic beverages.

**euphoria** A feeling of well-being or elation.

**eustress** A positive stress, which stimulates a person to function properly.

**euthanasia** A passive or active method of painlessly causing death for terminally ill patients.

**exhaustion** The final stage of the General Adaptation Syndrome, or stress response, in which the body can no longer maintain normal functioning.

**fallopian tubes** The pair of tubes that transport ova from the ovaries to the uterus; the usual site of fertilization.

**fat-soluble vitamin** A vitamin absorbed, with the aid of fats in the diet or bile from the liver, through the intestinal membrane and stored in the body.

**fertility awareness** A way of determining a woman's fertile period by observing changes in the consistency of mucus in the vagina; also called the mucus method.

**fertilization** The union of an ovum and a sperm.

**fetal alcohol syndrome** A condition distinguished by specific physical and mental abnormalities in infants born to mothers who drank heavily during pregnancy.

**fetus** The child in the uterus from the eighth week until birth.

**flexibility** The range of motion allowed by one's joints; determined by the length of muscles, tendons, and ligaments attached to the joints.

**follicle-stimulating hormone (FSH)** A hormone, produced by the pituitary gland, that stimulates the growth of ovarian follicles in females and sperm production in males.

**food allergy** A hypersensitivity to particular foods.

**gender** Maleness or femaleness as determined by a combination of anatomical, physiological, and psychological factors and learned behaviors.

**General Adaptation Syndrome (GAS)** The sequenced physiological response to a stressful situation; consists of three stages—alarm, resistance, and exhaustion.

**generic** Refers to products without trade names that are equivalent to other products protected by trademark registration.

**genes** The biologic units of heredity located on the chromosomes; transmitters of hereditary information.

**gonad** A sex organ: in women, the ovaries; in men, the testes.

**gonadotropins** The gonad-stimulating hormones produced by the pituitary gland.

**gonorrhea** A sexually transmitted disease caused by the bacteria *Neisseria gonorrhea;* symptoms in men include discharge from the penis; women may be asymptomatic.

**greenhouse effect** The warming of the earth's surface and atmosphere; caused by an accumulation of carbon dioxide.

**group therapy** A treatment in which participants interact using a variety of therapeutic methods, such as role playing and free conversation, to achieve goals.

**hallucinogen** A drug that causes hallucinations.

**health** Being sound in body, mind, and spirit.

**health maintenance organization (HMO)** An organization that provides health services on a fixed-contract basis.

**hemoglobin** The oxygen-transporting component of red blood cells.

**hepatitis** An inflammation and/or infection of the liver; caused by a virus; often accompanied by jaundice.

**hernia** The abnormal protrusion of an organ or body part through the tissues of the walls containing it.

**herpes simplex** A condition caused by one of the herpes viruses and characterized by lesions of the skin or mucous membranes; herpes virus Type 2 is sexually transmitted and causes genital blisters or sores.

**heterosexual** The sexual attraction to, and relationships with, persons of the other sex; a person who is attracted in such a way.

**heterozygous** Possessing different genes for a given inherited trait.

**history** The health-related information collected during the interview of a client by a health-care professional.

**holographic will** A will wholly in the handwriting of its author.

**homeostasis** The body's natural state of balance or stability.

**homophobia** The fear and dislike of homosexuals.

**homosexual** The sexual attraction to, and relationships with, persons of the same sex; a person who is attracted in such a way.

**homozygous** Possessing identical genes for a given inherited trait.

**hospice** A program of care, based either at home or in a home-like facility, that provides supportive care for terminally ill persons and their families.

**human chorionic gonadotropin (HCG)** A hormone produced by the chorionic villi.

**humanism** A philosophy concerned with human needs, human potential, and the importance of self-actualization.

**humor** The ability to laugh at oneself to handle stress and disappointment.

**hydrostatic immersion testing** The weighing of a person in water to distinguish buoyant fat from denser muscle.

**hypertension** High blood pressure.

**hypertrophy** To enlarge, as muscles do when lifting heavy weights.

**hypnotic** A drug that induces sleep or a trancelike state.

**hypoglycemia** An abnormal decrease of sugar in the blood, which results in feelings of weakness, confusion, irratation, and forgetfulness.

**hysterectomy** The surgical removal of the uterus.

**hysterotomy** The surgical opening of the uterus.

**id** In Freudian theory, one of the three divisions of the psyche; the primitive part of the unconscious, composed of unrestrained instincts for pleasure and survival.

**immune deficiency** Partial or complete inability of the immune system to respond to pathogens.

**immune system** The internal organs, tissues, cells, and mechanisms that protect the body against disease by producing antibodies against foreign bodies (antigens).

**immunization** The process of becoming immune; rendering someone immune.

**implantation** The embedding of the fertilized ovum in the uterine lining six to seven days after fertilization.

**impotence** A sexual difficulty in which a man is unable to achieve erection.

**incomplete protein** A protein that lacks one or more of the amino acids essential for protein synthesis.

**infertility** The inability to conceive a child.

**infiltration** A gradual penetration or invasion.

**inflammation** A localized response by the body to tissue injury; characterized by swelling and the dilation of blood vessels.

**influenza** A fairly common, highly contagious viral disease.

**informed consent** Permission given voluntarily, with full knowledge and understanding of the procedure or treatment, and its consequences.

**inhalant** A substance that produces vapors that has psychoactive effects when sniffed.

**insulin** A pancreatic hormone that is necessary for the metabolism of carbohydrates.

**intercourse** Sexual activity in which the penis repeatedly penetrates the vagina until orgasm and ejaculation occur.

**interval training** An aerobic conditioning method that involves repeated hard runs over a certain distance, with intervals of relaxed jogging in between.

**intimacy** The state of closeness between people; characterized by the desire and ability to share innermost feelings with each other.

**intramuscular** Into or within a muscle.

**intrauterine device (IUD)** A device inserted into the uterus to prevent pregnancy.

**intravenous** Into a vein.

**irradiation** The exposure to or treatment by some form of radiation.

**isokinetic** An exercise with specialized equipment that provides resistance through the whole range of motion.

**isometric** An increase in muscular tension without the muscle shortening in length, as when pushing an immovable object.

**isotonic** The repetition of an action to create muscular tension, as occurs in calisthenics.

**jaundice** A condition in which accumulation of pigments in the blood produces a yellowing of the skin.

**labia majora** The fleshy outer folds that border the female genital area.

**labia minora** The fleshy inner folds that border the female genital area.

**lacto-vegetarian** A person whose diet consists of dairy products and vegetables only.

**Lamaze method** See *psychoprophylaxis.*

**laparoscopy** A surgical sterilization procedure in which the fallopian tubes are first observed with a laparoscope inserted through a small incision and then ligated or occluded.

**laparotomy** A surgical sterilization procedure in which the fallopian tubes are ligated or occluded through an incision made in the abdomen.

**lipoprotein** A compound in the blood; made up of proteins and fat.

**long, slow distance (LSD) running** Noncompetitive running at a slow pace over fairly long distances.

**look-alike** A drug manufactured to look like real amphetamine and to mimic its effects.

**luteinizing hormone (LH)** A hormone, produced by the pituitary gland, that stimulates maturation of ovarian egg cells in the female and production of testosterone in males.

**lymph nodes** Storage sites for lymphocytes and macrophages.

**mainstream smoke** The smoke directly inhaled by a smoker.

**male menopause** A period of change and possible crisis for men at mid-life.

**malignant** Harmful; life-threatening.

**malpractice** The failure of a doctor or other health-care professionals to provide appropriate and skillful medical or surgical treatment.

**masturbation** Self-stimulation of the genitals, resulting in orgasm.

**menarche** The onset of menstruation at puberty.

**menopause** The period during which menstruation ceases and a woman's reproductive ability ends.

**menstrual extraction** The removal of uterine contents, usually performed to hasten the menstrual process or to eliminate possible pregnancy.

**mental health** The ability to perceive reality as it is.

**mescaline** A drug obtained from the mescal cactus; causes hallucinations, euphoria, and a heightened sense of awareness.

**metastasis** The spread of cancer cells beyond their site of origin in the body.

**migraine headache** A severe headache resulting from the dilation of blood vessels in the head; sometimes accompanied by vomiting and nausea.

**mineral** A naturally occurring inorganic substance; a small amount is essential to life.

**mini-pill** A type of oral contraceptive containing synthetic progestin.

**miscarriage** A pregnancy that terminates before the twentieth week of gestation.

**mononucleosis** An infectious viral disease characterized by an excess of white blood cells in the blood, fever, bodily discomfort, a sore throat, and kidney-liver complications.

**mons pubis** The rounded fleshy area over the junction of the pubic bones.

**multiphasic pill** A type of oral contraceptive that mimics the normal hormonal fluctuations of the menstrual cycle.

**mumps** A usually mild disease occurring most frequently in childhood.

**mutagen** An agent that causes alterations in the genetic material of living cells.

**mutation** A change in genetic material that can be transmitted to future generations and that is brought about by radiation, mutagenic chemicals, or natural causes.

**myocardial infarction (MI)** A condition characterized by dead-tissue areas in the myocardium; caused by interruption of the blood supply to those areas.

**myocardium** The cardiac muscle layer of the wall of the heart.

**narcotic** An addictive drug that relieves pain and induces sleep; derived from opium, or is chemically similar to such derivatives.

**negative conditioning** Teaching by means of punishment for undesired behavior.

**negligence** The failure to act in a way that a reasonable person would act.

**neoplasm** Any tumor, whether benign or malignant.

**neurosis** A mental disorder in which emotional conflict is either expressed openly in anxiety or hidden by complex compensating mechanisms in the personality.

**nicotine** A poisonous alkaloid found in tobacco; one of the most toxic of all poisons; used in concentrated amounts as a powerful agricultural insecticide.

**nonaerobic exercise** Exercise in which the activity does not require extra effort by the heart and lungs to take in more oxygen.

**nongonococcal urethritis (NGU)** Inflammation of the urethra; caused by organisms other than the gonorrhea bacteria.

**nutrient** A food element essential to life and that the body cannot produce on its own.

**nutrition** A science devoted to the study of the need for, and effects of, food on organisms.

**obesity** The excessive accumulation of fat in the body; a condition of being 20 percent or more above ideal weight.

**oncologist** A physician specializing in the treatment of cancer.

**opiate** A drug derived from opium.

**oral contraceptive** A preparation of synthetic hormones that inhibit ovulation; also referred to as the birth control pill or "the pill."

**organic** A term designating food produced with, or based on, fertilizer originating from plants or animals but without pesticides or chemically formulated fertilizers.

**osteoporosis** A condition common in older people, in which their bones become increasingly soft and porous, making them susceptible to injury.

**ovary** The female sex organ in which ova are produced.

**over-the-counter (OTC) drug** A medication that can be obtained legally without a prescription from a medical professional.

**ovo-lacto-vegetarian** A vegetarian who eats eggs as well as dairy products and vegetables.

**ovum** (plural: *ova*) the female gamete (egg cell).

**ozone** A form of oxygen ($O_3$) naturally present in the upper atmosphere, sometimes present in the lower atmosphere as a component of air pollution.

**ozone layer** An upper layer of the earth's atmosphere that protects the earth from harmful ultraviolet radiation from the sun.

**pacemaker** Compact battery-powered system that delivers a series of small electrical impulses to the heart.

**panic attack** An intense experience of fear, terror, and a sense of impending doom.

**Pap smear** A test in which cells removed from the cervix are examined under a microscope for signs of cancer; also called a Pap test.

**passive immunity** Temporary immunity acquired from the injection of antibodies produced by another person or animal.

**passive smoking** Living or working with people who smoke.

**passive stretching** See *static stretching.*

**pathogen** A microorganism that produces disease.

**PCB** Polychlorinated biphenyls; compounds—ranging from light, oily fluids to greasy or waxy substances—that have been widely used as industrial coolants and lubricants and in the manufacture of plastics, paints, and varnishes.

**pelvic inflammatory disease (PID)** An inflammation of the internal female genital tract; characterized by abdominal pain, fever, and tenderness of the cervix.

**penis** The organ of sex and urination in the male.

**perinatology** The medical specialty concerned with the diagnosis and treatment of pregnant women with high-risk conditions and their fetuses.

**perineum** The area between the anus and the vagina in the female and between the anus and the scrotum in the male.

**pesticide** Any toxic substance used to kill pests; types include insecticides, herbicides, fungicides, and others.

**phenylketonuria (PKU)** A genetic disorder in which a crucial liver enzyme is absent, resulting in severe mental retardation if not treated.

**phobia** A persistent, irrational fear of a specific object, activity, or situation; produces a compelling desire to avoid what is feared.

**physical dependence** The physiological attachment to, and need for, a drug.

**physical fitness** A state of well-being in which a person has enough energy to meet daily needs as well as unexpected challenges.

**pinch test** A simple method of checking for excess body fat by using the thumb and index finger to pinch the loose skin on the underside of the upper arm; more than an inch of loose skin indicates a need for exercise or weight loss.

**placenta** An organ that develops after implantation and to which the embryo attaches, via the umbilical cord, for nourishment and waste removal.

**plaque** A substance composed of cholesterol and other materials that builds up in blood vessels.

**platelet** A component of blood involved in clotting.

**pneumonia** An inflammation of the lungs; caused by infection or irritants.

**pollutant** A substance or agent that is the by-product of human industry or activity and that is injurious to human, animal, or plant life.

**pollution** The presence of pollutants in the environment.

**polyabuse** The use of more than one drug.

**positive conditioning** teaching by means of rewards for desired behavior.

**posttraumatic stress disorder** The repeated reliving of a trauma through nightmares or recollection.

**potentiating** Making more effective or powerful.

**pre-AIDS** A group of symptoms that develop in some individuals exposed to the AIDS virus.

**premature ejaculation** A sexual difficulty in which a man ejaculates so rapidly that his partner's satisfaction is impaired.

**premenstrual syndrome (PMS)** A disorder that causes physical discomfort and psychological distress prior to a woman's menstrual period.

**primary care** "First-contact" care provided by a health-care professional, usually in an office or clinic, without referral from a physician.

**progesterone** A hormone that stimulates the uterus, preparing it for the arrival of a fertilized egg.

**projection** Externalizing one's own anxieties, guilts, or aggressions and blaming them on other people or outside causes.

**proof** The alcoholic strength, measured as twice the percentage of alcohol present.

**prostate gland** A gland, wrapped around the male urethra, that provides a secretion that helps liquefy the semen from the testes.

**protein** A substance that is basically a compound of amino acids; one of the essential nutrients.

**psyche** The sum of mental activity, including the conscious and unconscious functions.

**psychedelic** A drug that produces a heightened sense of reality; visual hallucinations; and, in some instances, psychoticlike behaviors.

**psychoactive** Affecting mood and/or behavior.

**psychoanalysis** A system of psychotherapy, developed by Sigmund Freud, in which emotions, dreams, and behavior are analyzed in terms of repressed instinctual drives in the unconscious.

**psychological dependence** The emotional or mental attachment to the use of a drug.

**psychological health** A state of emotional and mental well-being.

**psychoprophylaxis** A method of childbirth preparation taught to expectant parents to help the woman cope with the discomfort of labor; combines breathing and psychological techniques.

**psychosis** A mental disorder in which there is gross impairment in reality perception.

**psychotherapy** A treatment designed to produce a response by psychological means (suggestion, persuasion, reassurance, and support) rather than physical means.

**pulmonary heart disease** A cardiovascular condition resulting from alterations in the blood vessels in the lungs.

**quackery** Medical fakery; unproven practices claiming to cure diseases or solve health problems.

**rape** Sexual penetration of a female or a male by means of intimidation, force, or fraud.

**rationalization** The creation of logical explanations for beliefs or actions that are really motivated by unconscious desires.

**reaction formation** Adopting a behavior pattern that, in fact, directly contradicts the desires of the unconscious.

**recessive trait** A specific trait, determined by a gene on a chromosome, that will not occur in offspring unless matched at fertilization by an identical gene on the pairing chromosome.

**refractory period** The period, following sexual intercourse, during which the male cannot ejaculate again.

**remission** A period during which a former victim of cancer or another disease shows no recurring symptoms.

**rep** In exercise, a single repetition, or performance, of a movement.

**repression** The act of pushing unhappy or painful thoughts out of the conscious mind and into the unconscious.

**resistance** The second stage of the General Adaptation Syndrome, or stress response, in which the body's internal activities return to normal and the energy focused on the stressor changes from physical to mental.

**response** A behavior or an action compelled by a stimulus.

**resting heart rate** The number of heartbeats per minute during inactivity.

**rhythm method** A type of birth control in which sexual intercourse is avoided during those days of the menstrual cycle in which fertilization is most likely to occur.

**rock** See *crack.*

**rubella** A disease similar to, but milder than, typical measles; also known as German measles.

**schizophrenic disorders** A general term for a variety of mental disorders involving a highly distorted sense of inner and outer reality that significantly impairs a person's perceptions, thinking, speech, and physical activity.

**scrotum** The sack of skin that holds the testes.

**sedative** A drug that depresses the central nervous system, resulting in sleep or a trancelike state.

**self-actualization** According to Abraham Maslow, a state of wellness and fulfillment that can be achieved after certain human needs are satisfied; living to one's full potential.

**semen** The viscous whitish liquid that is the complete male ejaculate; a combination of secretions from the prostate gland, seminal vesicles, and other glands.

**seminal vesicles** Glands in the male reproductive system that produce the major portion of the fluid of semen.

**set** A person's expectations or preconceptions about a situation or experience.

**set** In conditioning, a specified number of repetitions of the same movement or exercise.

**sex** Maleness or femaleness resulting from structural, functional, and genetic factors.

**sexual harassment** Unwanted sexual attention, including leering, pinching, patting, pressure for a sexual relationship, and lewd comments.

**sexually transmitted disease (STD)** Any of a number of diseases that are acquired through sexual contact.

**sexual orientation** One's preference in sexual partners; preference can be for the other sex, same sex, or both sexes.

**sickle-cell anemia** A debilitating genetic disorder of the blood characterized by sickle-shaped red blood cells, primarily affecting blacks.

**sidestream smoke** The smoke indirectly inhaled by a nonsmoker, usually as a result of being in the same room as a smoker.

**simple carbohydrate** A sugar; like all carbohydrates, provides the body with glucose.

**skin caliper** An instrument used to pinch skin folds at the arms, waist, and back to determine percentage of body fat.

**smog** A grayish or brownish fog caused by the presence of smoke and/or chemical pollutants in the air.

**sperm** Cells produced in the seminiferous tubules of the male reproductive system and ejaculated through the penis.

**spermatogenesis** The process by which sperm cells are produced.

**spiritual** Relating to the beliefs each of us has about the universe, human nature, and the significance of life and relationships.

**spontaneous abortion** See *miscarriage.*

**static stretching** A relaxed slow stretch held for 6 to 60 seconds.

**statutory rape** Unlawful sexual intercourse between a male over 16 years of age and a female under the age of consent.

**sterilization** A surgical procedure that causes infertility.

**stimulant** Any substance that excites the central nervous system.

**stimulus** An environmental factor able to evoke a response in an organism.

**strength** Physical power; the maximum weight one can lift, push, or press in one effort.

**stress** The nonspecific response of the body to any demands made upon it; may be characterized by muscle tension and acute anxiety or may be a positive force for action.

**stroke** See *cerebrovascular accident.*

**subcutaneous** Under the skin.

**subfertility** Difficulty conceiving a child.

**sublimation** The channeling of sexual energy or a socially unacceptable urge into socially acceptable activities.

**suction curettage** The removal of the contents of the uterus by means of suction and scraping.

**superego** In Freudian theory, one of the three divisions of the psyche; the internal voicing of messages from parents and society regarding morals, behavior, and goals.

**suppression** The conscious inhibition of certain thoughts or impulses.

**synergistic** Characterized by a combined effect that is greater than the sum of the individual effects.

**syphilis** A sexually transmitted disease caused by the bacteria *Treponema pallidum* and characterized by early sores, a latent period, and a final period of life-threatening symptoms, including brain damage and heart failure.

**systemic disease** A pathologic condition that spreads throughout the body.

**systole** The contraction phase of the cardiac cycle.

**systolic blood pressure** The force exerted on the walls of a blood vessel by the blood during contraction of the heart.

**tachycardia** An abnormally rapid heart rate, over 100 beats per minute.

**tar** A substance present in the smoke of burning tobacco; composed of combustion by-products.

**target heart rate** A rate 60 to 85 percent of the maximum heart rate; the heart rate at which one derives maximum benefit from aerobic exercise.

**Tay-Sachs disease** A genetic disorder resulting in death by age 5 or 6; occurs almost exclusively among Jews of Eastern European ancestry.

**tension headache** Pain and discomfort caused by involuntary contractions of the scalp, head, and neck muscles.

**teratogen** Any agent that causes defects or malformations in a fetus.

**terminal illness** The final stages of a fatal illness.

**testes** (singular: *testis*) The primary male sex organs that produce sperm.

**testosterone** The male sex hormone that stimulates male secondary sex characteristics.

**tetrahydrocannabinol (THC)** The primary psychoactive ingredient in marijuana and hashish.

**thrombosis** Blood-clot formation within a blood vessel.

**thrombus** A clot that is fixed or stuck to a vessel wall.

**tolerance** The capacity to endure the effects of a substance.

**toxicity** Poisonousness.

**toxic shock syndrome (TSS)** A disease characterized by fever, vomiting, diarrhea, and often shock; caused by bacteria that release toxic waste products into the bloodstream.

**training** See *conditioning.*

**transsexual** One who undergoes complex medical treatment to change genitals and secondary sex characteristics.

**tubal ligation** The suturing closed or tying shut of the fallopian tubes to prevent pregnancy.

**tubal occlusion** The blocking of the fallopian tubes to prevent pregnancy.

**tuberculosis (TB)** A highly infectious disease that primarily affects the lungs and is often fatal; caused by bacteria.

**ulcer** A lesion in, or an erosion of, the mucous membrane of an organ.

**ultraviolet radiation** The light rays of a specific wavelength emitted by the sun; most is screened out by the ozone layer in the upper atmosphere.

**unconscious** In Freudian theory, that part of mental activity, including repressed wishes and fears, of which a person is unaware.

**urethra** The canal through which urine from the bladder leaves the body; in the males, serves as the conduit for semen as well.

**uterus** The female organ that houses the fetus until birth.

**vaccine** A treatment containing weakened or inactive antigens; given to stimulate production of antibodies.

**vagina** The canal leading from the exterior opening in the female genital area to the uterus.

**vaginal contraceptive film (VCF)** A small dissolvable sheet saturated with spermicide.

**vaginal spermicide** A substance in the form of a cream, foam, jelly, or suppository that is inserted into the vagina to kill or neutralize sperm.

**vaginismus** A sexual difficulty in which a woman experiences painful spasms of the vagina during sexual intercourse.

**values** The criteria by which people evaluate themselves, others, and the events in life.

**vas deferens** The two tubes that carry sperm from the testes to the urethra.

**vasectomy** The cutting and tying shut of the vas deferens to stop the passage of sperm to the penis.

**vegan** A vegetarian who eats only vegetables—no dairy products, eggs, or other animal-derived foods.

**ventricle** Either of the two lower chambers of the heart, which pump blood out of the heart and into the arteries.

**villi** Short vascular projections attaching the fetus to the uterine wall.

**virus** A tiny pathogen consisting of either DNA or RNA surrounded by a protein coat.

**vital signs** Measurements of physiological functioning; specifically, temperature, blood pressure, pulse rate, and respiration rate.

**vitamin** An organic substance needed by the body in a very small amount; carries out a variety of functions in metabolism and nutrition.

**water-soluble vitamin** A vitamin used up or excreted in urine and sweat; must be replaced daily.

**wellness** A state of optimal health.

**zero population growth** The point at which the number of births equals the number of deaths.

**zygote** A fertilized egg.

# REFERENCES


## Chapter 1

1. "Constitution of the World Health Organization," *Chronicle of the World Health Organization,* 1947.
2. National Center for Health Statistics, Washington, D.C., interview.
3. Siegel, Bernie. *Love, Medicine and Miracles.* New York: Harper & Row, 1986.
4. Yankelovich, Daniel and Joel Gurin. "The New American Dream," *American Health,* March 1989.
5. Bozzi, Vincent. "A Healthy Dose of Religion," *Psychology Today,* November 1988.
6. Centers for Disease Control, interview.
7. "Mormon Lifestyle Credited with Low Death Rates," *American Medical News,* February 16, 1990.
8. Yankelovich, Daniel and Joel Gurin. "The New American Dream," *American Health,* March 1989.

## Chapter 2

1. Offer, Daniel and Melvin Sabschin. *Normality and the Life Cycle.* New York Basic Books, 1984.
2. Shapiro, Deane and Roger Walsh. *Beyond Health and Normalcy.* New York: Van Nostrand Reinhold, 1983.
3. Zimbardo, Philip. *Shyness.* Reading, MA: Addison-Wesley, 1977.
4. Brody, Jane. "New Techniques Help Millions of Wallflowers Overcome Their Fears," *New York Times,* November 16, 1989.
5. Hales, Robert E. "Exercise and the Treatment of Depression," *Depression Dialogue,* July 1987.
6. Schroepfer, Lisa. "Emotional Ills Come Out of the Closet," *American Health,* April 1989.
7. Kashani, J. et al. "Depression, Depressive Symptoms and Depressed Mood Among a Community Sample of Adolescents," *American Journal of Psychiatry,* July 1987.
8. "Doctors Are Said to Miss Diagnosing Depression Half of the Time," *New York Times,* December 19, 1989.
9. Goleman, Daniel. "Beliefs on Depression in Women Contradicted," *New York Times,* January 9, 1990.
10. Seligman, Martin. "Boomer Blues," *Psychology Today,* October 1988.
11. "Adolescent Suicide: Second Leading Death Cause," *Journal of the American Medical Association,* June 26, 1987.
12. *Facts About Teen Suicide,* Washington, D.C.: American Psychiatric Association, 1987.
13. *Ibid.*
14. *Facts About Anxiety Disorders,* Washington, D.C.: American Psychiatric Association, 1987.
15. *Facts About Phobias,* Washington, D.C.: American Psychiatric Association, 1987.
16. *Ibid.*
17. *Facts About Schizophrenia,* Washington, D.C.: American Psychiatric Association, 1987.
18. Media office, American Psychiatric Association.

## Chapter 3

1. London, Perry and Charles Spielberger. "Job Stress, Hassles and Medical Risk," *American Health,* March/April 1983.
2. Lazarus, Richard. "Little Hassles Can Be Hazardous to Health," *Psychology Today,* July 1981.
3. Syme, S. Leonard. "People Need People," *American Health,* July/August 1982.
4. Sherman, Carl. "The Ills of Unemployment," *American Health,* July/August 1982.
5. "Little Control = Lots of Stress," *Psychology Today,* April 1989.
6. Machlowitz, Marilyn. *Workaholics.* Reading, MA: Addison-Wesley, 1980.
7. Pines, Ayala and Eliott Aronson. *Burnout.* New York: Free Press, 1981.
8. Friedman, Meyer. "Changing Behavior Reduces Coronary Deaths," *American Heart Journal,* October 1986.
9. Miller, Laurence. "To Beat Stress, Don't Relax: Get Tough," *Psychology Today,* December 1989.
10. Eliot, Robert and Dennis Breo. *Is It Worth Dying For?* New York: Bantam Books, 1984.
11. "Gut Emotions," *Psychology Today,* March 1989.
12. "Ulcers and Stress: The Missing Link," *Psychology Today,* November 1989.
13. Borysenko, Joan. Author of *Minding the Body, Mending the Mind.* Reading, MA: Addison-Wesley, 1987. September 1987 telephone interview.
14. Elkind, David. *All Grown Up and No Place to Go: Teenagers in Crisis.* Reading, MA: Addison-Wesley, 1984.
15. "Dear Diary . . ." *American Health,* August 1987.
16. Squires, Sally. "The Immune System Responds to Health," *Washington Post,* March 31, 1987.
17. Bozzi, Vincent. "A Healthy Dose of Religion," *Psychology Today,* November 1988.

## Chapter 4

1. Barnett, Robert. "New AHA Guidelines: Reasons of the Heart," *American Health,* November 1986.

2. Brody, Jane. "More Benefit Seen in Certain Fats," *New York Times*, February 7, 1990.
3. American Medical Association Council on Scientific Affairs. "Saturated Fatty Acids in Vegetable Oils," *Journal of the American Medical Association*, vol. 263, no. 5, February 2, 1990.
4. Trevisan, M. et al. "Consumption of Olive Oil, Butter and Vegetable Oils and Coronary Heart Disease Factors," *Journal of the American Medical Association*, vol. 263, no. 5, February 2, 1990.
5. Burros, Marian. "Brand-Name Lean Beef: Is It Really Better?" *New York Times*, January 31, 1990.
6. Phillipson, Beverley et al. "Reduction of Plasma Lipids, Lipoproteins, and Apoproteins by Dietary Fish Oils in Patients with Hypertriglyceridemia," *New England Journal of Medicine*, May 9, 1985.
7. Kurtz, Theodore, W. et al. "'Salt-Sensitive' Essential Hypertension in Men: Is the Sodium Ion Alone Important?" *New England Journal of Medicine*, October 22, 1987.
8. Alabaster, Oliver. *What You Can Do to Prevent Cancer.* New York: Simon and Schuster, 1986.
9. Brody, Jane. "The Benefit of Oat Bran Is Challenged," *New York Times*, January 18, 1990.
10. Behan, Eileen. "Sweet Reason," *American Health*, December 1986.
11. Boffey, Philip. "Diet Sweetener Risk Is Being Reassessed after New Research," *New York Times*, August 31, 1984.
12. "The Taste That Failed," *American Health*, July/August 1983.
13. Jacobson, Michael and Sarah Fritschner. *The Fast Food Guide.* New York: Workman Publishing, 1986.
14. Leary, Warren. "Young Women Are Getting Fatter, Study Finds," *New York Times*, February 29, 1989.
15. Gurin, Joel. "Eating Goes Back to Basics," *American Health*, March 1990.
16. Andres, Reuben. Clinical director, National Institute on Aging, Baltimore, MD. Personal interview.
17. Saltman, Paul et al. *The California Nutrition Book.* Boston: Little, Brown, 1987.
18. Stunkard, Albert. "Eating Disorders," in R. E. Hales and A. Francis (eds.), *Annual Review of Psychiatry*, vol. 4, Washington, D.C.: American Psychiatric Press, 1984.
19. Stunkard, Albert. "Obesity," in *American Psychiatric Association Annual Review*, vol. IV, Washington, D.C.: American Psychiatric Press, 1985.
20. National Institutes of Health Consensus Development Conference Statement. *Health Implications of Obesity.* Bethesda, MD. February 1985.
21. Beck, Melinda. "The Losing Formula," *Newsweek*, April 30, 1990.
22. *Ibid.*
23. Wadden, T. A. et al. "Responsible and Irresponsible Use of Very-Low-Calorie Diets in the Treatment of Obesity," *Journal of the American Medical Association*, vol. 263, no. 1, January 5, 1990.
24. O'Neill, Molly. "Congressional Hearings on Diet Industry," *New York Times*, March 28, 1990.
25. Hall, Trish. "Diet: A Four-Letter Word for Healthy Eating Plan," *New York Times*, January 3, 1990.
26. *Exercise and Weight Control.* Washington, D.C.: The President's Council on Physical Fitness, 1986.


## Chapter 5


1. Brody, Jane. "Fitness Is," *New York Times Magazine*, September 28, 1986.
2. Cooper, Kenneth. *The Aerobics Program for Total Well-being*, New York: M. Evans, 1982.
3. Kiesling, Stephen. "Is Walking Enough?" *American Health*, October 1986; also Kiesling, Stephen. "Walk-shaping," *American Health*, October 1986.
4. Kaufman, Elizabeth. "The New Rhythms of Fitness," *American Health*, December 1989.
5. Hales, Dianne and Robert Hales. *U.S. Army Total Fitness Program*, New York: Ballantine, 1986.
6. Vaz, Katherine. "Shifting to Two Wheels," *Washington Post Health*, October 7, 1986.
7. Adrian, Marlene. "Jumping Rope, Again," *Washington Post Health*, January 29, 1986.
8. Rogers-Gould, Ginna. "Soft Aerobics," *American Health*, November 1985.
9. Williams, Linda. "America Goes Stair Crazy," *Time*, December 18, 1989.
10. Kaufman, Elizabeth. "The New Rhythms of Fitness," *American Health*, December 1989.
11. Kashkin, K. B. and H. D. Kleber. "Hooked on Hormones?" *Journal of the American Medical Association*, January 11, 1990.
12. Groves, David. "The Rambo Drug," *American Health*, September 1987.
13. "Anabolic Steroid Abuse," *FDA Drug Bulletin*, October 1987.
14. Bracciale, Donna and Edward Remmers. "Athletes & Steroids: A Losing Proposition," *News and Views*, New York: American Council on Science and Health, September/October 1987.
15. Blair, S. N. et al. "Physical Fitness and All-Cause Mortality," *Journal of the American Medical Association*, vol. 262, no. 17, November 3, 1989.
16. Siscovick, D. et al. "The Incidence of Primary Cardiac Arrest During Vigorous Exercise," *New England Journal of Medicine*, October 4, 1984.
17. Leon, Arthur et al. "Leisure-Time Physical Activity Levels and Risk of Coronary Heart Disease and Death," *Journal of American Medical Association*, November 6, 1987.
18. "Mix of Weights, Aerobics Called Best for Bones," *Washington Post Health*, August 20, 1986.
19. Carr, D. B. et al. "Physical Conditioning Facilitates the Exercise-Induced Secretion of Beta Endorphin and Beta-Lipotropin in Women," *New England Journal of Medicine*, September 3, 1981.
20. Frisch, R. E. et al. "Lower Prevalence of Breast Cancer and Cancers of the Reproductive System Among Former College Athletes Compared to Non-Athletes," *British Journal of Cancer*, vol. 52, 1985.
21. Hales, Dianne and Robert Hales. *U.S. Army Total Fitness Program*, New York: Ballantine, 1986.


## Chapter 6


1. Bureau of the Census. *Studies in Marriage and the Family: Singleness in America.* Washington, D.C.: Government Printing Office, 1989.
2. *Ibid.*
3. "Does Cohabitation Last?" *Psychology Today*, June 1989.
4. Grant, Eleanor. "Marriage: Practice Makes Perfect?" *Psychology Today*, November 1989.
5. Norton, Arthur and Jeanne Moorman. "Current Trends in Marriage and Divorce Among American Women," *Journal of Marriage and the Family*, February 1987.

6. National Opinion Research Center at the University of Chicago. American Association for the Advancement of Science. February 19, 1990, presentation.
7. Elias, Marilyn. "Role-Strained Couples," *American Health,* November 1987.
8. Greeley, Andrew. "Faithful Attraction," *Psychology Today,* March 1990.
9. Kiecolt-Glaser, Janice and Ronald Glaser. "Interpersonal Relationships and Immune Function," in L. Carstensen and J. Neale (eds.), *Mechanisms of Psychological Influence on Health.* New York: Wiley, 1988.
10. Cleminshaw, Helen. Personal interview.
11. "Staying Power," *Marin Independent Journal,* March 19, 1990.
12. Newberger, Carolyn et al. "The American Family in Crisis: Implications for Children," *Current Problems in Pediatrics,* vol. 18, no. 12, 1986.
13. Hales, Dianne. *The Family* (one volume in *The Encyclopedia of Health*). New York: Chelsea House Publishers, 1988.


## Chapter 7


1. Katzman, Barbara. "Menopause Poses No Problems for a Majority of Women, Says NIA Study," *News and Features from NIH,* July 1987.
2. Crooks, Robert and Karla Baur. *Our Sexuality, Fourth Edition.* Benjamin/Cummings, 1990.
3. Byrd, Robert. "Teen Girls Having Sex Sooner," *San Francisco Chronicle,* February 6, 1990.
4. Crooks, Robert and Karla Baur. *Our Sexuality, Fourth Edition.* Benjamin/Cummings, 1990.
5. Bell, Alan et al. *Sexual Preference: Its Development in Men and Women.* Bloomington: Indiana University Press, 1981.
6. *Ibid.*
7. Gail, M. H. "Projecting the Incidence of AIDS," *Journal of the American Medical Association,* vol. 263, no. 11, March 16, 1990.
8. Lemp, G. F. et al. "Projections of AIDS Morbidity and Mortality in San Francisco," *Journal of the American Medical Association,* vol. 263, no. 11, March 16, 1990.
9. National Opinion Research Center at the University of Chicago. American Association for the Advancement of Science; February 19, 1990; presentation.
10. Crooks, Robert and Karla Baur. *Our Sexuality, Fourth Edition.* Benjamin/Cummings, 1990.
11. Centers for Disease Control. "Update—Acquired Immune Deficiency Syndrome," *Journal of the American Medical Association,* vol. 263, no. 9. March 2, 1990.
12. Leary, Warren. "AIDS Risk Among College Students Is Real but Not Rampant, Tests Find," *New York Times,* May 23, 1989.
13. Wofsky, Constance. "Human Immunodeficiency Virus Infection in Women," *Journal of the American Medical Association,* April 17, 1987.
14. Peterman, Thomas et al. "Risk of Human Immunodeficiency Virus Transmission from Heterosexual Adults with Transfusion Associated Infections," *Journal of the American Medical Association,* vol. 259, no. 1, January 1, 1988.
15. "Coffee and Cigarettes: Facts on Helping and Hindering Sexual Potency," Impotence Information Center, January 1990.
16. Dolan, Barbara. "Do People Get Hooked on Sex?" *Time,* June 4, 1990.
17. Brownmiller, Susan. *Against Our Will: Men, Women, and Rape.* New York: Simon and Schuster, 1975.
18. Goleman, Daniel. "When the Rapist Is Not a Stranger," *New York Times,* August 29, 1989.
19. Carmody, Deidre. "Sexual Harassment on Campus: A Growing Issue," *New York Times,* July 5, 1989.


## Chapter 8


1. Kantrowitz, Barbara. "Kids and Contraceptives," *Newsweek,* February 16, 1987.
2. Shapiro, Samuel. "Oral Contraceptives: Time to Take Stock," *New England Journal of Medicine,* August 14, 1986.
3. Kolata, Gina. "For Those Concerned with Pill's Risk, a Look at the Choices," *New York Times,* January 12, 1989.
4. "Oral Contraceptive Use and the Risk of Breast Cancer: The Cancer and Steroid Hormone Study of the Centers for Disease Control and the National Institute of Child Health and Human Development," *New England Journal of Medicine,* August 14, 1986.
5. "Facts about Oral Contraceptives," in *The Search for Health.* Bethesda, MD: National Institutes of Health, 1987.
6. "The Pill and the Risks," in *The Search for Health.* Bethesda, MD: National Institutes of Health, 1987.
7. Linn, Shai et al. "Delay in Conception for Former Pill Users," *Journal of the American Medical Association,* February 5, 1982.
8. Lemonic, Michael. "Blocks and Barriers," *Time,* May 18, 1987.
9. "Barrier Birth Control Linked to Disease in Some Pregnancies," *San Francisco Chronicle,* December 18, 1989.
10. Louik, Carol et al. "Maternal Exposure to Spermicides in Relation to Certain Birth Defects," *New England Journal of Medicine,* August 20, 1987.
11. Warburton, Dorothy et al. "Lack of Association Between Spermicide Use and Trisomy," *New England Journal of Medicine,* August 20, 1987.
12. Massey, F. J. et al. "Vasectomy and Health," *Journal of the American Medical Association,* August 24/31, 1984.
13. Seligmann, Jean. "Abortion in the Form of a Pill," *Newsweek,* April 17, 1989.
14. Barringer, Felicity. "Waiting Is Over: Births Near 50's Level," *New York Times,* October 31, 1989.
15. Lemire, Ronald, J. "Neural Tube Defects," *Journal of the American Medical Association,* vol. 259, no. 4, January 22/28, 1988.
16. Rosenthal, Elisabeth. "When a Pregnant Woman Drinks," *New York Times,* February 4, 1990.
17. *Ibid.*
18. Hales, Dianne and Timothy R. B. Johnson. *Intensive Caring: New Hope for High-Risk Pregnancy.* New York: Crown Publishers, 1990.
19. *Ibid.*
20. *Ibid.*
21. *Ibid.*
22. "Teenage Pregnancy and Birth Rates Drop," *New York Times,* October 20, 1987.
23. Gardner, Maureen. "Prenatal Care Improves Pregnancy Outcome Among Adolescents," *NICHD News Notes,* August 1987.
24. Brody, Jane. "Research Casts Doubts on Need for Many Caesarean Births as Their Rate Soars," *New York Times,* July 27, 1989.
25. Notzon, Francis et al. "Comparison of National Cesarean Section Rates," *New England Journal of Medicine,* February 12, 1987.
26. "High Rate of Caesareans Among the Affluent," *New York Times,* July 27, 1989.

27. Hickey, Mary. "The Quiet Pain of Infertility," *Washington Post,* April 28, 1987.

## Chapter 9

1. "Rise in Nasal Inhaler Abuse Worries Officials," *New York Times,* September 22, 1985.
2. Barnett, Robert. "A Proper Cup," *American Health,* January/February 1990.
3. Brody, Jane. "Flurry of New Findings About Caffeine Stirs Hopes and Fears—As Well as General Confusion," *New York Times,* May 18, 1989.
4. Bennett, William et al. *Your Good Health.* Cambridge, MA: Harvard University Press, 1987.
5. "Amphetamines," *The Harvard Medical School Mental Health Letter,* vol. 6, no. 10, April 1990.
6. Kashkin, K. B. and H. D. Kleber. "Hooked on Hormones?" *Journal of the American Medical Association,* vol. 262, no. 22, January 11, 1990.
7. Groves, David. "The Rambo Drug," *American Health,* September 1987.
8. "Anabolic Steroid Abuse," *FDA Drug Bulletin,* October 1987.
9. Bracciale, Donna and Edward Remmers. "Athletes & Steroids: A Losing Proposition," *News and Views,* New York: American Council on Science and Health, September/October 1987.
10. Castro, Janice. "Battling the Enemy Within," *Time,* March 17, 1986.
11. Squires, Sally. "America's Drugs of Abuse," *Washington Post Health,* November 4, 1986.
12. *Drug Use Among American High School Students, College Students, and Other Young Adults.* Rockville, MD: National Institute on Drug Abuse, 1986.
13. Centers for Disease Control. April 1990.
14. Whitman, David. "The Streets Are Filled with Coke," *U.S. News and World Report,* March 5, 1990.
15. Isner, Jeffrey. "Acute Cardiac Events Temporally Related to Cocaine Abuse," *New England Journal of Medicine,* December 4, 1986.
16. Cregler, Louis and Herbert Mark. "Medical Complications of Cocaine Abuse," *New England Journal of Medicine,* December 4, 1986.
17. "The Neurologic Impact of Cocaine Abuse," *Emergency Medicine,* April 30, 1988.
18. Wallis, Claudia. "Cocaine Babies," *Time,* January 20, 1986.
19. Gross, Jane. "Rise in Cocaine Abuse Poses Threat to Infants," *New York Times,* February 3, 1986.
20. Kolata, Gina. "Experts Finding New Hope on Treating Crack Addicts," *New York Times,* August 24, 1989.
21. Carey, Benedict. "Cracking Crack with Acupuncture," *In Health,* January/February 1990.
22. "Amphetamines," *The Harvard Medical School Mental Health Letter,* vol 6, no. 10, April 1990.
23. Jackson, Jon. "Hazards of Smokable Methamphetamine," *New England Journal of Medicine,* vol. 321, no. 13, 1989.
24. Jones, Laurie. "New Drug Overtakes Hawaii, Threatens Mainland," *American Medical News,* November 10, 1989.
25. *Drug Use Among American High School Students, College Students, and Other Young Adults.* Rockville, Md.: National Institute on Drug Abuse, 1986.
26. Colburn, Don. "Update on Marijuana," *Washington Post Health,* November 17, 1987.
27. "Psychedelic Drugs," *The Harvard Medical School Mental Health Letter,* vol. 6, no. 8, February 1990.
28. *Drug Use Among American High School Students, College Students, and Other Young Adults.* Rockville, MD: National Institute on Drug Abuse, 1986.
29. "DEA Says Heroin Poses 'Huge Problem,'" *San Francisco Chronicle,* March 13, 1990.
30. Holmes, Steven. "Methadone Units Faulted in Report," *New York Times,* March 23, 1990.
31. Gallagher, Winifred. "The Looming Menace of Designer Drugs," *Discover,* August 1986.
32. "Psychedelic Drugs," *The Harvard Medical School Mental Health Letter,* vol. 6, no. 8, February 1990.
33. "Drugs and Driving," in *Clinical Research Notes.* Rockville, MD: National Institute on Drug Abuse, 1984.
34. Shenon, Philip. "The Score on Drugs: It Depends on How You See the Figures," *New York Times,* April 22, 1990.

## Chapter 10

1. "Alcohol Use Down, Cocaine Use Higher," *San Francisco Chronicle,* April 20, 1990.
2. *Seventh Special Report to the U.S. Congress on Alcohol and Health.* Department of Health and Human Services, 1990.
3. Pinkney, Deborah. "Alcohol Remains Most Widely Used Drug," *American Medical News,* February 16, 1990.
4. *Seventh Special Report to the U.S. Congress on Alcohol and Health.* Department of Health and Human Services, 1990.
5. Carmody, Deidre. "College Drinking: Changes in Attitude and Habit," *New York Times,* March 7, 1990.
6. Curtis, Diane. "Student Drinking a Serious Worry," *San Francisco Chronicle,* April 30, 1990.
7. "Twenty Percent of College Women Have a Drinking Problem," *San Francisco Chronicle,* April 18, 1990.
8. *Seventh Special Report to the U.S. Congress on Alcohol and Health,* Department of Health and Human Services, 1990.
9. Desmond, Edward. "Out in the Open," *Time,* November 30, 1987.
10. Vaillant, George. *The Natural History of Alcoholism.* Cambridge, MA: Harvard University Press, 1983.
11. Hales, Dianne and Robert Hales. "Alcohol: Better Than We Thought?" *American Health,* December 1986.
12. Schuckit, Marc. Psychiatrist; University of California, San Diego; San Diego. Personal interview.
13. Hales, Dianne and Robert Hales. "Alcohol: Better Than We Thought?" *American Health,* December 1986.
14. *Sixth Special Report to the U.S. Congress on Alcohol and Health from the Secretary of Health and Human Services.* Bethesda, MD: U.S. Department of Health and Human Services, 1987.
15. Kolata, Gina. "Study Tells Why Alcohol Is Greater Risk to Women," *New York Times,* January 11, 1990.
16. Toufexis, Anastasia. "Why Men Can Outdrink Women," *Time,* January 22, 1990.
17. Willet, Walter et al. "Moderate Alcohol Consumption and the Risk of Breast Cancer," *New England Journal of Medicine,* vol. 316, no. 19, 1987.
18. Graham, S. et al. "Alcohol and Breast Cancer," *New England Journal of Medicine,* vol. 316, no. 19, 1987.
19. Schatzkin, A. et al. "Alcohol Consumption and Breast Cancer in the Epidemiologic Follow-up Study of the First National Health and Nutrition Examination Survey," *New England Journal of Medicine,* vol. 316, no. 19, 1987.
20. Pinkney, Deborah. "Specialists Give New Definition of Alcoholism," *American Medical News,* May 11, 1990.

21. *Ibid.*
22. Vaillant, George. *The Natural History of Alcoholism.* Cambridge, MA: Harvard University Press, 1983.
23. *Seventh Special Report to the U.S. Congress on Alcohol and Health,* Department of Health and Human Services, 1990.
24. Seixas, Frank. "Alcoholism Treatment: A Descriptive Guide," *Psychiatric Annals,* April 1982.
25. Miller, Norma. "A Primer of the Treatment Process for Alcoholism and Drug Addiction," *Psychiatry Letter,* July 1987.
26. Council on Scientific Affairs, "Aversion Therapy," *Journal of the American Medical Association,* November 13, 1987.
27. Helzer, John et al. "The Extent of Long-Term Moderate Drinking Among Alcoholics Discharged from Medical and Psychiatric Treatment Facilities," *New England Journal of Medicine,* June 27, 1985.

## Chapter 11

1. American Cancer Society. *General Facts on Smoking and Health.* New York: American Cancer Society, 1987.
2. *Smoking and Health: A National Status Report.* Rockville, Md.: U.S. Department of Health and Human Services, 1990.
3. Ibid.
4. Ibid.
5. Ibid.
6. American Cancer Society. *General Facts on Smoking and Health.* New York: American Cancer Society, 1987.
7. Pinkney, Deborah. "War Mounts Against Cigarette, Liquor Ads," *American Medical News,* March 16, 1990.
8. Work, Clemens. "Where There's Smoke," *U.S. News and World Report,* March 5, 1990.
9. Blakeslee, Sandra. "Nicotine: Harder to Kick Than Heroin," *New York Times Magazine,* March 29, 1987.
10. American Psychiatric Association. *Diagnostic and Statistical Manual of Mental Disorders,* 3d ed., revised. Washington, D.C.: American Psychiatric Association, 1987.
11. *Smoking and Health: A National Status Report.* Rockville, MD: U.S. Department of Health and Human Services, 1990.
12. *The Health Consequences of Involuntary Smoking: A Report of the Surgeon General.* Rockville, MD: U.S. Department of Health and Human Services Office on Smoking and Health, 1987.
13. *The Health Consequences of Smoking: Cardiovascular Disease, A Report of the Surgeon General.* Rockville, MD: U.S. Department of Health and Human Services Office on Smoking and Health, 1984.
14. Abbott, Robert et al. "Risk of Stroke in Male Cigarette Smokers," *New England Journal of Medicine,* September 18, 1986.
15. American Cancer Society, 1990.
16. *Smoking and Health: A National Status Report.* Rockville, MD: U.S. Department of Health and Human Services, 1990.
17. *The Health Consequences of Smoking: Chronic Obstructive Lung Disease, A Report of the Surgeon General.* Rockville, MD: U.S. Department of Health and Human Services Office on Smoking and Health, 1984.
18. Fielding, Jonathan. "Smoking and Women: Tragedy of the Majority," *New England Journal of Medicine,* November 19, 1987.
19. Willett, Walter et al. "Relative and Absolute Excess Risks of Coronary Heart Disease among Women Who Smoke Cigarettes," *New England Journal of Medicine,* November 19, 1987.
20. *Smoking and Health: A National Status Report.* Rockville, MD: U.S. Department of Health and Human Services, 1990.
21. Squires, Sally. "Smoking Interferes with Drug Action, Pharmacists Warn," *Washington Post,* November 25, 1986.
22. "Health Secretary Assails Tobacco Firms," *San Francisco Chronicle,* February 21, 1990.
23. Bennett, William et al. *Your Good Health.* Cambridge, MA: Harvard University Press, 1987.
24. Ibid.
25. *The Health Consequences of Using Smokeless Tobacco: A Report of the Advisory Committee to the Surgeon General.* Bethesda, MD: Public Health Service, 1986.
26. Ibid.
27. Herzfeld, John. "Their Smoke in Your Lungs," *American Health,* November 1987.
28. Altman, Lawrence. "The Evidence Mounts on Passive Smoking," *New York Times,* May 29, 1990.
29. Ibid.
30. Ibid.
31. Cohen, Sheldon et al. "Debunking Myths about Self-quitting: Evidence from 10 Prospective Studies of Persons Who Attempt to Quit Smoking by Themselves," *American Psychologist,* November 1989.
32. Ferguson, Tom. *The Smoker's Book of Health.* New York: Putnam, 1987.
33. Blonston, Gary. "Quitting for Life," *American Health,* April 1987.
34. Hjalmarson, A. I. et al. "Effect of Nicotine Chewing Gum in Smoking Cessation," *Journal of the American Medical Association,* November 23/30, 1984.

## Chapter 12

1. Cohn, Victor. "Doctors on How to Cope with Doctors," *Washington Post Health,* September 1, 1987.
2. Carey, Benedict. "Do You Need a Physical?" *In Health,* March/April 1990.
3. Cramer, Joyce et al. "How Often Is Medication Taken as Prescribed?" *Journal of the American Medical Association,* vol. 261, no. 22, June 9, 1989.
4. Leary, Warren. "Generic Drugs: Are They As Good As the Original?" *New York Times,* October 12, 1989.
5. Strom, Brian. "Generic Drug Substitution Revisited," *New England Journal of Medicine,* June 4, 1987.
6. Faich, Gerald et al. "Reassurance about Generic Drugs," *New England Journal of Medicine,* June 4, 1987.
7. Avery, Caryl. "Can You Trust Generic Drugs?" *American Health,* April 1990.
8. Lunzer, Francesca. "Are Bargain Drugs Right for You?" *American Health,* July 1987.
9. Cohn, Victor. "Behind the Hospital Death Statistics," *Washington Post Health,* December 22, 1987.
10. Dunn, Si. "Fast Medicine: Doc in the Box," *American Health,* June 1985.
11. "Emergicenters: The McDonald's of Medicine," *Medical Month,* October 1983.
12. Friedman, Joanne. "Hospital Care Comes Home," *American Health,* June 1987.
13. Tuller, David and Lori Olszewski. "New Crisis in Health Care Insurance," *San Francisco Chronicle,* February 26, 1990.
14. Cassileth, Barrie et al. "Contemporary Unorthodox Treatments in Cancer Medicine," *Annals of Internal Medicine,* July 1984.

## Chapter 13

1. Pashkow, Fredric. "The 1980s: Ten More Years of Progress Against Heart Disease," *Heartline*, vol. 20, no. 1, January 1990.
2. *The Sixteenth Annual Report of the National Heart, Lung and Blood Advisory Council.* Bethesda, MD: National Institutes of Health, 1989.
3. "Blood Cholesterol," in *Facts About* . . . Bethesda, MD: National Institutes of Health, July 1987.
4. "The Great Cholesterol Debate," *American Health*, January/February 1990.
5. Kolata, Gina. "Major Study Aims to Learn Who Should Lower Cholesterol," *New York Times*, September 26, 1989.
6. Husten, Larry. "What's Your HDL Level?" *American Health*, January/February 1990.
7. Kolata, Gina. "Cholesterol Tests: What Your Blood Will Tell," *American Health*, January/February, 1988.
8. Husten, Larry. "What's Your HDL Level?" *American Health*, January/February 1990.
9. Kolata, Gina. "Report Urges Low-Fat Diet for Everyone," *New York Times*, February 28, 1990.
10. Leon, Arthur et al. "Leisure Time Physical Activity Levels and the Risk of Coronary Heart Disease and Death," *Journal of the American Medical Association*, November 6, 1987.
11. Grady, Denise. "Bad News Bellies," *American Health*, May 1989.
12. American Heart Association. March 1990.
13. "A New Role for the Wonder Drug," *Time*, April 2, 1990.
14. Blakeslee, Sandra. "Study Hints of Harm in Heart Operations," *New York Times*, February 28, 1990.
15. Pashkow, Fredric. "The 1980s: Ten More Years of Progress Against Heart Disease," *Heartline*, vol. 20, no. 1, January 1990.
16. Thompson, Larry. "Ten Years of Transplants," *Washington Post Health*, December 1, 1987.
17. Taylor, Frances. "Treating Stroke in the Year 2000," *NIH Healthline*, May 1990.
18. Taylor, Frances. "You Can Lower Your Risk of Stroke," *NIH Healthline*, May 1990.

## Chapter 14

1. Silverberg, Edwin et al. "Cancer Statistics, 1990," *Ca: A Cancer Journal for Clinicians*, vol. 40, no. 1, January/February 1990.
2. Rosenthal, Elisabeth. "The Cancer War: A Major Advance," *New York Times*, October 8, 1989.
3. Silverberg, Edwin et al. "Cancer Statistics, 1990," *Ca: A Cancer Journal for Clinicians*, vol. 40, no. 1, January/February 1990.
4. George, Leslie. "Playing Hide and Seek with the Sun—Safely," *American Health*, May 1989.
5. Faivelson, Saralie. "The Dark Truth about Tanning Salons," *American Health*, January/February 1988.
6. Barnett, Robert. "Give Me Five!" *American Health*, April 1989.
7. Rosenthal, Elisabeth. "The Cancer War: A Major Advance," *New York Times*, October 8, 1989.
8. Alabaster, Oliver. *The Power of Prevention.* New York: Simon and Schuster, 1986.
9. "Mammography Benefits," *FDA Drug Bulletin*, October 1987.
10. Eddy, David et al. "The Value of Mammography Screening in Women Under Age 50 Years," *Journal of the American Medical Association*, March 11, 1988.
11. "Mammography Benefits," *FDA Drug Bulletin*, October 1987.
12. Kolata, Gina. "Beating Cancer Can Sometimes Be Just the Start of the Fight," *New York Times*, November 24, 1988.
13. Rovner, Sandy. "Ulcers: A Medical Success Story for Most," *Washington Post Health*, October 13, 1987.
14. Dean, Cory. "Seat Belt Study Assesses Savings in Medical Costs and Injuries," *New York Times*, January 12, 1989.

## Chapter 15

1. Brody, Jane. "Flu Shots Are Recommended for Nearly Everybody, Even the Young and Healthy," *New York Times*, October 26, 1990.
2. Dunnett, Bill. "Drugs That Suppress Immunity," *American Health*, November 1986.
3. "Substance Blocks Cold Viruses in Test Tube," *New York Times*, March 1, 1990.
4. La Montagne, John. Researcher, National Institute of Allergy and Infectious Diseases. Personal interview.
5. Beck, Melinda. "Feeling Bad, Getting Worse," *Time*, February 5, 1990.
6. Dorfman, Andrea. "Laid Low by the Flu," *Time*, February 12, 1990.
7. Norton, Clark. "Not Just for Kids," *Hippocrates*, September/October 1989.
8. Brody, Jane. "Resurgence of Measles Across the Nation Prompts New Recommendations on Vaccinations," *New York Times*, January 11, 1990.
9. Talan, Jamie. "Deceptive Depression," *Psychology Today*, July/August 1989.
10. "Counterattack: Alpha-interferon Becomes the First Treatment for Hepatitis C," *Time*, December 11, 1989.
11. *Ibid.*
12. Schmitz, Anthony. "After the Bite," *Hippocrates*, May/June 1989.
13. "Update: Acquired Immunodeficiency Syndrome," *Journal of the American Medical Association*, vol. 263, no. 9, March 2, 1990.
14. Shilts, Randy. *And the Band Played On.* New York: St. Martin's Press, 1987.
15. "Update: Acquired Immunodeficiency Syndrome," *Journal of the American Medical Association*, vol. 263, no. 9, March 2, 1990.
16. *Ibid.*
17. Food and Drug Administration, January 1990.
18. Food and Drug Administration, January 1990.
19. Okie, Susan. "Study Faults Lab Accuracy in Testing for AIDS Infection," *Washington Post Health*, October 27, 1987.
20. "Boom in STDs Setting Off Alarms," *Medical World News*, August 22, 1988.
21. Hales, Dianne and Timothy Johnson. *Intensive Caring: New Hope for the High-Risk Pregnancy.* New York: Crown Publishers, 1990.
22. "Boom in STDs Setting Off Alarms," *Medical World News*, August 22, 1988.
23. Johnson, Dirk. "At Colleges, AIDS Alarms Muffle Older Dangers," *New York Times*, March 8, 1990.
24. "Condoms for Prevention of Sexually Transmitted Diseases," *Journal of the American Medical Association*, vol. 259, no. 13, April 1, 1988.
25. Levine, Joseph. "Syphilis: Ancient and on the Rise," *Emergency Medicine*, February 15, 1989.
26. Brock, B. V. et al. "Frequency of Asymptomatic Shedding of Herpes Simplex Virus in Women with Genital Herpes," *Journal of the American Medical Association*, vol. 263, no. 13, January 19, 1990.

27. "Virus Linked to Genital Cancers," *American Health*, April 1987.
28. Duncan, W. C. "Chancroid: Detection and Treatment," *Medical Aspects of Human Sexuality*, August 1989.
29. Schmid, G. P. et al. "Chancroid in the U.S.: Reestablishment of an Old Disease," *Journal of the American Medical Association*, vol. 258, no. 22, December 11, 1987.
28. Ehrlich, Paul and Anne Ehrlich. *The Population Explosion*. New York: Simon & Schuster, 1990.
29. Toufexis, Alexandra. "Our Violent Kids," *Time*, June 12, 1989.
30. Malcolm, Andrew. "Study of Domestic Violence Fails to Find Path to Killings," *New York Times*, February 5, 1990.
31. "The Subtle Shades of Abuse," *American Health*, April 1990.


## Chapter 16


1. Fisher, David. *Fire & Ice: The Greenhouse Effect. Ozone Depletion and Nuclear Winter.* New York: Harper & Row, 1990.
2. Linden, Eugene. "Now Wait Just a Minute," *Time*, December 18, 1989.
3. Weiner, Jonathan. *The Next One Hundred Years*. New York: Bantam Books, 1990.
4. Wald, Matthew. "How Dreams of Clean Air Get Stuck in Traffic," *New York Times*, March 11, 1990.
5. Sancton, Thomas. "The Fight to Save the Planet," *Time*, December 18, 1989.
6. "Higher Skin Cancer Rate Blamed on Ozone Layer," *San Francisco Chronicle*, March 27, 1990.
7. Carpenter, Betsy. "Greenhouse Redesign," *U.S. News & World Report*, June 18, 1990.
8. Stevens, William. "Study of Acid Rain Uncovers a Threat to Far Wider Area," *New York Times*, January 16, 1990.
9. Stevens, William. "Worst Fears on Acid Rain Unrealized," *New York Times*, February 20, 1990.
10. Raeburn, Paul. "The Switched-On House," *American Health*, March 1990.
11. Brodeur, Paul. *Currents of Death: Power Lines, Computer Terminals and the Attempt to Cover Up Their Threat to Your Health.* New York: Simon & Schuster, 1990.
12. Lemonick, Michael. "An Overblown Asbestos Scare?" *Time*, January 29, 1990.
13. "Study Finds Persistent Lead Peril," *San Francisco Chronicle*, March 6, 1990.
14. Schmitz, Anthony. "Should You Test for Radon?" *Hippocrates*, September/October 1989.
15. Browne, Malcolm. "Rat Study Reignites Dispute on Fluoride," *New York Times*, March 13, 1990.
16. Begley, Sharon. "Don't Drink the Water?" *Newsweek*, February 5, 1990.
17. Environmental Protection Agency, January 1990.
18. Purvis, Andrew. "Clean Bill for Agent Orange," *Time*, April 9, 1990.
19. "Public Health Statement on PCBs," Agency for Toxic Substances and Disease Registry, U.S. Public Health Service, 1990.
20. "Public Health Statement on Cadmium," Agency for Toxic Substances and Disease Registry, U.S. Public Health Service, 1990.
21. Beck, Melinda. "Buried Alive," *Newsweek*, November 27, 1989.
22. Mylander, Maureen. "Experts Meet on Noise and Hearing Loss," *NIH Healthline*, February 1990.
23. Leary, Warren. "Risk of Hearing Loss Is Growing, Panel Says," *New York Times*, January 25, 1990.
24. Browne, Malcolm. "Research on Noise Disappears in the Din," *New York Times*, March 6, 1990.
25. Hilts, Philip. "Higher Cancer Risk Found in Low-Level Radiation," *New York Times*, December 20, 1989.
26. Wald, Matthew. "New Estimates Increase Radiation Risk in Flight," *New York Times*, February 19, 1990.
27. Schmitz, Anthony. "Is This Any Way to Treat Your Food?" *Hippocrates*, November/December 1988.


## Chapter 17


1. U.S. Bureau of the Census, 1990.
2. Groch, Judith and Ruth Winter. "Biological Markers," *American Health*, May 1984.
3. Rowe, John. "Physiological Changes of Aging and Their Clinical Impact," *Psychosomatics*, December 1984.
4. Fitzgerald, Patrick. "Exercise for the Elderly," *Medical Clinics of North America*, vol. 69, no. 1, 1985.
5. Cooke, Patrick. "The Changes of Time," *Washington Post Health*, January 9, 1985.
6. Goleman, Daniel. "Studies Offer Fresh Clues to Memory," *New York Times*, March 27, 1990.
7. Blazer, Dan. "Epidemiology of Late-Life Depression and Dementia: A Comparative Study" in *Review of Psychiatry*. Washington, D.C.: American Psychiatric Press, 1990.
8. *Osteoporosis*, Washington, D.C.: National Osteoporosis Foundation, 1987.
9. Yudofsky, Stuart; Robert Hales; and Thomas Ferguson. *Psychiatric Drugs*. New York: Grove Weidenfeld, 1991.
10. Tomb, David. *Growing Old: A Handbook for You and Your Aging Parents*. New York: Viking, 1984.
11. Trafford, Abigail. "Growing Old in America," *Washington Post Health*, April 14, 1987.
12. Beck, Melinda. "Be Nice to Your Kids," *Newsweek*, March 12, 1990.
13. *Ibid.*
14. Trafford, Abigail. "Growing Old in America," *Washington Post Health*, April 14, 1987.
15. Talbott, John; Robert Hales and Stuart Yudofsky. *Textbook of Psychiatry*. Washington, D.C.: American Psychiatric Press, 1988.
16. "Alzheimer's Rise," *Time*, November 20, 1989.
17. Gelman, David. "The Brain Killer," *Newsweek*, December 18, 1989.
18. Cowley, Geoffrey. "Medical Mystery Tour," *Newsweek*, December 18, 1989.
19. *Ibid.*
20. Nissenson, Marilyn. "Therapy after Sixty," *Psychology Today*, January 1984.
21. Beck, Melinda. "The Search for the Fountain of Youth," *Newsweek*, March 5, 1990.
22. Fries, J. F. and L. M. Crapo. *Vitality and Aging*. San Francisco: Freeman, 1981.
23. Heynen, Jim. *One Hundred Over 100: Moments with One Hundred North American Centenarians*. San Francisco: Fulcrum Publishing, 1990.


## Chapter 18


1. Kubler-Ross, Elisabeth. *Death: The Final Stage of Growth*. Englewood Cliffs, NJ: Prentice-Hall, 1975.
2. *Aging and the Circumstances of Death*. Bethesda, MD: National Institute on Aging, 1981.

3. Gibbs, Nancy. "Love and Let Die," *Time,* March 19, 1990.
4. Margolick, David. "Patient's Lawsuit Says Saving Life Ruined It," *New York Times,* March 18, 1990.
5. Middleton, W. and B. Raphael. "Bereavement: State of the Art and State of Science," *Psychiatric Clinics of North America,* September 1987.
6. Irwin, Michael et al. "Immune and Neuroendocrine Changes During Bereavement," *Psychiatric Clinics of North America,* September 1987.
7. Bowling, Ann. "Mortality after Bereavement: A Review of the Literature on Survival Periods and Factors Affecting Survival," *Social Science in Medicine* vol. 24, no. 2, 1987.
8. "When Death Does Us Part: The Difference Between Widows and Widowers," *Psychology Today,* November 1989.
9. Talbott, John; Robert Hales; and Stuart Yudofsky. *The American Psychiatric Textbook of Psychiatry.* Washington, D.C.: American Psychiatric Press, 1989.
10. Goleman, Daniel. "New Studies Find Many Myths about Mourning," *New York Times,* August 8, 1989.
11. "Guide to the Living Will," *Hippocrates,* May/June 1988.

# RECOMMENDED READINGS


### Chapter 1

Barsky, Arthur. *Worried Sick.* Reading, MA: Addison-Wesley, 1989. An intriguing look at how too much concern about illness can interfere with feelings of wellness.

Ornstein, Robert and David Sobel. *Healthy Pleasures.* Reading, MA: Addison-Wesley, 1989. The latest scientific evidence that pleasures and positive attitudes are not only good in themselves, but good for you.

### Chapter 2

"Talking about . . ." American Psychiatric Association, 1500 K Street, Washington, D.C. An excellent series of brochures and fact sheets on mental health and specific mental disorders.

Cousins, Norman. *Head First: The Biology of Hope.* New York: E. P. Dutton, 1989. A fascinating exploration of the biological mechanisms of hope, faith, love, the will to live and good humor.

McKay, Matthew and Patrick Fanning. *Self-Esteem.* Oakland, CA: New Harbinger, 1987. An easy-to-follow approach designed to help readers disarm their internal critic and hear positive messages about themselves.

### Chapter 3

Friedman, Meyer and Diane Ulmer. *Treating Type A Behavior and Your Heart.* New York: Fawcett, 1984. The classic exploration of how Type A behavior can harm a person's heart and health.

Karasek, Robert and Tores Theorell. *Healthy Work: Stress, Productivity, and the Reconstruction of Working Life.* New York: Basic Books, 1990. An analysis of the relationships between work conditions and key indicators of stress, such as depression, anxiety, mental fatigue, and heart disease.

Langer, Ellen. *Mindfulness,* Reading, MA: Addison-Wesley, 1989. A guide to a psychological self-help technique for overcoming stress.

### Chapter 4

Christian, Janet and Janet Greger. *Nutrition for Living, Second Edition.* Redwood City, CA: Benjamin/Cummings, 1988. A comprehensive textbook, with many practical applications of the theories described.

Connor, Sonja and William Connor. *The New American Diet.* New York: Simon and Schuster, 1986. An eating plan for life, with a focus on lowering fat and cholesterol.

Berland, T. *Consumer Reports: Rating the Diets.* New York: Signet, 1990. A quick, sensible guide to the latest fads in dieting.

### Chapter 5

Anderson, Bob. *Stretching.* Bolinas, CA: Shelter Publications, 1980. The classic how-to book for safe, effective stretching.

Cooper, Kenneth. *The Aerobics Program for Total Well-being.* New York: M. Evans, 1982. A classic, comprehensive guide to shaping up your heart and lungs.

Sheehan, George. *Personal Best.* New York: Rodale/St. Martins, 1989. Essays, facts and advice on fitness.

### Chapter 6

Beck, Aaron. *Love Is Never Enough.* New York: Harper & Row, 1988. A guide to overcoming miscommunication and misunderstanding in marriage.

Scarf, Maggie. *Intimate Relations.* New York: Ballantine, 1989. Provocative discussion of couples, and how they can relate and communicate more effectively.

Schaeffer, Brenda. *Is It Love or Is It Addiction?* New York: Harper/Hazelden, 1987. A guide to identifying characteristics of addictive and healthy love, and moving toward more positive relationships.

### Chapter 7

Benderly, Beryl Lieff. *The Myth of Two Minds: What Gender Means and Doesn't Mean.* New York: Doubleday, 1987. An insightful, balanced analysis of the differences and similarities between the sexes.

Crooks, Robert and Karla Baur. *Our Sexuality, Fourth Edition.* Redwood City, CA: Benjamin/Cummings, 1990. An up-to-date, comprehensive textbook for college students.

Helmering, Doris. *Husbands, Wives and Sex.* Holbrook, MA: Bob Adams, 1990. A marital therapist's description of sexual patterns and problems in marriage.

### Chapter 8

Tribe, Laurence. *Abortion: The Clash of Absolutes.* New York: W. W. Norton & Company, 1990. A comprehensive, readable guide to the abortion controversy.

Rosen, Mortimer and Lillian Thomas. *The Cesarean Myth.* New York: Penguin Books, 1989. An obstetrician's challenge to the increase in cesarean deliveries, with advice for women who want to avoid cesareans.

### Chapter 9

____________. *Narcotics Anonymous, Fifth Edition.* Van Nuys, CA: Narcotics Anonymous, 1988. The basic recovery program used by Narcotics Anonymous groups and 38 stories of recovery.

Seymour, Richard and David Smith. *Drugfree: A Unique, Positive Approach To Staying Off Alcohol and Other Drugs.* New York: Facts on File, 1987. An overview of addictions and specific approaches for overcoming them.

Yoder, Barbara. *The Recovery Resource Book.* New York: Fireside Books, 1990. A comprehensive guide to programs, publications and places to turn for help in overcoming addictions and codependence.

### Chapter 10

Marshall, Shelly. *Young, Sober and Free.* New York: Harper/Hazelden, 1987. First-person stories of teenagers who've struggled with alcoholism or other addictions.

Wegscheider-Cruse, Sharon. *Another Chance: Hope and Health for the Alcoholic Family.* Palo Alto, CA: Science & Behavior Books,

1989. A practical approach to intervention and recovery from "the family disease" of alcoholism.

Beattie, Melody. *Codependent No More.* New York: Harper/Hazelden, 1987. A perennial best-seller that offers practical advice for loved ones of alcoholics and addicts.

Beattie, Melody. *Beyond Codependency.* New York: Harper/Hazelden, 1989. The sequel to *Codependent No More* deals with the art of self-care and self-nurturing.

## Chapter 11

Casey, Karen. *If Only I Could Quit: Becoming a Nonsmoker.* New York: Harper/Hazelden, 1987. Daily meditations and guidelines plus the stories of 24 ex-smokers.

Chandler, William. *Banishing Tobacco.* Washington, D.C.: Worldwatch Institute, 1986. A report on worldwide trends in tobacco use, its health consequences and costs to society.

## Chapter 12

Bennett, William et al. *Your Good Health: How to Stay Well, and What to Do When You're Not.* Cambridge: Harvard University Press, 1987. Well-documented advice on common health concerns from the editors of the *Harvard Medical Letter.*

Vickery, Donald and James Fries. *Take Care of Yourself, Fourth Edition.* Reading, MA: Addison-Wesley, 1989. The classic self-care guide; a must for every home.

Kemper, Donald, Kathleen McIntosh and Toni Roberts. *Healthwise Handbook.* Boise, ID: Healthwise Inc., 1989. A handy guide to prevention, home treatment and professional care for more than 130 medical problems.

## Chapter 13

Kwiterovick, Peter. *Beyond Cholesterol.* Baltimore, MD: Johns Hopkins Press, 1989. An authoritative nutritional guide to lowering risk of heart disease.

Moore, Thomas. *Heart Failure.* New York: Random House, 1989. A critical review of the national cholesterol education program.

Williams, Redford. *Great News About Type A Behavior.* New York: Times Books, 1989. An exploration of the complex links between personality, behavior and the risk of heart disease.

## Chapter 14

Columbia University College of Physicians and Surgeons. *Complete Home Medical Guide.* New York: Crown Publishers, 1989. An informative manual that provides descriptions of common medical problems and their treatment.

Rosenfeld, Isadore. *Symptoms.* New York: Simon & Schuster, 1989. A complete, reliable guide to what dozens of common symptoms may mean and when you should seek professional help.

———————. *Choices: Realistic Alternatives in Cancer Treatment.* New York: Avon, 1987. An excellent source book for cancer patients and their families.

## Chapter 15

Douglas, Paul and Laura Pinsky. *The Essential AIDS Fact Book.* New York: Pocket Books, 1987. A concise guide to protecting yourself and reducing the risks of HIV infection.

Shilts, Randy. *And the Band Played On.* New York: St. Martin's Press, 1987. A combination detective story and expose about the spread of HIV infection and AIDS, and how federal officials and the gay community failed to respond to the threat early and effectively.

Ulene, Art. *Safe Sex in a Dangerous World.* New York: Vintage, 1987. A concise, comprehensive guide to what all sexually active people should know about sexually transmitted diseases.

## Chapter 16

Earthworks. *50 Simple Things You Can Do to Save the Earth.* Berkeley: Earthworks Group/Publishers Group West, 1989. An easy-to-follow guide to making small changes that could have a big impact.

MacEachern, Diane. *Save Our Planet: 750 Everyday Ways You Can Help Clean Up the Earth.* New York: Dell Publishing, 1990. Practical, personal solutions to problems that endanger us all.

Weiner, Jonathan. *The Next One Hundred Years: Shaping the Fate of Our Living Earth.* New York: Bantam Books, 1990. A readable examination of the complex problems of ozone depletion and the greenhouse effect.

## Chapter 17

Berland, Ted. *Fitness for Life.* Washington, D.C.: American Association of Retired Persons, 1986. Exercise for men and women over age 50.

Henig, Robin. *The Myth of Senility.* Washington, D.C.: American Association of Retired Persons, 1986. A comprehensive and readable explanation of what happens to the brain as we age.

Tomb, David. *Growing Old: A Handbook for You and Your Aging Parents.* New York: Viking, 1984. A comprehensive guide to the physical, emotional, and financial problems of aging.

## Chapter 18

Callahan, Daniel. *Setting Limits.* New York: Simon & Schuster, 1987. A medical ethicist presents well-reasoned arguments why longer is not always better when it comes to life.

Kubler-Ross, Elisabeth. *Death: The Final Stage of Growth.* Englewood Cliffs, NJ: Prentice-Hall, 1975. The classic work by this noted psychiatrist on life's ultimate meaning.

Rollin, Betty. *Last Wish.* New York: Warner, 1986. The touching controversial story of a woman with terminal cancer, well told by the daughter who helped her commit suicide.

# PHOTO CREDITS

**p. 4** © Eunice Harris/Photo Researchers
**p. 8** © Bob Daemmrich/Stock Boston
**p. 9** © Ellis Herwig/Stock Boston
**p. 12** © Peter Menzel/Stock Boston
**p. 13** © Bob Daemmrich/Stock Boston
**p. 16** © Richard Pasley/Stock Boston
**p. 20** © Mike Mazzaschi/Stock Boston
**p. 25** © Roswell Angier/Stock Boston
**p. 28** © Susan Rosenberg/Photo Researchers
**p. 30** © Nik Kleinberg/Stock Boston
**p. 31** © Roswell Angier/Stock Boston
**p. 32** © Ron Nelson/Stock Boston
**p. 34** © Will and Deni McIntyre/Photo Researchers
**p. 37** © David Madison
**p. 42** © Bill Gallery/Stock Boston
**p. 44** © IFA/Peter Arnold
**p. 48** © Billy E. Barnes/Stock Boston
**p. 50** © Richard Hutchings/Photo Researchers
**p. 52** © Jim Weiner/Photo Researchers
**p. 59** © Lawrence Migdale/Stock Boston
**p. 62** © Yada Claasen/Jeroboam
**p. 65** © Bob Daemmrich/Stock Boston
**p. 73** © Herminia Dosal/Photo Researchers
**p. 75** © G. Mancuso/Stock Boston
**p. 77 left** Sara Hunsaker
**p. 77 right** © Tony Freeman/Photo Edit
**p. 79** © Eric Jaquier/Stock Boston
**p. 89** © Frank Keillor/Jeroboam
**p. 90 top** © David Madison
**p. 90 bottom** © Barbara Alper/Stock Boston
**p. 91 top and bottom** © David Madison
**p. 94** © Rocky Weldon/Jeroboam
**p. 101** © John Running/Stock Boston
**p. 103** © Mike Neveux
**p. 104** © Renee Lynn
**p. 108** © Olaf Kallstrom/Jeroboam
**p. 113** © Ginger Chih/Peter Arnold
**p. 114** © Rhoda Sidney/Stock Boston
**p. 116** © Matthew McVay/Stock Boston
**p. 123** © Charles Gupton/Stock Boston
**p. 129** © Peter Menzel/Stock Boston
**p. 136** © John Walsh/SPL Photo Researchers, Inc.
**p. 139** © Bob Daemmrich/Stock Boston
**p. 141** © Kit Hedman/Jeroboam
**p. 143** © Ericka Stone/Peter Arnold
**p. 145** © Bill Horsman/Stock Boston
**pp. 167, 169, 170 left, 171, 172, 173** © William Thompson
**p. 170 right** © SIU/Peter Arnold
**p. 186** © Photo Researchers
**p. 188** © Robert McElroy/Woodfin Camp
**p. 189** © Mike Malyszko/Stock Boston
**p. 192** © Frank Siteman/Stock Boston
**p. 196** © Laura Dwight/Peter Arnold
**p. 201** © A. Tannenbaum/Sygma
**p. 205** © Mary Kate Denny/Photo Edit
**p. 211** © Jean-Marc Giboux/Gamma Liaison
**p. 214** © Ken Sakamoto/Black Star
**p. 216** © Jon Feingersh/Stock Boston
**p. 219** © Sygma
**p. 222** © Marty Katz/Gamma-Liaison
**p. 223** © Rick Browne/Stock Boston
**p. 227** © Charles Gupton/Stock Boston
**p. 231** © Stacy Pick/Stock Boston
**p. 234** © Paul Conklin/Photo Edit
**p. 237** Streissguth, A.P., Clarren, S.K., and Jones, K.L., Natural History of the Fetal Alcohol Syndrome: A ten-year follow-up of eleven patients. *Lancet* 2 (July 1985): 85-92.
**p. 239** © B. Grunzweig/Photo Researchers
**p. 242** © Tony Freeman/Photo Edit
**p. 247** © Rob Nelson/Stock Boston
**p. 249** © Johannes Hofman/Photo Researchers
**p. 257** © Tony Freeman/Photo Edit
**p. 265** © Bohdan Hrynewych/Stock Boston
**p. 270** © Dion Ogust/Image Works
**p. 271** © Guy Gillette/Photo Researchers
**p. 275** © Blair Seitz/Photo Researchers
**p. 277** © Bob Daemmrich/Stock Boston
**p. 281** © Doug Menvez/Stock Boston
**p. 284** © Paul Biddle and Tim Maylon/ Photo Researchers
**p. 290** © Catherine Ursillo/Photo Researchers
**p. 293** © Ellis Herwig/Stock Boston
**p. 294** © Ed Reschke
**p. 297** © Richard Hutchings/Photo Researchers
**p. 298** © Tim Holt/Photo Researchers
**p. 304** © J.P. Laffont/Sygma
**p. 306** © Stacy Pick/Stock Boston
**p. 309** © John Greim/Medichrome
**p. 314** © Jean Claude Lejeune/Stock Boston
**p. 319** © Milton Feinberg/Stock Boston
**p. 327** © J.P. Laffont/Sygma
**p. 332** © Southern Living/Photo Researchers
**p. 334** © Sygma
**p. 335 left** © Lennart Nilsson/Boehringer Ingelheim International
**p. 335 right** © James D. Wilson/Woodfin Camp
**p. 345** © Will and Deni McIntyre/Photo Researchers
**p. 348** Centers for Disease Control/Biological Photo Service
**p. 349** © M. Abbey/Photo Researchers
**p. 357** © John Running/Stock Boston
**p. 360** © Seth Resnick/Stock Boston
**p. 363** © Norm Thomas/Photo Researchers
**p. 365** © Peter Menzel/Stock Boston
**p. 370** © Brock May/Photo Researchers
**p. 376** © Barbara Alper/Stock Boston
**p. 377** © F.B. Grunzweig/Photo Researchers
**p. 383** © Del Mulkey/Photo Researchers
**p. 390** © Randy Taylor/Sygma
**p. 392** © James D. Wilson/Woodfin Camp
**p. 399** © Oliver Rebbot/Stock Boston

**Chapter Opener Photos**

**Chapter 1** © Bob Daemmrich/Stock Boston
**Chapter 2** © Michael P. Godomski/ Photo Researchers
**Chapter 3** © Bill Gallery/Stock Boston
**Chapter 4** © Chuck O'Rear/Woodfin Camp
**Chapter 5** © Frank Keillor/Jeroboam
**Chapter 6** © Explore/Photo Researchers
**Chapter 7** © Julie Houck/Stock Boston
**Chapter 8** © Cary Groner
**Chapter 9** © Larry Kolvoord/Image Works
**Chapter 10** © Matthew Neal McVay/ Stock Boston
**Chapter 11** © Michael P. Gadomski/ Photo Researchers
**Chapter 12** © Dion Ogust/Image Works
**Chapter 13** © David Madison
**Chapter 14** © Bob Daemmrich/Stock Boston
**Chapter 15** © Jeffrey D. Smith/Woodfin Camp
**Chapter 16** © John Eastcott/Image Works
**Chapter 17** © Joe Sohm/Image Works
**Chapter 18** © Jack Spratt/Image Works

**Your Body: An Owner's Manual (color insert)**

**p. 1** (left) Magnum/Ernst Haas
**p. 1** (right) Photo Researchers/Dr. Clark Goff
**p. 2** Life Picture Service/Andreas Feininger
**p. 3** (left) Taurus Photos/Martin Rotker
**p. 3** (left) Photo Researchers/Richard Hutchings
**p. 4** (middle) Jeroboam/Kent Reno
**p. 4** (right) Sara Hunsaker
**p. 5** (top) Ed Reschka
**p. 5** (bottom left) Photo Researchers/ Catherine Ursillo
**p. 5** (bottom right) H. Armstrong Roberts/D. Corson
**p. 6** (bottom) Lennart Nilsson
**p. 7** (top) Peter Arnold/Manfred Kage
**p. 7** (bottom left) Sara Hunsaker
**p. 7** (bottom right) Stock, Boston/Malave
**p. 8** (left) Sara Hunsaker
**p. 8** (right) Taurus Photos/Alfred Pasieka
**p. 9** Photo Researchers/Nancy Pierce
**p. 10** Lennart Nilsson
**p. 11** (top) Peter Arnold/Ed Reschka
**p. 11** (bottom left) Peter Arnold/Werner Müller
**p. 11** (bottom right) Sara Hunsaker
**p. 12** (left) Peter Arnold/Steve Allen
**p. 12** (right) Peter Arnold/Manfred Kage
**p. 13** (top) Taurus Photos/Martin Rotker
**p. 13** (bottom left) Tom Stack/Doug Lee
**p. 13** (bottom right) Tom Stack/Dave Baird
**p. 14** (left) W. H. Freeman & Co. /Richard Kessel and Randy Kardon
**p. 14** (right) Biophoto Service/ W. Rosenburg
**p. 15** (top) Lennart Nilsson
**p. 15** (bottom) Sara Hunsaker
**p. 16** (top) Peter Arnold/Manfred Kage
**p. 16** (bottom left) Peter Arnold/Manfred Kage
**p. 16** (bottom right) Sara Hunsaker

---

# INDEX

Page numbers in bold indicate those pages where a term is defined; a page number followed by "t" indicates a table; a page number followed by "f" indicates a figure.